CANCER-ASSOCIATED GENODERMATOSES

CANCER-ASSOCIATED GENODERMATOSES

Edited by

Henry T. Lynch, M.D.

Professor and Chairman
Department of Preventive Medicine
Creighton University School of Medicine

and

Ramon M. Fusaro, M.D., Ph.D.

Professor and Chairman
Department of Dermatology
Creighton University School of Medicine
and
University of Nebraska College of Medicine

VNR VAN NOSTRAND REINHOLD COMPANY
NEW YORK   CINCINNATI   TORONTO   LONDON   MELBOURNE

Published by Van Nostrand Reinhold Company Inc.
135 West 50th Street, New York, N.Y. 10020

Van Nostrand Reinhold Limited
1410 Birchmount Road
Scarborough, Ontario M1P 2E7, Canada

Van Nostrand Reinhold Australia Pty. Ltd.
17 Queen Street
Mitcham, Victoria 3132, Australia

Van Nostrand Reinhold Company Limited
Molly Millars Lane
Wokingham, Berkshire, England

15 14 13 12 11 10 9 8 7 6 5 4 3 2 1

Library of Congress Cataloging in Publication Data

Main entry under title:

Cancer-associated genodermatoses.

    Includes index.
    1. Skin – Diseases – Genetic aspects. 2. Skin – Cancer – Genetic aspects.
3. Cancer – Diagnosis. 4. Cutaneous manifestations of general diseases.
I. Lynch, Henry T. II. Fusaro, Ramon M. [DNLM: 1. Skin diseases – Familial
and genetic. 2. Skin manifestations – Familial and genetic. 3. Skin neoplasms – Familial and genetic. 4. Neoplasms – Complications. 5. Skin
diseases – Etiology. 6. Neoplasms – Familial and genetic.]
RL72.C33   616.99'4042   81-14701
ISBN: 0-442-22471-0   AACR2

Foreword

When one is asked to review a monograph and to write its foreword, one finds a certain security if one can compare the text's strong and weak points with those of a comparable work. However, there seems to be no paradigm for this effort of Drs. Lynch and Fusaro and their coauthors. It represents a unique effort that will serve as a model to which future monographs on this subject may be compared.

This book, *Cancer-associated Genodermatoses,* covers all aspects of the subject. Its appeal is not limited to a few specialists at a highly sophisticated level of presentation, but because of clever editing it seduces the reader, be he neophyte or expert, to read further − to be challenged by the many questions and inconsistencies that are raised by the authors. There is no attempt to talk down to the beginner. On the contrary, the reader is subtly educated, becoming increasingly engaged while being led progressively through the complexity (clinical, cutaneous, radiologic, immune aspects) to its culmination in the biochemical knowledge of the cancer-related genodermatoses. This chapter is perhaps the most thorough coverage of the subject ever attempted.

The information presented is current and authoritative. Each author has made significant contributions to the field. The controversy concerning many disorders presented is meant to pique the readers' interest. The authors were instructed to ask questions of the readers in order to provoke investigation. I believe that they have succeeded.

Most pleasing to me was the completeness of coverage of the cancer-related genodermatoses. Regardless of how rare the disorder, one can count on its having been discussed and the apposite bibliography presented.

It was an exciting experience for me to read this monograph. I sincerely believe that it cannot fail to catalyze investigation into the mechanisms of single gene cancer.

ROBERT GORLIN, D.D.S., M.S.

Regents' Professor and Chairman,
Department of Oral Pathology and Genetics
Professor, Departments of Dermatology, Pathology, Pediatrics,
Obstetrics-Gynecology, and Otolaryngology
University of Minnesota
Schools of Dentistry and Medicine
Minneapolis, MN 55455

This book is dedicated to the countless physicians, medical record librarians, Departments of Vital Statistics, and other resource people who tirelessly aided our research in cancer genetics by providing the necessary genealogical, medical, and pathological data which enabled our interpretation of family pedigrees.

Acknowledgments

We wish to acknowledge the faithful care given to the typing of this book by our secretaries, Diane Stanley and Maggie Meston, as well as additional technical assistance provided by Georgia Race, Mary Markytan, and Jody Hargens. We also acknowledge our devoted librarian staff including its Director Marge Winarka, Sr. Rae Marie and their staff. Finally, any effort of this type eventually focuses upon the cooperation of individual patients and their relatives. Words cannot possibly express our gratitude for these countless individuals who labored so hard on our behalf through the collection of data and their submission to examinations in order that we might better understand the problems in cancer-associated genodermatoses.

Preface

Physicians have been curious about familial cancer for many centuries. Possibly the first report on the subject appeared in the Roman literature in 100 A.D. when a clinician marveled at the excess of breast cancer in the family of one of his patients. However, only in the past two decades has the problem been attacked systematically, thereby making possible recognition of an increasing number of hereditary cancer syndromes. The frustratingly slow progress to date has undoubtedly resulted in part from man's preoccupation with environmental causes of cancer, coupled with the physician's relative inattention to the potential wealth of information in the family history component of the history and physical examination.

Cutaneous signs have long been known to herald internal manifestations of major disease and, in some instances, their genetic transmission. With the exception of a handful of classical cancer-associated genodermatoses such as the phakomatoses and xeroderma pigmentosum (XP), surprisingly little attention has been devoted to them. This fact has motivated our attempt to evaluate more critically the general topic of heritable cancer syndromes with cutaneous manifestations. With the dedicated assistance of our several colleagues, we have sought to provide our readers with a treatise that will enable them to grasp the range of disorders regardless of their own field of specialization. The diversity of topics under consideration, their etiology, pathogenesis, carcinogenesis, and nosology, should provide a basis for rational critique.

Certain of the cancer-associated genodermatoses provide intriguing models for the study of genetic/environmental interaction. Classical ones are XP, in which sunlight strongly influences skin cancer development, or porphyria cutanea tarda and hemochromatosis, in which chronic alcoholism may trigger an underlying genetic susceptibility to primary liver cancer. These conditions display in high relief the need for cognizance of both genetics and the environment when studying cancer etiology.

Problems of genetic heterogeneity are rampant in these disorders, e.g., the several varieties of XP (complementation groups A through G and the XP varient).

Intriguing also is the finding of cancer excess in heterozygous carriers of the gene for ataxia telangiectasia and possibly XP. What other cancer-associated autosomal recessively inherited genodermatoses may show similar cancer association among heterozygotes?

After considerable investigation of the rapidly developing field of cancer genetics, particularly the cancer-associated genodermatoses, it soon became obvious that the tip of the iceberg had barely been exposed. If this monograph stimulates further exploration into cancer etiology, prevention, and control, its mission will have been more than adequately accomplished.

HENRY T. LYNCH/RAMON M. FUSARO

Contributors

Walter Burgdorf, M.D.
Assistant Professor
Department of Dermatology
University of Oklahoma Medical
 School
Oklahoma City, Oklahoma

Ramon M. Fusaro, Ph.D., M.D.
Professor and Chairman
Departments of Dermatology
Creighton University School of Medicine
University of Nebraska College of
 Medicine
Omaha, Nebraska

Roger K. Harned, M.D.
Professor
Department of Radiology
University of Nebraska Medical Center
Omaha, Nebraska

John A. Johnson, Ph.D.
Associate Professor
Department of Biochemistry
University of Nebraska College of
 Medicine
and Associate Professor
Department of Dermatology
Creighton University and the University
 of Nebraska Medical Center
Omaha, Nebraska

Henry T. Lynch, M.D.
Professor and Chairman
Department of Preventive Medicine and
 Public Health, and Professor of
 Medicine
Creighton University School of
 Medicine
Omaha, Nebraska

Jane F. Lynch, R.N.
Instructor
Department of Preventive Medicine and
 Public Health
Creighton University School of
 Medicine
Omaha, Nebraska

Patrick M. Lynch, J.D.,
Medical Student
Creighton University School of
 Medicine
Omaha, Nebraska

Judith Pester, M.D.
Former Assistant Professor
Department of Pathology
University of Nebraska Medical Center
Omaha, Nebraska
Currently in Private Practice
 in Pathology
Andrews, Texas

Richard J. Reed, M.D.
Department of Pathology
Tulane University School of Medicine
 and Charity Hospital
New Orleans, Louisiana

J. Corwin Vance, M.D.
Assistant Professor
Department of Dermatology
University of Minnesota Medical
 School
Minneapolis, Minnesota

Contents

CANCER-ASSOCIATED GENODERMATOSES

1
Genodermatoses and Cancer

Henry T. Lynch, M.D., and Ramon M. Fusaro, M.D., Ph.D.

INTRODUCTION

Historical Perspective

Scientific developments in the fields of genetics and oncology during the past two decades have been almost explosive; consequently, the informational content now available to these disciplines has become almost staggering. This has been particularly true for the cancer-associated genodermatoses, a pervasive area of inquiry linking genetics, molecular biology, dermatology, internal medicine, oncology, pathology, and clinical immunology.[1,2] This monograph has emerged in the midst of many exciting developments in these disciplines.

Historically, we find many examples which indicate that our clinical predecessors were extremely interested in the cancer-associated genodermatoses; however, because of limitations in the body of knowledge as well as the technology of their times, they were necessarily restricted to primary descriptive approaches to these disorders. This was clearly evidenced by the efforts of clinicians a century ago which led to their recognition of familial aggregation in such cancer-associated genodermatoses as von Recklinghausen's neurofibromatosis, tuberous sclerosis, xeroderma pigmentosum (XP), and others.[1,2] Attention throughout this monograph will be focused upon a concerted appraisal of those common denominators which best characterize the cancer-associated genodermatoses. Not only should this then aid in providing integration of the seemingly diverse and multifaceted contributions to the field, but it will also assist in syndrome identification, classification, and hopefully, early cancer diagnosis. Furthermore, it should also provide a more enlightened comprehension of current knowledge about the etiology of cancer-associated genodermatoses. The study of these diseases will certainly be stimulating, in that they present untold challenges because of their position at the crossroads of the basic and applied medical sciences. This presumption is amply fortified by the steady scientific progress which has taken place during the past several decades on the part of countless clinicians and basic scientists, and it has led to invaluable insights into the role of genetics, including those molecular mechanisms which may more clearly define relationships between host factors and environmental events in carcinogenesis. One important example pertains to the pioneering efforts of Cleaver,[3] emanating from his identification of defective DNA repair in XP, which had led to novel approaches to the study of cancer etiology and carcinogenesis in humans (see Chapter 10).

Statement of Position on Genetics

Research in the discipline of human cancer genetics has revealed a growing consensus regarding the manner in which particular genotypes contribute to the overall cancer burden. Cancer liability can be seen as a combination of genetic susceptibility and environmental exposure. The question becomes, What proportion of the *variance* in liability in a population can be attributed to the genetic component (heritability)? With rare exceptions (i.e., single gene defects or extraordinarily potent carcinogens), it is misleading to regard individual cases as being "due" to *genetic* or *environmental* factors since these effects are totally confounded in the majority of patients (Figure 1-1).[4]

Hereditary (single gene determined) forms of cancer play a primary role in the pathogenesis of approximately 5-10% of all human cancer, but even here, exogenous and endogenous factors, including suppressor genes, position effect, maternal and cytoplasmic effects, may temper gene penetrance and expressivity.

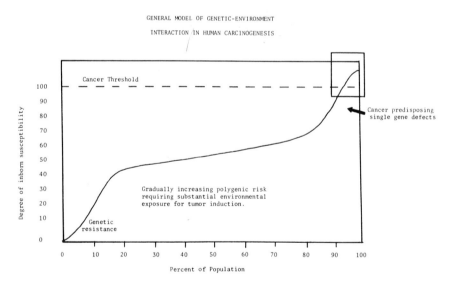

GENERAL MODEL OF GENETIC-ENVIRONMENT
INTERACTION IN HUMAN CARCINOGENESIS

Figure 1-1. Polygenic and simple genetic model for cancer resistance and cancer proneness in concert with environmental interaction. (From H.T. Lynch. Genetics, etiology, and human cancer. *Prev. Med.* 9:231-243, 1980.

Less clearly defined genotypes, including polygenic inheritance, predispose to as much as an additional 5-10% of the cancer load, but again, myriad exogenous and endogenous factors may be influential. Malignant neoplasms among hetero-zygous carriers of genes for ataxia telangiectasia (AT) may account for 3% of all patients with cancer. What other recessively inherited forms of cancer and/or precancer syndromes pose an increased risk for cancer in heterozygous carriers of the respective deleterious genes?

It is well recognized that primary genetic factors mediate the nature of the immune response and the susceptibility of individual cell types to viral infection (Chapter 7). In the case of immunodeficiency disease (several of which are cancer-associated genodermatoses, e.g., AT), the frequency of malignancy may be roughly 10,000 times greater than that of the general age-matched population.[5]

The fraction of cancer that is genetically induced is substantially greater in patients below age 40 and even higher in certain forms of childhood cancer. This aspect of the problem leads to a loss of productive patient-years that is remark-ably disproportional to sporadic varieties of cancer. These aspects of the problem are clearly characteristic of the cancer-associated genodermatoses. The predict-ability of such devastatingly early and multiple cancers in members of thousands of families nationwide is of as high, or higher, an order of magnitude as the pre-dictability of cancer in, for example, atomic bomb survivors, vinyl chloride and asbestos workers, or heavy cigarette smokers.[4]

DNA Repair: a Model for the Study of Etiology and Carcinogenesis

In contrast to early descriptive work, the already mentioned more recent recog-nition of defective DNA repair in XP, as well as other accomplishments in molec-ular biology, has promulgated a logarithmic advance toward fostering the com-prehension of etiology, pathogenesis, carcinogenesis and, ultimately, control in the cancer-associated genodermatoses. At the outset, therefore, we deem it im-portant for purposes of providing perspective to the subject, that we digress briefly into a consideration of DNA repair as a prototype model for certain of these scientific advances, even though this matter will be discussed in much greater detail in Chapter 10. In our opinion, these accomplishments have been virtually unparalleled in the fields of medicine, genetics, and oncology in general, and in the cancer-associated genodermatoses in particular. Specifically, the identifica-tion of a probable enzyme deficiency (possibly UV-endonuclease), observed in cultured skin fibroblasts from patients with XP, may ultimately have an enor-mous impact on biology and medicine.

Fibroblasts from XP patients were found to be *sensitive* to ultraviolet (UV) light, but interestingly, they were also observed to be *resistant* to the harmful effects on DNA repair by γ-radiation. However, in AT, the converse was observed; namely, fibroblasts from an AT patient in culture were found to be *sensitive* to γ-radiation, but *resistant* to UV exposure.[6] In addition, certain of the AT cells were found to be incapable of removing γ-induced damage to DNA. Later studies of skin fibroblasts from a patient with the D-deletion variety of retinoblastoma were found to be abnormally sensitive to γ-radiation.[7] The fibroblasts from this retinoblastoma-affected patient were not as sensitive as those from the AT patient, but nevertheless they showed significantly greater sensitivity to γ-radiation than fibroblasts from normal patients.

This particular model should lend itself well to investigations of many other cancer-associated genodermatoses and should facilitate the investigation of variable environmental influences upon DNA repair. It may also prove useful in the investigation of hybridization of cultured fibroblasts from XP patients and AT patients in order to determine whether mutual correction of these deficiencies in the subject genotypically distinct disorders may occur. For example, the investigations of fibroblasts from patients with Hurler's and Hunter's syndromes[8] have revealed that when grown together, they correct each other's defects. Each cell line secretes a degradative enzyme into the medium that the other lacks.

Such investigations as these provide a clear example of the manner in which practicing clinicians, who are adept at syndrome identification, can refer patients to medical geneticists and molecular biologists for definitive biological studies. Activities such as these should then expedite significant scientific advances which will mutually benefit the several respective disciplines; in turn, they may provide a practical basis for improved patient care.

Cancer Is More than a Problem of Physical Dimensions

Waldenstrom[9] has recently emphasized the need to look beyond malignant neoplastic lesions as merely localized collections of cells which have properties for invasion of adjacent tissues and which later may metastasize widely. He states that such mechanical effects of tissue destruction from tumors, which give rise to pain, bleeding, or pressure on organs and cause obstruction, have dominated our thinking in oncology. His plea is that we "get away from the purely morphologic viewpoint" and capitalize upon more recent evidence which shows clearly that cancer cells can produce chemicals which may ultimately be utilized as cancer signals. They may also provide clues to etiology and carcinogenesis. Many of these substances are polypeptides and are truly metabolic. These include catecholamines produced by cells of the adrenal medulla, 5-hydroxytryptamine elaborated by carcinoid tumors, and calcitonin produced by the parafollicular C cells in medullary thyroid carcinoma. Other examples of such chemical "cancer signals" pertain to the reawakening of fetal patterns of chemical synthesis such as that evidenced by carcinoembryonic antigen (CEA) and α-fetoprotein (AFP). For example, AFP may be found in the serum of newborns, only to reappear in certain patients manifesting hepatomas; similarly, CEA may also be a product of certain cancer cells. However, the etiology of these proteins is complex, and they may even be the result of gene-coding processes in certain hereditary cancer-associated disorders.[10]

Explanations for the "reawakening" of these oncodevelopmental proteins have included the assumption that they represent a derepression of dormant templates for protein synthesis. In this regard, Waldenstrom draws the analogy of such a reversion to uterine life with that of the growth of another fetal product, namely, abundant lanugo hair over the face, nose, and ears in certain cancer-affected patients.

Topic and ectopic humoral factors notwithstanding, Waldenstrom[9] considers the most conspicuous cancer signals in man to belong to the discipline of dermatology. He cites only one of countless examples, namely, that of the carcinoid patient manifesting transient ("flushing") erythema. Thus, such cutaneous signs as these should ". . . announce that the patient is carrying a cancer — but only to the *doctor who can read the signals*" (our italics). This latter admonition is clearly one of the primary objectives of this book. However, in the case of cancer-associated genodermatoses, additional clues to excess cancer proclivity may be provided through knowledge of the *family* history. We recently have shown that in 70% of cancer patients who had excess cancer in the family, this fact was not mentioned in the historical record of the patient.

It would be prudent when considering etiologic factors in cancer-associated genodermatoses that we follow closely the sage advice of Waldenstrom and "look beyond the cell"; we should "look beyond the skin" and encompass in our diagnostic reasoning systemic manifestations when they exist. We should also scrutinize pertinent aspects of physiology, biochemistry, immunology, virology, and pathology so that the full message of the *experimenta naturae* may be gleaned.

Catalogues of Cancer-associated Genodermatoses

Tables 1-1 to 1-3 provide, in a succinct form, the commonly accepted terminology for the cancer-associated genodermatoses, their mode of inheritance when known, major tumor associations, distinguishing cutaneous signs, and cardinal clinical manifestations. Figure 1-2 portrays diagrammatically the anatomic sites of cancer predilection in these diseases. Table 1-4 is an alphabetized listing of cancer-associated genodermatoses including numerical coding of cancer sites illustrated in Figure 1-2. Throughout this monograph, we shall describe in greater depth certain of these disorders, including several newly recognized syndromes, such as the familial atypical multiple mole-melanoma syndrome (we have ascribed the acronym FAMMM for this cancer-associated genodermatosis).[11]

While we talk glibly about cancer-associated genodermatoses as if these problems were clear-cut from the standpoint of etiology and classification, the problems are, in fact, exceedingly complex. In the strict sense, host factors play a lesser

Table 1-1. Autosomal Dominant Diseases.

NO.	NAME OF DISEASE	ASSOCIATED CANCER	CARDINAL CLINICAL MANIFESTATIONS
10940	Multiple nevoid basal cell carcinoma syndrome (basal cell nevus syndrome)	Numerous basal cell carcinomas skin (mean age onset — 15) on sun- and non-sun-exposed areas; medulloblastoma; astro-cytoma; ameloblastoma; ovarian carci-noma	Numerous basal cell nevi; palmar and plantar pits; mandibular prognathism; lateral displacement of the inner canthi; jaw cysts; kyphoscoliosis; fused ribs; bossing of the skull; characteristic lamellar calcification of the falx cerebri; ovarian fibromas; short 4th and/or 5th metacarpals
	Cheilitis glandularis	Epidermoid cancers of lips in 12-33%	Patulous openings of ducts and of mucous glands, cysts, and general enlargement of lips
12950	Hidrotic ectodermal dysplasia	Squamous cell cancer of palms and soles; also of nail bed	Normal sweating, total alopecia, severe dystrophy of nails, hyperpigmentation of skin — especially of the joints; occasionally mental retardation and seizures; palmar and plantar hyperkeratosis
13280	Multiple self-healing squamous cell cancer of the skin of the Ferguson-Smith type (keratoacanthoma)	These lesions may transform into squamous cell carcinoma of the skin	Rapidly growing tumor of the skin which usually reaches 1-2 cm with a central umbilication filled with a thick keratinous plug
13755	Giant pigmented nevus	Malignant melanoma	An extensive nevus cell nevus present at birth favoring the bathing trunk area; may be associated with café au lait spots, fibromas, and lipomas
	Familial hyperglucagonemia	Alpha-2-cell tumor of the islets of Langerhans (glucagonoma); in a single family, medullary thyroid cancer and pheochromocytoma	Necrolytic migratory erythema (dermatitis — exudative and pruritic), diabetes, weight loss, anemia, glossitis, immunoreactive glucagon with a molecular weight of 3,500-9,000 daltons; serum glucagon levels elevated

Table 1-1 (Cont.)

NO.	NAME OF DISEASE	ASSOCIATED CANCER	CARDINAL CLINICAL MANIFESTATIONS
14415	Hyperkeratosis lenticularis perstans (Flegel's disease)	Cutaneous squamous and basal cell carcinomas	Hyperkeratotic lesions of the lower extremities, trunk, thighs, arms, and dorsum of the hands; papules, pink or reddish-brown, 1-5 mm in size, occur in the 3rd and 4th decade
14800	Kaposi sarcoma	Malignant lymphoma, mycosis fungoides, Hodgkin's disease, lymphosarcoma, leukemia, and multiple myeloma (excess multiple primary cancer)	Multicentric origin, tumors of vascular and fibroblastic elements involving the skin and other tissues as well
14850	Keratosis palmaris et plantaris with esophageal cancer	Esophageal cancer	Diffuse thickening of the skin of the palms and soles — of later onset than genetic variety which is not cancer associated
	Bazex syndrome	Basal cell carcinomas of the face, 2nd to 3rd decade of life	Follicular atrophoderma; localized anhidrosis and/or generalized hypohidrosis
15270	Lupus erythematosus (systemic)	Malignant thymoma; lymphoma	Protean manifestations, including malar "butterfly" erythematous eruption, alopecia, photosensitivity, polyarthritis, intermittent fever, Raynaud's phenomenon, Sjogren's syndrome features (salivary gland involvement), nephritis, autoimmune hemolytic anemia, positive antinuclear antibodies
15340	Lymphedema with distichiasis	One case of fibrosarcoma in edematous leg	Lymphedema of the lower extremities usually at puberty; a double row of eyelashes and possibly webbed neck

Table 1-1 (Cont.)

NO.	NAME OF DISEASE	ASSOCIATED CANCER	CARDINAL CLINICAL MANIFESTATIONS
	Familial atypical multiple-mole melanoma syndrome (FAMMM)	Cutaneous malignant melanoma; intraocular malignant melanoma, carcinoma of breast and gastrointestinal tract, squamous cell carcinoma respiratory tract, lymphoreticular malignancy, sarcomas may be associated	Multiple, large, variable coloration (in some they are red to reddish-brown) moles with pigment leakage and irregular border located primarily on the trunk and arms; familial occurrences of malignant melanoma and associated cancer; histopathology variable and nondiagnostic
15835	Multiple hamartoma syndrome (Cowden's disease)	Carcinoma of the breast, colon, and thyroid; benign tumors of the thyroid, ovary, breast, gastrointestinal tract	Coexistence of multiple ectodermal, mesodermal, and endodermal nevoid neoplastic abnormalities; cutaneous lesions including dome-shaped, flat-topped papules, verrucous lesions, punctate keratoderma of the palms, multiple angiomas and lipomas; gingival and palatal papules, as well as scrotal tongue, may exist; abnormalities of the thyroid, breast, gastrointestinal tract, and CNS coexist
16220	Neurofibromatosis (von Recklinghausen's)	Malignant degeneration of the neurofibromas in 3-15% of cases; also sarcomas, intracranial and optic nerve gliomas, acoustic neuroma, optic neuroma, meningioma, and pheochromocytoma; lesions are often bilateral	Café au lait spots and fibromatous skin tumors; occasional features include multiple skeletal anomalies, i.e., scoliosis, pseudoarthrosis of tibia; mental retardation, hypertension, pulmonary involvement secondary to cystic lesions; peripheral variety shows multiple cutaneous signs and increased functional β-nerve growth factor (β-NGF) while central variety has paucity of cutaneous signs, excess CNS tumors (acoustic neuromas)

Table 1-1 (Cont.)

NO.	NAME OF DISEASE	ASSOCIATED CANCER	CARDINAL CLINICAL MANIFESTATIONS
16230	Multiple mucosal neuroma syndrome (MEN-III)	Pheochromocytoma, medullary thyroid carcinoma, possible parathyroid carcinoma	Pedunculated nodules on the eyelid margins, lip, and tongue have true neuromas; there are occasional cafe au lait spots; hyperplastic corneal nerves and rarely parathyroid disorders, eunuchoid habitus
17140	Sipple's syndrome (MEN-II)	Pheochromocytoma, medullary thyroid carcinoma, possible astrocytoma, and possible parathyroid carcinoma	Not considered a genodermatosis in the classical sense; may well qualify because of occasional association of neurofibromas and a recent report by Samaan wherein fibroepithelial polyps were found on skin and chest in a patient with this disease
	Maffucci's syndrome	Pituitary chromophobe adenoma, parathyroid adenoma, and malignant transformation of benign enchondromas or blood vessel tumors; chondrosarcomas 30%	Multiple hemangiomas of skin; skeletal dyschondroplasia which may result in shortening of bones and fractures, deformities from enchondromas
16730	Extramammary Paget's disease	Internal malignancy, particularly underlying adnexal, urinary, renal or rectal carcinoma	An eczematous eruption with weeping and crust formation, most often in anogenital region
17520	Intestinal polyposis II (Peutz-Jeghers syndrome)	Adenocarcinoma of the colon, small bowel (duodenum); granulosa cell tumors of ovaries; and possibly breast	Pigmented macular spots of the lips, buccal mucosa, conjunctiva, periorbital area, and digits; intestinal polyps which may lead to intussusception, bleeding

Table 1-1 (Cont.)

NO.	NAME OF DISEASE	ASSOCIATED CANCER	CARDINAL CLINICAL MANIFESTATIONS
17530	Intestinal polyposis III (Gardner's syndrome)	Malignant degeneration of colon, adenomatous polyps, sarcomas, thyroid cancer, periampullary malignancy, and adrenal cortical carcinoma	Polyps of the colon; sometimes in the stomach and small intestine; associated with bony and soft tissue tumors; globoid osteomata of the mandible with overlying fibromata are also characteristic; bony changes in the skull associated with fibromas of skull; also epidermoid cysts; retroperitoneal fibrosis, desmoids
17580	Porokeratosis of Mibelli	Squamous cell carcinoma within the lesion	Centrifugally spreading lesion with central atrophy and a narrow horny ridge at the periphery known as a cornoid lamellae; chromosomal breaks and rearrangements only in cells cultured from skin lesions, not from fibroblasts or lymphocytes
18160	Sclero-atrophic and keratotic dermatosis of limbs (sclerotylosis)	Skin cancer and bowel cancer	Atrophic fibrosis of the skin and limbs; hypoplasia of nails and keratoderma of the palms and soles; also linkage with MNS blood group locus
18840	DiGeorge's syndrome	Squamous cell carcinomas of upper respiratory tract	Congenital absence of the thymus and parathyroid glands; hypocalcemia and tetany; an absence of cellular immunity; patients are prone to acid fast, viral, fungal, and *Pneumocystis carinii* infections; deformities of ears, nose, mouth with abnormal facies; cardiac abnormalities including truncus arteriosus or interrupted aortic arch; failure to thrive is common

Table 1-1 (Cont.)

NO.	NAME OF DISEASE	ASSOCIATED CANCER	CARDINAL CLINICAL MANIFESTATIONS
19110	Tuberous sclerosis	Rhabdomyoma of the myocardium and mixed tumor of kidney; gliomas	A triad of angiofibroma, epilepsy, and mental retardation; also ash leaflet hypopigmented macules; shagreen patches; subungual fibromas; subcutaneous nodules and café au lait spots; phakomas occurred in 70%; skull X-ray shows intracranial calcification in 50% (CT scan of diagnostic benefit); marked variable expressivity of phenotype with frequent *forme fruste*
19330	von Hippel-Lindau's syndrome	Hemangioblastomas of cerebellum, spinal cord tumors, pheochromocytoma; hypernephroma of kidney	Vascular nevi of face; angiomas of retina; hemangiomas of spinal cord; cysts of pancreas, spleen, liver, and kidneys; polycythemia vera
	Neuroblastoma	Ganglioneurofibromas, neuroblastomas, pheochromocytomas	Café au lait spots and ganglioneuromas that may metastasize to the skin and resemble neurofibromas
	Cancer family syndrome (inclusive cutaneous signs of Torre's syndrome)	Multiple adenocarcinomas, predominantly of proximal colon, endometrium and ovary	Multiple sebaceous adenoma, carcinomas, and keratoacanthomas in rare patients, thereby integrating features of so-called Torre's syndrome
	Pigmented xerodermoid (possible dominant)	Basal and squamous cell carcinoma, malignant melanoma	Cutaneous signs same as xeroderma pigmentosum but with onset in adulthood; may be XP variant

Table 1-1 (Cont.)

NO.	NAME OF DISEASE	ASSOCIATED CANCER	CARDINAL CLINICAL MANIFESTATIONS
	Blue rubber bleb nevus syndrome	Medulloblastoma (in a single pt.), lymphocytic leukemia and renal cell carcinoma (double primaries in single patient)	Cutaneous distinctive hemangiomas, nipple or bladder-like, soft, bluish, erectile, easily compressible and slowly refill with blood after compression; may be pedunculated, sessile, and painful; angioma may involve mouth, lung, spleen, liver, kidney, adrenal, CNS, and muscle
17610	Porphyria, cutanea tarda	Hepatoma	Bullae and fragile skin in exposed areas, hyperpigmentation, hypertrichosis, photosensitivity, erosions, milia, occ. sclerodermoid areas
17620	Porphyria, variegata (South African type)	Hepatoma	Same as above with symptoms of acute intermittent porphyria
13170	Epidermolysis bullosa dystrophica	Squamous cell carcinoma	Life long history of bullae; phenotype not as severe as autosomal recessive forms

Table 1-2. Autosomal Recessive Diseases.

NO.	NAME OF DISEASE	ASSOCIATED CANCER	CARDINAL CLINICAL MANIFESTATIONS
14160	Hemochromatosis	Hepatocellular carcinoma in more than 10% of patients	Tetrad of cutaneous hyperpigmentation, cirrhosis of the liver, diabetes mellitus, and cardiac failure; genetic linkage to HL-A system
20210 20320	Albinism I Albinism II	Increased incidence of cutaneous malignancy (squamous and basal cell carcinomas, melanomas)	Lack of pigment in the skin; associated incomplete hypopigmentation of the ocular fundi; transluminate irides and horizontal congenital nystagmus, often associated with head movements; also myopia
20890	Ataxia telangiectasia (Louis-Bar syndrome)	Lymphocytic leukemia; Hodgkin's disease, reticulum cell sarcoma, lymphosarcoma and other lymphoma; also possible gliomas, medulloblastoma, and gastric carcinoma; increased cancer in heterozygotes	Progressive cerebellar ataxia, telangiectasia especially of the conjunctiva, progressive immune deficiency, both humoral and cell-mediated, and susceptibility to sino-pulmonary infection; chromosomal breakage; DNA repair deficiency to γ-radiation; decreased IgA
21090	Bloom's syndrome	High incidence of leukemia and lymphoma, squamous cell cancer of esophagus and adenocarcinoma of the colon	Dwarfism of the "low birth weight" type and a cutaneous photosensitivity to sunlight; chromatid breaks occur
21450	Chediak-Higashi syndrome	Malignant lymphoma	Decreased pigmentation of the hair and eyes, photophobia, nystagmus, abnormal susceptibility to infection, and death usually before 7 years of age

Table 1-2 (Cont.)

NO.	NAME OF DISEASE	ASSOCIATED CANCER	CARDINAL CLINICAL MANIFESTATIONS
22640	Epidermodysplasia verruciformis	Malignant degeneration of the wart-like lesions usually of the basal cell type; also Bowen's disease and squamous cell carcinoma	Lesions that resemble flat warts (verruca plana) usually 2-5 mm in size on the face, neck, and extremities, and characteristically do not respond to treatment; also keratosis palmaris may be present (*note*: This condition is caused by the human papovavirus; consanguinity of parents is common)
22660	Epidermolysis bullosa dystrophica	Basal and squamous cell carcinoma developing in the skin and cancer of mucous membrane	Condition may be present at birth or appears in infancy; involves the hands, feet, elbows, and knees; bullae develop at sites of trauma; also may involve mucous surfaces and even conjunctiva and cornea
22765	Fanconi pancytopenia (constitutional infantile panmyelopathy)	Leukemia 3 to 4 times the normal population — especially myelomonocytic; squamous cell carcinoma of mucocutaneous junctions, e.g., around mouth, tongue, vulva, and anus	All marrow elements affected with resulting anemia, leukopenia, and thrombopenia; reticulated hyper- and hypopigmentation of the skin occur along with malformations of the heart, kidney, and extremities; chromosomal breakage occurs; skeletal abnormalities
22785	Fanconi-like syndrome	Multiple cutaneous malignancies	Pancytopenia, recurrent infections, low IgA, chronic lung infections, bilateral pneumothroaces, osteomyelitis

Table 1-2 (Cont.)

NO.	NAME OF DISEASE	ASSOCIATED CANCER	CARDINAL CLINICAL MANIFESTATIONS
23500	Hemihypertrophy	Wilms' tumor, adrenal cortical carcinoma and hepatoblastoma	Enlargement of an entire side or specific region of the body; approximately 20–30% of the reported cases have hamartomatous lesions such as hemangiomas or various congenital defects, especially mental retardation, genitourinary abnormalities
26840	Rothmund-Thomson syndrome (poikiloderma congenitale)	Cutaneous malignancies	Cutaneous atrophy, hyper- and hypopigmentation, erythema, frequently accompanied by juvenile cataract in 50%, saddle nose, congenital bone defects (short stature), dystrophy of nails, alopecia, hypogonadism; photosensitivity to sunlight, predominantly in females
27630	Turcot syndrome (malignant tumors of the CNS associated with familial polyposis of the colon)	Malignant gliomas of the CNS and malignant polyposis of the bowel	Glioma and colon polyposis, multiple pigmented nevi, and café au lait spots
27770	Werner's syndrome	Sarcoma (osteogenic), hepatoma, adenocarcinoma of bile ducts, breasts, and thyroid; malignant melanoma; squamous cell carcinoma; meningiomas	Short stature, older appearance of face, high-pitched voice, beak-shaped nose, juvenile cataracts, diabetes mellitus, generalized atrophy of cutaneous tissue, hypogonadism, osteoporosis, premature atherosclerosis, and calcification of blood vessels and soft tissues

Table 1-2 (Cont.)

NO.	NAME OF DISEASE	ASSOCIATED CANCER	CARDINAL CLINICAL MANIFESTATIONS
27870	Xeroderma pigmentosum	Basal and squamous cell carcinomas of the skin, malignant melanoma, and bulbar squamous cell carcinoma	An exquisite photosensitivity to sunlight; excessive freckling in exposed areas in the first years of life; early degeneration of the skin leads to freckling, telangiectasia, keratoses, papillomas, and eventually to carcinomas and melanomas; the eyes may also be affected with photophobia, lacrimation and keratitis with resulting opacities; DNA repair deficiency to UV light
27880	DeSanctis-Cacchione syndrome	Basal and squamous cell carcinomas of the skin; malignant melanoma	Microcephaly, mental retardation, dwarfism, gonadal hypoplasia, retarded bone age, choreoathetosis, cerebellar ataxia, sensorineural deafness and shortening of Achilles tendon; DNA repair deficiency to UV light
	Sjogren's syndrome	Reticulum cell sarcoma, malignant lymphoma and adenocarcinoma of parotid gland	Keratoconjunctivitis sicca, disorders of lacrimal glands, xerostomia, rheumatoid arthritis, collagen vascular disorders, progressive systemic sclerosis, Raynaud's phenomenon, polyarthritis, chronic active hepatitis, primary biliary cirrhosis, features of SLE; possible genetic linkage to HL-A-B8
	Episodic lymphocytopenia with lymphocytotoxin (immunologic amnesia syndrome)	Reticulum cell sarcoma (one case)	Severe recurrent bacterial and viral infections; eczema is prominent; eczema herpetiformis has been described; episodic profound lymphocytopenia secondary to circulating lymphocytopenia; T-cell deficiency and combined immunodeficiency

Table 1-3. Sex-linked Recessive Diseases.

NO.	NAME OF DISEASE	ASSOCIATED CANCER	CARDINAL CLINICAL MANIFESTATIONS
30030	Agammaglobulinemia (Bruton type)	Lymphoreticular malignancies	A clinical picture resembling rheumatoid arthritis and an increased susceptibility to infection; dermatitis; B-cell deficiency, all immunoglobulin classes are reduced or absent
30040	Agammaglobulinemia, Swiss type (severe combined immunodeficiency; may be autosomal recessive)	Lymphomas	A propensity to bacterial, viral, fungal, and protozoal infections resulting from both decreased humoral and cell-mediated immunity; patients frequently die in infancy because of disseminating infection; low levels of serum immunoglobulins
30100	Wiskott-Aldrich syndrome	Lymphoreticular malignancies, malignant lymphoma, myelogenous leukemia, astrocytoma	Eczema, thrombocytopenia, bleeding problems, i.e., melena, epistaxis, purpura; susceptibility to infection of skin as impetigo, cellulitis, abscesses, furunculosis, otis media, pneumonia, meningitis, etc.; eczematous dermatitis may be present at birth
30500	Dyskeratosis congenita (Zinsser-Cole-Engman syndrome)	Squamous cell carcinoma, oral cavity, esophagus, nasopharynx, skin, anus, cervix, adenocarcinoma rectum	Reticulated hypo- and hyperpigmentation of the skin, dystrophy of nails, leukoplakia of the oral mucosa, continuous lacrimation due to atresia of lacrimal ducts, thrombocytopenia, anemia, and in most cases, testicular atrophy
	X-linked immunodeficiency with hyper-IgM	Lymphoproliferative malignancies	Recurrent pyogenic respiratory tract infections, extensive wart infection, neutropenia, hemolytic anemia, thrombocytopenia; have capacity to synthesize and secrete IgM, but fail to switch to IgG and IgA

Table 1-4.

Agammaglobulinemia (Bruton type) 20

Agammaglobulinemia, Swiss type (severe combined immunodeficiency); (may be autosomal recessive) 20

Albinism I 16B, 16M, 16S

Albinism II 16B, 16M, 16S

Ataxia telangiectasia (Louis-Bar syndrome) 1, 20, 21, 23, 27

Bazex syndrome 16B

Bloom's syndrome 14, 20, 21, 32

Blue rubber bleb nevus syndrome 5, 20, 25

Cancer family syndrome (inclusive of Torre's cutaneous signs) 16P, 28, 29, 30, 32, 34

Chediak-Higashi syndrome 20

Cheilitis glandularis 7

DeSanctis-Cacchione syndrome 16B, 16M, 16S

DiGeorge's syndrome 4

Dyskeratosis congenita (Zinsser-Cole-Engman syndrome) 4, 8, 12, 14, 16S, 31, 34, 35

Epidermolysis bullosa dystrophica
Dominant 16S
Recessive 8, 14, 16B, 16S

Epidermodysplasia verruciformis 16B, 16S

Episodic lymphocytopenia with lympho-cytotoxin (immunologic amnesia syndrome) 20

Extramammary Paget's disease (multiple potential internal sites)

Familial atypical multiple mole-melanoma syndrome (FAMMM) 2, 16M, 18, 20, 23, CT, GI

Familial hyperglucagonoma 11, 24, 27

Fanconi-like syndrome 16

Fanconi pancytopenia (constitutional infantile panmyelopathy) 7, 8, 21, 35, vulva

Giant pigmented nevus 16M

Hemihypertrophy 22, 24C, 25

Hemochromatosis 22

Hidrotic ectodermal dysplasia 16S*

Hyperkeratosis lenticularis perstans (Flegel's disease) 16B, 16S

Intestinal polyposis II (Peutz-Jeghers syndrome) 23, 26, 29, 32, 33

Intestinal polyposis III (Gardner's syndrome) 11, 24C, 26, 33, CT

Kaposi sarcoma 15, 20, 21, CT

Keratosis palmaris et plantaris with esophageal cancer 14

Lupus erythematosus (systemic) 13, 20

Lymphedema with distichiasis CT

Maffucci's syndrome 3, 12, 15, 17

Multiple hamartoma syndrome (Cowden's disease) 11, 18, 33

Multiple mucosal neuroma syndrome (MEN-III) 11, 12, 24M

Multiple nevoid basal cell carcinoma syndrome (basal cell nevus syndrome) 1, 5, 16B, 29

Multiple self-healing squamous cell cancer of the skin of the Ferguson-Smith type (keratoacanthoma) 16S

Neuroblastoma 1, 24M

Neurofibromatosis (von Recklinghausen's) 1, 2, 24M, CT

Pigmented xerodermoid (possible dominant) 16B, 16M, 16S

Porokeratosis of Mibelli 16S

Porphyria, cutanea tarda and variegata 22

Rothmund-Thomson syndrome (poikiloderma congenitale) 16

Sclero-atrophic and keratotic dermatosis of the limbs (sclerotylosis) 16, 28, 32

Sipple's syndrome (MEN-II) 1, 11, 24M

Sjogren's syndrome 9, 20

Tuberous sclerosis 1, 19, 25

Turcot syndrome 1, 10, 33

von Hippel-Lindau's syndrome 5, 6, 10, 24M, 25

Werner's syndrome 1, 11, 16M, 16S, 17, 18, 22, 30, CT

Wiskott-Aldrich syndrome 1, 20, 21

Xeroderma pigmentosum 2, 16B, 16M, 16S

X-linked immunodeficiency with hyper-IgM 20

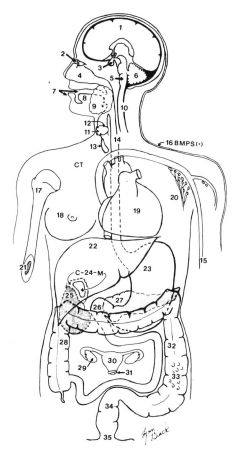

Figure 1-2. Schematic depicting anatomic location of cancer in the cancer-associated geno-dermatoses. (Code next page, Figure 1-2A).

or greater role in the etiology of *all* varieties of cutaneous stigmata and/or their cancer association; in turn, environmental factors will invariably interact in this process and thereby mediate expression of the phenotype. Therefore, events central to this critical genetic-environmental interphase may differentially en-hance the capacity for tumor induction and promotion in a given patient. The challenge to etiology and carcinogenesis lies in the comprehension of events at the *interphase* of this genetic-environmental interactive process.

Genetic Heterogeneity: Phakomatoses and Xeroderma Pigmentosum as Clinical Models

Phakomatoses. Any attempt at classification and critical assessment of cancer-associated genodermatoses, particularly in the midst of such dynamically evolving

CODE

1	Brain	19	Heart
2	Eye	20	Lymphatic system
3	Pituitary gland	21	Bone marrow
4	Upper respiratory tract	22	Liver
5	Medulla oblongata	23	Stomach
6	Cerebellum	24C	Adrenal cortex
7	Lips and mucous membranes	24M	Adrenal medulla
8	Tongue	25	Renal
9	Parotid gland	26	Duodenal loop
10	Spinal cord	27	Pancreas
11	Thyroid gland	28	Colon, proximal segment
12	Parathyroid glands	29	Ovary
13	Thymus	30	Uterus
14	Esophagus	31	Uterine cervix
15	Venous system	32	Colon, distal segment
16	Skin	33	Multiple colonic polyposis
16B	Basal cell carcinoma	34	Colon, rectosigmoid segment
16M	Malignant melanoma	35	Mucocutaneous junction
16P	Pilosebaceous carcinoma	GI	Multiple sites in gastrointestinal
16S	Squamous cell carcinoma		tract, no specific localization
16(*)	Carcinoma, palms and soles	CT	Connective tissue sarcoma
17	Bone		
18	Breast		

Figure 1-2A. Code for numerical designations of anatomic sites of cancer depicted in Figure 1-2.

clinical/pathologic investigations as are now possible, must necessarily be tentative. Nevertheless, it is imperative that we continue to study this broad subject as systematically as we possibly can, so that we might more effectively build upon its rapidly emerging superstructure. Therefore, in order to provoke further inquiry, certain liberties will be taken by us and our contributors throughout this monograph, in terms of the manner in which we perceive the cancer-associated genodermatoses from an etiologic, nosologic, and pathologic point of view. This will be particularly important from the classification standpoint. Possibly, it will even strike at the essence of syndrome delineation/identification. For example, it may appear that we should be *lumping* when we are splitting or, contrariwise, we may be *splitting* when we should be lumping. Emerging problems in the recognition of genetic heterogeneity mandate that a fresh view be given to this entire subject. The following discussion of this important concept, using the phakomatoses as a model, should lend perspective to the all-encompassing issue of genetic heterogeneity.

The term "phakomatoses" was introduced in 1923 by Van der Hoeve[12,13] to describe a heredofamilial group of diseases whose primary clinical features included disseminated hamartomas. Six diseases are so characterized. These include autosomal dominantly inherited tuberous sclerosis (Bourneville's disease), Sturge-Weber syndrome (no clear evidence of heredity established), autosomal recessively inherited ataxia telangiectasia (Louis-Bar syndrome), von Hippel-Lindau's syndrome (autosomal dominant), von Recklinghausen's neurofibromatosis (autosomal dominant), and Wyburn-Mason syndrome (arteriovenous communication of retina and brain – etiology unknown).[14] The clinical features of von Recklinghausen's neurofibromatosis and tuberous sclerosis are attributed primarily to ectodermal abnormalities, while those in von Hippel-Lindau's syndrome, Louis-Bar syndrome, Wyburn-Mason syndrome, and Sturge-Weber syndrome are believed to involve primarily mesoderm.

Tishler,[15] and subsequently Thomas, Schwartz, and Gradoudas[16] studied ten members of a large family wherein clinicopathological features of either von Hippel-Lindau's syndrome or von Recklinghausen's neurofibromatosis were present. Three of the ten individuals studied were found to manifest retinal angiomas (von Hippel's disease) in association with ocular and systemic evidence of neurofibromatosis. It was of interest that one of the affected members of the family with retinal angiomas had a combined syndrome showing neurofibromatosis, café au lait spots, pheochromocytomas, cerebellar hemangioblastoma, renal cell carcinoma, and pancreatic cysts. A review of the literature disclosed only two other patients showing concurrent neurofibromatosis and retinal angiomas. A case was made for the existence of overlapping manifestations of the differing phakomatoses in support of a common etiology.[15] Genetic heterogeneity must also be considered as a likely possibility in the explanation of these clinical phenomena.

The spectrum of anomalies in von Recklinghausen's neurofibromatosis involves the central nervous system (CNS), bones, skin, eyes, and endocrine glands. Cafe au lait spots and cutaneous neurofibromas provide some of the more striking aspects of the phenotype. Recent work has now subclassified neurofibromatosis into a central and peripheral variety based in part upon clinical and laboratory findings of nerve growth factor.[17]

Xeroderma Pigmentosum. Xeroderma pigmentosum provides another excellent clinical example of genetic heterogeneity (Chapter 10). As already mentioned, the main biochemical defect in XP is believed to be the failure of excision repair of UV damage in DNA of fibroblasts from the skin of such patients. This aberration is believed to be associated with a UV-endonuclease which initiates excision.[18-21] It is now believed that XP may involve defects in enzymatic steps in multiple systems and that comprehension of its biochemistry and clinical aspects may be exceedingly complex.[19] Indeed, cells from different patients with XP may show variation in the excision defect ranging between 0 and 90% of normal. Siblings are usually similar to each other in the degree of repair replication; heterozygotes are generally indistinguishable from normal patients with respect to dimer excision and repair replication.[18] These observations indicate genetic heterogeneity in XP-affected patients,[19] since cells from affected members of a given family generally show the same amount of repair replication. It is likely that the level of DNA repair is inherited as a distinct genetic trait.[18] In vitro hybridization of cells from XP patients has revealed seven distinct complementation groups (A to G) with the excision repair defective XP syndrome. A deoxyribonucleotide excision proficient form also has been described.[18-21] The frequency distribution of these groups shows variability in different populations throughout the world. The incidence of XP is estimated to occur with a frequency of 1 to 4 per million births. Robbins[22] has extensively reviewed the subject with specific reference to repair of human DNA. Eighteen patients with this disease have been evaluated at the National Institutes of Health, several others were from Europe and the Middle East, and 70 have been reported from Japan. It is believed that the literature may contain as many as 150 XP strains which have been the subject of DNA repair studies.

Evidence reviewed by Robbins[22] has supported the hypothesis that normal functioning of DNA repair processes prevents not only sunlight-induced neoplasia but also premature death of neurons in all healthy humans. It has been further suggested that the XP pigmentation abnormalities and neoplastic sequelae might arise from somatic mutations induced by the UV radiation in sunlight which causes photochemical damage in the DNA of human cells, and that the mutation frequency per dose of UV radiation is higher in XP cells than in normal cells. The mechanisms leading to the clinical manifestations in XP remain elusive, in spite of the knowledge that XP aberrations may result from photochemical damage in the DNA of these patients. The excisional defect is believed to be present in all XP cells which are capable of division, and it has been demonstrated in epidermal cells, conjunctival cells, peripheral blood lymphocytes, and Epstein-Barr virus-transformed lymphocyte lines.

The neurological abnormalities of XP, as observed in the DeSanctis-Cacchione syndrome, have been considered by Robbins[22] to be the result of an abnormal aging of the human nervous system. These abnormalities include mental deterioration, microcephaly, sensorineural deafness, areflexia, choreoathetosis, ataxia, extensor plantar reflexes, spasticity, and a neuropathologic electromyogram and abnormal muscle biopsy. Robbins[22] suggests that there is sufficient evidence of neurologic abnormalities in each of the several group A patients from four kindreds and patients from all five confirmed group D kindreds to indicate that the subject patients inherited deoxyribonucleotide sequences defining groups A and D, respectively, and that these may possibly determine the occurrence of the neurologic abnormalities in these patients.

Among the 18 XP patients clinically evaluated by Robbins,[22] it was not possible to relate the degree of the patient's accelerated solar skin degenerations to any in vitro tests of DNA repair. He suggested that any such correlation which might exist would be obscured by the absence of accurate quantitation of the patient's previous sun exposures. However, Robbins did find a correlation between the patient's post-UV colony forming abilities and the presence or absence of a history of acute sun sensitivity. He concluded that the acute sun sensitivity experienced by some XP patients apparently results from excessive killing or damage of cells in their skin as a result of inadequate DNA repair.

Robbins[22] considers XP to be the first human disease which has been conclusively shown to be caused by inherited defects in processes required for the repair of damaged DNA. He suggests that when more is known about the pertinent molecular defects and abnormal DNA repair dependent processes of XP, we shall then better comprehend how damage to DNA results in somatic mutations that can cause cancer in humans.

Problems of genetic heterogeneity will be encountered throughout this monograph. Discussion of genetic heterogeneity in the phakomatoses and in XP is presented to depict the ramifications of genetic heterogeneity as these may relate to other cancer-associated genodermatoses.

SIGNIFICANCE OF CUTANEOUS SIGNS

Genetic and Sporadic Varieties

One may encounter classical hereditary presentations of certain genodermatoses within families with either variable or rather constant cancer associations. An identical phenotype of a cancer-associated genodermatoses may also be encountered in a given patient wherein there is a complete *absence* of other occurrences in the family. This may result from a fresh germinal mutation (and, therefore, be of primary genetic etiology) or it may represent a *phenocopy*, i.e., a phenotype with features identical to its genetic counterpart, but whose etiology is unknown. The fact of the matter is, it may be impossible to discriminate clinically, biochemically, or pathologically between the *genetic* and the *sporadic* (phenocopy) varieties. In turn, there may well exist differences in cancer rates and/or sites in the genetic and sporadic forms. Unfortunately, very little information is currently at hand on this important but presently enigmatic subject.

Categories of Cutaneous Signs and Internal Cancer

Perry, Kiley and Moertel[23] have classified cutaneous changes which are associated with internal malignant disease into three general categories: (1) those cutaneous changes which are indicative of a specific type of malignant neoplasm, (2) those cutaneous changes that might indicate the presence of malignant neoplasms involving various organ systems, and (3) those cutaneous changes that are suggestive of the presence of lymphoreticular forms of cancer.

Paget's Disease and Malignant Carcinoid Syndrome:
Sporadic Models

An example of a lesion in the first category, namely, those cutaneous clues which are indicative of a specific malignant tumor, is Paget's disease of the nipple. In this example, the presence of an often unilateral, slightly elevated, eczematous or smooth plaque found about the areola, which on histological examination shows typical Paget's cells, should lead the clinician to consider that an intraductal carcinoma of the breast is present. This tumor must be pursued even when physical examination or mammography is negative. Appropriate action at this point would be mastectomy and meticulous histologic study of the entire breast.

By the same token, extramammary Paget's disease of the skin, as evidenced by the presence of nonhealing banal eczematous plaques located in the anogenital or axillary regions, oral cavity, ear canal, cheek, and lip regions, also necessitates biopsy of the lesion so that a search for the presence of Paget's cells can be made. When confirmed, one must then consider the high probability of an underlying malignant neoplasm, particularly an adnexal, urinary, genital, or rectal carcinoma.

So far as we have been able to determine, genetic factors do *not* appear to play a primary etiologic role in most occurrences of Paget's disease. Therefore, this specific cutaneous clue to internal cancer, while of inestimable value to the clinician in his cancer diagnostic armamentarium, will not pertain in a direct way to the cancer-associated genodermatoses under consideration in this monograph. However, these lesions are important in the differential diagnosis and serve as useful clinical examples in that they clearly illustrate the association between cutaneous signs and the presence of internal cancer.

The malignant carcinoid syndrome, characterized by the constellation of valvular lesions on the right side of the heart, diarrhea, and episodic cutaneous flushing, particularly of the face, neck, and upper chest, should alert the physician to the presence of a carcinoid tumor, usually primary to the small bowel, with hepatic metastases. These signs and symptoms may also be elicited by primary bronchial carcinoids without liver involvement and by carcinoids which are limited to the ovary. Certain noncarcinoid tumors may also elicit this syndrome. These include oat cell carcinomas of the lung, medullary carcinomas of the thyroid, and adenocarcinomas of the pancreas. As in Paget's disease, the malignant carcinoid syndrome does not appear to emanate from a primary genetic etiology; nevertheless, it is an exceedingly important indication of internal cancer and systemic disease, and thereby poses a problem in differential diagnosis of cancer-associated genodermatoses.

Genetic Models

In contrast to the above examples, disorders discussed in Tables 1-1 to 1-3 such as von Recklinghausen's neurofibromatosis, von Hippel-Lindau's syndrome, multiple mucosal neuroma syndrome, Gardner's syndrome, and others, provide specific examples of cancer-associated genodermatoses, wherein cutaneous clues coupled with family history should provide highly predictive information indicative of the risk for and/or the presence of malignant neoplastic lesions. As seen in Tables 1-1 to 1-3, in each of these cancer-associated genodermatoses one may observe the association of certain specific histologic varieties of cancer involving predictable anatomic target organs and systems (Figure 1-2). These disorders will be discussed in greater detail throughout this monograph.

General Cutaneous Clues to Internal Cancer

In the second category, namely the presence of cutaneous clues which may be *suggestive* of malignant neoplasms of internal origin, we find such conditions as arsenical keratoses, acanthosis nigricans, Bowen's disease, erythema perstans, multicentric reticulohistiocytosis, pachydermoperiostosis, acquired universal hypertrichosis lanuginosa, and the Leser-Trelat sign. Primary genetic factors do *not* appear to be characteristic of these disorders. However, this category does include the bulk of the cancer-associated genodermatoses which do show internal malignant neoplasms and/or systemic disease (Tables 1-1 to 1-3).

In the third category, namely the presence of cutaneous clues which are suggestive of malignant lymphoreticular disease, we find pruritis, herpes-varicella infections, and purpura. Again, these disorders are usually not associated with primary genetic factors; however, there are several genodermatoses (Tables 1-1 to 1-3), including Bloom's syndrome, ataxia telangiectasia, Wiskott-Aldrich syndrome, Chediak-Higashi syndrome, systemic lupus erythematosus, and Fanconi aplastic anemia, which harbor associations with this category in light of their association with lymphoreticular cancer.

Primary Cancer of the Skin: Genetics and Environment

Primary cancer of the skin is the most common malignant neoplastic lesion affecting Caucasians. Worldwide incidence figures vary greatly. In part, this variation in incidence is a function of latitude, i.e., there is a greater frequency of skin cancer in individuals of fair complexion, light eye color, light original hair, and poor ability to tan, especially when they reside in areas which are in closer proximity to the equator. The racial and ethnic makeup of the population also contributes to increased incidence of cutaneous malignancy. Specifically, these individuals, who are often of Celtic origin, are at greatest risk for the development of squamous and basal cell carcinomas of the skin as well as malignant melanoma.

Because of the fact that cancer of the skin is such a common affliction of man, with its incidence further confounded by the above-mentioned racial and ethnic considerations, it is not surprising that one will frequently encounter families showing an apparent excess of this disease. In addition, in certain cultures, many of these individuals will be found to be sun worshippers; they may also have a history of exposure to other potential skin carcinogens. These facts pose difficulty in comprehending fully the relative role of primary genetic factors which are operating in concert with these environmental carcinogenic interactions.

These problems notwithstanding, there are a number of primary hereditary disorders wherein skin cancer has been an integral feature of the particular condition. These include autosomal dominantly inherited multiple nevoid basal cell carcinoma syndrome, several hereditary disorders showing variable associations with cutaneous malignant melanoma, and finally, several hereditary conditions wherein squamous cell carcinoma is a prominent feature, i.e., autosomal recessively inherited xeroderma pigmentosum, albinism, epidermolysis bullosa dystrophica (this disorder may be inherited as an autosomal dominant or autosomal recessive), autosomal recessively inherited epidermodysplasia verruciformis, autosomal dominantly inherited porokeratosis of Mibelli, and X-linked dyskeratosis congenita. Finally, another condition, namely autosomal dominantly inherited keratoacanthoma, also referred to as self-healing squamous cell carcinoma, is characterized by multiple cutaneous lesions developing over most areas of the body at about the fourth decade. These lesions are histologically indistinguishable from squamous cell carcinoma, but of great interest is the fact that the overwhelming majority of them spontaneously regress a few months after their appearance, leaving residual scarring. Keratoacanthoma has also been reported in association with a variety of visceral carcinomas, including those of the colon, esophagus, duodenum, larynx, breast, endometrium, and ovary. This disorder has been referred to in the literature as Torre's syndrome (Chapter 8). However, our own recent investigations have suggested that this disorder may be a component of the autosomal dominantly inherited cancer family syndrome. Each of these diseases are presented succinctly in Tables 1-1 to 1-3 and will be discussed in greater detail throughout this monograph.

CANCER RISK TO CERTAIN HETEROZYGOTES

The magnitude of cancer in the general population which might be contributed to by the cancer-associated genodermatoses may be great. This is evidenced by the implications of heterozygous carriers in ataxia telangiectasia[24] and in xeroderma pigmentosum.[25]   An excess cancer risk for Fanconi anemia heterozygotes had been considered, but recent data have failed to substantiate that supposition.[26]

In accord with the Hardy-Weinberg principle, heterozygotes for certain rare autosomal recessive cancer-predisposing disorders should be relatively common in the general population. Swift,[24] in reviewing the subject, found that homozygotes with AT may occur as often as 1 in 40,000 live births, and from this, he estimated that heterozygotes would appear in about 1% of the general population. In the case of Werner's syndrome, a rare disorder wherein homozygotes would only occur once in 1,000,000 patients, the heterozygotes for this syndrome would nevertheless appear in about 0.2% of the population.

With the exception of recent studies by Auerbach and Wolman[27,28] in Fanconi aplastic anemia, there are no readily available methods which enable the detection of individuals who are heterozygous for these relatively rare cancer-associated genodermatoses. However, once homozygotes are recognized, then the study of their families, wherein heterozygotes would be common among close relatives of the affected homozygotes (parents of a homozygous affected individual would be obligate heterozygous carriers of the deleterious gene), should then be informative.

In the relatives of patients with AT, Swift observed an increase in deaths from all types of malignancies.[24]   These were primarily in young individuals. Of 329 deaths from all causes in 27 AT families, there were 59 deaths from malignant neoplasms (42.6 expected) in individuals below age 75. In those below age 45, 15 of the deaths were from cancer (5.2 expected). It was of interest that there were fewer cancer deaths than expected among those individuals dying after age 75, and fewer cancer deaths were observed than expected among spouse controls in these families. While the possibility that familial, rather than genetic factors in AT, could have been responsible for the increased deaths, the goodness-of-fit tests revealed that a model which assumed an increased risk associated with the AT gene fit the observed data better than did a model which assumed that the entire population sample harbored an increased risk of dying from cancer or leukemia.

Swift has provided estimates for the proportion of all cancer and leukemia patients who are heterozygous carriers of AT genes. This estimate is based upon the product of the relative risk and the heterozygote frequency. If the interpretation of the AT family data is correct, Swift estimates that over 5% of *all* individuals dying before age 45 from cancer of any anatomic site, may be heterozygous for the AT gene.

Swift and Chase[25] studied 31 families with XP and observed that a significantly greater number of blood relatives as opposed to spouse controls had manifested nonmelanoma skin cancer. These investigators concluded that heterozygous carriers of the deleterious XP genes may predispose such individuals to skin cancer, particularly in those who have inordinate exposure to sunlight.

Swift's observations should be tested on *all* of the recessively inherited disorders in Tables 1-2 and 1-3. This task will be expediated once appropriate markers for heterozygosity are identified. Search for recognition of heterozygous carriers of these rare disorders should be given a high priority because of their implications for genetic counseling and cancer control, as well as for their potential role in the comprehension of facts about etiology and carcinogenesis.

Cytogenetics

Fanconi anemia (FA) is one of the several genodermatoses (AT and Bloom's syndrome are others) in which chromosomal instability has been associated with an increased susceptibility to cancer and has resulted in these disorders being referred to as *chromosome-breakage syndromes.*[29] Lymphocytes from FA homozygotes show an increased incidence of chromosomal aberrations following exposure to alkylating agents[30,31] or to ionizing radiation.[32]

Auerbach and Wolman[27,28] have shown that baseline breakage rates for FA cell strains varied from 0.20 to 0.36 break per cell. However, after carcinogen treatment, these rates were increased three- to fivefold. In addition, treatment with the same carcinogens did not show a clastogenic effect on normal, XP, or trisomy-18 fibroblasts. These investigators[28] were also able to distinguish FA heterozygote strains from normals following exposure of the cells to the difunctional alkylating agent diepoxybutane (DEB), an active mutagen and carcinogen. The most frequent findings were chromatid breaks. Normal cells utilized as controls in this study, in contrast to the FA heterozygote cells, did not show chromosome breakage.

The observations by Auerbach and Wolman[27,28] indicate that utilization of a clastogenic agent in an in vitro stress system may be a valuable method for determination of the presumptive heterozygous status for FA. In discussing their findings, these investigators speculate that FA heterozygous cells may have a reduced capacity for repairing DNA, although this will not be apparent except under the stress of increased damage.

Finally, Auerbach and Wolman[27,28] suggest that utilization of an in vitro system based on extended exposure to low levels of carcinogen may also provide an effective stress test for the detection of other genes which predispose patients to cancer.

VARIABLE EXPRESSIVITY OF PHENOTYPE

Dominantly inherited disorders frequently show marked variability in the expression or severity of manifestation of a penetrant gene or genotype. This is referred to as *variable expressivity.* It refers specifically to the degree of expression of a trait controlled by a particular penetrant gene which may produce different degrees of expression in different patients. Therefore, expressivity of a particular penetrant gene in any single individual may show a range from slight to severe and may be characterized qualitatively and/or quantitatively. Certain genes show variable expressivities in different individuals while others are relatively consistent in their manifestations from one individual to the next. Phenotypic variation may be prominent within and/or between families.

Examples of significant variable expressivity of phenotype occurring in two of the mentioned phakomatoses, namely, autosomal dominantly inherited von Recklinghausen's neurofibromatosis and tuberous sclerosis, will be discussed briefly. A patient with von Recklinghausen's neurofibromatosis with only minimal cutaneous expression, as evidenced by multiple café au lait spots but an absence of neurofibroma of the skin (Figure 1-3), presented with a posterior fossa intracranial neurofibrosarcoma at age 17. This lesion was inoperable and the patient died several months following craniotomy. His family history was significant for expression of minimal signs of neurofibromatosis in many of the relatives through multiple generations. This patient most probably represents the so-called

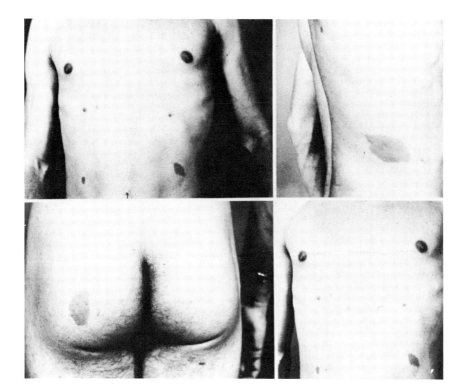

Figure 1-3. Patient showing neurofibromatosis with minimal cutaneous lesions (café au lait spots) who subsequently expired from a posterior fossa neurofibrosarcoma at age 17. This demonstrates the central variety of this disease.

central form of this disease which is characterized by an excess nerve growth factor (NGF) as measured by radioimmunoassay.[17]. In a second patient (Figure 1-4), we see a 65-year-old lady with severe cutaneous manifestations of neurofibromatosis as evidenced by hundreds of neurofibromas and cafe au lait spots covering most surfaces of her body. Her past history revealed an absence of cancer. This patient died of a myocardial infarction at age 65 and at autopsy did not show any evidence of cancer. This patient represents the *peripheral* form of this disease wherein there is an excess of the functional form of β-NGF as measured by radioreceptor assay. It will now be important to perform family studies on a

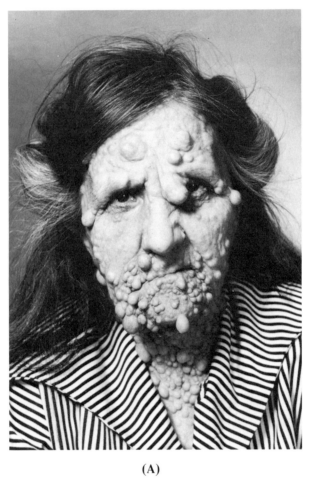

(A)

Figure 1-4. Patient with neurofibromatosis showing extensive cutaneous phenotypic findings consistent with peripheral variety of this disease.

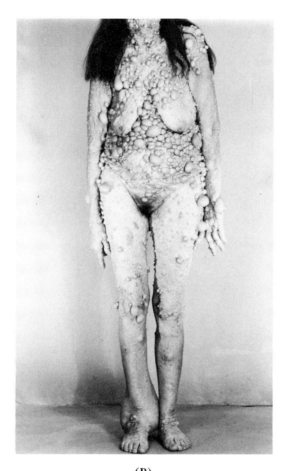

(B)

Figure 1-4. (Continued)

sufficient number of patients with the central and peripheral forms of neurofibromatosis in order to determine if phenotypic overlap occurs or whether these
are genetically distinct disorders.   Determination of β-NGF functional activity
should aid significantly in this endeavor.[17]

In a second example, namely, tuberous sclerosis, certain patients represent
the so-called *forme fruste* of this disease evidenced only by angiofibromas of the
face.   Others, however, may manifest angiofibromas, severe mental retardation,
convulsive disorders, subungual fibromas, shagreen plaques, white leaf-shaped
macules (which may be present at birth, with recognition facilitated by a Wood's
light), phakoma in any part of the retina, pulmonary cystic lesions, angiomyo-

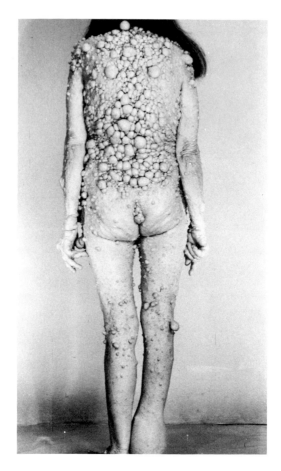

(C)

Figure 1-4. (Continued)

lipomas of the kidney, rhabdomyomas of the heart, tubers, and subependymal nodules of the brain (see Chapter 2).[1,2]

It is important in studying cancer-associated genodermatoses that the clinician recognize the extent of variable expressivity of the phenotype in these disorders. Failure to fully comprehend this clinical-genetic phenomenon could lead to misdiagnoses as well as to confusion in the interpretation of the mode of genetic transmission of the specific disorders.[1]

Theoretical Aspects of Hereditary Cancer:
Susceptibility and Resistance

Intensive studies of cancer in pedigrees could provide clues which might be broadly applied to the cancer problem. Matsunaga[33] studied distribution of hereditary retinoblastoma phenotypes in 231 families. A comparison of segregation ratios was made for the three possible phenotypes (bilaterally affected, unilaterally affected, or unaffected) among offspring of obligate carrier parents. These data indicated that penetrance and expressivity of the retinoblastoma genotype was correlated within families. The observed results were consistent with a multifactorial basis for host resistance in gene carriers, with two thresholds corresponding to the unilateral and bilateral phenotypes. The heritability of host resistance was estimated to be on the order of 90%. Penetrance of the retinoblastoma gene was estimated to be about 87%.

Given the relatively high frequency of resistant carriers of the retinoblastoma gene, Matsunaga[33] suggested that genes determining host resistance to retinoblastoma are nonspecific and may affect the growth of tumor cells in general. If this were the case, one might expect penetrance and expressivity of the retinoblastoma gene within families to be correlated with the frequency of cancer of all sites among relatives. In other words, these observations are consonant with the hypothesis that patients at high cancer risk may harbor in their genotype an array of cancer-resistant genes (so-called suppressor genes) which could have a major effect on penetrance of the phenotype (cancer). This hypothesis, therefore, suggests the presence of polygenic systems independent of the major cancer-predisposing gene which has a more general effect on cancer susceptibility or resistance. The cutaneous markers characteristic of the cancer-associated genodermatoses should prove invaluable for the testing of Matsunaga's genetic hypothesis relevant to cancer resistance and susceptibility.

DESIGN OF THE MONOGRAPH

This monograph has been designed primarily to meet the needs of practicing clinicians so that they might appreciate more fully the significance of those cutaneous signs which could then ideally provide a "window" to aid them in recognizing a wide variety of cancer-associated disorders that harbor a hereditary etiology. Following closely on this objective, the subject matter has been extensively annotated and interpreted by us so that it might also be more profitable to clinical investigators, geneticists, biologists, and interested social scientists. Controversy has been purposely provoked, particularly in those areas where we believe fresh and imaginative research is sorely needed. With such a variable readership in mind, we have attempted to organize the subject matter as conveniently as possible, through emphasis upon those clinical features which can best elucidate problems epitomizing the cancer-associated genodermatoses.

We realize fully that investigations of the cancer-associated genodermatoses are still in their infancy. If this monograph compels some of its readers to inquire into the subject in greater depth, then its mission will be fulfilled.

REFERENCES

1. Lynch, H.T.: *Skin, Heredity, and Malignant Neoplasms.* Flushing, NY: Medical Examination Publishing Co., 1972.
2. Lynch, H.T.: *Cancer Genetics.* Springfield, IL: Charles C. Thomas Publishing Co., 1976, 630 pp.
3. Cleaver, J.E.: Defective repair replication of DNA in xeroderma pigmentosum. *Nature* 218:652-656, 1968.
4. Lynch, H.T.: Genetics, etiology, and human cancer. *Prev. Med.* 9:231-243, 1980.
5. Lynch, H.T., and Frichot, B.C.: Skin, heredity, and cancer. *Sem. Oncol.* 5:62-83, 1978.
6. Paterson, M.C., Smith, B.P., Lohman, P.H., et al.: Defective excision repair of Y-ray-damaged DNA in human (ataxia telangiectasia) fibroblasts. *Nature* 260:444-447, 1976.
7. Weichselbaum, R.R., Nove, J., and Little, J.B.: Skin fibroblasts from a D-deletion type retinoblastoma patient are abnormally X-ray sensitive. *Nature* 266:726-727, 1976.
8. Fratantoni, J.C., Hall, C.W., and Neufeld, E.F.: The defect in Hurler's and Hunter's syndromes: faulty degradiation of mucopolysaccharide. *Proc. Natl. Acad. Sci. USA* 60:699-706, 1968.
9. Waldenstrom, J.: Cancer signals and the metabolic outlook in oncology. *Am. J. Med.* 66:720-722, 1979.
10. Lynch, H.T., Guirgis, H.A., Harris, R.E., Lynch, P.M., Lynch, J.F., Elston, R.C., and Kaplan, E.: Clinical, genetic, and biostatistical progress in the cancer family syndrome. In: (P. Rozen, ed.) *Frontiers of Gastrointestinal Research,* pp. 142-150, Basel, Karger, 1979.
11. Lynch, H.T., Frichot, B.C., and Lynch, J.F.: Familial atypical multiple mole-melanoma syndrome. *J. Med. Genet.* 15(5):352-356, 1978.
12. Van der Hoeve, J.: Eye diseases in tuberous sclerosis of the brain and in von Recklinghausen's disease. *Trans. Ophthal. Soc. UK* 43:534-541, 1923.
13. Van der Hoeve, J.: Doyne Memorial lecture: eye symptoms in phakomatoses. *Trans. Ophthal. Soc. UK* 52:380-401, 1932.
14. Yanoff, M.T., and Fine, B.S.: *Ocular Pathology – A Text and Atlas* (1st ed.) New York: Harper & Row, 1975, pp. 30-38.
15. Tishler, P.V.: A family with coexistent von Recklinghausen's neurofibromatosis and von Hippel-Lindau's disease: diseases possibly derived from a common gene. *Neurology* 25:840-844, 1975.
16. Thomas, J.V., Schwartz, P.L., and Gradoudas, E.S.: Von Hippel's disease in association with von Recklinghausen's neurofibromatosis. *Br. J. Ophthal.* 62:604-608, 1978.

17. Fabricant, R.N., Todaro, G.J., and Eldridge, R.: Increased levels of a nerve growth factor cross-reacting protein in "central" neurofibromatosis. *Lancet* 1:4-7, 1979.
18. Bootsma, D.: Defective DNA repair and cancer. In: *Research in Photobiology* (A. Castellani, Ed.). New York: Plenum, 1977, pp. 455-468.
19. Andrews, A.D., Barrett, S.F., and Robbins, J.H.: Relation of DNA repair processes to pathological ageing of the nervous system in xeroderma pigmentosum. *Lancet* 1:1318-1320, 1976.
20. Arlett, C.F., and Lehmann, A.R.: Human disorders showing increased sensitivity to the induction of genetic damage. *Ann. Rev. Genet.* 12:95-115, 1978.
21. Takebe, H., Miki, Y., Kozuka, T., Furuyara, J.I., and Akiba, H.: DNA repair characteristics and skin cancers of xeroderma pigmentosum patients in Japan. *Cancer Res.* 37:490-495, 1977.
22. Robbins, J.H.: Significance of repair of human DNA: evidence from studies of xeroderma pigmentosum. *JNCI* 61(3):645-656, 1978.
23. Perry, H.O., Kiley, J.M., and Moertel, C.G.: Cutaneous clues to internal malignant disease. In: *Skin, Heredity, and Malignant Neoplasms* (H.T. Lynch, ed.). Flushing, NY: Medical Examination Publ. Co., 1972, pp. 29-35.
24. Swift, M.: Malignant neoplasms in heterozygous carriers of genes for certain autosomal recessive syndromes. In: *Genetics of Human Cancer* (J.J. Mulvihill, R.W. Miller, and J.F. Fraumeni, Eds.). New York: Raven Press, 1977.
25. Swift, M., and Chase, C.: Cancer in families with xeroderma pigmentosum, *JNCI* 62: 1415-1421, 1979.
26. Swift, M., Caldwell, R.J., and Chase, C.: Reassessment of cancer predisposition of Fanconi anemia heterozygotes. *JNCI* 65: in press, 1980.
27. Auerbach, A.D., and Wolman, S.R.: Susceptibility of Fanconi's anemia fibroblasts to chromosome damage by carcinogenesis. *Nature* 261:494-496, 1976.
28. Auerbach, A.D., and Wolman, S.R.: Carcinogen-induced chromosome breakage in Fanconi's anemia heterozygous cells. *Nature* 271:69-71, 1978.
29. German, J.: Genes which increase chromosomal instability in somatic cells and predispose to cancer. *Prog. Med. Genet.* 8:61-101, 1972.
30. Remsen, J.F., and Cerutti, P.A.: Deficiency of gamma ray excision repair in skin fibroblasts from patients with Fanconi's anemia. *Proc. Natl. Acad. Sci. USA* 73: 2419-2423, 1976.
31. Schuler, D., Kiss, A., and Fabian, F.: Chromosomal peculiarities and "in vitro" examinations in Fanconi's anemia. *Humangenetik* 7:314-332, 1969.
32. Kigurashi, M., and Conen, P.E.: In vitro chromosomal radiosensitivity in Fanconi's anemia. *Blood* 38:336-343, 1971.
33. Matsunaga, E.: Hereditary retinoblastoma: delayed mutation or host factor resistance? *Am. J. Hum. Genet.* 30:406-424, 1978.

2
Cancer-associated Genodermatoses and Internal Manifestations

Henry T. Lynch, M.D., Ramon M. Fusaro, M.D., Ph. D., and Jane Lynch, R.N.

INTRODUCTION

Cutaneous manifestations of systemic disorders, including cancer, pose an extremely important area of concern to the dermatologist, pediatrician, family practice specialist, surgeon, oncologist, and in certain circumstances, the medical geneticist.[1] In the study of cancer-associated genodermatoses, the surface has barely been scratched regarding the genetic relationship between skin signs, benign systemic manifestations, and cancer. Consequently, new information is implicating an increasing number of organs and systems in the respective syndromes. The classification of these disorders, particularly as it pertains to "lumping" or "splitting" must take full cognizance of problems of genetic heterogeneity. Thus, any rigid or "final" classification of the cancer-associated genodermatoses is not only difficult, but also premature.[2]

Several sources[1-3] have focused upon systemic manifestations of cutaneous diseases. In spite of this recent surge of attention, only marginal interest has been given to the role of host factors (genetics) in these disorders.[2]

Physicians have long been intrigued with any variation in the skin which may herald internal disease.[3] The integument, because of its accessibility to inspection, was particularly scrutinized by our physician predecessors in the hope of relating the tangible findings to the relatively inscrutable internal disease manifestations. This was only natural for clinicians who lacked the many technological capabilities in laboratory medicine now taken for granted. They were compelled to depend heavily upon historical findings in conjunction with physical diagnosis during their bedside evaluation of patients.

More than 30 years ago, Weiner urged physicians to give greater attention to the skin in the quest for clues to internal manifestations of diseases, including cancer.[3] He used the term *dermadromes* to denote the skin component of a particular syndrome which was accompanied by varied internal manifestations.

Diagnostic and prognostic information, gleaned through critical scrutiny of the skin, can be embellished even more significantly through a detailed family history. When this is coupled with a knowledge of genetics and hereditary cancer syndrome identification, the gain may become even more bountiful. In the case of cancer-associated genodermatoses, a valuable opportunity is at hand for the incorporation of genetic principles, physical diagnosis, and syndrome identification, in the office or at the bedside, thereby enabling the enactment of a more comprehensive management program; thus, in certain circumstances, cancer prevention and/or improved control can be maximized.[1,2]

The chief concern in this chapter will be with those cancer-associated genodermatoses which harbor systemic manifestations. It is not intended to provide a detailed discussion of each of these disorders, since many of them will be discussed in other contexts throughout this monograph. Bloom's syndrome, systemic lupus erythematosus, Sjogren's syndrome, blue rubber bleb nevus syndrome, familial malignant melanoma, DiGeorge's syndrome, Cowden's disease, and others will be discussed briefly as clinical prototypes. The primary message to be conveyed in this chapter is that the physician must rely heavily upon his skills in physical diagnosis, particularly in the recognition of the significance of cutaneous signs, and his knowledge about cancer genetic syndromes, so that internal manifestations of the cancer-associated genodermatoses might be identified correctly.

Bloom's Syndrome

In 1954, Bloom[4] described a patient whose clinical findings were utilized for the subsequent portrayal of a syndrome that now bears his name. Clinical features which characterized this syndrome include: (1) photosensitive congenital telangiectatic erythema, located primarily on the butterfly area of the face, and (2) retardation of growth (short stature and slenderness, with fine-featured facies).[5] The head is often doliocephalic (Figure 2-1). Additional features have included café au lait spots and hypogonadism in males.[6]

The spectrum of internal manifestations in Bloom's syndrome may be greater than heretofore recognized. Recently, Ahmad and associates[7] reported two brothers with Bloom's syndrome who manifested endocrine abnormalities and myopathy. In addition to the well-known finding of growth retardation, hypoglycemia failed to elicit a rise in growth hormone in one brother (age 14), while it did evoke this response in the second brother who was older (age 17). Serum TSH (thyroid-stimulating hormone) was elevated in the older brother. This individual also showed values of FSH (follicle-stimulating hormone) and LH (luteinizing hormone) which were above the normal range. Finally, the younger brother was found to manifest myopathy. This was characterized by marked dilitation of the sarcoplasmic reticulum. Significant reduction in muscle strength and ul-

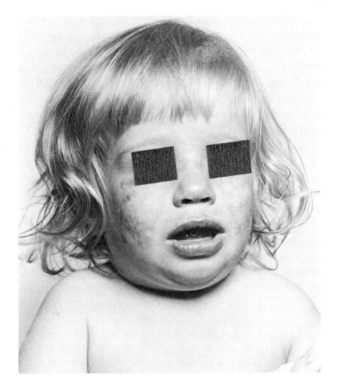

Figure 2-1. Bloom's syndrome showing distribution of an erythematous scaling eruption on patient's face. (From C.H. Dicken et al., *Arch. Derm.* 114:755, 1978)

trastructural alteration of the mitochondria and myofibrils were present in the older brother.

German and associates[8] described families with multiple affected siblings and an increase in parental consanguinity as well as an excess of this disease in Ashkenazi Jews. They concluded that this disorder was the result of an autosomal recessive pattern of inheritance. Cytogenetic studies revealed that affected patients had a chromosomal instability characterized by chromosome breaks and rearrangement.[9]

These same types of chromosomal aberrations also occur in Fanconi anemia and in ataxia telangiectasia. They likewise occur following exposure to certain cytotoxic chemicals, radiation, viruses, and mycoplasma. While these findings are therefore nonspecific, there has recently been a cytogenetic observation of unusual interest which was found in almost all chromosome preparations from patients with Bloom's syndrome. Specifically, this was the finding of quadriradial configurations resulting from the exchange of material between chromatids of homologous chromosomes. Dicken and associates,[10] utilizing recently developed techniques for sister chromatid exchanges (SCE), showed a nine- to tenfold increase in the frequency of spontaneous sister chromatid exchange in Bloom's syndrome (Figure 2-2). This has not been observed in other heritable syndromes of chromosome instability, and it appears to be restricted to the homozygous state of the deleterious gene. The greatly increased frequency of sister chromatid exchange in some or possibly all cells of some patients with Bloom's syndrome may be specific for this disease. Therefore, certain patients who would have been rejected earlier on clinical grounds alone can now be confidently diagnosed as harboring Bloom's syndrome.[11,12]   In four obligate heterozygote patients (parents of Bloom's syndrome-affected children), there was no evidence for an increase in the frequency of spontaneous sister chromatid exchange.[10]

The chromosome aberrations in this disorder are of interest, in that affected patients show a markedly increased susceptibility to cancer. These malignant lesions include leukemia, lymphoma, and gastrointestinal tract cancer, often occurring at significantly early ages.[11]   German et al.[12] reported findings from their Bloom's syndrome registry which comprises 71 individuals with this rare genetic disorder. A major objective of the registry is surveillance of cancer in both affected homozygotes and heterozygotes. Of the 71 individuals in the registry, 66 constitute the denominator for estimating the cancer incidence in this disease. Within this group, 12 of the 66 developed 13 cancers. These were as follows: six patients manifested acute leukemia; two had lymphosarcoma; one had reticulum cell sarcoma; one had squamous cell carcinoma of the tongue; two had adenocarcinoma of the sigmoid colon (one of these patients had a second primary, namely squamous cell carcinoma of the esophagus). The mean age at the time cancer was diagnosed was age 20. German et al. concluded that with the exception of skin cancer in xeroderma pigmentosum, Bloom's syndrome may have the greatest predisposition to cancer of all known recessively transmitted diseases affecting man. It was of interest that one of their patients with Bloom's syndrome – namely, a male who developed adenocarcinoma of the sigmoid colon at age 37 – is alive at 43 and may be cured of his cancer. He received early detection of this lesion even though his symptoms were only trivial. Significantly, the early detection resulted from his physician's awareness of the patient's genetic predisposition to cancer.

DiGeorge's Syndrome

DiGeorge's syndrome is an example of isolated T-cell deficiency resulting from embryologic aberrations in organs derived from the third and fourth embryologic pouches. It is characterized by a congenital absence of the thymus and parathyroid glands; it follows logically, therefore, that affected patients would develop hypocalcemia and tetany, and that there would be an absence of cellular immunity.

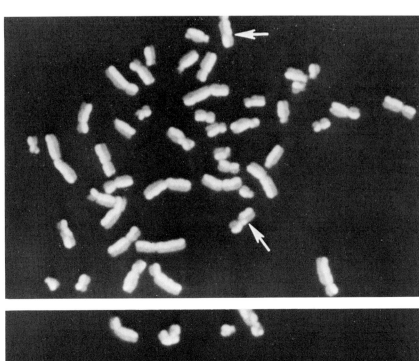

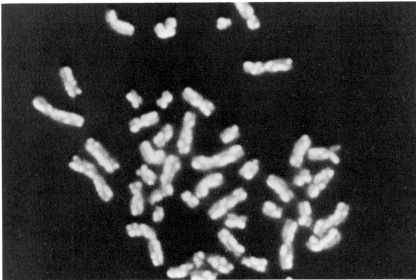

Figure 2-2. *TOP:*   Bloom's syndrome – normal metaphase of BrdU-treated preparation stained with acridine orange, showing differential fluorescence of sister chromatids. Thirteen SCE are present, two are indicated by arrows. *BOTTOM:* Similarly prepared metaphase from patient with Bloom's syndrome. One hundred twenty-four SCE are present. (From C.H. Dicken et al., *Arch. Derm.* 114:755, 1978)

The latter predisposes affected patients to infections, including those to acid-fast, viral, fungal, and cystitis *Pneumocystis carinii* organisms. Associated anomalies have included congenital defects of the heart and great vessels, abnormal ears, shortened philtrum, and hypertelorism.

Total lymphocyte counts may be normal, although the overwhelming majority will be B cells. In certain carefully conducted autopsies, a very small histologically normal thymus, usually in an ectopic location, has been observed. This may explain the fact that a few patients with DiGeorge's syndrome have developed normal T cells. Affected patients have also received transplants of fetal thymus, and subsequently developed normal cell-mediated immunity and T cells of host origin.

DiGeorge's syndrome may be inherited as an autosomal dominant though the matter remains tenuous at this time.[13] Predominant cancers are of squamous cell origin and involve the upper respiratory tract.[14]

Systemic Lupus Erythematosus

Systemic lupus erythematosus (SLE) is a multisystem disease with protean manifestations which may be extremely variable from one patient to another. Findings may include intermittent fever, arthritis, arthralgia, arteritis, phlebitis in the central nervous system, renal disease (lupus nephritis), and a variety of cutaneous manifestations. The latter include the characteristic malar erythema of the so-called butterfly area of the face (Figure 2-3).[1]

Immunological factors in this disease have been the subject of immense interest. A possible relationship between immunological deficiency, lymphoma, and connective tissue disease in a patient with SLE, dysgammaglobulinemia, and lymphoma has been described by Smith and associates.[15] In their review, they included eight additional patients with SLE and lymphoma. These investigators suggested that a spectrum of immune abnormalities exists in patients with SLE, and they further postulated the existence of a selected immunoglobulin deficiency in connective tissue diseases in general, associated with cancer or lymphoma; other connective tissue diseases in this category included dermatomyositis and Sjögren's syndrome.

The patient who was the subject of the report by Smith and associates[15] was of interest because of manifestations of a high titer of IgM antinuclear antibodies, profuse development of extracellular hematoxylin material, and cryoglobulinemia, which might have been related predominantly to the presence of IgM. Histopathological findings in the patient showed the concurrent presence of connective tissue disease, dysgammaglobulinemia, and lymphoma, all of which implied the likelihood of an immunopathogenetic relationship between the disorders.

Larsen[16-18] demonstrated increased concentrations of IgG in relatives of probands with SLE. Subgroups of the probands with SLE were selected according

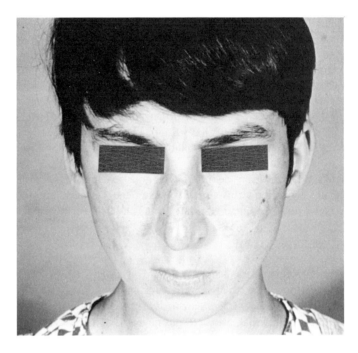

Figure 2-3. A 20-year-old male patient with subacute lupus erythematosus with the classic butterfly eruption.

to clinical and serological criteria. It was of interest that a significant difference in distribution of IgG concentrations was found between relatives of SLE probands with lupus nephritis and relatives of those without lupus nephritis.

Specifically, relatives of probands without lupus nephritis showed increased frequency of IgG concentrations greater than 174 mg/100 ml. The distribution of serum gamma globulin concentrations in SLE probands with, or who had previously developed, lupus nephritis did not differ from those without. SLE probands manifesting lupus nephritis, but who did not display uremia, showed significantly lower IgG concentrations than SLE probands without. Larsen concluded that these findings may indicate that patients with SLE who develop lupus nephritis are less prone to produce persistently high levels of IgG. He also showed an aggregation of increased IgG concentrations in relatives of SLE probands when compared with their spouses.[17, 18]

Larsen and Godal,[19] in another investigation, studied thyroid antibodies in relatives of SLE patients and observed that familial aggregation of thyroid antibodies was less marked than that of other autoantibodies. However, they did find that thyroid disease and thyroid antibodies were closely related in female relatives and in SLE probands and their relatives. In still another investigation, Larsen[16] studied rheumatoid factors in relatives and spouses of patients with SLE. A significant familial aggregation of rheumatoid factors was found in SLE probands and in their blood relatives.

Salivary gland scintigraphy employing radionuclides has been found to be accurate and reproducible for the demonstration of salivary gland involvement in Sjogren's syndrome. Clinical signs of Sjögren's syndrome did not necessarily correlate with abnormal scintiscans. Katz et al.[20] performed a prospective study utilizing these techniques in 24 consecutive patients who were diagnosed as manifesting SLE, 78 consecutive patients who were diagnosed as having classic or definite rheumatoid arthritis, and 18 control patients. Greatly abnormal scintiscans were found consistently in patients with SLE who were seronegative for rheumatoid factor. These investigators concluded that salivary gland scintigraphy may ultimately serve as an adjunctive procedure for the diagnosis of this disease.

These observations correlate closely with prior studies showing clinical features of SLE in patients with Sjögren's syndrome. It has been established that clinical examination alone may be insufficient to establish a diagnosis of Sjögren's syndrome in patients with SLE. Radionuclide scintigraphy appears to be more sensitive than parotid injection sialography for the diagnosis of Sjögren's syndrome. An abnormal scintiscan may have diagnostic importance when a clinical diagnosis of SLE is being considered. Discrepancies between clinical signs and severity of abnormality of salivary scintiscan may be of value in differential diagnosis. The investigators concluded that ". . . it is for this reason that the need for a full study, including salivary gland biopsy, seems to be obviated when the scan is meant to help discriminate between rheumatoid arthritis and SLE, not necessarily when the diagnosis of Sjögren's syndrome is at issue."

Singsen and associates[21] studied the onset and course of SLE in 100 children. Interestingly, they observed more black patients than expected from hospital population statistics. In addition, there was a surprising predominance of males with onset of the disease at less than 12 years of age, and there was a large number of familial cases. Signs and symptoms in the children differed from those observed in adults; specifically, affected children showed a greater degree of reticuloendothelial involvement and a possible greater propensity to change renal biopsy category. A major contributor to death in both children and adults was diffuse proliferative renal lesions. However, the importance of extrarenal mortality factors and the greater proportion of male deaths were emphasized in this childhood cohort.

The mode of inheritance in SLE has not been clearly delineated. However, several studies have suggested the probability of an autosomal dominant gene in certain families.[22-24] Recently, Beckman and associates[25] have reported their observations on 340 patients with SLE wherein demographic data, history of other illnesses, and pedigrees were obtained. Interestingly, 41 (12%) of the 340 patients with SLE had affected relatives. A careful evaluation of individual pedigrees showed examples of possible autosomal dominant, autosomal recessive, and sex-linked dominant and recessive modes of genetic transmission. When all of the pedigrees were considered as a group, however, multifactorial inheritance was suggested.

Additional evidence supporting a familial/hereditary etiology of SLE has included: abnormal serologic patterns in relatives of patients affected with SLE[26-29] and dermatoglyphic similarities in patients with SLE as compared to controls. However, in spite of these findings, it should be noted that these lines of evidence have not been sufficient for some investigators to conclude strongly, that there does, in fact, exist a high familial prevalence of SLE.[30,31]

SLE patients show an increased proclivity to the development of lymphomas and thymic tumors.[32-34] Distinction between the clinical features of SLE and the rheumatic manifestations of cancer may be difficult. In the case of lymphomas, the problem is further compounded by certain histological and serological similarities to SLE.[35]

Green and associates[36] described four women with lymphomas which developed 2 months to 12 years after the onset of SLE. Their literature review disclosed that an association between the two diseases had been recorded in 14 cases. In six of these, lymphoma either preceded or was diagnosed at the same time as the autoimmune disease. These investigators suggest that a common factor underlying the association could be immunodeficiency since patients with primary immunodeficiency disorders have an incidence of malignancy which is 10,000 times greater than expected, and interestingly, in a high proportion of these patients, the malignant neoplasms are lymphomas.[37]

Green et al.[36] reviewed the pertinent literature supporting an immunological-genetic axis for SLE and cancer, particularly lymphoma. They describe data showing that delayed hypersensitivity and T- and B-cell function are impaired in SLE and that genetic lesions which are located in the major histocompatibility complex adjacent to the suggested immune response genes produce a disease similar to SLE. In the case of NZB/BL mice, we also find that they spontaneously acquire an SLE-like disease and that they, in turn, have a high incidence of lymphomas. It is further stated that current concepts "favor suppressor-T-cell dysfunction as the primary lesions in SLE, predisposing to abnormal B-cell proliferation in response to an extrinsic antigen or autoantigen. Most non-Hodgkin's lymphomas are thought to be of B-cell origin."[36] These investigators also reviewed evidence for the role of a virus infection, either as an initiator or as the antigenic stimulator of an opportunistic or latent infection, leading to oncogenesis of the primed lymphoid cells. They reviewed studies showing virus-like particles in SLE lesions and increased Epstein-Barr virus titers in patients with SLE, as well as in those manifesting Hodgkin's disease and other lymphomas. In animal investigations, they observed reports linking a murine virus with an SLE-like disease and lymphoma in neonatal mice. They concluded that since SLE is not a rare disease, it is surprising that lymphomas are not more often observed. They suggest that the relationship of SLE to subsequent development of lymphoma may be considered as ". . . facilitation of the neoplastic process by the autoimmune disorder, however the former was initiated. It is even possible that chronic autoimmune and lymphoreticular neoplasms are all manifestations of one basic underlying pathological process — perhaps virus infection in a genetically susceptible host. Benign lymphadenopathy in autoimmune disease, immunoblastic lymphadenopathy, and lymphoma could then be regarded as forming a spectrum of diseases with a common aetiology."[36]

It is clear that because of the association between lymphoma and SLE, patients presenting with signs of SLE should undergo early biopsy of suspect lymph nodes. Advances in chemotherapy, radiation therapy, and surgery are now providing cures for these diseases, particularly when there is favorable histology and early staging.

Maternal Effect and Systemic Lupus Erythematosus. Jackson and Gulliver[38] have described a patient who manifested neonatal lupus erythematosus (LE) and at age 13 developed SLE. The mother of this child manifested SLE herself at the time of delivery.

This observation of neonatal LE progressing to SLE is purportedly the first of its kind. The authors review several clear examples of neonatal LE (none were known to have progressed to SLE), although the observation time of these cases was limited.

A multigene system acting in concert with environmental and maternal influences has recently been postulated as an explanation for neonatal LE.[39] SLE has been associated with two distinct histocompatibility antigens, namely HL-A1 and HL-A8, a factor which tends to support the multigene theory of this disease.[29] Many of the mothers of children with neonatal LE have had active or latent collagen vascular disease. (Paternal influences have also been suspected as being of major importance in the pathogenesis of neonatal LE.) It was of interest that in one of the cases of neonatal LE, the father of the affected child was himself affected. Familial non-neonatal cases of LE have been reported in a father and his offspring. Early on, a passive placental transfer of the LE factor from mother to fetus was believed to be etiologic in neonatal LE.[39,40] Other theories have included transplacental viral infection[41] or the passage of antibodies other than the LE factor.[42] A most remarkable occurrence of clinical and serologic abnormalities of SLE was observed in household dogs of two families with verified multiple SLE relatives.[43] A transmissible factor was postulated.

In light of increasing interest in possible maternal influence on hereditary disease,[44] i.e., in neurofibromatosis,[45] myotonia dystrophica,[46] and the familial tumor complex of sarcoma, brain tumors, breast cancer, leukemia, lung and laryngeal carcinoma, and adrenal cortical carcinoma (SBLA) syndrome,[47] it would seem prudent that more attention be given to the study of potential maternal influence in the phenotypic expression of all hereditary disorders including SLE.

Sjögren's Syndrome

The association of keratoconjunctivitis sicca, disorders of lacrimal and salivary glands, xerostomia (dryness of the mouth), and rheumatoid arthritis was described in a series of patients in 1933 by Sjögren, a Swedish ophthalmologist.[48] Subsequent observations of new cases have clearly provided evidence that these findings constitute a syndrome, which now bears the name of Sjögren. However, the spectrum of physical findings in this disease has increased remarkably and includes collagen vascular disorders, progressive systemic sclerosis, Raynaud's phenomenon, polyarteritis, polymyositis, chronic active hepatitis, primary biliary cirrhosis, and systemic lupus erythematosus.[34]   An extensive review of this subject has recently been presented by Kassan and Gardy.[49]   These investigators consider Sjögren's syndrome, once a medical curiosity, to be a disorder which is at the "... crossroads of a number of areas of major interest – the *autoimmune* disorders, lymphoproliferative malignancies, and the dysproteinemias." They suggest that the potential for unraveling these particular relationships, while conjectural at this time, is nevertheless too great to be ignored.

Primary signs and symptoms in this disease include dryness and atrophy of the mucous membranes, particularly of the mouth, conjunctiva, nose, throat, perianal area, and occasionally the urinary bladder and vagina. Severe ocular manifestations may occasionally present as corneal ulceration and loss of visual acuity. Salivary glands may be palpably enlarged, inflamed, and tender to touch. Anemia and achlorhydria may occur. Granuloma annulare has been described in rare cases. The fingernails may be brittle and the scalp may be dry. Alopecia is a frequent finding. Dental hygiene may be poor, with many carious teeth. Osteoporosis occurs frequently.[50]

Hypergammaglobulinemia is a frequent finding in this disorder. The rheumatoid factor, antinuclear factors, precipitating antibodies, and anti-IgM may also occur. Indeed, these associations have now led to the considerations by many that this disorder represents an autoimmune disease.[51]

Cancer has occurred in excess in patients with Sjögren's syndrome. In one series of 58 patients affected with Sjögren's syndrome, three developed reticulum cell sarcoma.[52] Other tumors have included malignant lymphoma of the salivary glands[53, 54] as well as adenocarcinoma of the parotid gland.[55]

Only a limited amount of information has been available concerning the role of heredity in Sjögren's syndrome.[50] Reasons for considering a hereditary predisposition are that Sjögren's syndrome is frequently associated with other collagen diseases wherein hereditary factors have been implicated, and because of certain findings established in laboratory animal models. For example, the inbred New Zealand Black/White F_1 hybrid mouse has provided an excellent model for systemic lupus erythematosus,[56] as well as for Sjögren's syndrome.[57] Since genetics plays a significant role in the development of autoimmune diseases in the New Zealand mouse model, this has logically led to further interest in the possible genetic etiology of Sjögren's disease. Family studies[54] have also been helpful wherein autosomal recessive inheritance has been suggested. More studies are obviously needed.

Further credence for a genetic etiology has been provided by studies of histocompatibility cell typing in patients with Sjögren's disease, a phenomenon first reported by Gershwyn and associates,[58] wherein an association between Sjögren's syndrome and HL-A-B8 was observed. These investigations have been confirmed by Fye and associates,[59] Chused and associates,[60] and by Sengar and Terasaki.[61] The latter investigators reviewed associations of HL-A-B8 and found that, the relative risk of persons with B8 are approximately 4.4 times (from combined data) more likely than persons without B8 to develop Sjögren's syndrome. In addition, their review of the literature indicated that the corresponding relative risk for B8 in patients with other associated diseases were: juvenile diabetes – 2.1, Reye's disease – 3.6, chronic active hepatitis – 3.6, dermatitis herpetiformis – 4.3, myasthenia gravis – 4.5, coeliac disease – 11.1, and idiopathic Addison's disease – 12.0. These authors reasoned that because B8 is the only HL-A antigen occurring in high frequency in several suspected autoimmune diseases, it seemed more logical that a genetic locus in linkage dysequilibrium with HL-A-B8 might predispose to these disorders. They stressed the unlikelihood that genes controlling each of these diseases had by mere chance come to be in linkage dysequilibrium with HL-A-B8 alone and not with any of the other HL-A specificities. They therefore postulated that this putative autoimmunity gene, genetically linked to B8, could express itself through a wide variety of mechanisms for the generation of autoimmune diseases.

Werner's Syndrome

Werner[62] studied a family of four siblings with a combination of short stature, cataracts, skin changes (which include atrophy, hyperkeratosis, tautness, and ulceration of the feet and hands) muscle and joint changes, early menopause, early graying of the hair, and premature progressive senility. These observations are now known to be characteristic of the disorder (Werner's syndrome) bearing the name of this investigator. Epstein[63] reviewed the subject and included 122 additional cases. He also described three members of a sibship affected with Werner's syndrome. Primary features of this disorder, based upon this review, are described as follows:

... symmetrical retardation of growth with absence of the adolescent growth spurt, graying of the hair, atrophy and hyperkeratosis of the skin, generalized loss of hair, alteration of the voice, cataracts (subcapsular and cortical, usually posterior), ulcerations of the feet, and mild diabetes in about half of the cases ... atrophy of the muscle, fat, and bones of the extremities, vascular calcification, and generalized osteoporosis .... "Hypogonadism" ... (in both sexes) was frequently present.

An additional physical finding was the presence of a beak-shaped nose. Furthermore, it was found that approximately 10% of these patients manifested cancer. The predominant varieties of malignant neoplasms were sarcomas, as opposed to carcinomas. Meningiomas also occurred with increased frequency.

Tri and Combs[64] have called attention to cardiovascular involvement, including precocious generalized arteriosclerosis and coronary artery disease. In addition, they described a 17-year-old boy who manifested congestive cardiomyopathy as an additional feature of this syndrome. It was of interest that the coronary arteries in this 17-year-old boy were free of disease. They suggested that myocardial cellular atrophy and fibrosis contributed to the congestive cardiomyopathy and that these were primary manifestations of the Werner's syndrome.

The basic metabolic defect in Werner's syndrome is unknown. Possible etiologies have included defects in ectoderm as well as primary endocrinopathies, implicating the parathyroid or pituitary glands.[65] Enzymatic defects have also been considered in this disease.[65-67] In spite of the fact that atrophy of the gonads and diabetes millitus occur in Werner's syndrome (thereby suggesting endocrinologic events), Riley and associates[68] have presented evidence opposing the theory of an endocrinologic basis for this disease. More recently, Nakao and associates,[69] in a study of endocrine function in three patients with Werner's syndrome, could not find definite evidence of generalized hypopituitarism or impaired function of hormone secretion. They did suggest a possible alteration of diverse proteins affecting hormone receptors.

One of the diagnostic difficulties in Werner's syndrome is the fact that the disease cannot usually be diagnosed until the patient is past the age of 30. However, knowledge of the presence of the disease in the family could provide clues for its earlier diagnosis in a given patient.

Werner's syndrome is inherited as an autosomal recessive. The tumor association with this disease has been well documented[63,70-77] and has included sarcomas, thyroid and breast cancer, hepatomas, hemangiomas, and acute leukemia.[78]

The Glucagonoma Syndrome

In 1942, Becker and associates[79] reported a patient with pruritic exudative dermatitis, weight loss, anemia, glossitis, and an abnormal glucose tolerance test, in association with an islet cell carcinoma of the pancreas. This may have been the first report of the glucagonoma syndrome.

The glucagonoma syndrome is associated with alpha-2-cell tumors of the islets of Langerhans and is now recognized as a member of the APUD system. The term APUD is derived from the initial letters of their most characteristic cytochemical features, i.e., Amine, Precursor, Uptake, and Decarboxylation.

Higgins and associates[80] have reviewed extensively the glucagonoma syndrome. While attributing the first report of this disorder to Becker et al.,[79] they stated that the symptom complex was nevertheless not fully documented until 1966. The three patients which they described, plus those which they reviewed from the literature, comprised a total of 47 case reports of the syndrome. The age span of these patients was from 23 to 73 years, and the sex ratio was 28 females to 19 males.

Major features of the syndrome include diabetes mellitus, characteristic skin lesions, glossitis, normochromic normocytic anemia, and weight loss with associated elevations in the plasma level of immunoreactive glucagon.

Dermatologic manifestations of the syndrome were described by Wilkinson[81] as being those of a necrolytic migratory erythema. The following description by Higgins and associates[80] reflects their extensive review of cutaneous manifestations in this disorder:

Necrolytic migratory erythema is the distinctive skin eruption of the glucagonoma syndrome, and this eruption led to the diagnosis in many of the cases reported. There is a characteristic evolution of each individual lesion over 7 to 14 days. The center of the individual erythematous macules or papules rapidly becomes pale or purpuric, which blisters or easily rubs off, and if extensive, may be mistaken for scalded skin syndrome. Serious oozing from the resultant central erosions produces crusts, while the erythematous margin spreads peripherally and is accompanied by central clearing. In some lesions, central scales develop on the inner margins of the erythema and a collarette of scale develops. Adjoining lesions may coalesce, giving circinate or gyrate configurations. Crops of lesions result in waves of extending annular, circinate, gyrate, or if superimposed, serpiginous erythema. Superinfection with yeast, fungus, or bacteria is common. In any one lesion, by the 7th to 14th days, erosions heal, crusts fall off, and scales clear with no scar formation. Frequently, a distinctive bronze coloration remains.

Lesions occur most frequently in areas of friction, such as buttocks, perineum, groin, perianal area, natal cleft, lower legs, hands, feet, or perioral area, although scattered lesions may occur anywhere on the body. Microscopically, the stratum corneum shows focal parakeratosis. In the superficial granular layer, and at times in the upper half of the epidermis, there are swollen, pale, vacuolated cells with pyknotic nuclei.

The mechanism of production of the characteristic skin changes is unknown. In only five of the detailed case reports were there no skin manifestations. Increased awareness of the characteristic skin lesions should lead to earlier diagnosis, thereby enabling more successful surgical treatment.

Glossitis or stomatitis was noted in one-third of the case reports; however, this feature was not commented upon in most of the remainder.

In 30 of the patients, characteristics of the tumors suggested their origin in the body and tail of the pancreas, while in 12 the tumor was so extensive that localization in the pancreas was not possible. The primary occurred in the head and neck of the pancreas in four patients. In one, the primary could not be found because of extensive metastases. The majority of the primary tumors were at least 3 cm in diameter at the time of the operation, somewhat larger than most insulinomas. It was also suggested that the majority of the lesions harbor malignant characteristics since there was a high incidence of metastases. Finally, in all reports having careful microscopic studies, the tumors were of the alpha-2 type of islet cell. Secretory granules described by electron microscopy were found to be membrane bound with a dense core, and they were frequently eccentrically placed in the organelle and were surrounded by a dense halo, characteristic of granules of the alpha-2 type.

Forty-four of the patients in the review by Higgins et al.[80] had either clinical evidence of diabetes mellitus or an abnormal glucose tolerance test. Ketoacidosis was not observed even in the face of the fact that two of the patients were insulin resistant. The majority of patients were controlled by diet, small doses of oral agents, or insulin.

While details pertaining to the metabolic function of glucagon are not fully comprehended, its primary role nevertheless pertains to the regulation of plasma glucose concentration. While increased insulin will decrease the plasma glucose level, an increase in glucagon leads to an increase in the plasma glucose concentration.

Elevation of the plasma immunoreactive glucagon concentration was reported in 33 of the patients reviewed by Higgins et al.[80] Elevations of glucagon level in the tumor were observed in an additional four patients, while in the remaining ten the glucagon levels were not reported. Of the reported findings of the molecular weight substrata of glucagon, the major plasma component has been a molecule of 9,000 to 20,000 daltons as compared to the molecular size of 3,500 daltons observed in normal subjects.

For diagnostic purposes, the most obvious clinical manifestation of the glucagonoma syndrome is the distinctive skin eruption (necrolytic migratory erythema). Thus, any diabetic patient exhibiting these skin signs should undergo further study, and when an elevated plasma immunoreactive glucagon level is observed, there is then justification for further studies to localize a pancreatic lesion. The findings of weight loss, anemia, and glossitis, characteristics of the glucagonoma syndrome, will not prove helpful unless there are other manifestations which might lead to a high index of suspicion of the syndrome. Recent developments with untrasonography and computerized tomography now make it possible to visualize relatively small pancreatic lesions. Selective celiac axis ateriography also enables diagnosis of pancreatic lesions.

Treatment of the glucagonoma syndrome may be curative through surgical resection when the tumor is localized. However, this was only possible in 15 of the 47 patients in the series reported by Higgins et al.[80] In at least three of these patients, recurrent tumor developed postoperatively. However, as in the case for other islet cell tumors, these lesions, even when malignant, tend to be very slow growing. Treatment with chemotherapy utilizing streptozotocin has been shown to be effective. Other drugs, including diaminotriazenoimidazole carboximide (DTIC), have also been tried and shown to be successful in a patient who did not respond to streptozotocin. Better recognition of the syndrome, coupled with earlier diagnosis, should provide for improved prognosis through surgical resection of the tumor.

Boden and Owen[82] studied a family in which four relatives of a paitent with glucagonoma had elevated plasma concentrations of immunoreactive glucagon that persisted throughout multiple observations over several weeks (Figure 2-4). The proband with the glucagonoma syndrome manifested a glucagon-secreting carcinoma of the pancreas and a medullary carcinoma of the thyroid. Because of the presence of a glucagon-secreting carcinoma of the pancreas in the proband, an alpha-cell tumor or alpha-cell hyperplasia was considered to be a likely cause

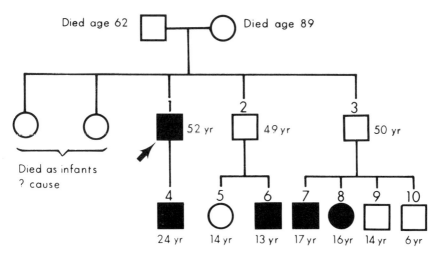

Figure 2-4. Family showing proband with glucagonoma syndrome and medullary thyroid carcinoma.   His son, nephew, and niece showed hyperglucagonemia and other lesions suggestive of a link with Type II multiple endocrine adomatosis. (From G. Boden, *N. Eng. J. Med.* 296:534, 1977)

for the elevated concentrations of immunoreactive glucagon in the remaining four relatives. This was hypothesized in spite of the failure to visualize a pancreatic tumor or hepatic metastases by angiography, pancreatic ultrasound studies, and liver scans, since microadenomatosis or hyperplasia cannot be detected by these studies. A genetic nonneoplastic disturbance in glucagon biosynthesis was also considered a possible explanation for the occurrence of hyperglucagonemia in these relatives. A finding of hyperglucagonemia in the father (the proband), his 24-year-old son, and the three remaining relatives was compatible with a possible autosomal dominant mode of genetic transmission. Finally, the 17-year-old nephew of the proband showed biochemical evidence of a pheochromocytoma in addition to hyperglucagonemia. A link with Type II multiple endocrine adenomatosis was therefore suggested.

Cowden's Disease (Multiple Hamartoma Syndrome)

The cardinal clinical manifestations of Cowden's disease include facial papules, oral papillomas, fibromas, and keratoses involving the acral portions of the limbs, and multiple trichilemmomas[83] (Figures 2-5 and 2-6). Additional skin manifestations include angiomas, lipomas, vitiligo, café au lait spots, and cutaneous squamous cell carcinoma. Mucocutaneous lesions, including smooth or verrucous hyperkeratotic papular lesions, may also occur. Cancer is a significant component of this autosomal dominantly inherited disease; it has included carcinoma of the breast, thyroid, colon, malignant melanoma, and the aforementioned squamous cell carcinoma of the skin.

Internal manifestations in this disease abound. Nuss[84] provides a detailed listing of abnormalities associated with Cowden's disease, including those involving internal organs. These include thyroid adenoma, goiter, hypothyroidism, uterine leiomyomas, and virginal hypertrophy of the breast, often with severe bilateral cystic disease of the breast.

Porphyria Cutanea Tarda (Hepatic-Cutaneous Type)

The porphyrias can be classified conveniently into two main categories, namely hepatic and erythropoietic;[85] a convenient division may be based upon the principal site of formation of abnormal porphyrins and their precursors.[86] Hepatic porphyria may present clinically as a cutaneous type as seen in porphyria cutanea tarda (PCT), rare examples of which have demonstrated autosomal dominant inheritance.[34, 87]

Primary attention shall be focused upon PCT. This is the most common variety of the porphyrias. Patients with this disorder show an increased fecal excretion of coproporphyrin and protoporphyrin. The urine may be colored orange or red, and may contain large amounts of uroporphyrin and lesser amounts of coproporphyrin.[88]

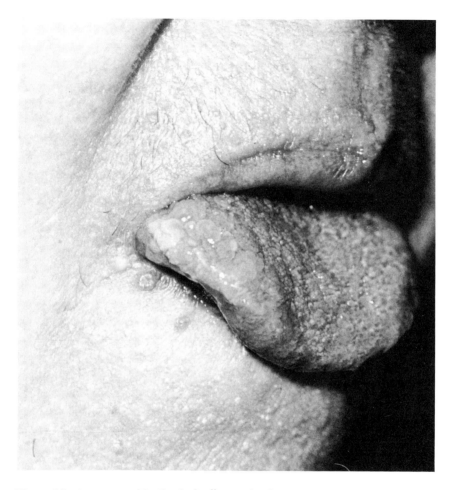

Figure 2-5. A woman with Cowden's disease showing cutaneous trichilemmomas and papillomas of the tongue. This lady had carcinoma of the endometrium and also exhibited the sign of Leser-Trelat. *(Courtesy of D. Reese, M.D., and J.C. Vance, M.D., University of Minnesota School of Medicine, Minneapolis, MN)*

The cardinal cutaneous manifestations consist of bullae, easy bruisability, hypertrichosis, and increased pigmentation. Patients may show crops of vesicles, which may be mixed with bullae. These occur primarily on exposed areas, including the face, neck, and hands. Sunlight, heat, and other types of local trauma may incite their appearance.[76] The skin abrades easily and when it heals, it may show depigmented scars on sun-exposed areas, particularly the hands. A few patients show extensive skin damage which is sclerodermoid in character. Photo-

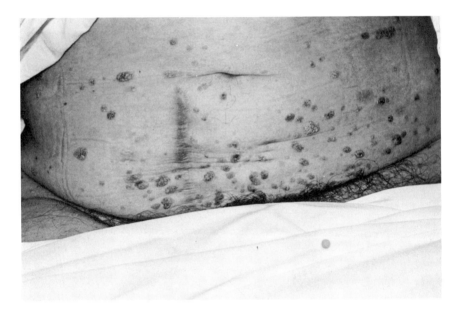

Figure 2-6. Patient in Figure 2-5 with Cowden's disease who also shows the sign of Leser-Trelat. *(Courtesy of D. Reese, M.D., and J.C. Vance, M.D., University of Minnesota School of Medicine, Minneapolis, MN)*

sensitivity in this disease is believed to result from preformed porphyrins in the liver.

Certain drugs may precipitate an acute attack and thereby should be used prudently when considering the diagnosis of PCT. Affected patients, in time, develop excessive iron deposition in the liver, not unlike findings described in hemochromatosis. During acute attacks, internal manifestations in patients with variegate porphyria include abdominal colic, motor paralysis, and jaundice. It should be noted that PCT features are an integral component of the variegate type of porphyria.

Cancer occurs frequently in this disease. These are primarily carcinomas of the liver.[88,89] PCT may give rise to some of the rare cutaneous manifestations of benign, malignant, or metastatic hepatic cancer. Malformations of the liver associated with PCT may predispose the patient to hepatocellular carcinoma. Liver scan is therefore indicated in patients with PCT. This includes those showing manifestations over a long duration who, in turn, have an unexplained exacerbation of their disease. This subject has been recently reviewed by Grossman and Bickers[89] and by Perry.[90] Hepatic tumors in this disease were also described by Rimbaud and coworkers.[91] Four of their patients had primary hepatomas, two had secondary metastatic cancer to the liver, and in one patient, the secondary nature of the tumor could not be determined. One of the previously reported patients manifested a benign adenoma of the liver. Waddington[92] reported a patient manifesting PCT of 10 years' duration who died from primary carcinoma of the liver with metastases. Most patients reported with PCT and cancer have been elderly and have had histories of chronic alcoholism.[89-92]

Ziprowski et al.[93] and Kishner et al.[94] considered PCT to be acquired and often secondary to alcoholic liver disease. On the other hand, this disorder may well represent a genetic susceptibility to the trait, with signs and symptoms triggered by an environmental factor such as chronic alcoholism. Benedetto et al.[95] described PCT in three generations of a family, consistent with an autosomal dominant factor.

Blue Rubber Bleb Nevus Syndrome

Bean[96] described the blue rubber bleb nevus syndrome (BRBNS) as a disorder with distinctive hemangiomas of the skin, mucous membranes, gastrointestinal tract, and other systemic manifestations. The cutaneous hemangiomas may occur anywhere on the skin. They may be nipple- or bladder-like, soft, bluish, erectile, easily compressible, and slowly refill with blood when pressure is applied and then released. They may be pedunculated or sessile and, in certain patients, exquisitely painful (Figure 2-7A and B). Occasionally, there may be spontaneous pain and sweating of the angioma. The angiomas have been described in the mouth, lungs, spleen, liver, kidneys, adrenals, central nervous system, and muscles.[34]

Recently, Waybright and associates[97] described a 19-year-old male who showed dermatological features of the BRBNS and who presented with focal seizures and lateralized neurological signs. Computerized tomography revealed a high density in the region of the vein of Galen. Postmortem findings revealed that this density was a clot within a malformation of the vein of Galen. Hemangiomas grossly resembling the skin lesions of the BRBNS were seen on the cerebral surface. Many were thrombosed and overlay patchy zones of infarction.

Berlyne and Berlyne[98] described a patient with the BRBNS who had iron deficiency anemia. He had complained of bleeding hemorrhoids and had undergone surgery for massive hematemesis. He was found to have numerous cavernous hemangiomata in the rectal mucosa which would prolapse on straining. It was of interest that this syndrome was manifested through five generations of this patient's family, consistent with an autosomal dominant mode of genetic transmission.

The BRBNS should be distinguished from the Osler-Weber-Rendu syndrome. A detailed differential diagnosis of the BRBNS is provided in Bean's monograph.[96]

Medulloblastoma has been observed in a patient with the BRBNS.[99]   While this observation could have been fortuitous, attention should be called to the fact that medulloblastoma has been found in other hereditary disorders, including the multiple nevoid basal cell carcinoma syndrome, an autosomal dominantly inherited cancer-associated genodermatosis.[34]   Hoffman et al.[100] described a patient with the BRBNS who showed typical findings of B-cell chronic lymphocytic leukemia and renal cell carcinoma.   While these reports are not sufficient to link the BRBNS unequivocally as a cancer-associated genodermatosis, they nevertheless should prompt further inquiry into this possibility.

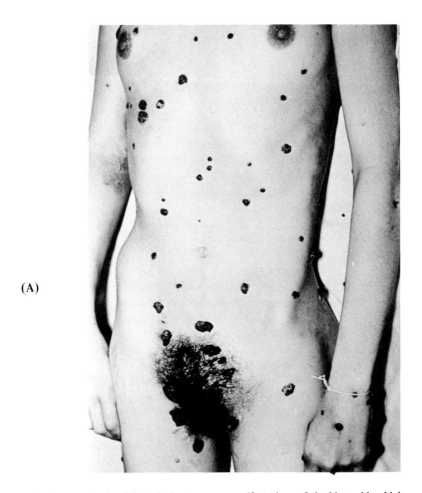

(A)

Figure 2-7A and B.   Female with typical cutaneous manifestations of the blue rubber bleb nevus syndrome. (From J. Sidney Rice, *Arch. Derm.* 86:503, 1962)

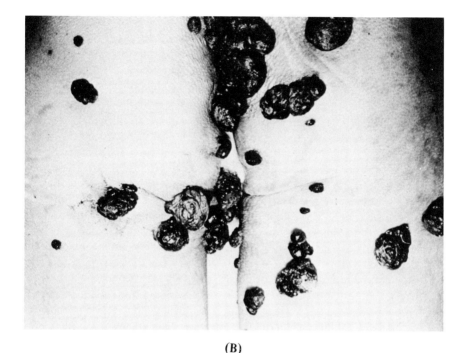

(B)

Figure 2-7. (Continued)

Bazex Syndrome

There are four primary components to the Bazex syndrome: (1) localized anhidrosis and/or generalized hypohidrosis, (2) hypotrichosis, (3) follicular atrophoderma, and (4) basal cell carcinomas. Bazex and associates[101] initially described this syndrome and, in a subsequent report, published the disorder under the title "Follicular Atrophoderma, Basal Cell Carcinomas, and Hypotrichosis."[102] This study included six affected members of a single family with hypotrichosis; some also had generalized hypohidrosis and anhidrosis of the face.

Viksnins and Berlin[103] described findings of this rare syndrome in seven members of a single family. Basal cell carcinoma developed on the skin of the face in five of seven of these patients between the ages of 15 and 26. They were most commonly distributed on the central facial area, including the eyelids. The basal cell carcinomas were morphologically and histologically identical to lesions found in the multiple nevoid basal cell carcinoma syndrome, a disorder which is high on the list of differential diagnoses for the Bazex syndrome. It was also of interest that facial eczema occurred soon after birth and became severe in several of the patients with Bazex syndrome.

Internal manifestations included hay fever in three of the seven patients, rheumatoid arthritis in one, and diabetes mellitus in another. One of the patients had scoliosis. These findings could be fortuitous and need to be studied in additional families. In contrast to Bazex's original description, none of the patients of Viksnins and Berlin[103] showed hypotrichosis.

These investigators believe that the follicular atrophoderma, as it occurs in this disorder, should not be confused with any other entity. These skin lesions have been variously described as ice-pick marks or dimples, which make the skin look vermiculate, or as depressions appearing in a funnel shape around the pilosebaceous orifices. The term *multiple ice-pick markers* has been used to describe multiple lesions occurring in a single area, while the term *exaggerated follicular funnels* has been used to describe individual lesions. It was of interest that in each of the seven patients described by Viksnins and Berlin,[103] the follicular lesions were restricted to the dorsum of the hands and elbows. Pedigree analysis showed vertical transmission of the syndrome consistent with a dominant pattern of inheritance. However, an X-linked dominant inheritance pattern could not be excluded in that all of the daughters of affected male subjects were affected, while none of the sons of the affected male subjects were affected.

There was no evidence of male-to-male transmission in the pedigree reported by Bazex and associates[102] which would lend further support to a possible X-linked dominant pattern of inheritance. However, the numbers involved are too small to provide conclusive support of an X-linked dominant pattern so that the more common autosomal dominant pattern of inheritance must also be given strong consideration. Further genetic studies of this syndrome are strongly indicated.

Finally, certain features of this disorder suggest that in addition to the multiple nevoid basal cell carcinoma syndrome, one must consider Conradi's disease in the differential diagnosis. However, Conradi's disease is inherited as an autosomal recessive.

Familial Malignant Melanoma

The most common site of malignant melanoma is the skin. Familial factors i· this heterogeneous disease are discussed in detail elsewhere in this book (Chapter 9). While malignant melanoma of the skin may metastasize to virtually any organ or bodily system, thereby giving rise to internal manifestations secondary to metastases (as is true in metastases from any type of malignant lesions), one should not lose sight of the fact that malignant melanoma may rarely arise in primary sites other than the skin. Intraocular melanoma is one such example. DasGupta and associates[104] have reported such unusual sites of primary melanoma as the meninges, adrenal glands, liver, esophagus, vagina, rectum, gallbladder, lung, breast, urinary bladder, small intestines, and ovary. Smith and Opipari[105] added to this list by presenting the first reported case of primary melanoma of the pleura.

Hemochromatosis

Hemochromatosis, also referred to as "bronze diabetes," is an iron storage disease. The genetics of this disease have only recently been clarified.[106,107] Specifically, in a pioneering venture, Cartwright et al.[106] and Beaumont et al.[107] showed how genetic-linkage studies could be used to clarify the mode of inheritance and to identify the presence of the gene for hemochromatosis. Prior to their investigation, the mode of inheritance of hemochromatosis was unclear, with both autosomal recessive and autosomal dominant factors having been invoked. However, these investigators discovered that patients with hemochromatosis had a higher frequency of HL-A-A3 and HL-A-B14 antigens when compared to unaffected individuals from appropriate control populations. It was concluded that the susceptibility to hemochromatosis is inherited as an autosomal recessive trait. Since the HL-A region is known to exist on chromosome 6, it was thereby inferred that the locus for the autosomal recessive trait for hemochromatosis is tightly linked to the HL-A region on the subject chromosome. This correlation among the hemochromatosis patients was explained by linkage dysequilibrium. The studies by Cartwright et al.[106] and Beaumont et al.[107] were combined with findings by a group from France (Lipinski and associates), quoted by these investigators, and when the three studies were considered collectively, there was found to be only about 1% recombination between the locus for hemochromatosis and the HL-A-A locus. This provided a lod score of 10 wherein odds favoring tight linkage were observed to be 10.[10]

Persons homozygous for the susceptibility allele showed severe iron overload, while those who were heterozygous showed wide clinical variability.

One of the advantages of linkage studies of this type is the fact that the hemochromatosis genotype of an individual can be determined prior to the onset of clinical symptoms. Hence, it is now possible, using this methodology, to develop laboratory tests which might enable the identification of homozygotes as well as heterozygotes. This will also allow investigators to study environmental factors, including alcohol, in the pathogenesis of this disease. Females, because of loss of blood during menstruation and pregnancy, show apparent incomplete penetrance of the deleterious gene.[108,109] Family studies involving asymptomatic relatives of patients with hereditary hemochromatosis have shown that approximately one-half of adult male siblings and male offspring of affected individuals over age 15 had abnormally high serum iron levels and coefficients of iron saturation.[108]

Hemochromatosis is a multisystem disease whose major target organ is the liver. Powell and Kerr[110] evaluated liver pathology in 125 patients with hemochromatosis and observed a greater frequency of hepatoma than in patients manifesting cirrhosis, but without an iron overload. Edmonson[111] found that hepatoma complicated 18% of the cases of hemochromatosis.

The liver is involved in virtually all patients affected with hemochromatosis; it is palpably enlarged in 93% of the patients, while the spleen is palpable in about one-half of affected patients. Approximately one-third of the patients develop cardiac symptoms. While multiple organs are involved in hemochromatosis, approximately 80% of the patients present with the triad of pigmentation of the skin, diabetes mellitus, and cirrhosis of the liver.[112] About 90% of the patients with hemochromatosis will show skin pigmentation at the time the diagnosis is established. It is believed that the pigmentation results from a deposition of both iron and melanin. Pigmentation is often diffuse and generalized. It is more prominent on the face, neck, and extensor surfaces of the distal forearms and the dorsum of the hands. The pigmentation is also increased on the lower portion of the legs, in the genital region, and in scars. The slate bluish-gray appearance of the skin is believed to result from increased melanin. Approximately 10-15% of affected patients will have pigmented mucous membranes. Manifestations also include diabetes, heart disease, hypogonadism, and arthropathy.

As in porphyria cutanea tarda, hemochromatosis seems to be exacerbated by alcoholism. The differential diagnosis between alcoholic hemochromatosis and idiopathic hemochromatosis may be exceedingly difficult. Finally, heavy ingestion of iron over prolonged periods of time may result in hemochromatosis, particularly in individuals who are genetically predisposed to this disease.

The diagnosis of hemochromatosis must be considered in any patient with increased pigmentation of the skin, enlarged liver, and diabetes mellitus. Diagnostic tests are based, in part, on the demonstration of abnormal iron metabolism.

Therapy for hemochromatosis is comprised primarily of phlebotomies alone or in combination with chelating agents.

Epidermal Nevus Syndrome

While no genetic basis has been established to date for the epidermal nevus syndrome, it shall be presented here briefly, for heuristic reasons. The syndrome consists of congenital nevi, associated multiorgan defects involving skeletal, dental, neurologic, ocular, vascular, and cardiac systems. Malignant neoplasms occur with increased frequency in this disease.[113] McAuley[114] described a patient with the epidermal nevus syndrome who presented with dysphasia, transient left hemiparesis, and sensory symptoms resulting from an occlusion of the right internal carotid artery. In addition, she had abnormal retinal vessels and Raynaud's phenomenon. These investigators suggested that the arterial occlusion may have been caused by a dysplastic artery. The patient had an older brother who reportedly had a foot anomaly requiring amputation. Unfortunately, no further history on the patient's brother or family is provided.

Thus, we see a disorder with striking cutaneous manifestations, cancer association, and multisystem disease, but whose etiology is unclear. Patients with this disorder, in addition to detailed medical and dermatologic study, should have their family histories carefully scrutinized. Personal study of close relatives should be made in the search for anomalies consistent with the syndrome.

Von Recklinghausen's Neurofibromatosis

The fact that brain and skin share a common ectodermal derivation makes it understandable that there should be a group of disorders having neurologic manifestations associated with cutaneous signs. Because of its frequency in the population and its multifaceted internal manifestations, von Recklinghausen's neurofibromatosis will serve as a prototype for primary neurological cancer-associated genodermatoses. While skin and neurological manifestations have predominated in historical accounts of this disease, endocrine, skeletal, ocular, vascular, and other visceral manifestations are also of paramount concern.[1,2,34]

Von Recklinghausen's neurofibromatosis is usually easy to diagnose,[115-117] particularly in the presence of multiple neurofibromas of the skin (sessile or pedunculated) and café au lait spots (originally thought to require more than six spots, with each one being at least 1.5 cm or greater in size), as well as axillary freckles.[115,117] However, there is considerable phenotypic variation in this disease, a fact already discussed in our introductory chapter. The café au lait spots are brown-pigmented macules which show varying size and shape. It has been stated that the presence of giant melanosomes in the pigmented spots is peculiar to neurofibromatosis.[116] However, recent evidence casts doubt on the specificity of giant melanosomes in café au lait spots in neurofibromatosis.[118] Perhaps more firmly associated are the axillary freckles, also referred to as Crowe's sign.[115,117] These are considered by some to be pathognomonic of this disease.

Recent evidence has disclosed that there are two forms of neurofibromatosis, a central and a peripheral variety, distinguishable clinically and by laboratory methods. The *peripheral* variety is characterized by multiple café au lait spots and neurofibromas of the skin in addition to a variety of internal manifestations.[2] This form is associated with a β-nerve growth factor (β-NGF) which is present in normal concentrations by radioimmunoassay but which shows increased functional activity by radioreceptor assay. *Central* neurofibromatosis is a clinical variant whose hallmark is bilateral acoustic neuromas and a paucity of cutaneous findings. This variety shows low to normal levels of functional NGF by radio-receptor assay, but increased NGF antigenic activity by radioimmunoassay (see Chapter 1).

Neurological manifestations of neurofibromatosis are many and exceedingly variable. For example, any of the cranial nerves may be affected, though optic and vestibulo-cochlear nerves are commonly involved with tumor (optic glioma and acoustic neurinomas, respectively, the latter frequently bilateral). Acoustic neurinomas may produce deafness, cerebellar signs, facial palsy, and loss of the corneal reflex.

Tumors involving spinal nerves may grow through the intervertebral foramen, and as a result of pressure on the spinal cord, paraplegia may occur. Meningiomas may also occur in this disease. For example, Dellman and associates,[119] recently reported a family in which four members in two generations had meningiomas without evidence of neurofibromatosis. However, another member of the family had multiple meningiomas and bilateral acoustic neurinomas. Still another member had café au lait spots. This particular kindred introduces an exceedingly interesting clinical feature of multiple neurofibromatosis, namely the fact that in certain families, the cutaneous manifestations may be exceedingly minimal despite more ominous disease, including central nervous system neoplasms, both benign (meningiomas) and malignant (gliomas); this is consistent with the already mentioned concept of a central form of neurofibromatosis. This feature of neurofibromatosis has also been discussed by Lee and Abbott,[120] who reported a family with neurofibromatosis whose affected patients manifested meningiomas and sarcomas, but with as few as one or two café au lait spots. We therefore believe that the previous criterion of a minimum of six café au lait spots, 1.5 cm or greater in size, must be reassessed.

As mentioned, neurofibromatosis may also occur in the orbit, resulting in unilateral proptosis; glioma of the optic nerve is common in children. It is also of interest that superficial neurofibromas seldom undergo malignant change; however, neurogenic sarcoma or fibrosarcoma may arise from deeply situated tumors.[121]

Skeletal manifestations are extremely common in this disease. These include hypertrophy as well as underdevelopment of bone, congenital pseudoarthrosis, kyphosis, and scoliosis. Intraosseous cystic lesions have also been reported.[115] Osteomalacia in association with congenital renal tubular defect has been reported in neurofibromatosis by Saville and associates.[122] Findings of retardation of sexual maturation, suggestive of panhypopituitarism, have also been described.[115]

Patients with multiple neurofibromatosis may present with hypertension secondary to pheochromocytoma,[123] a tumor which has a relatively high incidence in this disease. Hypertension may also occur secondary to renal ischemia, resulting from involvement of the renal arteries by an adjacent neurofibroma.[124]

Intestinal obstruction with intussusception and/or melanin of stool secondary to involvement by neurofibroma in the intestine, may also occur in this disease.[125]

Pulmonic involvement has also been described. Specifically, patients may present with exertional dyspnea, cough, fever, and hemoptysis secondary to cystic lesions of the lung.[126] Vascular lesions, particularly benign capillary hemangiomas, are known to occur with increased frequency.[127] A patient with von Recklinghausen's neurofibromatosis died from an intracerebral hemorrhage resulting from metastatic angiosarcoma. The primary site of the malignant neoplasm was a peripheral nerve which microscopically showed both angiosarcoma and neurofibromatosis.

This brief review shows clearly the extent of systemic involvement as a result of probable pleiotropy of a single deleterious autosomal dominant gene in von Recklinghausen's neurofibromatosis. Undoubtedly, the spectrum of internal manifestations in this multisystem disease will be shown to be even greater as more patients and/or families are investigated.[34]

Family Study. The proband (Figure 2-8, IV-1) is a 14-year-old, mildly retarded, white male with a known history of von Recklinghausen's neurofibromatosis. He had previously excision of multiple neurofibromas and is deaf in the right ear. He was admitted to the hospital with an abdominal mass which was allegedly first noted only two weeks prior to admission. He complained of pain in his left leg with some numbness over the left thigh. The patient had numerous subcutaneous neurofibromas over the upper extremities and trunk. There was one large neurofibroma on the medial aspect of the right knee. There were also numerous large café au lait spots on the posterior trunk, bilateral axillary freckling, and anterior truncal freckling. At surgery, a massive tumor of the left abdomen with invasion of the psoas muscle was excised (Figure 2-9). Histologic diagnosis was low to moderate grade malignant schwannoma.

We subsequently examined several of the patient's relatives in an attempt to identify other family members with the stigmata for neurofibromatosis.

The proband's mother (Figure 2-8, III-3) had marked facial freckling, present since early childhood. She reported that she had a large neurofibroma removed from her leg at age 14. A basal cell carcinoma was removed from her lower eyelid at age 8. On examination, she was noted to have a 3 X .5 cm café au lait spot on her back and a 4 X 1 cm café au lait spot on her thigh. The remainder of her examination was essentialy negative.

The proband's maternal grandmother (Figure 2-8, II-2) had a mottled, tannish, giant pigmented nevus, present since birth, which covered the T4-L-3 area and stopped at the midline in front and back. There was also a 10 cm café au lait spot on her left arm.

Examination of the proband's maternal uncle (Figure 2-8, III-5) showed a large dermal nevus on his back and a 2 cm scapular subcutaneous mass representing either a lipoma or an epithelial cyst.

Café au lait spots were noted in two other relatives (Figure 2-8, II-7 and IV-7) whom we examined. The maternal great-grandmother (Figure 2-8, I-4) had cutaneous stigmata of neurofibromatosis by history.

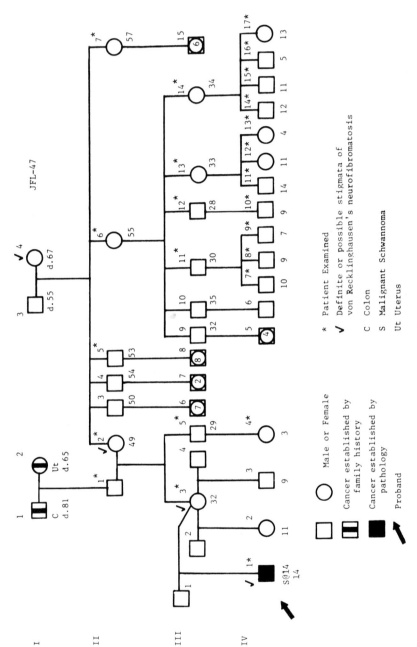

Figure 2-8. Pedigree of family with neurofibromatosis in four generations.

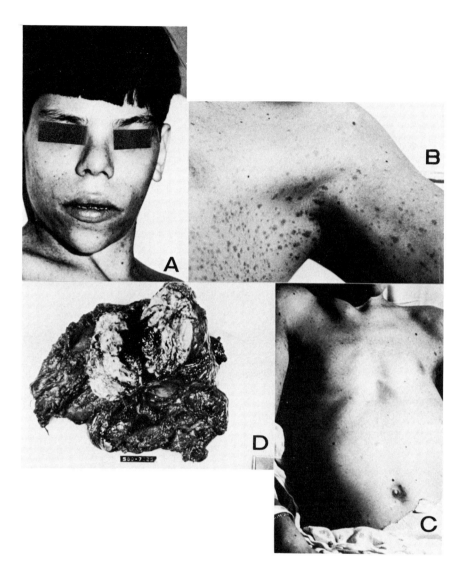

Figure 2-9. (A) The proband, a 14-year-old boy, from Figure 2-8, with mild mental retardation; (B) typical axillary freckling; (C) evidence of a mass lesion filling most of the right abdomen; (D) tumor weighing more than 2,000 grams excised from the right abdomen which histologically was a malignant schwannoma.

The only other finding of interest was in a 4-year-old second cousin of the proband (Figure 2-8, IV-13), who showed bilateral vitiliginous areas containing ianugo hairs. This probably represented a nevus depigmentosis.

Tuberous Sclerosis

The triad of angiokeratoma (adenoma sebaceum), epilepsy, and mental retardation characterize tuberous sclerosis (Bourneville's disease), an autosomal dominantly inherited disorder. However, sporadic occurrences of this disease are common.[128, 129]

This disorder, like multiple neurofibromatosis, is characterized by multisystem involvement. The major skin manifestaions, however, are more varied than those of von Recklinghausen's neurofibromatosis. Both conditions share café au lait spots as a common manifestation, although they appear to be less numerous in tuberous sclerosis. The most common skin manifestation is angiokeratoma, and it is believed by some that 100% of the affected patients over 35 years of age, and approximately 50% of the patients under 5 years of age will manifest this lesion[130] (Figure 2-10). Another skin sign which may aid in diagnosis early

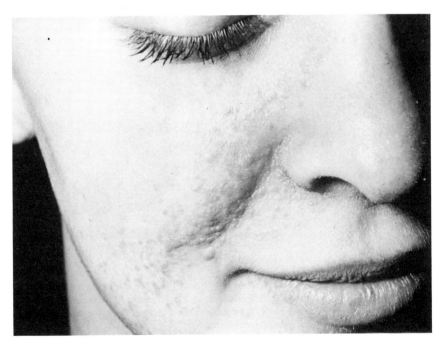

Figure 2-10. Patient with tuberous sclerosis showing papules which are the classical angiokeratomas of this disorder.

in life is the presence of a white ash leaf-shaped macule. This lesion differs from vitiligo in that depigmentation is not complete and the patches are more likely to be oval or lancet-shaped as opposed to being irregular. Examination with a Wood's light aids in their detection. Another cutaneous lesion is the shagreen plaque (Figure 2-11). These elevated lesions show transverse wrinkling, like the skin of a shark, and are rough. Subungual fibromas may also occur (Figure 2-12).

Neurologic manifestations are common, the most frequent of which are convulsions. Ocular findings, including optic atrophy, papilledema (secondary to brain lesions), and phakomas, also characterize this disease.[129]   Intracranial lesions, described as tubers ("potato-like lesions") may involve the cortex (Figure 2-13) and/or the intraventricular system (Figure 2-14).

Internal manifestations are frequent in tuberous sclerosis. These may involve the lungs, heart, and kidneys. Pulmonary cystic lesions, similar to those occurring in neurofibromatosis, may also be observed. This complication may give rise to progressive exertional dyspnea.[129]   Pleural effusion has also been described in this disease.[131]

Renal involvement in tuberous sclerosis is often manifested by enlarged cystic kidneys (necessitating differentiation from polycystic kidney disease and renal cancer), flank pain, and episodic hematuria with progressive renal failure.[132]

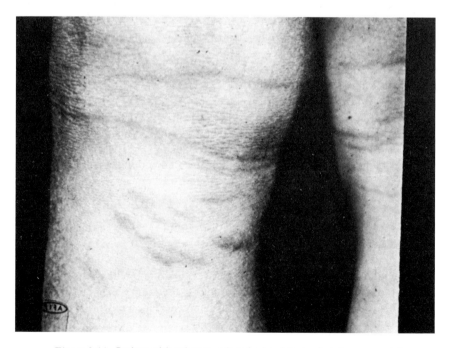

Figure 2-11. Patient with tuberous sclerosis showing classical shagreen patch.

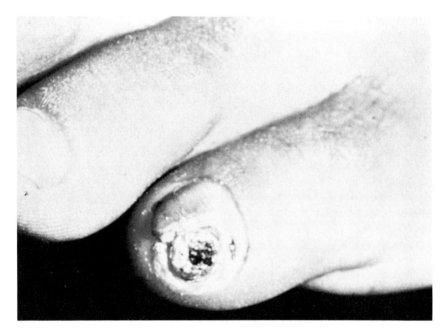

Figure 2-12. Patient with tuberous sclerosis showing typical subungual fibroma.

Angiomyolipomatous hamartomatous transformation (Figure 2-15) may lead to renal failure and may, in certain patients, present as the *forme fruste* of tuberous sclerosis, being the sole clinical expression of this disease.[133]

While initial reports of tuberous sclerosis emphasize its neurologic and skin manifestations, it is important to note that kidney involvement was reported by Lynne and associates in 40-80% of affected patients.[134] These investigators report a patient with tuberous sclerosis who presented with renal failure secondary to bilateral angiomyolipoma. Of further interest was the fact that the angiomyolipoma was associated with polycystic kidney disease, having a focus of renal cell carcinoma.

In reviewing the literature dealing with renal involvement in tuberous sclerosis, Lynne and associates[134] state that less than ten cases have been reported in the literature wherein renal failure has occurred. The angiomyolipoma is usually benign and no cases of metastases have been reported in the literature. However, adjacent tissues and lymph nodes surrounding the kidney may be involved by multicentric involvement of the tumor, as opposed to local extension or metastases. Only three examples of associated renal cell carcinoma and angiomyolipoma have been reported.[135-137]

Finally, it is important to note that on plain abdominal x-ray films or intravenous pyelography, the angiomyolipoma may be mistaken for polycystic kid-

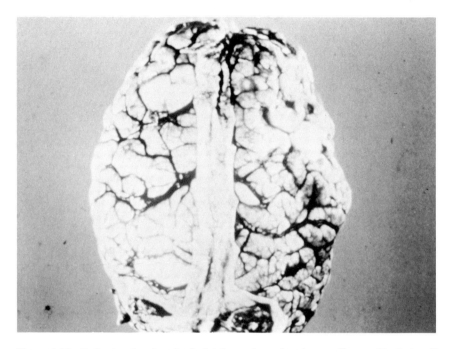

Figure 2-13. Brain showing the classical tubers, also referred to as "potato-like lesions."

ney disease. Renal angiography may be used to distinguish these two lesions since polycystic kidney disease will have a relatively avascular pattern. Thus, the case reported by Lynne and associates is unique in that in addition to the full spectrum of the disease, the unusual combination of angiomyolipoma, polycystic kidney disease, and renal cell carcinoma was observed.

Rhabdomyosarcomas of the heart have also been described as showing an excess association with this disease.[138]

Computerized axial tomography has been found to be a very sensitive diagnostic tool in tuberous sclerosis,[139] particularly in early cases and incomplete forms of the disease.

Von Hippel-Lindau's Syndrome

Von Hippel-Lindau's syndrome is inherited as an autosomal dominant. This disorder is characterized by malignant neoplasms involving multiple organ systems. The most frequently found tumors are cerebellar hemangioblastomas and retinal angiomatosis. In varying combinations, one may also observe medullary and spinal hemangioblastomas, pheochromocytomas, angiomas of the liver and kidney, adenomas and cysts of the kidneys, epididymis, and pancreas, and renal cell car-

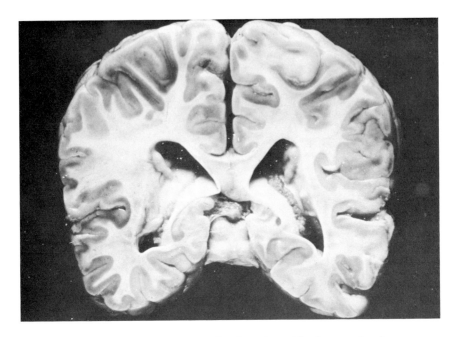

Figure 2-14. Intraventricular tubers in patient with tuberous sclerosis.

cinoma.[140] Secondary internal manifestations include polycythemia, hypertension, and syringomyelia. One of the most extensive reviews of the clinical and pathological aspects of this disease has been provided by Horton and associates.[141] In that series, retinal angiomatosis was observed in over half the patients, about one-fifth of whom were asymptomatic. Thus, in the screening of a family, it would be prudent to have meticulous ophthalmologic examinations performed for these early lesions on all relatives at high risk.

The natural history of retinal angiomatosis is not well understood, and of course, this should compel the investigation of these lesions and others in every new patient and his relatives. It should be noted that if left untreated, retinal angiomatosis can lead to blindness, but when treated early, it can be halted.

The lesion of greatest morbidity and mortality is cerebellar hemangioblastoma. In Horton's study, it was found in one-third of those individuals known to have been affected with von Hippel-Lindau's syndrome. Other reports suggest that this particular lesion may occur in 50-60% of affected individuals. The mean age at diagnosis in Horton's study was 31 years, and there was a slight male predominance. As is true for all familial varieties of cancer, familial hemangioblastoma occurs at an earlier age than so-called sporadic hemangioblastoma.

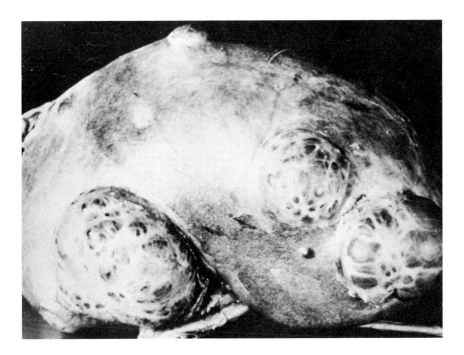

Figure 2-15. Multiple angiomyolipomas of kidney from patient with tuberous sclerosis.

Medullary and spinal hemangioblastomas occur in less than 5% of the affected individuals, but autopsy data suggest that these lesions may go unrecognized clinically. Pheochromocytoma is said to occur in 10% of affected individuals, though it is not distributed evenly among different families. The reason for this is not clear, but it could be due to heterogeneity of the major genetic disease. However, when pheochromocytoma occurs, it tends to occur bilaterally, as it does in other hereditary disorders.

Approximately one-fourth of the patients studied by Horton et al. had renal cell carcinoma. It was metastatic in half of these cases, and it led to death in nearly one-third. Again, its onset is earlier than that for sporadic varieties, though chronologically, it is the latest manifestation of von Hippel-Lindau's syndrome.

Findings of epididymal cysts or adenoma may be specific enough to diagnose this syndrome in an otherwise unaffected male who is a high risk member of a family with this disease. Cutaneous manifestations, including café au lait spots or hemangiomas, are considered to be too nonspecific to establish the diagnosis in high risk patients, though they certainly should be used to suggest the possibility of the disease. It is rare to see all the manifestations of the syndrome in any one individual.

A major consideration in the management of patients at high risk for von Hippel-Lindau's syndrome is the fact that it is not possible to describe an age at which a family member is no longer at risk. For example, in one family,[141] a patient developed renal cell carcinoma at age 61 and another developed visual loss from retinal hemangiomatosis at age 67.

While treatment can alter the course of the various tumors in this disease, there is nevertheless a disturbing tendency for recurrence of tumors arising either from incomplete resection or at new sites. Thus, if a single lesion is excised and "cured," the patient will still be at risk for other manifestations of the disorder. Hence, early detection and periodic screening is extremely important in all members at high risk.

Screening of high risk members should include indirect ophthalmoscopic examination, nephrotomography, VMA determination (preferably serum cathecholamines), and brain scan but more preferably, computerized axial tomography.[141]

Family Study. The proband (Figure 2-16, III-1) at age 21 presented with problems of ataxia of gait and progressive headache of several months duration. Diagnostic studies indicated a cerebellar mass lesion. Evaluation by an ophthalmologist showed no evidence of retinal angiomatosis. Craniotomy was performed and a cerebellar hemangioblastoma was excised. This patient had an uneventful postoperative course and has recovered without any sequelae. She was reexamined by us in September 1980 when she was age 23.

Cutaneous examination showed a 2 × .5 cm café au lait spot at the level of L-1 on the back and a second café au lait spot measuring 2 × 1 cm was noted on the left medial thigh. The remainder of the physical examination, including a detailed neurological evaluation, was within normal limits.

Because of the possibility of other sequelae of von Hippel-Lindau's syndrome, including pheochromocytoma and renal cell carcinoma, the patient was counseled and told of the need for lifetime surveillance.

The proband's maternal aunt (Figure 2-16, II-7) had been hospitalized at age 28 because of severe headaches. Extensive neurologic evaluation including EEG, brain scan, pneumoencephalography as well as parotid angiography were all within normal limits. She also had a history of transitory slight weakness of the left side of her face, but these findings subsided. Her headaches resolved within one month and she had no further difficulty until her second hospital admission when she was age 32. Three days prior to this admission she developed severe generalized headaches which were more severe when she was upright. She also developed a subjective numbness of the left extremity. She was not aware of any precipitating cause of these symptoms. She stated that she felt relatively comfortable when lying supine.

Past medical history revealed that she had suffered from migraine headaches since age 12. These were of a characteristic type, usually left sided and associated

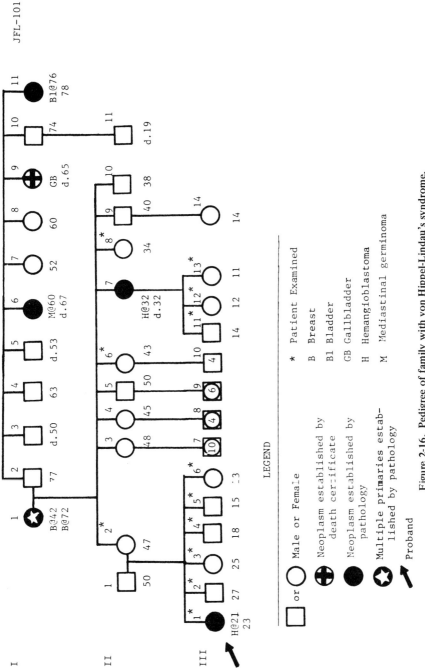

Figure 2-16. Pedigree of family with von Hippel-Lindau's syndrome.

with visual phenomena. These headaches would occur every three to four months. She could usually obtain relief by resting quietly in bed for several hours. She stated that her present headaches were not similar to her migraine headaches.

At the time of her admission, physical examination as well as a detailed neurological evaluation showed no definite abnormalities. The optic disks were well outlined and flat, and showed an absence of hemorrhages or exudates. There was no notation on her medical chart relative to the presence or absence of retinal angiomatosis. Despite the sensation of numbness over the left extremities, there was only very mild hemihypesthesia. Proprioception and stereognosis were intact and no weakness was noted. Clinical laboratory chemistries including SMA-12, urinalysis, and complete blood count were all within normal limits. An EEG was interpreted as being compatible with a migraine syndrome. A brain scan was normal.

Throughout the patient's hospitalization, she continued to complain of rather severe headaches. On the thirteenth and fourteenth day of hospitalization, the patient began to complain of nausea and she became slightly confused. On the fourteenth day, the patient became suddenly apneic and expired.

Autopsy showed positive findings which were restricted to the brain. Specifically, there was a small tumor rising from the medulla which proved histologically to be an hemangioblastoma with a small cystic cavity (Figure 2-17). There was considerable edema in and about the medulla and also in the cerebrum itself. These findings were compatible with a syringobulbia.

There were mutiple cystic follicles in both ovaries; however, there was no evidence of cystic formation in any other organs. No other pathologic abnormalities were noted.

On examination of her three children (Figure 2-16, III-11 to III-13), no specific stigmata of this disorder were identifiable. However, her 14-year-old son (Figure 2-16, III-11) had a syncopal episode one week ago and is currently being evaluated for this event.

The proband's 47-year-old mother (Figure 2-16, II-2) has been treated for "labile" hypertension and, for several years, has experienced "sick headaches" which were consistent with migraine cephalalgia. Physical examination showed no evidence of von Hippel-Lindau's syndrome. She will be under careful surveillance.

A 43-year-old aunt of the proband (Figure 2-16, II-6) has a history of possible migraine cephalalgia. Physical examination was entirely within normal limits, and was noteworthy for an absence of any cutaneous signs.

The proband's maternal aunt (Figure 2-16, II-8) was a 34-year-old lady who had had frequent headaches which she ascribes to being secondary to "sinusitis." Physical examination showed evidence of distinct unilateral axillary freckling present in the right axilla (Figure 2-18). The remainder of the physical examination was negative.

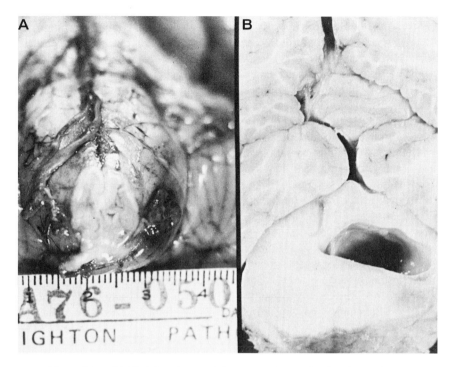

Figure 2-17. (A) Medullary hemangioblastoma; (B) associated syringobulbia.

All of the proband's siblings (Figure 2-16, III-2 to III-6) had café au lait spots of varying size, the largest (6 cm) was noted on the 27-year-old brother (Figure 2-16, III-2). The other spots did not exceed 3 cm or six in number. In addition, examination of the 18-year-old brother (Figure 2-16, III-4) revealed a giant pigmented nonhairy nevus extending over the right deltoid into the right back with clear demarcation at the midline halfway down the back and extending over the pectoralis muscle irregularly and down the entire dorsum of the right arm to the wrist (Figure 2-19). This lesion was nonuniformly pigmented and showed varying shades with nevi within it. There was definite axillary freckling on the right side with an absence of axillary freckling in the left axilla.

Funduscopic examination without dilation was performed on all of the individuals we examined. No evidence of retinal angiomatosis was observed.

The finding of cerebellar hemangioblastoma in the proband and the rarely occurring hemangioblastoma of the medulla in her maternal aunt, lesions known to be associated with von Hippel-Lindau's syndrome, is of interest. The primary question is, What is the likelihood that these two lesions might occur in this family and not result from primary genetic factors related to von Hippel-Lindau's syndrome? Unfortunately, in the absence of additional pathognomonic signs or biomarkers, we cannot provide an unequivocal answer to this important question. There were no stigmata of this disease in the proband's mother. It is known that patients with von Hippel-Lindau's syndrome may show reduced penetrance of this deleterious gene. Variable expressivity of its clinical phenotypic manifestations is also common in this as well as in many other autosomal dominantly inherited disorders. Therefore, in spite of our inability to answer the above question definitively, it will still be exceedingly important to monitor very carefully the proband's mother since, if in fact, we are dealing with von Hippel-Lindau's syndrome in this family, then this woman must necessarily harbor the genotype. In turn, all of the siblings of the proband including the progeny of the proband's affected aunt would be at 50% risk for this disease.

The significance of unilateral axillary freckling in the proband's maternal aunt (Figure 2-18) and that of giant pigmented nonhairy nevus observed in the proband's brother (Figure 2-19) remain elusive. We have not previously observed unilateral axillary freckling, either in the literature or in clinical experience. Therefore, we wonder whether one or both of these findings might possibly be an expression of the gene for von Hippel-Lindau's syndrome.

We describe this family primarily to provoke interest among our readers, some of whom might possibly have seen similar findings associated with von

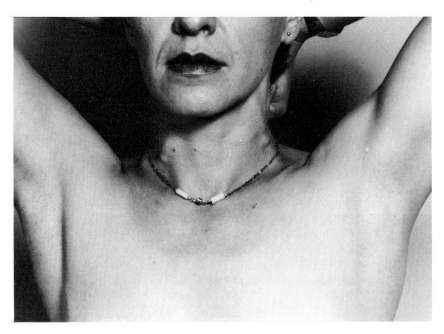

Figure 2-18. Unilateral axillary freckling (in right axilla) in family member of Figure 2-16.

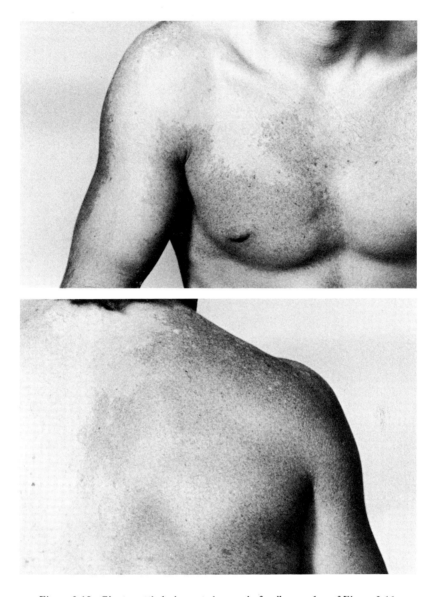

Figure 2-19. Giant mottled pigmented nevus in family member of Figure 2-16.

Hippel-Lindau's syndrome. We are dealing with a potentially lethal condition, particularly with respect to neoplastic involvement of the central nervous system as well as to the presence of renal cell carcinoma and pheochromocytoma. It, therefore, is extremely important that a fuller delineation of clinical and/or pathological features of this disease be identified so that more targeted surveillance programs might be enacted on high risk patients.

Ataxia Telangiectasia (Louis-Bar Syndrome)

Louis-Bar, in 1941, described a patient with progressive cerebellar ataxia and oculocutaneous telangiectasia.[142]   This complex of findings has now become well known as a clearly defined syndrome termed ataxia telangiectasia (AT; also referred to as Louis-Bar syndrome).   An additional manifestation of recurrent severe sinopulmonary infection was provided by Boder and Sedgwick.[143] These investigators subsequently suggested that this syndrome had a familial etiology.[144,145]

The first sign of this disease is usually cerebellar ataxia which may be recognized when the affected child first learns to walk.   Choreic and athetoid movements,[146] as well as pseudopalsy of the eyes resembling oculomotor apraxia, may also occur.[147, 148]   By age 5 or 6, one may observe findings of telangiectasia of the bulbar conjunctivae (Figure 2-20), which may later extend to the eyelids, ears (Figure 2-21), and butterfly area of the face, including the bridge of the

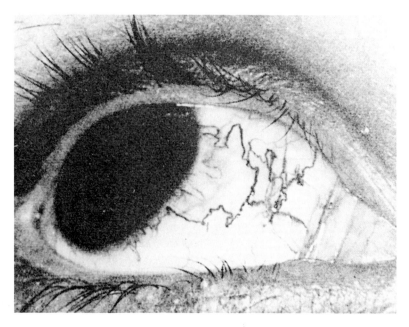

Figure 2-20. Illustration of telangiectasia of eye in patient with ataxia telangiectasia.

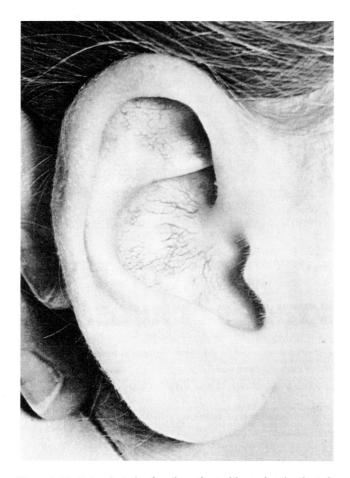

Figure 2-21. Telangiectasia of ear in patient with ataxia telangiectasia.

nose, and to the periorbital area.[149] Affected patients often show an absence of IgA immunoglobulin,[150] perhaps accounting for the susceptibility to repeated sinopulmonary infection. Autopsy studies have revealed thymic aplasia and dysplasia with deficiencies of lymphocytes in Hassall's corpuscles.[151-153] Lymph nodes are often abnormal, with poorly developed lymphoid cuffs about the germinal centers. Recticulum cell hyperplasia or lymphopenia may also occur.

Endocrine abnormalities in AT have included ovarian dysgenesis, follicular agenesis, male hypogonadism, and anterior pituitary pathology.[154, 155]

In a review of 64 families with AT, no affected children had affected parents.[156] There was an equal sex ratio. Affected sibs of index cases approximated the

25% expectation for an autosomal recessive gene. Consanguinity was highly reported, a not unexpected event for an autosomal recessive disorder.

Glucose intolerance and insulin resistance have also been described in this disease. In a study of two AT-affected siblings with insulin resistance, Bar et al.[157] postulated an inhibitor to insulin binding.

Patients with AT show an excess of cancer involving lymphoid tissue and the stomach.[153] Haerer et al.[152] studied gastric carcinoma in a mother (obligate heterozygote) and in two of her five affected offspring. Ages of onset of gastric cancer in the AT-affected patients were unusually young (19 and 21 years). Finally, carcinoma of the ovary,[158, 159] basal cell carcinoma,[160] and central nervous system malignant neoplasms[161] have also been described. However, further investigation will be required in order to determine the significance of these tumor associations. The matter of cancer excess in patients who are heterozygous carriers of the deleterious AT gene has been addressed in Chapter 1.

Celiac Disease (Nontropical Sprue, Gluten-induced Enteropathy)

Celiac disease may be inherited in certain families. MacDonald et al.[162] have suggested an autosomal dominant gene with increased penetrance as an explanation for multiple case families. More recently, Stokes et al.[163] have noted disparities among several of the reported kindreds and have therefore proposed a multifactorial model to explain its inheritance. Since women are affected twice as frequently as men, sex influence must also be considered.

The relationship between celiac disease and cancer, particularly intestinal reticulosis, was identified by Gough et al.[164] and confirmed by Harris et al.[165] in an investigation of 202 patients with celiac disease and idiopathic steatorrhea. They observed that approximately 7% of the patients with celiac disease developed either lymphoma or carcinoma of the gastrointestinal tract (predominantly carcinoma of the esophagus). There was an interval from the first appearance of symptoms of celiac disease to the cancer diagnosis of approximately 21.2 years for patients with lymphoma, and approximately 38.5 years for those who developed gastrointestinal tract cancer. The cancer association with this disease has been confirmed by other investigators.[166-169]

When steatorrhea occurs with malignant lymphoma, the lesion is more often located in the proximal small intestine. Harris et al.[165] stated that as a general rule, lymphoma is more likely to develop in a male with celiac disease who is over age 50, who has manifested this disorder for more than ten years, and who is *NOT* on a gluten-free diet. Whether or not a gluten-free diet will really diminish the cancer risk is not known with certainty.[169]

The primary cutaneous manifestation in this disease is eczema. Treatment with a gluten-free diet will frequently improve not only the malabsorption, but also the cutaneous manifestations.[170]

Epidermolysis Bullosa

Epidermolysis bullosa (EB) is a group of genetically determined cutaneous diseases characterized by blistering following minor trauma to the skin. Affected patients often show large eroded or ulcerated areas on the skin. In those individuals manifesting severe forms of EB, particularly autosomal recessive dystrophic EB, epidermoid carcinomas may develop in those areas showing chronic cutaneous ulcerations.[171]

Systemic manifestations in EB are evidenced by its involvement of the gastrointestinal tract.[172,173] Rochman and associates[174] have studied carcinoembryonic antigens (CEA) in 18 patients with various forms of EB. Marked elevations of CEA were observed in the plasma of four of six patients with recessive dystrophic EB and in one of two patients with recessive EB letalis. Patients with dominantly inherited forms of EB, namely dominant EB simplex and dominant dystrophic EB showed normal levels of CEA. In the patients with recessive EB, the plasma levels of CEA appeared to correlate with the severity of cutaneous involvement. These investigators concluded that CEA may be genetically linked to certain forms of recessive EB or it may be part of a pleiotropic effect of the gene which codes for this disease.

These observations of CEA elevation in recessive forms of EB are extremely interesting in light of recent evidence of CEA elevation in the cancer family syndrome[175] and in hereditary adenomatosis,[176] and of the elevation of both CEA and α-fetoprotein in ataxia telangiectasia.[177] These observations will require further study and should include evaluation of affected members and other relatives, particularly heterozygous carriers of the recessive EB gene. Spouses of affected patients should also be investigated in quest of possible communicable effects as suggested in the target theory of Guirgis et al.[175]

Nevoid Basal Cell Carcinoma Syndrome (Gorlin's Syndrome)

Gorlin and Sedano[178] have extensively reviewed the multiple nevoid basal cell carcinoma syndrome. Pedigree findings in this syndrome are consistent with the inheritance of an autosomal dominant trait.[179] This is truly a multifaceted disease wherein the original triad of multiple nevoid basal cell carcinoma, jaw cysts, and skeletal anomalies has been greatly expanded to include intracranial calcification, ovarian fibromas, lymphomesenteric cysts, medulloblastoma, and a number of minor associated anomalies.[179] The multiple nevoid basal cell carcinomas usually appear at puberty, though they may occur as early as the second year of life. They may involve both exposed and unexposed cutaneous areas. In some patients, they may never appear. Indeed, Gilhuus-Moe and associates[180] stated that in large kindreds wherein meticulous examination for all stigmata of this disease has been performed, only about half of the affected individuals 20 years of age or older manifested skin tumors.

The facies in this disease are often characteristic, though again, as in the case of cutaneous lesions, stigmata may be lacking in certain affected patients. Frontal and temporoparietal bossing is often marked. This gives the skull a pagetoid appearance. There may be well-developed supraorbital ridges giving a sunken appearance to the eyes. Prognathism may be present. Multiple wormian bones may be observed in the lambdoidal sutures. Broad nasal root is common and this may be associated with true ocular hypertelorism. Skeletal anomalies at other sites may be present in 60–70% of affected individuals. More common anomalies are splayed and/or bifurcated ribs. Bifurcation may involve several ribs and may be bilateral. Kyphoscoliosis and spina bifida occulta as well as Sprengel's deformity have also been described. Figure 2-22 shows a patient with several of these features, including pectus excavatum and exotropia, which also have been observed in this disease.

Recently, Burket and Rauh[181] described an adolescent with the syndrome who showed bilateral ovarian fibromas — a finding which emphasizes the importance of these lesions in young women. It also indicates the need for careful pelvic examinations beginning at early ages in these high risk women.

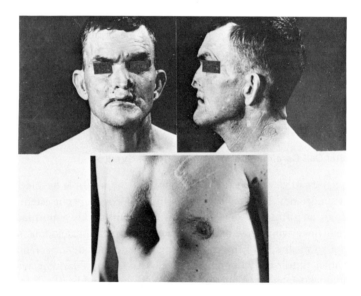

Figure 2-22. Patient with multiple nevoid basal cell carcinoma syndrome showing several striking phenotypic characteristics of this disease. Note ophthalmoplegia, hypertelorism, prognathism, pectus excavation, and evidence of excision of many basal cell cancers.

Peutz-Jeghers Syndrome

The clinical manifestations of the Peutz-Jeghers syndrome include multiple intestinal polyposis and a distinctive type of melanin pigmentation of the oral mucosa, occasionally of the vaginal mucosa, and the distal portion of the fingers (Figures 2-23 and 2-24). Polyps, which usually are hamartomas, may be found at any level of the gastrointestinal tract, exclusive of the esophagus.[182]

Utsunomiya and asssociates[183] studied 222 patients with the Peutz-Jeghers syndrome who were found in Japan between 1961 and 1974. Presenting complaints in 170 patients included obstruction in 42.8%, abdominal pain in 23.4%, rectal bleeding in 13.5%, and extrusion of a polyp in 7.2%. Intussusception occurred in 46.9% of the patients and, in these cases, it was most often in the small intestine. Polyps occurred in the stomach in 46%, in the small intestine in 64%, in the colon in 63%, and in the rectum in 32% of the patients. Among the 222 patients, cancer was varified in 28. Of 15 early cancers, 3 were in the stomach, 8 in the small intestine, and 4 in the colon, while 11 advanced cancers included 3 in the stomach, 1 in the small intestine, and 6 in the colon. A single patient manifested both colon and small intestinal carcinoma. It was of interest

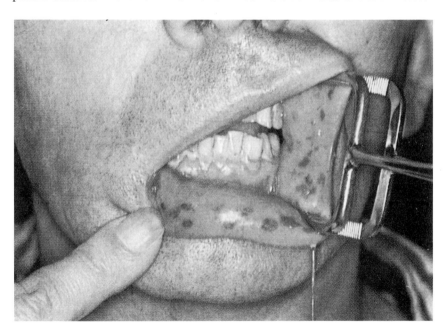

Figure 2-23. Patient with Peutz-Jeghers syndrome illustrating intraoral pigmentary lesions.

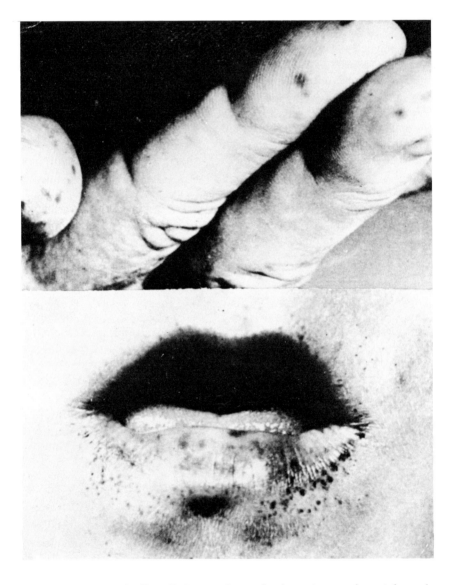

Figure 2-24. Patient with Peutz-Jeghers syndrome showing cutaneous pigmented macules of the lips, perioral area, and the distal portions of the fingers. (Reprinted from Thomas Butterworth and Lyon P. Strean, *Clinical Genodermatology*, with permission of Williams and Wilkins Co.) 1962.

that mortality was lower than that found in patients with familial polyposis coli, but was higher than that occurring in the general population.

Peutz-Jeghers syndrome is inherited as an autosomal dominant. Unfortunately, for too long, this disease has not been considered to predispose affected patients to carcinoma. However, data during the past decade have unequivocally documented this disorder as a cancer-associated genodermatosis wherein primary predilection to cancer involves target tissues in the gastrointestinal tract and ovary. In the latter, granulosa theca cell tumor[184] and papillary adenocarcinoma have been described.[185]

Wiskott-Aldrich Syndrome

The triad of infections, purpura, and eczema was discussed by Wiskott[186] in 1937. This was a report of a family in which three brothers were affected, all of whom died within the first five years of life. In 1854, Aldrich and associates[187] reported a family in which these same findings were manifested in three generations. A sex-linked recessive mode of inheritance was postulated. This disease now carries the eponym of Wiskott-Aldrich syndrome. Clinical features associated rather constantly with this disease are thrombocytopenia and an inordinate susceptibility to bacterial infections; occurrences of diarrhea, low serum levels of IgM, and variable levels of serum IgA, along with a depressed cell-mediated immune function in vitro, have also been described. Recently, Mackie and associates[188] employed transfer factor as a treatment modality in a male infant with the subject disorder. This led to improvement in the hematological aspects of the disease, but unfortunately, it was also accompanied by exacerbation of the cutaneous lesions.

Shapiro et al.[189] designed a stress test for the purpose of demonstrating a consistent abnormality in platelets from cariers of the Wiskott-Aldrich syndrome gene. Specifically, 2-deoxy-D-glucose (DDG), an inhibitor of glycolysis, completely inhibited second wave adrenaline-induced aggregations of platelets from ten carriers of this disease. This test had no effect on the response of control platelets. The authors thus considered the DDG stress test to provide a simple, reproducible assay for detection of carriers of this disease. Figures 2-25 through 2-28 show a patient and family with the Wiskott-Aldrich syndrome who have been investigated by N.C. Nevin, M.D.

The prognosis for children with Wiskott-Aldrich syndrome appears to be uniformly poor. The majority of these youngsters die prior to puberty from infection, hemmorrhage, or lymphoreticular cancer. Patients with Wiskott-Aldrich syndrome have a 10% chance for the development of cancer, with lymphoreticular neoplasia or leukemia predominating.[190, 191]

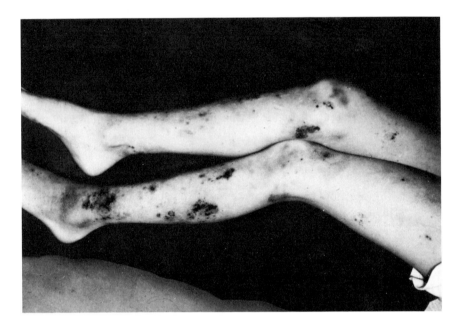

Figure 2-25. Patient with Wiskott-Aldrich syndrome showing hemorrhage into areas of eczema. (Reproduced by permission of N.C. Nevin in H.T. Lynch, *Cancer Genetics,* Charles C. Thomas Co., 1975)

Gardner's Syndrome

In 1912, Devic and Bussey[192] described a woman with multiple polyposis of the colon, sebaceous cysts of the scalp, subcutaneous lipomas, and osteomas of the mandible. Several isolated cases have been reported which were somewhat similar to that of Devic and Bussy.[193-194] Eldon Gardner was the first investigator to characterize these findings as a hereditary syndrome[195-197] and to show that it was an autosomal dominantly inherited disease which included the combination of polyposis coli,[198, 199] osteomas,[200-201] and cutaneous manifestations.[196] By 1967, approximately 118 cases of this syndrome had been reported in the world literature.[202] Watne[203] has provided some of the most recent descriptions of the syndrome, many of these having been based upon his own study of several large unrelated kindreds.

Diagnostic features of the syndrome vary widely when families are carefully studied. Sebaceous cysts of the skin represent the most common soft tissue tumors in this syndrome. Indeed, Gardner and Richards have emphasized the relationship between the sebaceous cysts and polyps of the colon.[196] The occurrence of large cysts around the face and neck is considered an important clinical characteristic of the syndrome (Figures 2-29 and 2-30).

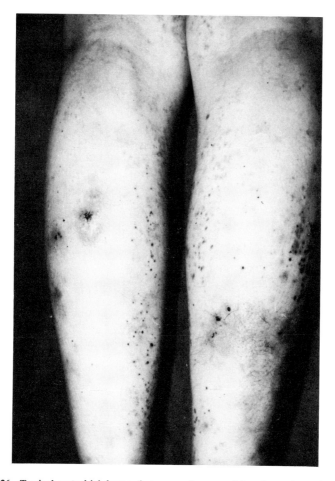

Figure 2-26. Typical petechial hemorrhages on dorsum of legs in patient with Wiskott-Aldrich syndrome. (Reproduced by permission of N.C. Nevin in H.T. Lynch, *Cancer Genetics*, Charles C. Thomas Co., 1975)

Benign osteomatoses are the most frequently observed bone abnormalities in this disease. These comprise dense, bony proliferations, variable in size, which may involve almost all areas of the skeletal system. Localized cortical thickening of the long tubular bones was the most common abnormality found in a bone survey of Gardner's syndrome families.[204] The frontal bone was the most frequent site of osteoma in the skull. Dental abnormalities have also been described including supernumerary and unerupted teeth.

Gardner's syndrome is inherited as an autosomal dominant. Danes[205] has described significantly increased in vitro tetraploidy in skin cultures from affected as well as high risk patients for Gardner's syndrome.

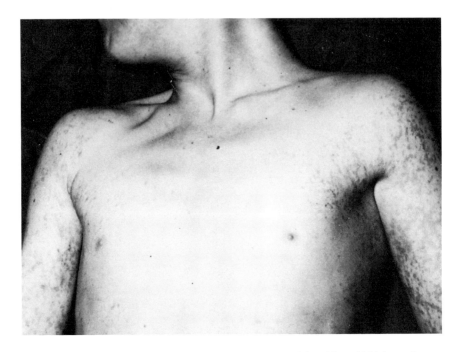

Figure 2-27. Eczema involving upper arms in patient with Wiskott-Aldrich syndrome. (Reproduced by permission of N.C. Nevin in H.T. Lynch, *Cancer Genetics,* Charles C. Thomas Co., 1975)

It is believed that there is virtually 100% potential for malignant degeneration of polyps in patients with Gardner's syndrome if they are untreated, just as has been postulated for simple multiple polyposis coli.[203] When cancers develop, they are typical adenocarcinomas and are often multiple. One such patient[206] developed five synchronous colon carcinomas at age 14, and four years later developed adenocarcinoma of the ampulla of Vater. Thirteen years after his initial colon surgery, he developed a transitional cell carcinoma of the bladder.

Other lesions in Gardner's syndrome have included anaplastic carcinoma of the mandible[207] and fibrous tumor of the parotid gland in a 9-year-old patient.[208] Camiel and associates[209] reported pigmented nevi in one of their patients with the syndrome who developed thyroid carcinoma nine years prior to the diagnosis of Gardner's syndrome. This patient's father had colorectal polyposis and a brain tumor. Retroperitoneal fibrosis and fibrodysplasias have also been described in Gardner's syndrome.[203] The retroperitoneal fibrosis and the development of desmoid tumors and fibrosarcomas following colon surgery have posed a serious complication and are a significant aspect of Gardner's syndrome.[203] Surgery is the treatment of choice for these tumors; radiation has not proved to be of any

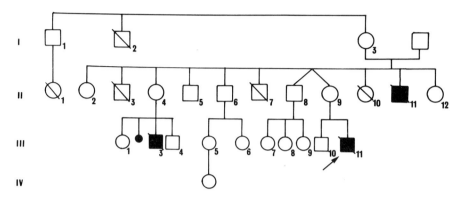

Figure 2-28. Pedigree of family with Wiskott-Aldrich syndrome showing a sex-linked mode of inheritance. (Reproduced by permission of N.C. Nevin in H.T. Lynch, *Cancer Genetics*, Charles C. Thomas Co., 1975)

value.[210]   To treat colonic polyposis, Watne recommends subtotal colectomy with ileoproctostomy immediately upon diagnosis, subject of course to the degree of involvement and the dependability of the patient. Watne had never observed spontaneous regression of the colon polyps without some type of surgical intervention.[203]   When the rectum is extensively involved with polyps and/or cancer, there is no regression of rectal polyps following ileoproctostomy. Total proctocolectomy with ileostomy is strongly recommended.

GENERAL COMMENTS

While the skin provides a convenient "looking glass" for the detection of a wide variety of systemic disorders, its significance in cancer-associated genodermatoses is virtually unparalleled.[1,2,34]   In certain circumstances, cutaneous signs may be recognizable at birth, i.e., sebaceous cysts in Gardner's syndrome.[2] Most important, knowledge of the family history and of hereditary cancer syndromes should alert the clinician to the significance of variable cutaneous and other associated stigmata, so that appropriate measures might be exercised for early detection of cancer of specific anatomic target organs. Indeed, in some cases, prevention might be possible as in total colectomy for the multiple adenomatous polyposis coli component of Gardner's syndrome.[34]

Cancers of internal organs and systems, whether sporadic or genetic, are frequently accompanied by a wide variety of cutaneous manifestations. Certain of these are nonspecific skin reactions which are (only on occasion) found to be associated with internal malignancy. Other nonspecific cutaneous manifestations may be highly suggestive of cancer of internal organs. Finally, certain specific cutaneous signs may be comprised of cancer cells which have metasta-

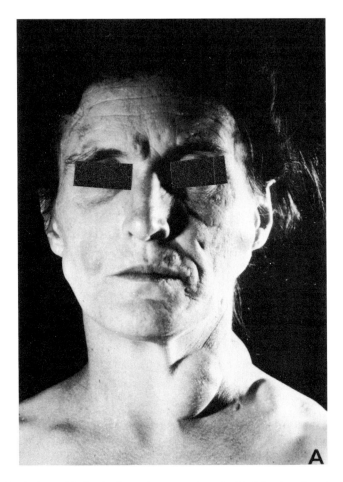

Figure 2-29. Patient with Gardner's syndrome: (A) typical facial and neck cysts; (B) cysts of arms.

sized to the skin. These observations — while pertaining to cancer in general — are, nevertheless, critical diagnostic clues in cancer-associated genodermatoses.[2]

Nonspecific cutaneous lesions associated with internal cancer include pruritis, reactive erythemas (as in carcinoid syndromes), and an increased susceptibility to skin infection. Those nonspecific skin conditions which are more frequently associated with internal varieties of cancer include acanthosis nigricans, Bowen's disease, digital hypertrophic osteoarthropathy (clubbing), particularly in association with carcinoma of the lung, the acquired variety of hypertrichosis languinosa, and sudden onset of multiple seborrheic keratoses (sign of Leser-Trelat). Other evidence of underlying malignant neoplasms may be the superior vena cava

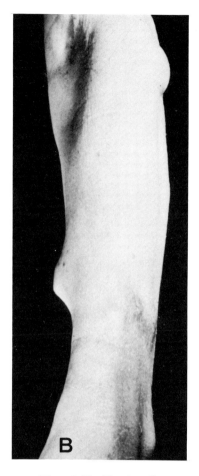

Figure 2-29. (Continued)

syndrome, characterized by edematous swelling of the face, especially of the periorbital area, erythema and/or cyanosis involving the head and neck, and dilitation as well as engorgement of the superficial cervical and thoracic veins. In certain situations, nonpitting edema may be manifested in the upper extremities. The most frequently occurring malignant neoplasms associated with the superior vena cava syndrome are lymphomas with mediastinal involvement and bronchogenic carcinoma.

In those skin manifestations of internal cancer, we find that metastatic cancer to the skin has been estimated to occur in about 2% of the cases. The majority of these lesions occur above the waist, with a predilection for the face and scalp area. These often present as painless discrete papules or nodules which may ultimately enlarge to plaques and then may ulcerate.

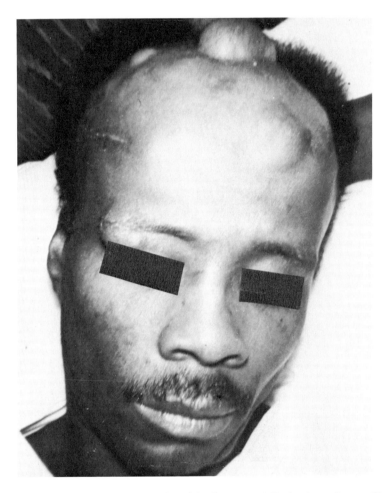

Figure 2-30. Black patient showing soft and hard tumors of Gardner's syndrome. (Reproduced by permission of E.J. Dunning and K.S. Ibrahim, *Ann. Surg.* 161:565, 1965)

Our brief review has clearly shown that internal manifestations in many of the cancer-associated genodermatoses abound. Undoubtedly, we will learn much more about associated systemic manifestations commensurate with the attention given to these disorders. We have selected several of the cancer-associated genodermatoses as prototype examples of disorders with internal manifestations. As already mentioned, it has not been the purpose of this chapter to document and discuss internal manifestations occurring in all of the cancer-associated genodermatoses. Such an exercise is clearly beyond our scope and could easily result in a monograph itself. The important message revolves around the necessity to consider the skin in hereditary disorders as a "beacon" for providing clues to internal disease manifestations. When integrated with the family history and coupled with knowledge of genetic transmission, a more clear understanding of the protean manifestations of the disease should then be forthcoming. The natural sequel of such an exercise would then lead to hereditary cancer syndrome identification. Comprehension of cancer etiology and pathogenesis will then be facilitated through a more thorough recognition of the salient aspects of internal manifestations in the cancer-associated genodermatoses. Indeed, recognition of certain of the internal manifestations may contribute in a major way toward the initiation of concerted cancer control measures which can be targeted to cancer of specific anatomic sites.

Unfortunately, the unraveling of the chronology and pathogenetic significance of signs and symptoms of the cancer-associated genodermatoses may not be clear-cut, and one may arrive at an impasse when attempting to integrate the patient's internal milieu with cancer etiology. Specifically, in certain circumstances, we may be led to the proverbial riddle of the chicken and the egg, i.e., do cancer occurrences in certain of these diseases elicit internal and/or external manifestations, or vice versa? Does the immunological deficiency per se, in the several disorders wherein this component is prevalent (e.g., autosomal recessively inherited ataxia telangiectasis, Chediak-Higashi syndrome, Fanconi aplastic anemia, sex-linked inherited agammaglobulinemia of the Bruton-type, agammaglobulinemia of the Swiss-type, or Wiskott-Aldrich syndrome), create a milieu which *causes* cancer induction and/or its *promotion* as suggested in the aforementioned discussion? Or on the other hand, has early development of cancer in certain of the genodermatoses contributed to and/or exaggerated the patient's immunodeficiency response? Solution of these dilemmas could lead to the development of methodologies for the prevention and/or control of cancer. High risk patients who are members of families manifesting these presumptive inborn errors could provide an invaluable resource for the pursuance of the elucidation of etiology and carcinogenesis.

In conclusion, it is obvious that the discerning clinician will be constantly challenged by a variety of skin manifestations in his patients. In some, these may represent phenotypic characteristics of cancer-associated genodermatoses. In others, they may result from underlying cancer per se, which may be of primary genetic or sporadic (unknown) etiology. In the former, the benefit of lead time provided by knowledge of family history may be used profitably for cancer prevention and control.

REFERENCES

1. Lynch, H.T.: *Skin, Heredity, and Malignant Neoplasms.* Flushing, NY: Medical Examination Publishing Co., 1972, 299 pp.

2. Lynch, H.T., and Frichot, B.C., III: Skin, heredity, and cancer. *Semin. Oncol.* **5**:67–84, 1978.

3. Weiner, K.: *Skin Manifestations of Internal Disorders.* St. Louis, MO: C.V. Mosby, 1947, 690 pp.

4. Bloom, D.: Congenital telangiectatic erythema resembling lupus erythematosus in dwarfs. *Am. J. Dis. Child* **88**:754–758, 1954.

5. Bloom, D.: The syndrome of congenital telangiectatic erythema and stunted growth. *J. Pediatr.* **68**:103–113, 1966.

6. German, J.: Bloom's syndrome. I. Genetical and clinical observations in the first twenty-seven patients. *Am. J. Hum. Genet.* **21**:196–227, 1969.

7. Ahmad, U., Fisher, E.R., Danowski, T.S., Nolan, S., and Stephan, T.: Endocrine abnormalities and myopathy in Bloom's syndrome. *J. Med. Genet.* **14**:418–421, 1977.

8. German, J., Archibald, R., and Bloom, D.: Chromosomal breakage in a rare and probably genetically determined syndrome of man. *Science* **148**:506–507, 1965.

9. German, J. (Ed.): *Chromosomes and Cancer.* New York: John Wiley & Sons, 1974, pp. 601–617.

10. Dicken, C.H., Dewald, G., and Gordon, H.: Sister chromatid exchanges in Bloom's syndrome. *Arch. Dermatol.* **114**:755–760, 1978.

11. Landsu, J.W., Sasaki, M.S., Newcomer, V.D., and Norman, A.: Bloom's syndrome. The syndrome of telangiectatic erythema and growth retardation. *Arch. Dermatol.* **94**:687–694, 1966.

12. German, J., Bloom, D., and Passarge, E.: Bloom's syndrome. V. Surveillance for cancer in affected families. *Clin. Genet.* **12**:162–168, 1977.

13. Steele, R.W., Limas, C., Thruman, G.B., Schuelein, M., Baur, H., and Bellanti, J.A.: Familial thymic aplasia. Attempted reconstruction with thymus in a millipore diffusion chamber. *N. Engl. J. Med.* **287**:787–791, 1972.

14. Tewfik, H.H., Ptacek, J.J., Krause, C.J., and Latourette, H.B.: DiGeorge syndrome associated with multiple squamous cell carcinomas. *Arch. Otolaryngol.* **103**:105–107, 1977.

15. Smith, C.K., Cassidy, J.T., and Bole, G.G.: Type I dysgammaglobulinemia, systemic lupus erythematosus, and lymphoma. *Am. J. Med.* **48**:113–119, 1970.

16. Larsen, R.A.: Family studies in systemic lupus erythematosus (SLE) – VI. Presence of rheumatoid factors in relatives and spouses. *J. Chronic. Dis.* **25**:191–203, 1972.

17. Larsen, R.A.: Family studies in systemic lupus erythematosus (SLE) – VII. Serum immunoglobulins: IgG concentrations in relatives and spouses. *J. Chronic. Dis.* **25**:205–213, 1972.

18. Larsen, R.A.: Family studies in systemic lupus erythematosus (SLE) – VII. Serum immunoglobulins: IgG concentrations in relatives of selected SLE probands. *J. Chronic. Dis.* **25**:215–223, 1972.

19. Larsen, R.A., and Godal, T.: Family studies in systemic lupus erythematosus (SLE) – IX. Thyroid diseases and antibodies. *J. Chronic. Dis.* **25**:225–233, 1972.

20. Katz, W.A., Ehrlich, G.E., Gupta, V.P., and Shapiro, B.: Salivary gland dysfunction in systemic lupus erythematosus and rheumatoid arthritis. *Arch. Int. Med.* **140**:949–951, 1980.

21. Singsen, B.H., Bernstein, B.H., King, K.K., and Hanson, B.: Systemic lupus erythematosus in childhood: correlations between changes in disease activity and serum. *J. Pediatr.* **89**:358–365, 1976.

22. Brunjes, S., Zike, K., and Julian, R.: Familial systemic lupus erythematosus. A review of the literature with a report of ten additional cases in four families. *Am. J. Med.* **30**:529–536, 1961.

23. Leonhardt, T.: Family studies in systemic lupus erythematosus. *Acta Med. Scand.* (Suppl. 416) **176**:1–156, 1964.

24. Pollak, V.E.: Antinuclear antibodies in families of patients with systemic lupus erythematosus. *N. Engl. J. Med.* **271**:165–171, 1964.

25. Buckman, K.J., Moore, S.K., Ebbin, A.J., Cox, M.B., and Dubois, E.L.: Familial systemic lupus erythematosus. *Arch. Intern. Med.* **138**:1674–1676, 1978.

26. Dubois, E.L. (Ed.): *Lupus Erythematosus. A Review of the Current Status of Discoid and Systemic Lupus Erythematosus and Their Variants.* (2nd ed.). Los Angeles, CA: University of Southern California Press, 1974.

27. Fraga, A., Armendares, S., Mintz, G., Mora, J., and Cortes, R.: Dermatoglyphic patterns in systemic lupus erythematosus (SLE) and their changes in patients with increased fetal wastage. *J. Rheumatol.* (Suppl. 1):35, 1974.

28. Dubois, R.W., Weiner, J.M., and Dubois, E.L.: Dermatoglyphic study of systemic lupus erythematosus. *Arthritis Rheum.* **19**:83–87, 1976.

29. Arnett, F.C., and Shulman, L.E.: Studies in familial systemic lupus erythematosus. *Medicine* **55**:313–322, 1976.

30. Ansell, B.M., and Lawrence, J.S.: A family study in lupus erythematosus, abstracted. *Arthritis Rheum.* **6**:260, 1963.

31. Bywaters, E.G.: Family studies of rheumatoid arthritis and lupus erythematosus in Great Britain. In: *The Epidemiology of Chronic Rheumatism* (J.H. Kellgren, Ed.). A symposium organized by the Council for International Organizations of Medical Sciences. Vol. 1. Philadelphia, PA: Davis, 1963, pp. 249–258.

32. Barnes, R.D.: Thymic neoplasms associated with refractory anaemia. *Guy Hosp. Rep.* **114**:73–82, 1965.

33. Beickert, A.: Lupus-erythematosus-syndrome bei lymphogranulomatose. *Schweiz. Med. Wschr.* **88**:668–669, 1958.

34. Lynch, H.T. (Ed.): *Cancer Genetics.* Springfield, IL: Charles C. Thomas, 1976.

35. Calabro, J.J.: Cancer and arthritis. *Arthritis Rheum.* **10**:553–567, 1976.

36. Green, J.A., Dawson, A.A., and Walker, W.: Systemic lupus erythematosus and lymphoma. *Lancet* **2**:753–755, 1978.

37. Gatti, R.A., and Good, R.A.: Occurrence of malignancy in immunodeficiency diseases. A literature review. *Cancer* **28**:89–98, 1971.

38. Jackson, R., and Gulliver, M.: Neonatal lupus erythematosus progressing into systemic lupus erythematosus. A 15-year follow-up. *Br. J. Dermatol.* **101**:81–86, 1979.

39. Brustein, D., Rodriguez, J.M., Minkin, W., and Rabhan, N.B.: Familial lupus erythematosus. *JAMA* **238**:2294–2296, 1977.

40. Jackson, R.: Discoid lupus in a newborn infant of a mother with lupus erythematosus. *Pediatrics* **33**:425–430, 1964.

41. Tuffanelli, D.J.: Lupus erythematosus. *Arch. Dermatol.* **106**:553–566, 1972.

42. Vonderheid, E.C., Koblenzer, P.J., Ming, P.M., and Burgoon, C.F.: Neonatal lupus erythematosus. Report of four cases with review of the literature. *Arch. Dermatol.* **112**:698–705, 1976.

43. Beaucher, W.N., Garman, R.H., and Condemi, J.J.: Familial lupus erythematosus. Antibodies to DNA in household dogs. *N. Engl. J. Med.* **296**:982–984, 1977.

44. Lynch, J.T.: Genetics, etiology, and human cancer. *Prev. Med.* **9**:231–243, 1980.

45. Miller, M., and Hall, J.G.: Possible maternal effect on severity of neurofibromatosis. *Lancet* **2**:1071–1073, 1978.

46. Harper, P.S., and Dyken, P.R.: Early-onset dystrophia myotonica. Evidence supporting a maternal environmental factor. *Lancet* **2**:53–55, 1972.

47. Lynch, H.T., and Guirgis, H.A.: Childhood cancer and the SBLA syndrome. *Med. Hypotheses* 5:15-22, 1979.
48. Sjogren, H.: Zur kenntnis der keratoconjuctivitis sicca (Keratitis filiformis bei hypofunktion der tranendrusen). *Acta Ophthalmol.* (Suppl.) 2:1-151, 1933.
49. Kassan, S.S., and Gardy, M.: Sjogren's syndrome: an update and overview. *Am. J. Med.* 64:1037-1046, 1978.
50. Sinkovics, J.G., Trujillo, J.M., Pienta, R.J., and Ahern, M.J.: Leukemogenesis stemming from autoimmune disease. In: *Genetic Concepts and Neoplasia. A Collection of Papers Presented at the Twenty-third Annual Symposium on Fundamental Cancer Research.* Baltimore, MD: Williams and Wilkins, 1970, pp. 138-190.
51. Denko, C.W., and Bergenstal, D.M.: The Sicca syndrome (Sjogren's syndrome). A study of sixteen cases. *Arch. Intern. Med.* 105:849-858, 1960.
52. Talal, N., and Bunim, J.J.: The development of malignant lymphoma in the course of Sjogren's syndrome. *Am. J. Med.* 36:529-540, 1964.
53. Rothman, S., Block, M., and Hauser, F.V.: Sjogren's syndrome associated with lymphoblastoma and hypersplenism. *Arch. Derm. Syph.* 63:642-643, 1951.
54. Lichtenfeld, J.L., Kirschner, R.H., and Wiernick, P.H.: Familial Sjogren's syndrome with associated primary salivary gland lymphoma. *Am. J. Med.* 60:286-292, 1976.
55. Delaney, W.E., and Balogh, K., Jr.: Carcinoma of the parotid gland associated with benign lymphoepithelial lesion (Mikulicz's disease) in Sjogren's syndrome. *Cancer* 19:853-860, 1966.
56. Howie, J.B., and Helyer, B.J.: The immunology and pathology of NZB mice. In: *Advances in Immunology* (F.J. Dixon, Jr., and H.G. Kinkel, Eds.). New York: Academic Press, 1968, pp. 215-266.
57. Kessler, H.S.: A laboratory model for Sjogren's syndrome. *Am. J. Pathol.* 52:671-685, 1968.
58. Gershwin, M.E., Terasaki, P.I., Graw, R., et al.: Increased frequency of HL-A8 in Sjogren's syndrome. *Tissue Antigens* 6:342-346, 1975.
59. Fye, K.H., Terasaki, P.I., Moutsopoulos, H., et al.: Association of Sjogren's syndrome with HLA-B8. *Arthritis Rheum.* 19:883-886, 1976.
60. Chused, T.M., Kassan, S.S., Opelz, G., and Moutsopoulos, H.M.: Sjogren's syndrome associated with HLA-Dw3. *N. Engl. J. Med.* 296:895-897, 1977.
61. Sengar, D.P., and Terasaki, P.I.: A semimicro mixed leukicyte culture test. *Transplantation* 11:260-267, 1971.
62. Werner, O.: *Ueber Katarakt in Verbinduna mit Sklerodermie.* Doctoral dissertation, Kiel University: Schmidt & Klaunig, 1904.
63. Epstein, C.J., Martin, G.M., Schultz, A.L., and Motulsky, A.G.: Werner's syndrome. A review of its symptomatology, natural history, pathologic features, genetics and relationship to the natural aging process. *Medicine* 45:177-221, 1966.
64. Tri, T.B., and Combs, D.T.: Congestive cardiomyopathy in Werner's syndrome. *Lancet* 1:1052-1053, 1978.
65. Oppenheimer, B.S., and Kugel, V.H.: Werner's syndrome; heredofamilial disorder with scleroderma, bilateral juvenile cataract, precocious graying of hair, and endocrine stigmatization. *Trans. Assoc. Am. Physicians* 49:358-370, 1934.
66. Boyd, M.W., and Grant, A.P.: Werner's syndrome (progeria of the adult). Further pathological and biochemical observations. *Br. Med. J.* 2:920-925, 1959.
67. Petrohelos, M.A.: Werner's syndrome. A survey of three cases, with review of the literature. *Am. J. Ophthalmol.* 56:941-953, 1963.
68. Riley, T.R., Wieland, R.G., Markis, J., and Hamwi, G.J.: Werner's syndrome. *Ann. Int. Med.* 63:285-294, 1965.

69. Nakao, Y., Kishihara, M., Yoshimi, H., Inoue, Y., Tanaka, K., Sakamoto, N., Matsukura, S., Imura, H., Ichihashi, M., and Fujiwara, Y.: Werner's syndrome. In vivo and in vitro characteristics as a model of aging. *Am. J. Med.* **65**:919-932, 1978.

70. Epstein, C.J.: Werner's syndrome. *Ann. Int. Med.* **63**:343-345, 1965.

71. Ellison, D.J., and Pugh, D.W.: Werner's syndrome. *Br. Med. J.* **2**:237-239, 1955.

72. Muller, L., and Andersson, B.: Werner's syndrome. A survey based on two cases. *Acta Med. Scand.* (Suppl. 283) **146**:3-17, 1953.

73. Agatson, S.A., and Gartner, S.: Precocious cataracts and scleroderma (Rothmund's syndrome; Werner's syndrome). Report of a case. *Arch. Ophthalmol.* **21**:492-496, 1939.

74. Jacobson, H.G., Rifkin, H., and Zucher-Franklin, D.: Werner's syndrome. A clinical-roentgen entity. *Radiology* **74**:373-385, 1960.

75. Boatwright, H., Wheeler, C.E., and Cawley, E.P.: Werner's syndrome. *Arch. Intern. Med.* **90**:243-249, 1952.

76. McKusick, V.A.: Medical genetics 1962. *J. Chron. Dis.* **16**:457-634, 1963.

77. Swift, M.: Malignant disease in heterozygous carriers. *Birth Defects* **12**:133-144, 1976.

78. Schimke, R.N.: *Genetics and Cancer in Man.* New York: Churchill Livingstone, 1978, 108 pp.

79. Becker, S.W., Kahn, D., and Rothman, S.: Cutaneous manifestations of internal malignant tumors. *Arch. Derm. Syph.* **45**:1069-1080, 1942.

80. Higgins, G.A., Recant, L., and Fischman, A.B.: The glucagonoma syndrome: surgically curable diabetes. *Am. J. Surg.* **137**:142-148, 1979.

81. Wilkinson, D.S.: Necrolytic migratory erythema with carcinoma of the pancreas. *Trans. St. Johns Hosp. Dermatol. Soc.* **59**:244-250, 1973.

82. Boden, G., and Owen, O.E.: Familial hyperglucagonemia – an autosomal dominant disorder. *N. Engl. J. Med.* **296**:534-538, 1977.

83. Brownstein, M.H., Wolf, M., and Bikowski, J.B.: Cowden's disease: a cutaneous marker of breast cancer. *Cancer* **41**:2393-2398, 1978.

84. Nuss, D.D., Aeling, J.L., Clemons, D.E., and Weber, W.N.: Multiple hamartoma syndrome (Cowden's disease). *Arch. Dermatol.* **114**:743-746, 1978.

85. Goldberg, A.: Diagnosis and treatment of porphyrias. *Proc. R. Soc. Med.* **61**:193-196, 1968.

86. Stanbury, J.B. (Ed.): *The Metabolic Basis of Inherited Disease.* New York: McGraw Hill, 1960.

87. Topi, G., and Gandolfo, L.D.: Inheritance of porphyria cutanea tarda. Analysis of 14 cases in 5 families. *Br. J. Dermatol.* **97**:617-627, 1977.

88. Butterworth, T., and Stream, L.P.: *Clinical Genodermatology.* Baltimore, MD: Williams & Wilkins, 1962.

89. Grossman, M.E., and Bickers, D.R.: Porphyria cutanea tarda. A rare, cutaneous manifestation of hepatic tumors. *Cutis* **21**:782-784, 1978.

90. Perry, H.O.: Less common skin markers of visceral neoplasms. *Int. J. Dermatol.* **15**:19-25, 1976.

91. Rimbaud, P., Meynadier, J., and Guilhou, J.J.: La porphyrie cutanée tardive. A propos de deux observations associees a un cancer hepatique. *Sem. Hop. Paris* **49**:719-725, 1973.

92. Waddington, R.T.: A case of primary liver tumor associated with porphyria. *Br. J. Surg.* **59**:653-654, 1972.

93. Ziprowski, L., Krakowski, A., Crispin, M., and Szeinberg, A.: Porphyria cutanea tarda hereditaria. *Isr. J. Med. Sci.* **2**:338-343, 1966.

94. Kushner, J.P., Lee, G.R., and Nacht, S.: The role of iron in the pathogenesis of porphyria cutanea tarda. An in vitro model. *J. Clin. Invest.* **51**:3044-3051, 1972.

95. Benedetto, A.V., Kushner, J.P., and Taylor, J.S.: Porphyria cutanea tarda in three generations of a single family. *N. Engl. J. Med.* **298**:358-362, 1978.

96. Bean, W.B.: *Vascular Spiders and Related Lesions of the Skin.* Springfield, IL: Charles C. Thomas, 1958, pp. 178-185.

97. Waybright, E.A., Selhorst, J.B., Rosenblum, W.I., and Suter, C.G.: Blue rubber bleb nevus syndrome with CNS involvement and thrombosis of a vein of Galen malformation. *Ann. Neurol.* **3**:464-467, 1978.

98. Berlyne, G.M., and Berlyne, N.: Anaemia due to "blue rubber-bleb" naevus disease. *Lancet* **2**:1275-1277, 1960.

99. Rice, J.S., and Fischer, D.S.: Blue rubber-bleb nevus syndrome. Generalized cavernous hemangiomatosis or venous hamartoma with medulloblastoma of the cerebellum: case report and review of the literature. *Arch. Dermatol.* **86**:503-511, 1962.

100. Hoffman, T., Chasko, S., and Safai, B.: Association of blue rubber bleb nevus syndrome with chronic lymphocytic leukemia and hypernephroma. *Johns Hopkins Med. J.* **142**:91-94, 1978.

101. Bazex, A., Dupre, A., and Christol, B.: Genodermatose complex de type indetermine associant une hypotrichose, un etat atrophodermique generalise et des degenerescences cutanees multiple (epitheliomasbaso-cellulaires). *Bull. Soc. Fr. Derm. Syph.* **71**:206, 1964.

102. Bazex, A., Dupre, A., and Christol, B.: Atrophodermie folliculaire, proliferations baso-cellulaires, et hypotrichose. *Ann. Derm. Syph.* **93**:241-254, 1966.

103. Viksnins, P., and Berlin, A.: Follicular atrophoderma and basal cell carcinoma. *Arch. Dermatol.* **113**:948-951, 1977.

104. DasGupta, T.K., Brasfield, R.D., and Paglia, M.A.: Primary melanomas in unusual sites. *Surg. Gynecol. Obstet.* **128**:841-848, 1969.

105. Smith, S., and Opipari, M.I.: Primary pleural melanoma. A first reported case and literature review. *J. Thorac. Cardiovasc. Surg.* **75**:827-831, 1978.

106. Cartwright, G.E., Edwards, C.Q., Kravitz, K., Skolnick, M., Amos, D.B., Johnson, A., and Buskjaer, L.: Hereditary hemochromatosis. Phenotypic expression of the disease. *N. Engl. J. Med.* **301**:175-179, 1979.

107. Beaumont, C., Simon, M., Fauchet, R., Hespel, J.P., Brissot, P., Genetet, B., and Bourel, M.: Serum ferritin as a possible marker of the hemochromatosis allele. *N. Engl. J. Med.* **301**:169-174, 1979.

108. Debre, R., Dreyfus, J.C., Frezal, J., Labie, D., Lamy, M., Maroteaux, P., Schapira, F., and Schapira, G.: Genetics of haemochromatosis. *Ann. Hum. Genet.* **23**:16-30, 1958.

109. Johnson, G.B., Jr., and Frey, W.G., III: Familial aspects of idiopathic hemochromatosis. *JAMA* **179**:747-751, 1962.

110. Powell, L.W., and Kerr, J.F.: The pathology of the liver in hemochromatosis. *Pathobiol. Annu.* **5**:317-337, 1975.

111. Edmondson, H.A., and Steiner, P.E.: Primary carcinoma of the liver. A study of 100 cases among 48,900 necropsies. *Cancer* **7**:462-503, 1954.

112. Finch, S.C., and Finch, C.A.: Idiopathic hemochromatosis, an iron storage disease. A. Iron metabolism in hemochromatosis. *Medicine* **34**:381-430, 1955.

113. Solomon, L.M., and Esterly, N.B.: Epidermal and other congenital organoid nevi. *Curr. Prob. Pediatr.* **6**:1-56, 1975.

114. McAuley, D., Isenberg, D.A., and Gooddy, W.: Neurological involvement in the epidermal naevus syndrome. *J. Neurol. Neurosurg. Psychiatry* **41**:466-469, 1978.

115. Crowe, F.W., Schull, W.J., and Neel, J.V.: *A Clinical, Pathological, and Genetic Study of Multiple Neurofibromatosis.* Springfield, IL: Charles C. Thomas, 1956.
116. Benedict, P.H., Szabo, G., Fitzpatrick, T.B., and Sinesi, S.J.: Melanotic macules in Albright's syndrome and in neurofibromatosis. *JAMA* **205**:618-626, 1968.
117. Crowe, F.W.: Axillary freckling as a diagnostic aid in neurofibromatosis. *Ann. Int. Med.* **61**:1142-1143, 1964.
118. Silvers, D.N., Greenwood, R.S., and Helwig, E.B.: Café au lait spots without giant pigment granules. Occurrence in suspected neurofibromatosis. *Arch. Dermatol.* **110**: 87-88, 1974.
119. Delleman, J.W., DeJong, J.G., and Bleeker, G.M.: Meningiomas in five members of a family over two generations, in one member simultaneously with acoustic neurinomas. *Neurology* **28**:567-570, 1978.
120. Lee, D.K., and Abbott, M.L.: Familial central nervous system neoplasia. *Arch. Neurol.* **20**:154-160, 1969.
121. Yakovlev, P.I., and Guthrie, R.H.: Congenital ectodermoses (neurocutaneous syndromes) in epileptic patients. *Arch. Neurol. Psychiatry* **26**:1145-1194, 1931.
122. Saville, P.D., Nassim, J.R., Stevenson, F.H., Mulligan, L., and Carey, M.: Osteomalacia in von Recklinghausen's neurofibromatosis. Metabolic study of a case. *Br. Med. J.* **1**:1311-1313, 1955.
123. Halpern, M., and Currarino, G.: Vascular lesions causing hypertension in neurofibromatosis. *N. Engl. J. Med.* **273**:248-252, 1965.
124. Lipton, S., and Zuckerbrod, M.: Familial enteric neurofibromatosis. *Med. Times* **94**:544-548, 1966.
125. Massaro, D., Katz, S., Matthews, M.J., and Higgins, G.: Von Recklinghausen's neurofibromatosis associated with cystic lung disease. *Am. J. Med.* **38**:233-240, 1965.
126. Krucke, W.: Pathologie der peripheren nerven. In: *Handbuch der Neurochirurgie* (H. Oliverona, W. Tonnis, and Krenkel, W. Eds.). Vol. 7, Part 3. Berlin: Springer-Verlag, 1974.
127. McAuley, R.A.: Neurofibrosarcoma of the radial nerve in von Recklinghausen's disease with metastatic angiosarcoma. *J. Neurol. Neurosurg. Psychiatry* **41**:474-478, 1978.
128. Bundey, S., and Evans, K.: Tuberous sclerosis: a genetic study. *J. Neurol. Neurosurg. Psychiatry* **32**:591-603, 1969.
129. Harlan, W.L., and Okazaki, H.: Neurocutaneous disease. In: *Skin, Heredity, and Malignant Neoplasms* (H.T. Lynch, ed.). Flushing, NY: Medical Examination Publishing Co., 1972, pp. 104-148.
130. Chao, D.H.: Congenital neurocutaneous syndromes in childhood. II. Tuberous scleorsis. *J. Pediatr.* **55**:447-459, 1959.
131. Ashbury, H.E., Wilding, J.G., and Rogers, F.T.: Roentgenological report of chest examinations. Made of registrants at the United States Army Induction Station, No. 6, 3d Corps Area, Baltimore, Maryland, May 1, 1941 to March 31, 1942. *AJR* **48**: 347-351, 1942.
132. O'Callaghan, T.J., Edwards, J.A., Tobin, M., and Mookerjee, B.K.: Tuberous sclerosis with striking renal involvement in a family. *Arch. Intern. Med.* **135**:1082-1087, 1975.
133. Thelmo, W.L., Lefkowitz, M., and Seemayer, T.A.: Renal failure secondary to angiomyolipoma. Case of *forme-fruste* tuberous sclerosis. *Urology* **11**:389-392, 1978.
134. Lynne, C.M., Carrion, H.M., Bakshandeh, K., Nadji, M., Russel, E., and Politano, V.A.: Renal Angiomyolipoma, polycystic kidney, and renal cell carcinoma in patient with tuberous sclerosis. *Urology* **14**:174-176, 1979.
135. Kavaney, P.B., and Fielding, I.: Angiomyolipoma and renal cell carcinoma in the same kidney. *Urology* **6**:643-646, 1975.

136. Hyman, A.: The association of hypernephroma with tuberose brain sclerosis and adenoma sebacecum. *J. Urol.* **8**:317–321, 1922.
137. Jochimsen, P.R., Braunstein, P.M., and Najarian, J.S.: Renal allotransplantation for bilateral renal tumor. *JAMA* **210**:1721, 1969.
138. Nevin, N.C., and Pearce, W.G.: Diagnostic and genetical aspects of tuberous sclerosis. *J. Med. Genet.* **5**:273–280, 1968.
139. Racy, A., Barakat, A.Y., and Cochran, W.E.: Computerized axial tomography in family members of patients with tuberous sclerosis. *Clin. Pediatr.* **17**:883–885, 1978.
140. Peterson, G.J., Codd, J.E., Cuddihee, R.E., and Newton, W.T.: Renal transplantation in Lindau-von Hippel disease. *Arch. Surg.* **112**:841–842, 1977.
141. Horton, W.A., Wong, V., and Eldridge, R.: Von Hippel-Lindau disease: clinical and pathological manifestations in nine families with 50 affected members. *Arch. Intern. Med.* **136**:769–777, 1976.
142. Louis-Bar (Mme.): Sur un syndrome progressif comprenant des telangiectasies capillaires cutanees et conjonctivales symetriques, a disposition naevoide et des troubles cerebelleux. *Confinia Neurol.* **4**:32–42, 1941.
143. Boder, E., and Sedgwick, R.P.: Ataxia-telangiectasia. A familial syndrome of progressive cerebellar ataxia, oculocutaneous telangiectasia, and frequent pulmonary infection. *Pediatrics* **21**:526–554, 1958.
144. Boder, E., and Sedgwick, R.: Ataxia-telangiectasia: a familial syndrome of progressive cerebellar ataxia, oculocutaneous telangiectasia, and frequent pulmonary infection. *Arch. Dermatol.* **78**:402–405, 1958.
145. Boder, E., and Sedgwick, R.P.: Ataxia telangiectasia. A review of 101 cases. In: *Little Club Clinics in Developmental Medicine* (G. Walsh, ed.). No. 8. London: Heinemann Medical Books, 1963, pp. 110–118.
146. Wells, C.E., and Shy, G.M.: Progressive familial choreoathetosis with cutaneous telangiectasia. *J. Neurol. Neurosurg. Psychiatry* **20**:98–104, 1957.
147. Smith, J.L., and Cogan, D.G.: Ataxia-telangiectasia. *Arch. Ophthalmol.* **62**:364–369, 1959.
148. Aguilar, M.J., Kamoshita, S., Landing, B.H., Boder, E., and Sedgwick, R.P.: Pathological observations in ataxia-telangiectasia. A report on 5 cases. *J. Neuropath. Exp. Neurol.* **27**:659–676, 1968.
149. Peterson, R.D., Kelly, W.D., and Good, R.A.: Ataxia-telangiectasia. Its association with a defective thymus, immunological-deficiency disease, and malignancy. *Lancet* **1**:1189–1193, 1964.
150. Levin, S., Gottfried, E., and Cohen, M.: Ataxia telangiectasia: a review – with observations on 47 Israeli cases. *Pediatrician* **6**:135–146, 1977.
151. Peterson, R.D., Cooper, M.D., and Good, R.A.: Lymphoid tissue abnormalities associated with ataxia-telangiectasia. *Am. J. Med.* **41**:342–359, 1966.
152. Haerer, A.F., Jackson, J.F., and Evers, C.G.: Ataxia telangiectasia with gastric adenocarcinoma. *JAMA* **210**:1884–1887, 1969.
153. Jackson, J.F.: Ataxia telangiectasia. In: *Skin, Heredity, and Malignant Neoplasms* (H.T. Lynch, Ed.). Flushing, NY: Medical Examination Publishing Co., 1972, pp. 94–103.
154. Bowden, D.H., Danis, P.G., and Sommers, S.C.: Ataxia-telangiectasia. A case with lesions of ovaries and adenohypophysis. *J. Neuropath. Exp. Neurol.* **22**:549–554, 1963.
155. Miller, M.E., and Chatten, J.: Ovarian changes in ataxia telangiectasia. *Acta Paediatr. Scan.* **56**:559–561, 1967.

156. Tadjoedin, M.K., and Fraser, F.C.: Heredity of ataxia telangiectasia (Louis-Bar syndrome). *Am. J. Dis. Child* **110**:64-68, 1965.

157. Bar, R.S., Levis, W.R., Rechler, M.R., Harrison, L.C., Siebert, C., Podskalny, J., Roth, J., and Muggeo, M.: Extreme insulin resistance in ataxia telangiectasia. Defect in affinity of insulin receptors. *N. Engl. J. Med.* **298**:1164-1171, 1978.

158. Swift, M., Sholman, L., Perry, M., and Chase, C.: Malignant neoplasms in the families of patients with ataxia-telangiectasia. *Cancer Res.* **36**:209-215, 1976.

159. Dunn, H.G., Meuwissen, H., Livingstone, C.S., and Pump, K.K.: Ataxia telangiectasia. *Can. Med. Assoc. J.* **91**:1106-1118, 1964.

160. Reed, W.B., Epstein, W.L., Boder, E., and Sedgwick, R.: Cutaneous manifestations of ataxia telangiectasia. *JAMA* **195**:746-753, 1966.

161. Sedgwick, R.P., and Boder, E.: Ataxia-telangiectasia. In: *Handbook of Clinical Neurology* (P.J. Vinken and G.W. Bruyn, Eds). Vol. 14, New York: American Elsevier, 1972, pp. 267-339.

162. MacDonald, W.C., Dobbins, W.O., III, and Rubin, C.E.: Studies of the familial nature of celiac sprue using biopsy of the small intestine. *N. Engl. J. Med.* **272**:448-456, 1965.

163. Stokes, P.L., Ferguson, R., Holmes, G.K., and Cooke, W.T.: Familial aspects of coeliac disease. *Q. J. Med.* **45**:567-582, 1976.

164. Gough, K.R., Read, A.E., and Naish, J.M.: Intestinal reticulosis as a complication of idiopathic steatorrhoea. *Gut* **3**:232-239, 1962.

165. Harris, O.D., Cooke, W.T., Thompson, H., and Waterhouse, J.A.: Malignancy in adult coeliac disease and idiopathic steatorrhoea. *Am. J. Med.* **42**:899-912, 1967.

166. Gupte, S.P., Perkash, A., Mahajan, C.M., Aggarwal, P.K., and Gupta, P.R.: Acute myeloid leukemia in a girl with celiac disease. *Am. J. Dig. Dis.* **16**:939-941, 1971.

167. Spracklen, F. (for Tonkin, R.D.): Reticulosis of small bowels as a late complication of idiopathic steatorrhoea. *Proc. R. Soc. Med.* **56**:167-168, 1963.

168. Whitehead, R.: Primary lymphadenopathy complicating idiopathic steatorrhoea. *Gut* **9**:569-575, 1968.

169. Holmes, G.K., Stokes, P.L., Sorahan, T.M., Prior, P., Waterhouse, J.A., and Cooke, W.T.: Coeliac disease, gluten-free diet, and malignancy. *Gut* **17**:612-619, 1976.

170. Friedman, M., and Hare, P.J.: Gluten-sensitive enteropathy and eczema. *Lancet* **1**: 521-524, 1965.

171. Didolkar, M.S., Gerner, R.E., and Moore, G.E.: Epidermolysis bullosa dystrophica and epitheolioma of the skin. Review of published cases and report of an additional patient. *Cancer* **33**:198-202, 1974.

172. Orlando, R.C., Bozymski, E.M., Briggaman, R.A., and Bream, C.A.: Epidermolysis bullosa: gastrointestinal manifestations. *Ann. Int. Med.* **81**:203-206, 1974.

173. Sehgal, V.N., Rege, V.L., Ghosh, S.K., and Kamat, S.M.: Dystrophic epidermolysis bullosa. Interesting gastro-intestinal manifestations. *Br. J. Dermatol.* **96**:389-392, 1977.

174. Rochman, H., Cooper, M., Esterly, N.B., and Bauer, E.A.: Carcinoembryonic antigen: increased plasma levels in recessive epidermolysis bullosa. *J. Inves. Dermatol.* **72**:262-263, 1979.

175. Guirgis, H.A., Lynch, H.T., Harris, R.E., and Vandervoorde, J.P.: Genetic and communicable effects on carcinoembryonic antigen expressivity in the cancer family syndrome. *Cancer Res.* **38**:2523-2528, 1978.

176. Alm, T., and Wahren, B.: Carcinoembryonic antigen in hereditary adenomatosis of the colon and rectum. *Scan. J. Gastroenterol.* **10**:875-879, 1975.

177. Sugiomoto, T., Sawada, T., Tozawa, M., Kidowaki, T., Kusunoki, T., and Yamaguchi,

N.: Plasma levels of carcinoembryonic antigen in patients with ataxia-telangiectasia. *J. Pediatr.* **92**:436–439, 1978.

178. Gorlin, R.J., and Sedano, H.O.: The multiple nevoid basal cell carcinoma syndrome revisited. In: *Skin, Hereditary, and Malignant Neoplasms.* (H.T. Lynch, Ed.). Flushing, NY: Medical Examination Publishing Co., 1972, pp. 149–164.

179. Gorlin, R.J., and Goltz, R.W.: Multiple nevoid basal cell epithelioma, jaw cysts, and bifid rib syndrome. *N. Eng. J. Med.* **262**:908–912, 1960.

180. Gilhuus-Moe, O., Haugen, L.K., and Dee, P.M.: The syndrome of multiple cysts of the jaws, basal cell carcinomata, and skeletal anomalies. *Br. J. Oral Surg.* **6**:211–222, 1968.

181. Burket, R.L., and Rauh, J.L.: Gorlin's syndrome: ovarian fibromas at adolescence. *Obstet. Gyn.* **47**(1):42s–46s, 1976.

182. Lynch, H.T.: Hereditary factors in carcinoma. In: *Recent Advances in Cancer Research.* (P. Rentchnil, Ed.). Vol. 12. Berlin: Springer-Verlag, 1967.

183. Utsunomiya, J., Gocho, H., Miyanaga, T., Hamaguchi, E., and Kashmure, A.: Peutz-Jeghers syndrome: its natural course and management. *Johns Hopkins Med. J.* **136**(2):71–82, 1975.

184. Christian, C.D., McLoughlin, T.G., Cathcart, E.R., and Eisenberg, M.M.: Peutz-Jeghers syndrome associated with functioning ovarian tumor. *JAMA* **190**:157–159, 1964.

185. Humphries, A.L., Shepherd, M.H., and Peters, H.J.: Peutz-Jeghers syndrome with colonic adenocarcinoma and ovarian tumor. *JAMA* **197**:138–140, 1966.

186. Wiskott, A.: Familiarer angeborenes morbus werlhofii. *Monatsschrift für Kinderheilkunde* **68**:212, 1937.

187. Aldrich, R.A., Steinberg, A.C., and Campbell, D.C.: Pedigree demonstrating a sex-linked recessive condition characterized by draining ears, eczematoid dermatitis, and blood diarrhoea. *Paediatrics* **13**, 133, 1954.

188. Mackie, R.M., Alcorn, M.J., Stevenson, R.D., Cochran, T., and McSween, R.N.M.: Wiskott-Aldrich syndrome with partial response to transfer factor. *Br. J. Derm.* **98**:567–571, 1978.

189. Shapiro, R.S., Perry, G.S., Krivit, W., Gerrard, J.M., White, J.G., and Kersey, J.H.: Wiskott-Aldrich syndrome: detection of carrier status by metabolis stress of platelets. *Lancet* **1**:121, 1978.

190. Ten Bensel, R.W., Stadlan, E.M., and Krivit, W.: The development of malignancy in the course of the Aldrich syndrome. *J. Paed.* **68**:761, 1966.

191. Model, L.M.: Primary reticulum cell sarcoma of the brain in Wiskott-Aldrich syndrome. *Arch. Neurol.* **34**:633, 1977.

192. Devic, A., and Bussy, P.: Un cas de polypose adenomateuse generalisee a tout l'intestin. *Arch. Mal. App. Digest* **6**:278–299, 1912.

193. Fitzgerald, G.M.: Multiple composite odontomes coincidental with other tumorous conditions. Report of a case. *J. Am. Dent. Assoc.* **30**:1408–1417, 1943.

194. Guptill, P.: Familial polyposis of the colon: two families, five cases. *Surgery* **22**:286–304, 1947.

195. Gardner, E.J.: Followup study of family group exhibiting dominant inheritance for syndrome including intestinal polyps, osteomas, fibromas, and epidermal cysts. *Am. J. Hum. Genet.* **14**:376–390, 1962.

196. Gardner, E.J., and Richards, R.C.: Multiple cutaneous and subcutaneous lesions occurring simultaneously with hereditary polyposis and osteomatosis. *Am. J. Hum. Genet.* **5**:139–147, 1953.

197. Gardner, E.J.: Inherited multiple neoplasia syndrome. Genetics today. *Proc. XI Intern. Cong. Genet.* **1**:287, 1963.

198. Gardner, E.J., and Stephens, F.E.: Cancer of the lower digestive tract in one family group. *Am. J. Hum. Genet.* **2**:41–48, 1950.
199. Gardner, E.J.: A genetic and clinical study of intestinal polyposis, a predisposing factor for carcinoma of the colon and rectum. *Am. J. Hum. Genet.* **3**:167–176, 1951.
200. Gardner, E.J., and Plenk, H.P.: Hereditary pattern for multiple osteomas in a family group. *Am. J. Hum. Genet.* **4**:31–36, 1952.
201. Plenk, H.P., and Gardner, E.J.: Osteomatosis (leontiasis ossea): hereditary disease of membranous bone formation associated in one family with polyposis of the colon. *Radiology* **62**:830–840, 1954.
202. MacDonald, J.M., Davis, W.C., Crago, H.R., and Berk, A.D.: Gardner's syndrome and wperiampullary malignancy. *Am. J. Surg.* **113**:425–430, 1967.
203. Watne, A.: Gardner's syndrome. In: *Skin, Hereditary, and Malignant Neoplasms* (H.T. Lynch, Ed.). Flushing, NY: Medical Examination Publishing Co., 1972, 299 pp.
204. Chang, C.H., Piatt, E.D., Thomas, K.E., and Watne, A.L.: Bone abnormalities in Gardner's syndrome. *Am. J. Roentgen.* **103**:645–652, 1968.
205. Danes, B.S.: The Gardner syndrome: increased tetraploidy in cultured skin fibroblasts. *J. Med. Genet.* **13**:52–56, 1976.
206. Moore, T.L., Kupchik, H.Z., Marcon, U., and Samcheck, N.: Carcinoembryonic antigen assay in cancer of the colon and pancreas and other digestive tract disorders. *Am. J. Dig. Dis.* **16**:1–7, 1971.
207. Fader, M., Kline, S.N., Spatz, S.S., and Zubrow, H.J.: Gardner's syndrome (intestinal polyposis, osteomas, sebaceous cysts) and a new dental discovery. *Oral Surg.* **15**: 153–172, 1962.
208. O'Brien, J.P., and Wels, P.: The synchronous occurrence of benign fibrous tissue neoplasia in hereditary adenosis of the colon and rectum. *NY J. Med.* **55**:1877–1880, 1955.
209. Camiel, M.R., Mule, J.E., Alexander, L.L., and Benninghoff, D.L.: Association of thyroid carcinoma with Gardner's syndrome in siblings. *N. Eng. J. Med.* **278**:1056–1058, 1968.
210. Schweitzer, R.J., and Robbins, G.F.: A desmoid tumor of multicentric origin. *Arch. Surg.* **80**:489–494, 1960.

3
Cutaneous Signs of Cancer-associated Genodermatoses

Ramon M. Fusaro, M.D., Ph.D., and Henry T. Lynch, M.D.

The skin represents a unique, external means of observing the cells of the body. Certain defects which are coded into our genetic makeup can be manifested in the skin in the epithelial, appendageal, vascular, neural, and connective tissue elements. There are approximately 50 genodermatoses which are associated with familial malignancies. These genodermatoses by definition will have some cutaneous expression which may serve as a sign for recognition of a malignant state. The identification of these signs and their proper interpretation can aid immeasurably in the early diagnosis of malignant disease not only in the patient but in his immediate family and the entire kindred as well. In this chapter, we will focus upon the cutaneous findings in the genodermatoses which are discussed by various contributors to this book.

Infantile X-linked Agammaglobulinemia[1-4]

The patient with infantile X-linked agammaglobulinemia (Bruton type) has repeated episodes of pyoderma, usually starting in the second year of life. These male patients have recurrent and severe episodes of furunculosis, usually caused by *Staphylococcus aureus*. They usually can handle viral infection well because of their intact cellular immunity. In addition, they appear to have a higher than normal occurrence of dermatomyositis, rheumatoid arthritis, and atopic eczema.

Severe Combined Immunodeficiency Agammaglobulinemia[2,5,6]

Patients with the X-linked Swiss type of agammaglobulinemia are usually sickly infants to whom death occurs in the first few years of life. They have repeated episodes of pyoderma and thrush, and are plagued by bacterial, viral, fungal, and protozoal infections. They may manifest massive candidiasis or vaccinia. Other cutaneous findings include seborrheic dermatitis, epidermal necrolysis, and a nonspecific morbilliform eruption.

DiGeorge's Syndrome[3,7,8]

This is a genetically transmitted disorder that manifests itself because of a failure to develop the thymus. There is a lymphopenia secondary to absence or hypoplasia of cellular immune response. The parathyroids are also absent, which leads to neonatal tetany and hypocalcemia. Patients are prone to viral and mycotic infections, and have extensive chronic, cutaneous, and oral moniliasis. Their susceptibility to viral infections can result in a severe hemorrhagic varicella. If vaccinated, a fatal progressive gangrenosa will occur. They also may have a persistent morbilliform eruption as a result of either a measles infection or a graft vs host reaction (runting syndrome).

Ataxia Telangiectasia[9-16]

Ataxia telangiectasia (AT) is an autosomal recessive disorder characterized by progressive cerebellar ataxia, oculocutaneous telangiectasia, and recurrent sinopulmonary infections. Immunologic studies have indicated a defect involving both B- and T-cell development. The evaluation of humoral immunity showed the frequent occurrence of reduced IgA levels, low molecular weight IgM, and undetectable or reduced levels of IgE. Measurements of cellular immunity by skin test antigens show deficiencies, and in patients who had been autopsied, the thymus was absent or atrophic. Resistance to skin and pulmonary infection (bacterial, viral, fungal) is reduced. AT also shows consistent elevation of α-fetoprotein and carcinoembyonic antigen (see Chapter 2).

Ocular telangiectasia usually appears between the ages of 3 and 6 years, and involves the temporal/nasal aspects of the bulbar conjunctivae while sparing the inferior and superior areas. The palpebral conjunctivae may be involved. Telangiectasia occurs later over the butterfly area of the face, external ear, necklace region of the neck, popliteal and antecubital fossae, retroauricular areas, and dorsum of the hands and feet. The sun-exposed areas are more prominently affected. The damaged skin shows a mottled pattern of hypopigmentation and hyperpigmentation with cutaneous atrophy and telangiectasia. The skin appears to be poikilodermic. AT patients have a higher than normal incidence of basal cell epitheliomas, and they show fibroblasts in culture which are sensitive to x-ray in that DNA repair is altered.

Cutaneous infections (pyoderma) are common occurrences in these individuals. The majority of patients also have other changes of the skin and hair with diffuse poliosis, café au lait spots, dryness of skin, seborrheic dermatitis, follicular keratosis, and hirsutism of the extremities.

Bloom's Syndrome[15,17-22]

This rare syndrome has three cardinal features: congenital facial telangiectatic erythema, photosensitivity, and dwarfism with dolichocephaly with narrow and characteristic facies. Within the first three years of life, a facial erythema develops involving the butterfly region of the face, forehead, lips, ears, and margins of the eyelids. The dorsum of the forearms and hands may be involved. The eruption consists of telangiectatic macules and papules with scaling. The erythema may be exacerbated by sunlight exposure with an action spectrum in the sunburn region. Prolonged exposure to light causes more intense photoreaction with vesiculation, crusting, and exfoliation. Atrophy can develop on the nose and cheeks. Other cutaneous defects noted are café au lait spots, lichen pilaris, ichthyosis, hypertrichosis, and acanthosis nigricans. Several patients were reported to have abnormally low concentrations of serum IgA and IgM.

In Bloom's syndrome, there are chromosomal abnormalities such as an increase in breaks, rearrangements, sister chromatid exchanges, and quadriradial configuration. There is also a decrease in RNA replication. The chromosomes are more sensitive than normal to radiation, and cultured cells are slightly more sensitive to UV light.

Fanconi Pancytopenia[23-34]

This disorder is characterized by a pancytopenia, genital hypoplasia (20–48%), microcephaly (33–43%), skeletal deformities (60%), stunted growth (56–67%), renal abnormalities (28%), hypoplasia of the thumb (75%), and abnormal pigmentation (20–75%). The brownish pigmentation or hyperpigmentation (local or diffuse) is the most frequent finding. The area of color change may be of varying sizes and a patchy distribution. It is prominent in the anogenital region, axillae, trunk, and neck. There may be depigmented areas within the hyperpigmented regions. The chromosomes cultured from lymphocytes show nonspecific structural abnormalities such as gaps, breaks, chromatid exchange, and endoreduplication. There is a deficiency in excising UV-induced pyrimidine dimers from DNA in some patients, but unscheduled DNA synthesis and single strand breaks function are intact, thereby lessening the probability of a deficiency of ligase, endonuclease, and DNA polymerase. Cells are more susceptible to DNA cross-links produced by mitomycin C, and there are increased chromosomal aberrations of several kinds.

Fanconi-like Syndrome[35]

There is only a single family consisting of two brothers reported in this syndrome. One had a pancytopenia, immunologic deficiencies, and cutaneous malignancies of squamous and basal cell carcinomas. He also had a protracted course of recurrent infections and multiple pneumothoraces. The immunologic deficiencies included very low levels of IgA, elevated IgG with an abnormal γ-globulin, and defective cellular immunity which was demonstrated at autopsy by absence of a thymus gland. The other brother had only a pancytopenia.

Dyskeratosis Congenita[36-45]

This rare congenital syndrome, which manifests itself before puberty, is characterized by the predominant cutaneous triad of oral leukokeratosis, nail dystrophy, and hyperpigmentation. In this extensive disorder, ectodermal, endodermal, and mesodermal tissues are affected. Pancytopenia is an important clinical aspect. The earliest expressions, in order of occurrence, are cutaneous hyperpigmentation, nail dystrophy, oral leukoplakia, epiphora, anemia, and bullous lesions.

Hyperpigmentation occurs in all cases and is the pathognomonic feature of the disorder. It is a fine telangiectatic maculopapular or linear reticulated lesion, gray to brown in color, surrounded by 1–3 cm or more of round or ovoid non-pigmented areas. The color changes start on the face, neck, and upper trunk, and spread to the extremities. The dystrophic nails are short and thin with longitudinal grooves and ridges. When loss of the nail occurs, it is replaced by an atrophic, wrinkled epidermis. The soles and palms are hyperkeratotic and hyperhidrotic, and in some patients, bullae develop after trauma.

The hair distribution is sparse and lusterless. Alopecia may occur in late childhood. Eyebrows and eyelashes may be absent. Premature graying of the hair occurs.

Mucosal lesions on the oral, vaginal, urethral, and conjunctival tissues are seen as glazed white patches with the most prominently involved areas in the oral cavity being the buccal and lingual regions. Oral ulcerations do occur and are recurrent. Ulcerations may appear as early as 5 years of age.

Eye findings may occur shortly after birth with epiphora resulting from obstruction of the lacrimal duct leading to continuous lacrimation, conjunctivitis, blepharitis, and ectropion.

Dental abnormalities are poorly defined but are multiple (caries, gingivitis, poorly aligned teeth, etc.).

The following findings occur in these frequencies: hyperpigmentation (100%), hyperhidrosis of palms and soles (89%), dystrophic nails (98%), wrinkled atrophic skin of extremities (93%), hyperkeratosis of palms and soles (72%), bullae after trauma (78%), acrocyanosis (55%), leukoplakia (78%), dental abnormalities (63%), hair changes (51%), epiphora (78%), low intelligence (42%), and dysphagia (59%).

In some patients, absence of delayed hypersensitivity, thymic aplasia, or low levels of immunoglobulins have been noted. Other data suggest chromosomal instability. Chromosomes of these patients show a greater increase in sister chromatid exchange after exposure to psoralens and UV light than do cells from normal individuals. These cells show delayed excision of psoralen-DNA cross-linking photoadducts.

Intracranial calcifications were seen in two male patients and consisted of symmetric dense masses in the gray matter of the basal ganglia, dentate nuclei, and cortex.

There appear to be two genetic forms of this disorder: (1) Zinsser-Cole-Engman type and (2) Scoggins type. The former is an X-linked recessive, while the latter is an autosomal dominant. The vast majority of the cases reported are males. The dominant cases are few and their clinical manifestations are similar to the X-linked recessive.

Wiskott-Aldrich Syndrome[2,9,46-50]

This is a rare sex-linked recessive disorder totally confined to males and characterized by thrombocytopenia, eczema, and multiple infections with all classes of microorganisms. The eczema usually starts on the scalp, face, buttocks, and flexural areas of the extremities. It may resemble atopic or seborrheic dermatitis and may be purpuric in nature. Superficial infections such as impetigo, furunculosis, and conjunctivitis are the most common of the recurrent infections; however, other sites of infection in lung, ears, and sinuses are common.

This disorder is one of the most severe immunologic deficiencies. The patient usually dies early in life. The affected males have abnormal cellular immunity, decreased platelet survival, abnormal platelet function, and decreased antibody response to carbohydrate antigens. The latter is the hallmark of this form of immunodeficiency. There are both cellular and humoral immunologic defects. The IgE levels are usually about the highest clinically recorded. There is abnormal ATP metabolism which may relate to the immunodeficiency state. Recently, the disorder has been treated successfully with allogeneic bone marrow transplants.

Rothmund-Thomson Syndrome[51-56]

This is a recessive disorder characterized by congenital poikiloderma of the skin, juvenile cataracts (50% of patients), and the development of bowenoid changes in the epidermis which may lead to invasive malignancy. The skin is apparently normal at birth, but within six months, a mild erythema appears on the face, ears, and dorsum of the hands. These areas develop a reticulated pattern of telangiectasia with hypopigmentation, atrophy, and surrounding hyperpigmentation, which assumes a marmoreal appearance. Later, the eruption spreads from the face and hands to the arms, lower extremities, buttocks, and trunk. The skin lesions do not progress after the age of 3–5 years, but they persist throughout life. The individual is extremely photosensitive and may develop bullae on exposure to sunlight. The syndrome is marked by short stature with small hands, stubby fingers, and saddle nose. Other features are anomalies of the hair (sparse and prematurely gray, alopecia totalis), disturbances in sweating, dystrophy of the nails (rough, ridged, heaped, small, atrophic), hypogonadism, and skeletal defects. Defective dentition occurs in less than 15% of the affected individuals.

Epidermolysis Bullosa Dystrophica (Recessive)[57-62]

This is the common form of epidermolysis bullosa which can lead to cancer. Onset of the cutaneous signs occurs at birth or in early infancy, and it becomes confined, usually to the extremities, in later years. One sees bullae and erosions which are large, flaccid, and occasionally hemorrhagic on any traumatized surface. Because of slow healing and repeated cycles of trauma healing, one sees atrophic scars. The hands and feet can be enclosed in a pseudowebbing of scar tissue with skeletal atrophy. Alopecia and hypotrichosis are common. Mucosal erosion and healing leads to scarring problems in the oral and anal regions. Even conjunctival scarring may occur. Both basal and squamous cell carcinoma have been reported in this disorder. The mucous membranes have developed leukoplakia and squamous cell carcinoma. The defect in this disorder is with the anchoring fibrils below the epidermis in the dermis. There may be an aberration in collagenase function.

Epidermodysplasia Verruciformis[63-70]

This is a rare, virus-induced, verrucous polymorphic eruption which infects a genetically susceptible host (autosomal recessive) with immunologic abnormalities. The papovavirus has been identified and there may be two subgroups of this clinical disorder with one group at a high risk for cutaneous cancer. The persistent process develops early in childhood and is resistant to usual wart therapy. The lesions are papular, warty and flat topped, and occasionally form plaques. They are usually found symmetrically on the exposed areas of the face, neck, and dorsum of the hands, but are seen also on the trunk and elsewhere. They remain unchanged, with no evidence of spontaneous regression. After a number of years, there is a 20–25% chance for malignant transformation.

Porokeratosis[71-79]

Porokeratosis has at least five clinical presentations: solitary plaque, disseminated eruptive form, disseminated superficial actinic porokeratosis, hypertrophic keratosis, and linear porokeratosis. One of these, the rare autosomal dominant form known as "classic porokeratosis of Mibelli," has had maligant degeneration occur in a significant number of patients — either squamous cell carcinoma or Bowen's disease. In two instances, basal cell epitheliomas have been described.

The clinical lesion begins as a reddish-brown or gray keratotic papule that persists and slowly enlarges into an irregular lesion with a raised, furrowed, or hyperkeratotic border (moat), and a depressed central, dry, and smooth area in which the normal skin markings are diminished. The eruptions may be few or many and usually start in early childhood. The sites of predilection are the extremities (especially the hands and feet), but also the face, neck, and genitalia. The mucous membranes may be involved. A mutant clone of epidermal cells has been proposed for the cornoid lamella. Cultured fibroblast studies from patients with porokeratosis of Mibelli have shown chromosomal instability.

Hyperkeratosis Lenticularis Perstans (Flegel's Disease)[80-83]

This disorder is characterized by asymptomatic inflammatory keratotic papules on the extremities, with concomitant palmar and plantar papules and pits. These keratotic papules measure less than 0.5 cm and are usually present on the dorsal aspects of the feet and lower legs. The lesions can occur elsewhere; nearly half of the patients will have lesions on the arms. The colors of the primary lesions are yellowish-brown to reddish-brown. The palms and soles show pinpoint keratotic papules and depressions. Most cases are seen in males, especially in the 30-50 year age group. The primary occurrence is the formation of hyperkeratotic papules in a normal-appearing epidermis. This inborn error of keratinization shows a lack of keratinosomes (Odland bodies) in small areas of the epidermis. After abrasion or shave excision, the lesions do not recur, which suggests that the defect is limited to small clones of keratinocytes. In one reported family, there was a high incidence of mainly squamous cell carcinomas which did not necessarily arise at the site of lesions of Flegel's disease.

Multiple Self-healing Keratoacanthoma (Ferguson-Smith Type)[84-93]

This dominant trait becomes manifest after puberty and starts with multiple papules which develop into nodules with a central, horn-filled crater which heals after a variable period of time (months) with a scar. The new lesions can appear at any cutaneous site; various authors differ as to whether the face or the extremities have unusually large numbers of lesions. These lesions can destroy underlying structures, such as bone or cartilage. New lesions continue to occur over many years with a diminished propensity for spontaneous remission.

The histologic classification of this tumor as a benign pseudomalignancy or a squamous cell carcinoma is difficult. This is an example of histologic appearance not reflecting biologic function. Ferguson-Smith's original patient died at age 37 years of causes other than his primary disease. Lever feels that it is doubtful that keratoacanthoma ever changes into a classical squamous cell carcinoma with metastatic potential. No case of the Ferguson-Smith type has ever been reported to have metastases; however, the local destructive potential places it in the biological behavior class of malignancy.

Multiple Trichoepithelioma (Epithelioma Adenoides Cysticum — Brooke)[94-102]

This dominant trait is characterized by the occurrence of many small cutaneous tumors, with more than 75% occurring on the face, especially the nasolabial fold, upper lip, and eyelids, but occasionally on the scalp, neck, and trunk. The lesions first develop in early childhood or at puberty as flesh-colored or pink papules measuring from 2-5 cm in diameter with occasional telangiectasia. After they increase in size for a few years, they remain stationary and few appear after the third decade. Groups of small lesions may coalesce to form larger lesions.

Associated cutaneous tumors are cylindroma and syringoma, the former more often than the latter. The cylindromas can vary in size from a few millimeters to several centimeters, and can undergo malignant degeneration with metastasis. The question has been raised about malignant degeneration of trichoepitheliomas into basal cell epitheliomas, as there can be histologic difficulty in separating them. Howell and Anderson reviewed the literature and feel that Brooke's disease does not break down into multiple (more than five) basal cell epitheliomas in any one patient. If these do occur, they are more likely to be examples of multiple nevoid basal cell carcinoma syndrome. Those patients who have one, two, or up to five lesions which break down into ulcerative processes are patients with trichoepithelioma. There is a question whether Brooke's tumors can degenerate because of size or inadequate blood supply being compromised rather than being a basal cell carcinoma. Of course, some could be malignant cylindromas.

Basal Cell Nevus Syndrome[103-111]

This syndrome is a complex disorder which has as its hallmark the onset of multiple basal cell epitheliomas in association with abnormalities of skin, bone, nervous system, eye, and reproductive systems. The basal cell epitheliomas are nevoid and occur between puberty and the mid-thirties; however, they can appear well before puberty. The early lesions appear as brownish or flesh-colored papules with a marked tendency for the central facial area, especially the nose, upper lips, cheeks, periorbital regions, and eyelids, but they also occur on the trunk. The appearance at the latter site of upper trunk and upper limbs is suggestive of the disorder. These nevoid tumors are biologically as destructive and invasive as the regular basal cell epitheliomas and have been known to metastasize to brain and lung.

The cutaneous lesions also include palmar and plantar pits, which are 1-3 mm shallow holes, both discrete and confluent. Over 70% of the patients have these lesions. Further cutaneous lesions are milia, epithelial cysts, comedone, lipomas, and café au lait pigmentation. Further abnormalities are listed in Table 3-1.

Chelitis Glandularis[112-116]

This rare dominant trait manifests as a diffuse enlargement of the lower lip, with firm nodularity. A mucous substance is exuded from the dilated orifices of the mucous gland. The condition is a hypertrophy of the mucous glands and

Table 3-1. Findings in Basal Cell Nevus Syndrome.

Cutaneous	Oral
Basal cell carcinomas	Multiple jaw cysts
Epithelial cysts	Fibrosarcomas of the jaw
Milia	Prognathism
Palmar and plantar pits	Cleft palate and lip
Comedones	Defective dentition
Café au lait	Ameloblastoma
Central nervous system	Osseous
Seizures	Bifid, synostic, splayed
Mental retardation	rudimentary ribs
Agenesis of corpus callosum	Spina bifida occulta
Medulloblastoma	Fusion of vertebra
Congenital hydrocephalus	Scoliosis
Nerve deafness	Bridging of sella
Lamellar calcification of falx	Frontal, temporoparietal bossing
	Oligodactyly or syndactyly
Ocular	Pes planus, hallux valgus
Dystopia canthorum	Defective clavicle
Hypertelorism	Pectus excavatum or carinatum
Strabismus, internal	Brachymetacarpals, 4th
Congenital blindness	Sprengel's deformity of scapula
cataracts	
glaucoma	Miscellaneous
coloboma	Renal malformations
	Inguinal hernias
Endocrine	lymphatic mesenteric cysts
Pelvic calcification	
Ovarian fibromas and cysts	
Hypogonadism	

ducts. Varying amounts of acute and chronic inflammatory processes occur with the resulting damage to tissue.

There is controversy concerning the reported 20% malignancy rate (squamous cell carcinoma) in these patients. One group of authors[113,114] feels that the squamous cell carcinoma develops from the glandular structure, while others[115,116] regard them as solar keratoses. The controversy possibly implicates different mechanisms for the cause of these cancers.

Hereditary Hidrotic Ectodermal Dysplasia (Touraine)[117-124]

There are two forms of ectodermal dysplasia, hidrotic type and anhidrotic type. The former, with which we are concerned, is usually dominant in its genetic expression, while the latter is usually X-linked recessive. This ectodermal defect shows nail dystrophy, a generalized hypotrichosis, and palmoplantar keratoderma.

The nail changes are varied (thick, slow-growing, discolored), but never characteristic. The body hair may be sparse or absent, and the scalp hair is minimal. The sweat glands and teeth are invariably normal in contrast to the anhidrotic type. Some patients have lower than normal intelligence. A generalized hyperpigmentation has been noted with some accentuation over certain joints. Commonly, there is a fine nodular character to palms and soles. Recently, histologic examination has shown this to be diffuse eccrine poromatosis. There are examples in the literature of squamous cell carcinoma of the nail bed and hands. Recently, demonstrations of defects in sulfur metabolism of polypeptides, and the formation of proteins of abnormally low molecular weight in the tissue, suggest a defect in structural genes of the matrix polypeptides.

Follicular Atrophoderma with Basal Cell Epitheliomas and Hypotrichosis (Bazex Syndrome)[125-129]

This very rare, newly described entity is an autosomal dominant trait which has follicular atrophoderma, localized anhidrosis, and basal cell carcinomas. The follicular atrophoderma, which is found especially in the elbows, on the dorsum of the hands and feet, and on the face (cheeks), is described as many ice-pick marks. These occur as sharply outlined plaques with 1–2 mm dimples without lanugo hairs. The areas of skin between the lesions appear normal. Hypotrichosis was not a constant feature, as a later report by Viksnius and Berlin notes. In Bazex's original description, the hypotrichosis was mainly localized to the first cervical vertebra region and the auriculotemporal regions. Anhidrosis and hypohidrosis of the face were observed. Multiple basal cell epitheliomas of the face, especially the upper and lower eyelids, develop in the second and third decades.

Pachyonychia Congenita (Jadassohn-Lewandowsky Syndrome)[130-137]

This autosomal dominant trait is characterized by dystrophy of the nails, hyperkeratosis palmaris et plantaris, follicular keratosis about the elbows and knees, hyperhidrosis, and a leukokeratosis of the mucous membranes. The dystrophic changes have been observed in the hair and in the cornea. Bullous lesions on the feet do occur. The cutaneous and oral lesions may be present at birth or become apparent soon after birth. Confusion occurs with respect to the white patches on the mucous membranes. These patches are not dyskeratotic or leukoplakic, but are probably a spongy nevus and do not become malignant.

Albinism[138-157]

Albinism is characterized as a hereditary recessive disorder of melanin synthesis which affects the skin and eyes. The clinical expression consists of white skin color (or shades thereof), white hair, nystagmus, and photophobia. There are six forms of oculocutaneous albinism: (1) tyrosinase-negative (albinism-I), (2) tyrosinase-positive (albinism-II), (3) yellow-mutant, (4) Hermansky-Pudlak syndrome, (5) Cross-McKusick-Breen syndrome, and (6) Chediak-Higashi syndrome. In albinism, the melanocyte is present and the hypopigmentation is a biologic functional defect in melanin synthesis.

Patients with albinism-I have snow-white hair, pink-white skin, gray to blue-gray and (diaphanous) irides, red reflex, photophobia, nystagmus, and poor visual acuity. The defect is an inability to synthesize tyrosinase; therefore, the melanosomes stop in their development at stage II. The skin, hair color, and eye changes persist throughout life.

Patients with albinism-II have the second most common form of the disorder in the United States. They have some melanin pigmentation, and the severity of the clinical features is inverse to the amount of pigment produced. Later in life these individuals may appear to be darker than many Caucasians. The hair will become yellow, yellow-white, light brown, or red. The eyes may be brown, hazel, gray-blue, or yellow. The red reflex is not as prominent as in albinism-I. Electron microscopy (EM) shows many melanosomes of stage I and II, some stage III, and rarely some stage IV. The enzyme tyrosinase is present, but the defect in function of pigmentation is not known.

The yellow-mutant patient resembles the tyrosinase-negative albino at birth. At about 6 months to 1 year of age, they develop yellow-red hair and fair skin. The irides become pigmented during infancy, and some retinal pigment is present. In comparison to the tyrosinase-positive individuals, they have a lesser manifestation of nystagmus and photophobia and better visual acuity. The melanosomes are seen in different stages, such as rounded, elongated, and unevenly or partially pigmented.

The Hermansky-Pudlak syndrome is a rare form of albinism with a hemorrhagic diathesis. These patients' skin and hair color can be fair to dark. The melanosomes can be found in stages I, II, and III with a rare occasional IV. The hemorrhagic episodes are the hallmark of this disorder. The bleeding is caused by a decreased amount of an adenine nucleotide in platelets and almost virtual absence of platelet-dense bodies.

The Cross-McKusick-Breen syndrome affects individuals with hypopigmentation, microphthalmia, nystagmus, opaque cornea, athetosis, oligophrenia, and severe mental retardation. The color of the skin is white, and the hair is blond with a yellow-gray sheen. Gingival fibromatosis is also present. This syndrome is tyrosinase-positive with hair bulb incubation.

The last type of oculocutaneous albinism is Chediak-Higashi syndrome, which is characterized by a partial albinism associated with neurologic and hematologic abnormalities. There is a dilution of pigment in skin, hair and eyes. The color of the skin varies from light tan to even gray. Hair color can be blond to brunette.

Irides may be brown to blue. EM studies show giant melanosomes (stage IV) which are not transferred properly to keratinocytes. Patients may have peripheral neuropathy, mental retardation, and seizures. There are definite hematologic problems such as neutropenia, anemia, and thrombocytopenia. The leucocytes from these patients have giant azurophilic staining granules. These patients have recurrent bacterial infections during infancy.

Patients with albinism have a higher incidence of cutaneous malignancies (squamous cell carcinoma, basal cell epithelioma, and malignant melanoma), with squamous cell carcinoma being the most common. It is not known what the susceptibility to cancer is in the yellow-mutant and the Cross-McKusick-Breen syndromes, but all other types of albinism have degrees of cutaneous neoplasia, probably because of their variable lack of pigment or because the presence of the biologic intermediates of melanin in abnormal amounts may be detrimental.

Melanin is considered the major defense of the skin against acute and chronic effects of sun exposure, with protection being directly proportional to degree of melanization. The gradation of pigment in albinism with its propensity to skin neoplasia is an attestation to the protective qualities of melanin. Still, in patients with vitiligo or piebaldism, where there is a complete absence not only of melanin but also of the melanocyte, the incidence of cutaneous malignancies is, to everyone's surprise, quite low. Solar keratoses are rarely seen. It has also been reported that there is less epidermal damage when vitiliginous skin is irradiated, compared to normal, lightly pigmented skin. Clearly, there are other factors than melanin which are significant in the protection of skin from radiation.

Giant Pigmented Nevi[158-166]

This condition is, in the vast majority of cases, an isolated congenital process. The nevus is present at birth, and in only two reports is there mention of an autosomal dominant inheritance. The giant nevi are usually greater than 930 cm^2 (or a new criteria, greater than 20 cm in diameter), but individuals can have multiple nevi of smaller size, usually exceeding 1.5 cm in diameter. The giant lesion can be unilateral, but is usually bilateral and symmetrical. Locations are usually the trunk and distal part of the upper and lower extremities. There is a tendency toward dermatome distribution. The pigmentation is highly variable but is usually dark brown to black. The lesions can be extremely verrucous and hairy. Growth of the nevi parallels that of the child.

These giant nevi may be associated with other external manifestations such as many smaller pigmented nevi, fibromas, lipomas, and café au lait spots. There is a relationship of importance between large congenital nevi and leptomeningeal melanocytosis with certain neurologic complications (seizures, mental retardation, hydrocephalus), especially if the giant pigmented nevi is present on head or neck.

The incidence of degeneration of these cutaneous lesions has varied from 1.8 to 13.0% (about 4% may be precise). The risk decreases exponentially below 20 cm diameter lesion as the size decreases. Those patients who develop malignant melanoma within their lesion usually die of same. These nevi should be excised as early as possible in childhood as many develop melanoma before age 10. Malignant transformation of the leptomeningeal tissue is known.

Familial Rosacea-like Eruption with Intraepidermal Epithelioma (Haber's Syndrome)[167]

This autosomal dominant syndrome, which was first recognized by Haber and reported by Sanderson and Wilson, is characterized by a persistent rosacea-like eruption of the face, occurrence in the second to third decade of life, a red follicular scaling eruption on trunk and extremities, a prolonged unremitting course, and wart-like lesions on the trunk that have histologic resemblance to Bowen's disease. It is the latter that are called intraepidermal epithelioma. The true cancerous potential is not known.

Xeroderma Pigmentosum[168-181]

Xeroderma pigmentosum (XP) is a rare autosomal recessive disorder which is characterized by excessive xerosis with areas of hypo- and hyperpigmentation and cutaneous malignancies on the sun-exposed area. Children are born normal but soon develop the earliest signs — conjunctivitis and photophobia. Shortly thereafter, on the sunexposed areas, the skin becomes erythematous and scaly with freckles and hypopigmented areas. By 3–4 years of age, telangiectasia, atrophy, and scarring are apparent. Later, cutaneous signs of malignant degeneration appear: actinic keratosis, keratoacanthoma, basal cell epithelioma, squamous cell carcinoma, malignant melanoma, and tumors of the mesoderm.

There are two basic forms of this disorder: (1) the common form with at least seven excision repair deficient complementation groups, A through G, and (2) a postreplication repair deficiency (XP variant). Within certain of the A–G groups are patients with the following neurologic abnormalities: microcephaly, progressive mental deterioration, areflexia, choreoathetosis, ataxia, eventual quadriparesis with Achilles tendon shortening, deafness, retarded skeletal growth, and hypogonadism (the DeSanctis-Cacchione type). Patients in the D group, some in the A group, none in the C group, and one in the XP variant develop severe XP-associated neurological abnormalities. In addition, patients with XP cells fail to excise damage by carcinogenic aromatic amines, polycyclic aromatic hydrocarbons, and other known carcinogens that bind to DNA.

Pigmented xerodermoid (PX) is possibly a form of XP, but the cutaneous manifestations do not appear until the middle part of life rather than in the first and second decades. However, PX is a dominant trait as opposed to XP which is recessive. For genetic counseling, the disorders must be handled as separate entities. These patients have somewhat similar cutaneous problems as those with XP, however excision repair is normal and DNA synthesis after UV exposure is markedly prolonged, suggesting that postreplication repair is abnormal.

It is apparent that the understanding of the disorder is further away than initially suspected; this will be discussed in Chapter 10. Protection of these patients from UV light, especially UVB, is paramount. Lynch et al. have shown that cutaneous malignancies can be prevented with a protective medical program and cooperative patients.

Keratosis Palmaris et Plantaris with Esophageal Cancer (Howell-Evans Syndrome) [182-185]

This very rare, autosomal dominant trait has only been recorded in a few families. It is a diffuse keratoderma of the palms and soles with a delayed onset (between the ages of 5 and 15 years). When any of these family members have the cutaneous findings, they have a 95% chance of developing cancer of the lower third of the esophagus before the age of 60 years.

Multiple Hamartoma Syndrome (Cowden's Disease) [186-193]

This is an autosomal dominant disorder with a complex mixture of endodermal, ectodermal, and mesodermal hamartomatous lesions involving many organs. The disorder can appear as early as 5 years of age. Recognition is important not only for the problems created by the hamartomatous tissue, but also for the associated visceral malignancies such as adenocarcinoma of the colon, carcinoma of the breast (females), cervical carcinoma (uterus), follicular cell carcinoma (thyroid), malignant melanoma, and squamous cell carcinoma (skin). The following visceral tumors have been reported: bone cysts, fibrocystic disease of the breasts (female), fibromas of the esophagus, stomach, and colon, hemangiomas, hepatic hamartomas, lipomas, meningiomas, neuromas, ovarian cysts, retinal gliomas, thyroid adenomas, uterine leiomyomas, and endometrial carcinomas.

The cutaneous lesions are many and include, especially on the face, flesh-colored, dome-shaped papules or flat-topped lichenoid papules with a central keratotic plug (facial trichilemmomas). There is a punctate acrokeratosis of the palms. Verrucous lesions are present and are very similar to verruca vulgaris or plana. The oral findings are papular and papillomatous lesions of the lips and gingiva with less involvement in buccal mucosa, tongue, and palate. These oral lesions are asymptomatic.

Intestinal Polyposis II (Peutz-Jeghers Syndrome)[194-198]

This syndrome is characterized by cutaneous pigmentation and generalized intestinal polyposis. This particular form of hereditary intestinal polyposis was once considered by many clinicians to be a disorder without malignant potential. However, gastrointestinal and ovarian malignancies have been reported in over 10% of the patients. In one series of 102 cases, 60% of the deaths over 30 years of age resulted from neoplasia, while 42% of the deaths before age 30 resulted from nonmalignant polyposis complications.

The cutaneous lesions are macular and pigmented with sharp margins and a color variation from brown through blue-black. These lesions appear in infancy or early childhood, and characteristically occur around the mouth, on the lips (especially the lower), and on the buccal mucosa. Pigmentation appears punctate and can occur on the fingers, palms, and toes. Less frequently, the macules are seen about the nostrils, hard and soft palate, tongue, and eyes. They can also occur on the conjunctiva and sclera. These macules are rarely seen elsewhere but have occasionally been found on the forearms, on the periumbilical area, under the fingernails, and in the rectal mucosa. They show a tendency toward grouping that permits a differentiation from the more disseminated clinical entity of ephelides, with which they are histologically identical. The skin lesions tend not to coalesce, while remaining about 2 mm in diameter. After puberty, the skin lesions disappear while the mouth lesions remain. This phenomenon becomes an important diagnostic sign.

Intestinal Polyposis III (Gardner's Syndrome)[199-209]

This autosomal dominant disorder is characterized by multiple diffuse intestinal polyposis, fibromas, osteomas, epidermal cysts, and systemic malignancy in one-third of the patients. The symptoms are insidious and start early in life. Epidermal cysts can be present at birth. Usually they arise on the scalp and face but can be observed elsewhere. They reach a certain size and terminate their growth, but they tend to appear in advance of the occurrence of polyposis, which has been reported as early as 4 years of age. Bony abnormalities occur in approximately 50% of the patients. Globoid osteomas of the mandible with overlying fibromas are characteristic of the disorder. Less than 50% of the patients have fibrous tissue abnormalities which include desmoid tumors, fibrosarcomas, and fibromas. Dental abnormalities are seen and include many supernumerary teeth, embedded teeth, cystic odontomas, and follicular odontomas. Examination of the teeth by x-ray is an important early diagnostic tool. Malignancies have been reported and include adenocarcinomas of the colon, sarcomas, thyroid cancer, periampullar cancer, adrenal cortical carcinoma, and tumors of the CNS. In patients at high risk, the search for malignancy should start in early childhood. Skin fibroblast cultures show increased tetraploidy.

Turcot Syndrome[210-212]

This is a very rare autosomal recessive disorder which belongs to the gastro-intestinal polyposis syndromes; however, its dermatologic manifestations are minimal. This does not diminish its importance as central nervous system malignancies and colonic cancers do occur. Cafe au lait spots and multiple pigmented nevi have been described. Polyposis of the colon has been associated with only three patients. The autosomal recessive inheritance of this disease is what clearly sets it apart from the other polyposis disorders.

Familial Hyperglucagonemia[213-219]

Glucagonoma is a very rare disorder. The cutaneous lesions seen are a polymorphous group with a characteristic distribution of intensely pruritic lesions, usually in the perioral and paragenital regions. Trauma seems to play a significant role in the precipitation of the eruption. The rash begins innocently as an erythematous area which develops into a vesiculopustular eruption with crusts. The lesions tend to spread in a peripheral annular pattern which coalesces into gyrate configurations which heal with pigmentation. The process takes several weeks. It extends with a prominent migratory erythema that advances into the intertrigingous areas with maceration and necrosis of the skin. Thus, the name "necrolytic migratory erythema" is appropriate. Any intertriginous areas can be involved. The oral lesions include mucosal erosions with a beefy and painful tongue which is never atrophic. There may be intermittent diarrhea with hypokalemia in association with the flare of the integument. Serum iron values may be low and a normocytic, normochromic anemia frequently accompanies relapses of the skin eruption. The patients are usually diabetic. The duration of symptoms is often prolonged and may extend over many years. The cutaneous process characteristically waxes and wanes and responds poorly to treatment of any type. It is this latter behavior coupled with the clinical characteristics that should bring to mind the diagnosis. In our own experience several years ago, we had a 40-year-old male patient with a chronic, undiagnosed cutaneous eruption which failed to respond to any therapy. We had considered the following diagnoses: tinea, chronic mucocutaneous candidiasis, pemphigus foliaceus, Hailey and Hailey disease, psoriasis vulgaris, pustular psoriasis, seborrheic dermatitis, acrodermatitis enteropathica, subcorneal pustular dermatosis of Sneddon-Wilkinson, erythema multiforme, erythema annulare centrifugum, and toxic epidermal necrolysis. A high serum glucagon level quickly resolved the issue. The x-ray arteriography demonstrated a tumor mass in the region of the pancreas. Subsequent surgical intervention established the diagnosis of alpha-cell tumor of the pancreas. Prompt recognition of the cutaneous signs of this syndrome can lead to early removal of the pancreatic tumor. Recently, two patients with necrolytic migratory erythema without glucagonoma have been reported.

Sclerotylosis (Sclero-atrophic and Keratotic Dermatosis of the Limbs)[220-222]

This is an autosomal dominant genodermatosis of the extremities which is associated with cutaneous squamous cell carcinoma and bowel cancer. The cutaneous eruption almost always occurs on the feet and hands and is symmetrical. There is a mild lamellar keratoderma on the palms and soles. The hands have a diffuse atrophy which varies from an atrophic erythrocyanotic area to sclerodactyly, and the nails have a hyperplastic dystrophy of varying intensity. The disorder is seen at birth and remains stationary during adult life.

Tuberous Sclerosis (Epiloia)[223-236]

In one-third of the reported cases, this is an autosomal dominantly inherited disorder of ectodermal and endodermal tissue which has the classic triad of angiokeratoma (adenoma sebaceum), mental deficiency, and epilepsy. Adenoma sebaceum of Pringle is the classic term for what is now referred to as an angiokeratoma. Over 80% of the patients have these lesions, which appear at approximately age 5–6 years. The lesions appear as reddish nodules with a waxy surface and are symmetrically scattered over the face in a butterfly pattern, especially on the nose, cheeks, chin, and nasolabial fold. However, other areas of the face may be involved. The lesions usually remain discrete and grow in size until puberty.

Ash leaf macules are present at birth in 85% of the patients. These oval lesions are of diagnostic importance. They can be visualized more easily under a Wood's light as white areas since they lack melanin. These macules may be the ONLY early cutaneous sign. Examination of these areas by the electron microscope allows differentiation of these hypopigmented macules from other hypopigmented lesions seen at birth. These EM findings present at birth display characteristic melanosomal alterations on ultrastructural examination.

Periungual or subungual fibromas (Konen's tumors) are present in approximately one-fourth of the patients. Varying from smooth papules to elongated nodules, they are positioned at the base of the nail or subungually. If they grow large enough, the nail bed and plate will be distorted. They are multiple, flesh-colored, and found on all four extremities.

The connective tissue nevus which commonly occurs in the lumbosacral region is known as a shagreen patch. It may have smaller lesions peripheral to the central one. These lesions appear as flat or slightly elevated with a shark-skin texture. Other, less frequently noted lesions include café au lait spots, mucosal fibromas, port-wine hemangiomas, and multiple skin tags on the axillae and neck.

The central nervous system manifestations are common and important. Mental retardation occurs in 70% of all patients, even as early as childhood. Epilepsy is present in all patients with mental deficiency and in many with normal intelligence (over 80% have abnormal EEGs). The CNS lesions are hamartomastous tubers. The latter calcify in 50% of the patients. Computerized tomographic scans reveal characteristic abnormalities which include multiple, scattered, subependymal, and periventricular densities indicative of calcification. This finding is virtually specific for the disease and can be found as early as 8 months of age.

With respect to retinal gliomas, there are two types: (a) nodular, mulberry-like lesions near the optic head, and (b) the flat, white, circular peripheral lesions. These gray and yellow plaques (phakomas) occur in 50% of the patients. Renal lesions (cystic in children and angiomyolipomas in adults) occur in two-thirds of the patients. They are usually bilateral. Cardiac lesions occur as multiple discrete rhabdomyomas causing numerous problems depending upon the anatomic location and size in the muscle. The lungs and skeletal system are not commonly involved. In 10% of the patients, oral nodules, fibromas, and papillomas are present, with the most common site being the anterior gingiva of the maxillary jaw.

Von Hippel-Lindau's Syndrome[237-239]

This disorder has no distinguishing cutaneous marker even though reports of vascular nevi of the face have been described (see Chapter 2). Systemic tumors associated with this disorder are: hemangioblastomas of the cerebellum, pheochromocytoma, hypernephroma of the kidney, and adenocarcinoma of the pancreas.

Neuroblastoma[240-242]

This rare, dominant disorder has no cutaneous signs except possibly café au lait lesions and metastatic ganglioneuromas that resemble neurofibromas.

Neurofibromatosis (von Recklinghausen's Disease)[243-256]

This is an autosomal dominantly inherited disorder, in which neural tissue, endocrine glands, skin, eyes, bone, and other organs are affected with a variety of congenital abnormalities and tumors. Until recently, this disorder was not compartmentalized, even though its clinical manifestations were varied, with multiple organ system involvement. At the present time, because of new research, we now divide the entity into a peripheral and central type. The central type has a circulating nerve growth factor which can be demonstrated in the serum in high concentrations; however, it has been shown to be low or normal in biologic function when measured. We are just beginning to appreciate that the two types, peripheral and central, have somewhat different clinical manifestations. The peripheral type has more cutaneous stigmata, while the central has a relative or almost absolute absence of cutaneous manifestations with higher occurrences of central nervous system pathology (e.g., acoustic neuromas and astrocytomas). The peripheral type has the plethora of cutaneous stigmata with a relatively lower incidence of CNS pathology.

The cardinal clinical features of neurofibromatosis are café au lait macules, neurofibromas, and iris hamartomas (Lish nodules). Other clinical signs are occasional mental retardation and seizures, macrocephaly, congenital pseudoarthrosis, kyphoscoliosis, pheochromocytomas (10%), and CNS tumors (10%, e.g., astrocytomas). Cutaneous neurofibromas vary greatly in size, shape, and consistency. They are mostly concentrated on the trunk and are normal flesh color. Characteristically, when pressed into the cutaneous surface, they invaginate through a dermal defect, "buttonholing." Tumors also occur in the oral mucosa. These neurofibromas quite characteristically occur on the nipple and appear postpubertally. The iris nodules are not areas of hyperpigmentation, but are iris hamartomas. They are unique to this disease and very diagnostic. Subcutaneous tumors are either firm, discrete nodules or large masses (plexiform neuromas). There is an associated cutaneous hyperpigmentation with these plexiform neuromas, especially when the tumor approaches or reaches the midline of the body. It appears to indicate that the tumor could be aggressive and/or involve the spinal cord. Other neurological manifestations include optic and acoustic nerve tumors, astrocytomas, and neurofibromas which affect neural functions centrally or peripherally depending upon their location and growth. Bone tissue abnormalities include bone cysts, kyphosis, and scoliosis. Endocrine tissue involvement has been manifested by cretinism, acromegaly, Addison's disease, sexual precocity, and hyper- or hypothyroidism.

Hyperpigmentation can appear at any cutaneous site and usually occurs shortly after birth. Café au lait macules may vary greatly in size and are flat (macular), discrete, and light tan or brown in color. It has been shown in a large series (223 patients) with neurofibromatosis that 95% of the patients had at least one cafe au lait spot, while 78% had at least six with at least one exceeding 1.5 cm in diameter. Because of this, the number six and the size (1.5 cm) became important criteria in the diagnosis of neurofibromatosis. However, in patients with the central type of this disorder, this number is no longer valid and patients may have none, one, or just several cafe au lait spots and still have neurofibromatosis. Café au lait spots have been estimated to occur in 10% of the normal population and in numbers less than six; however, in light of the new definition of the central type of neurofibromatosis and its spontaneous occurrence, this number will have to be reevaluated. It should be realized, of course, that the counting of cafe au lait on any one patient has no predictable value, as the statistics of their occurrence are applicable only to groups of individuals. Café au lait spots have macromelanosomes in the epithelium, on examination by electron microscopy. Café au lait spots also increase in size and number during childhood in patients with neurofibromatosis, and they can occur on the mucous membranes. Two-toned cafe au lait spots have been observed. Axillary (Crowe's sign) or perineal freckling is considered a pathognomonic sign of the disorder.

Multiple Mucosal Neuroma Syndrome (MEN-III)[257-261]

This autosomal dominant genodermatosis is characterized by the association of multiple mucosal neuromas with medullary thyroid carcinomas and pheochromocytomas. The patient develops the neuromas either at birth or in the first few years of life. The neuromas may precede the clinical manifestations of the neoplastic lesions associated with this disorder. These neuromas present as multiple pedunculated flesh- or pink-colored nodules which are usually present on the anterior surface of the tongue and the lips. However, lesions may occur on the buccal, gingival, nasal, and conjunctival mucosa as well as on other sites. The involvement of the face is pathognomonic as the patient has rather large, blubbery lips and pseudoprognathism. The skeletal structure and the body build of the patient may show an almost Marfanoid appearance. Hypotonia is commonly seen along with other musculoskeletal alterations such as lordosis, kyphosis, pes cavus, genu valgum, and a generalized joint laxity. Megacolon, probably secondary to intestinal neuromas, has been reported. There have been patients who have had true neurofibromas, and there has been an association with cutaneous pigmentation such as café au lait spots and diffuse lentiginous pigmentation. The mucosal neuromas and other physical abnormalities help differentiate this syndrome from MEN-II.

Sipple's Syndrome (MEN-II)[262]

The cutaneous findings are lacking in this syndrome; however, one report by Samaan was of a patient who had cutaneous neurofibromata on the trunk. It is possible that this case was one of MEN-III.

Werner's Syndrome (Adult Progeria)[263-267]

This autosomal recessive trait has as its characteristic clinical finding a premature aging which takes place in the second to third decades of life. The consistent characteristic feature is a prematurely aged-looking individual whose skin appears to be that of a very old person, short stature, a high-pitched voice, a beak- or sharp-shaped nose, a generalized atrophy of muscle and subcutaneous tissue, juvenile cataracts, high incidence of diabetes mellitus, osteoporosis, premature atherosclerosis, hypogonadism, and calcification of the blood vessels and connective tissues. There is a high association of systemic neoplasms with this disorder; however, despite the aged appearance of the skin, there is no evidence of any increase in cutaneous carcinoma. The life expectancy of these individuals is greatly reduced.

The cutaneous findings consist of baldness and premature canities, a sclerodermic bird-like facies with radial ridges at the corners of the mouth and eyes, scleroderma-like plaques (usually localized to the dorsum of the feet), hyperkeratosis of the soles and of the bony prominences (separation of these calluses either deliberately or spontaneously is followed by painful persistent ulceration), generalized hypotrichosis, acromicria, hyper- and hypopigmentation changes in the skin, telangiectasia (which, in addition to the sclerodermoid appearance, gives the features of poikiloderma), dystrophic changes in the nails (ranging from longitudinal striations to brittleness and complete loss of nails), and calcinosis cutis.

Other systemic features of Werner's syndrome include angina pectoris, myocardial infarctions, and congenital congestive heart failure. Prostatic hypertrophy is not seen in this disorder. The cause of death is usually from a malignancy, cerebrovascular accident, or cardiac decomposition.

There are no specific laboratory tests which are diagnostic of this disorder. Chemical changes occur in the scleroderma-like plaques on the dorsum of the feet which show an increase in hydroxyproline and relative increases in hexosamines. The fractionation of the glycosaminoglycans reveals an increase in the dermatan sulfate in the ground substance. This is in contrast to normal aging where these same substances are decreased. Cultures of skin fibroblasts show an abnormally increased proportion of the enzymes 6-phosphogluconate dehydrogenase (6-PGD) and hypoxanthine guanine phosphoribosyl transferase (HGPRT).

Hemihypertrophy (Klippel-Trenaunay-Weber Syndrome; Osteohypertrophic Angioectasia)[268-272]

This is a syndrome which is characterized by hypertrophy of the soft tissue and bone, usually unilateral, by hemangiomas generally of the nevus flammeus type, and by congenital phlebectasias and arteriovenous aneurysms. Children who have this disorder have a high risk of the development of several malignancies, including Wilms' tumor, hepatoblastomas, and adrenal cortical neoplasia.

The outstanding clinical finding is the hemihypertrophy of the soft tissue and skeleton, usually of one side and of the lower extremities; however, the upper extremities are also reported to be involved. The hypertrophy affects not only the length but also the circumference of the extremity. Usually, the hypertrophy begins very early in childhood and progressive enlargement continues for years.

The cutaneous abnormalities are usually vascular. Usually at birth or shortly thereafter, a nevus flammeus type of hemangioma involving the extremity or a portion of the trunk is present. Other vascular abnormalities then develop. These consist of congenital arteriovenous aneurysms, capillary and cavernous hemangiomas, congenital varicosities, lymphangiomas, and any combination thereof, along with the nevus flammeus. Other complications which occur are phlebitis, thrombosis, edema, stasis dermatitis, ulceration of the skin, skeletal dysfunction secondary to the skeletal hypertrophy, and decalcification of the involved bones. In addition, syndactylism and polydactylism have been reported. Epithelial nevi have been reported associated with this syndrome.

Porphyria Cutanea Tarda and Variegata[273-278]

These two hepatic porphyrias, which can be inherited as dominant traits, have identical cutaneous findings. Clinically, these patients have small blisters and erosions arising from trauma to the exposed areas, hands, face, V of the neck, and forearms. The patients complain of fragile skin. The erosions crust and heal slowly with scars and milia. In rare cases, the damage to the skin caused by photosensitivity to long UV light (symptoms can occur through window glass) can produce a sclerodermoid skin. The exposed skin develops brownish hyperpigmentation. Facial hypertrichosis occurs in two-thirds of the patients and is a major cosmetic problem for the female. Liver scan in patients with or without alcohol ingestion may reveal hepatoma. Those patients with familial occurrences of the disorder are at high risk and need careful evaluation.

Systemic Lupus Erythematosus[279-281]

The cutaneous findings in systemic lupus erythematosus (SLE) are many and varied, but represent a fraction of the clinical manifestations of the various affected organs of the body in which multiple autoantibodies participate in immunologically mediated tissue damage. The vast majority of patients have cutaneous involvement in some stage of their disease.

Probably because of the photosensitivity, there is the classic "butterfly" eruption involving the cheeks and nose. This blush is an erythematous edematous eruption which may precede other symptoms by weeks or months. When it fades, it does not scar or leave pigmentation. Another common erythematous eruption consists of maculopapular lesions which frequently occur after sunlight exposure. This is usually seen on exposed areas, especially on the upper part of the body, and if it persists, may become crusted and cause mild cutaneous atrophy. A third characteristic lesion seen in SLE is the classical discoid lesion with its erythematous, fine scaling, sharp borders, follicular plugging, and atrophy. About one-fifth of the individuals affected with SLE have chronic discoid lesions and also a high incidence of photosensitivity and Raynaud's phenomenon. Discoid lesions are commonly seen on the scalp. Because of their scarring nature, permanent alopecia occurs. A diffuse alopecia can occur in acute cases, but this "toxic effluvium" or the fracturing of frontal hair ("lupus hair") represents a generalized vascular reaction rather than the localized type described above.

The cutaneous vasculitis results in livedo reticularis (especially common on the lower extremities), painful erythematous nodules of the digits and palms, ulcerations of the lower legs and digits, gangrene of the digits, palpable purpura, bullae, splinter hemmorhage, urticaria, erythema multiforme-like lesions, pete-chiae, and ecchymoses. Subcutaneous nodules which are persistent occur as periarticular nodules most commonly on the extensor surfaces of the elbow. In contrast to these tender lesions, the firm discrete nodules of lupus panniculitis are relatively asymptomatic and occur on the face, trunk, and extremities.

The mucous membranes of the eyes, mouth, and vagina are involved in approximately one-tenth of the patients. The oral cavity shows shallow painful ulcers with a gray base and erythematous borders. The nasal septum may perfo-rate from the erosions. Laryngeal involvement can be life threatening. The pathology of the eyes causes a keratoconjunctivitis sicca. The familial occurrence of SLE, depending on the pedigree, includes many examples of different inheri-tance patterns.

Extramammary Paget's Disease[282,283]

This autosomal dominant trait usually appears in adult life, primarily in the anogenital area, but may be found on any part of the body where apocrine glands are present. Multiple lesions can occur. The lesion characteristically is a sharply marginated erythematous area which may be eczematous, crusted, or ulcerative. Typically, the correct diagnosis is rarely made by physicians since the clinical picture may mimic many other dermatologic entities. However, its hallmark is the failure of the lesion to respond to topical therapy. At this point, a histologic examination of the skin reveals the correct diagnosis. The hidden carcinoma usually arises from the cutaneous apocrine glands and their structure. However, other cancers, especially adenocarcinoma, are associated.

Sjögren's Syndrome[284-291]

This autoimmune classical triad consists of xerostomia, keratoconjunctivitis sicca, and rheumatoid arthritis. The sicca complex may be associated with scleroderma, systemic lupus erythematosus, periarteritis nodosa, chronic active hepatitis, polymyositis, and primary biliary cirrhosis. The disorder usually affects middle-aged females; HL-A-B8 antigen occurs in 58% of these patients as compared to a normal distribution of 21%.

The dermatologic manifestations include both cutaneous and mucosal abnor-malities. Xerosis with decreased sweating and pruritis are common complaints by the patient. Xerostomia and dryness of nasal passages with crusting cause symptoms with respect to taste and smell. Keratoconjunctivitis sicca is a common finding manifesting as photophobia, inability to tear, a "gritty feeling" in the eyes, and burning/itching of the eyes. A minority of patients complain of vaginal dryness associated with dyspareunia, burning, and pruritis.

Many patients have hyperpigmented freckle-like lesions in the exposed areas of the body; however, both localized hypopigmented and hyperpigmented areas occur. In approximately one-fifth of the patients, there is cold intolerance — Raynaud's phenomenon. Cryoglobulinemia is very common. Hypergammaglobulinemia is observed in up to four-fifths of the patients and may be monoclonal. About one-fifth of the patients have cutaneous vasculitis with clinical lesions ranging from petechiae, and palpable purpura, to ecchymoses.

Hemochromatosis[292-298]

Hemochromatosis is an autosomal recessive disorder; however, it has also been reported to be a dominant trait. Generalized hyperpigmentation results from melanin and not iron in the skin. The latter is emphasized by patients who remain depigmented in their vitiliginous skin when they develop hemochromatosis. The hypermelanosis varies in color from bronze or brown-black to blue-gray and is usually accentuated in the sun-exposed areas of the body. The pigmentation is also intense in the area of body folds and genitalia. About 15% of the patients have mucous membrane involvement. Cutaneous and mucous membrane involvement may resemble Addison's disease and may precede the cirrhosis and diabetes mellitus by years. In addition to hyperpigmentation, other cutaneous skin signs include loss of body hair, fine hair with female distribution pattern, soft and atrophic skin, xerosis, palmar erythema, and spider angiomata.

Maffucci's Syndrome (Dyschondroplasia with Hemangiomas)[299-301]

In this autosomal dominant disorder, the child is born normal. Clinical disease becomes manifest during ages 1–12 years. The abnormalities consist of dyschondroplasia and hemangioma. The vascular lesions consist of phlebectasias, cavernous hemangiomas, and cystic lymphangiomas. Phleboliths occur in the phlebectasias and hemangiomas. These lesions can develop anywhere, but are most common on the extremities.

The dyschondroplasia is seen as hard nodules appearing on the fingers and toes and spreading to other areas of the extremities. Skeletal deformities then ensue with bone distortions, spontaneous fractures, poor healing, bone thickening, exostoses near the epiphyses and multiple enchondromata. These changes are seen mostly in the peripheral skeleton. The end result of these changes is a grotesque distortion of the body.

Blue Rubber Bleb Nevus Syndrome[300,302-305]

This autosomal dominant trait has cutaneous and gastrointestinal hemangiomas associated with malignancies in the CNS, kidneys, and lymphatic system. The cutaneous lesions have the characteristic appearance and texture of bluish, cyanotic rubber nipples which are compressible and promptly refill on absence of external pressure. There are three forms of these hemangiomas: large cavernous angiomas, blue rubber bleb, and an irregular blue coloring of the skin. The lesions appear at birth and in early infancy, and increase in size and number with passing years. They may be singular or numerous and usually have a predilection for the trunk and upper extremities; however, they can occur over the entire integument. They range in size from a few millimeters to several centimeters. The hues of color vary from red to blue to black. They can thrombose and calcify. Lesions may be painful. Vascular lesions can occur throughout the gastrointestinal tract and may cause severe bleeding and anemia. Pulmonary hypertension may be present.

Kaposi Sarcoma[306-314]

This is a multifocal neoplastic disorder which primarily expresses itself as multiple vascular nodules in various tissues, including the skin. There is no agreement as to the histogenesis of this neoplasm.

Clinically, this is a disease predominantly seen in males. However, in immunosuppressed patients, the percentage of women is very greatly increased. The skin lesions are multiple and occur as papules, plaques, nodules, and tumors. Their color varies over a range of red to purple and, with time, becomes brownish. The consistency on palpation is variable. The number of lesions are variable, and the size may be as great as 10-15 cm or more in diameter. The skin may become atrophic, break down, and ulcerate. Other lesions can be verrucous and fungating. The lesions may be anywhere on the cutaneous surface but most commonly start on the lower extremities and spread centripetally. The lower legs can develop edema, and involvement may be severe enough to restrict use of the lower extremities.

The internal findings are extremely varied, depending upon which organ is involved and to what extent. The disorder may be almost exclusively internal with little cutaneous expression. There are four clinical types with some variation in expression (see Table 3-2).

Epidermolysis Bullosa Dystrophica (Dominant)[315]

This is a rare dominant type of EBD. The dominant form is very much less common and less severe than the recessive EBD. Recently, Schwart et al.

Table 3-2. Clinical Behavior of Kaposi Sarcoma.

CLINICAL TYPE	BEHAVIOR	AGE GROUP	BONE INVOLVE-MENT	LYMPH NODE INVOLVE-MENT	PREDOMINANT CUTANEOUS SIGN
Nodular	Indolent	>25	Rare	Rare	Nodules, plaques
Lymphad-enopathic	Disseminated aggressive	<25	Rare	Always	Nodules
Florid	Locally aggressive	>25	Often	Rare	Fungating
Infiltrative	Locally aggressive	>25	Always	Rare	Diffuse, infiltrat-ing

reported a pedigree in which two first cousins (one male and one female) developed squamous cell carcinoma in ulcers in the legs.

These patients have a lifelong history of blisters from minimal cutaneous trauma. Although the extremities are the main sites of lesions, they occur all over the body, especially at sites of bony prominences. These sites are covered by cigarette paper scars. The fingernails and toenails are lost and the hands and feet are covered by a mitten-like deformity secondary to scarring, atrophy and contractures. Both patients in this kindred with other members affected had long standing ulcers which on repeated histologic examination showed pseudo-epithelial hyperplasia. These same sites eventually developed squamous cell carcinoma.

Previous electron microscopic studies have shown the primary abnormality as a defect in the anchoring fibrils beneath the basal lamina but in this dominant pedigree the defects were not only in the anchoring fibrils but there was a marked disruption of the basal lamina with deposits of an amorphous substance.

Dermatofibroma, Familial[316]

Roberts, et al. described a 47 year old man who had a history of skin nodules, subsequently proven to be dermatofibromas, with onset in his teens and progression throughout life. At age 47, he presented with a history of left-sided chest pain and dysphagia, and one year following his initial chest symptoms, he expired. At autopsy, there was a large tumor in the left upper lobe of the lung which encircled the arch of the aorta, perforated the tracheal bifurcation, and projected into the left main bronchus. It caused erosion of the middle third of the esophagus. Tumor nodules of said similar malignant histologic character were·present in the rest of both lungs and were extensively distributed over both pleural surfaces, in the liver, the heart, the thoracic nodes, and the mesentery.

The lung biopsy specimen showed a pattern of atypical spindle-cells in a fibrous stroma that bore a definite resemblance to his skin tumors. This contained bizarre giant cells. The tumor was anaplastic and had many atypical mitoses. There were occasional areas of blood vessel proliferation. A myxoid or storiform pattern predominated.

The proband had 5 sons and 2 daughters. Four of his sons were affected and in his own sibship of 9, a brother was affected. The lesions in all of his relatives were restricted to skin. Inheritance pattern was consistent with an autosomal dominant factor, but it was of interest in this pedigree that only males were affected. However, in his review of the literature, Roberts found 4 other families wherein the dermatofibromas were restricted to the skin. In these families, mothers and daughters were also found to be affected.

Thus, we have evidence of a probable new, albeit rare, cancer-associated genodermatosis. In the natural history of this inherited form of dermatofibroma or fibrous histiocytoma of the dermis, the onset appears to be in the teens with progression of the lesions throughout life. While the malignant neoplastic transformation rate appears to be low in this disorder, it would be important that other investigators critically evaluate family history in their affected patients and be cognizant of the possibility of malignant degeneration.

COMMENT

We have emphasized in this chapter the descriptive aspects of the cutaneous expressions of the genodermatoses. The spectrum of the cutaneous stigmata of the cancer-associated genodermatoses is both complex and extremely varied. One can easily be overwhelmed by the plethora of cutaneous findings in each of those disorders, and collectively they become of unimaginable enormity. As yet, order and clarity remain elusive, a problem which in a major way is a reflection of the complex structure and origin of the integument, both ectodermal and mesodermal. Not only does the glabrous epidermis have its own unique character, but its appendageal structures such as pilosebaceous, apocrine, and eccrine glands magnify almost geometrically the genetic expressions that can be observed. In addition, the epidermis has a unique melanocytic population, along with the other tissues of neural origin, and the expression of this unusual pigmented cell population in clinical disorders is very varied and complex.

The dermal-mesodermal component of the skin with its neural segments, connective tissue elements (both fibrous and nonfibrous), vascular tree, lymphatic system, and immunologic apparatus extends the expressivity of genetic and environmental influences to produce a multiplicity of aberrations. For example, the barrier function of the skin is very dependent on its immunologic integrity and any malfunction will result in a host of infectious disorders as a cutaneous marker for genodermatoses.

It is timely to focus attention on the biomolecular aspects of genodermatoses. The skin represents a unique window to the continuous monitoring of metabolic functions of the body. We can observe directly both extracellular and intracellular tissue functions diagnostically, therapeutically, and investigationally. For example, in patients with Multiple Endocrine Neoplasia, type III, there is a significant increase in the diameter of cutaneous nerves at all levels of the dermis. In addition, there are abnormal histologic findings in the nerves of some of these patients. They also have an abnormal histamine skin test response in that there is either a diminished or no flare around the wheal as described recently by Carney et al.[317] Further study will be needed to define the abnormal histamine response and the hypertrophy of the nerves. This observation should be tested in all of the neural crest (neurocristopathies) derived cancer associated genodermatoses. We tend to forget that the sampling of skin tissue is almost a benign and undisturbing act. The acquisition of just a few micrograms of connective tissue for fibroblast cultures can help us identify precise complementation groups in such disorders as xeroderma pigmentosum. It can identify γ-radiation sensitivity in ataxia telangiectasia, a problem now clearly verified clinically by severely untoward response to radiation therapy in those patients. We can observe in the skin the metabolic function of protein, fat, and carbohydrate metabolism. The research potential for investigation of the various genodermatoses will be accelerated when the cutaneous sampling of tissue is more clearly appreciated.

Finally, the study of abnormalities in the skin might one day provide clues to pathogenesis and carcinogenesis in the several disorders which are believed to have their origin in tissues of the neural crest. Among cells believed to originate in the neural crest are the melanocytes and the parafollicular cells — the former migrating primarily to the skin where they may appear as café au lait spots in von Recklinghausen's neurofibromatosis or as malignant melanoma in the familial atypical multiple mole-melanoma syndrome, the latter migrating to the thyroid gland to give rise to the characteristic medullary thyroid carcinoma with amyloid deposition in MEN-II and MEN-III. Many other systems with similar implications could be listed.

Obviously we have barely begun to exploit scientifically the potential wealth of the skin in comprehending the extant mysteries of genetics and carcinogenesis. We implore our readers to become involved in the fascinating ventures which we can visualize awaiting discovery on the horizon.

REFERENCES

1. Fraumeni, J.F., and Hoover, R.: Immunosurveillance and cancer: epidemiologic observations. In: Epidemiology and Cancer Registries. *NCI Monog.* **47**, 1976.
2. Gatti, R.A., and Good, R.A.: Occurrence of malignancy in immunodeficiency diseases. *Cancer* **28**:89–98, 1971.
3. Shackelford, G.D., and McAlister, W.H.: Primary immunodeficiency diseases and malignancy. *Am. J. Roetg.* **123**:144–153, 1975.

4. Rosen, F.S., and Janeway, C.A.: Agammaglobulinemia. In: *Dermatology in General Medicine* (T.B. Fitzpatrick et al., Eds., 2nd ed.) Ch. 2. New York: McGraw-Hill, pp. 1053–1062.

5. Hoyer, J.R., Cooper, M.D., Gabrielsen, A.H., and Good, R.A.: Lymphopenic forms of congenital immunologic deficiency: clinical and pathologic patterns. In: *Immunologic Deficiency Diseases in Man* (D. Bergsma, Ed.). Vol. IV. New York: National Foundation, 1968, pp. 81–103.

6. O'Laughlin, J.M.: Disorders of immunity, hypersensitivity, and inflammation. In: *Dermatology*. (S.L. Moschella et al. Eds.).Vol. 1, Ch. 4. Philadelphia, PA: W.B. Saunders, 1975, pp. 199–218.

7. Hathaway, W.E., et al.: Graft vs. host reactions following a single blood transfusion. *JAMA* 201:1015–1020, 1967.

8. Kersey, J.H., Gajl-Peczalska, K., and Nesbit, M.E.: The lymphoid system: abnormalities in immunodeficiency and malignancy. *J. Ped.* 84:789–796, 1974.

9. Waldmann, T.A., Strober, W., and Blaese, R.M.: Various immunologic deficiencies of man and the role of immune processes in the control of malignant disease. *Ann. Int. Med.* 77:605–628, 1972.

10. Reed, W.B., Epstein, W.L., Boder, E., and Sedgwick, R.: Cutaneous manifestations of ataxia-telangiectasia. *JAMA* 195:126–133, 1966.

11. Biggar, D., Lapointe, N., et al.: IgE in ataxia telangiectasia and family members. *Lancet* 2:1089, 1970.

12. Kumar, G.K., Al Saadi, A., Yang, S.S., and McCaughey, R.S.: Ataxia telangiectasia and hepatocellular carcinoma. *Am. J. Med. Sci.* 278:157–160, 1979.

13. Sugimoto, T., Sawada, T., Tozawa, M., et al.: Plasma levels of carcinoembryonic antigen in patients with ataxia telangiectasia. *J. Ped.* 92:436–439, 1978.

14. Waldmann, T.A., and McIntyre, R.A.: Serum alpha-fetoprotein levels in patients with ataxia telangiectasia. *Lancet* 2:1112–1115, 1972.

15. Setlow, R.B.: Repair deficient human disorders and cancer. *Nature* 271:713–717, 1978.

16. Boder, E., and Sedgwick, R.P.: Ataxia telangiectasia: a review of 101 cases. *Clin. Develop. Med.* 8:110–119, 1963.

17. Bloom, D., and German, J.: The syndrome of congenital telangiectatic erythema and stunted growth. *J. Ped.* 68:103–113, 1966.

18. Sawitsky, A., Bloom, D., and German, J.: Chromosomal breakage and acute leukemia in congenital telangiectatic erythema and stunted growth. *Ann. Int. Med.* 65:487–495, 1966.

19. Bloom, D., and German, J.: The syndrome of congenital telangiectatic erythema and stunted growth. *Arch. Derm.* 103:545–546, 1971.

20. German, J.: Genetic disorders associated with chromosomal instability and cancer. *J. Inves. Derm.* 60:427–434, 1973.

21. Dicken, C.H., Dewald, G., and Gordon, H.: Sister chromatid exchanges in Bloom's syndrome. *Arch. Derm.* 114:755–760, 1978.

22. German, J., Bloom, D., and Passarge, E.: Bloom's syndrome. V. Surveillance for cancer in affected families. *Clin. Genet.* 2:162–168, 1977.

23. Fanconi, G.: Familial constitutional panmyelocytopathy, Fanconi's anemia (FA). I. Clinical aspects. *Sem. Hemat.* 4:233–240, 1967.

24. Boivin, P.: La maladie fanconi et les aplasies medularies congenitalis. *Act. Ped.* series 1, 94–104, 1959.

25. Nilsson, L.R.: Chronic pancytopenia with multiple congenital abnormalities (Fanconi's anaemie). *Acta Paed. Scand.* 49:518–529, 1960.

26. Gmyrek, D., and Syllm-Rapoport, I.: Zur Fanconi-Anamie (FA). Analyse von 129 beschriebenen Fallen. *Z. Kinderheilk.* 91:297–337, 1964.

27. Bloom, G.E., et al.: Chromosome abnormalities in constitutional aplastic anemia. *N. Eng. J. Med.* **274**:8–14, 1966.

28. Esparaza, A., and Thompson, W.R.: Familial hypoplastic anemia with multiple congenital anomalies (Fanconi's syndrome): report of three cases. *RI Med. J.* **49**:103–110, 1966.

29. Swift, M.R., and Hirschorn, K.: Fanconi's anemia, inherited susceptibility to chromosome breakage in various tissues. *Ann. Int. Med.* **65**:495–503, 1966.

30. Bernstein, M.S., et al.: Hepatoma and peliosis hepatitis developing in a patient with Fanconi's anemia. *N. Eng. J. Med.* **284**:1135–1136, 1971.

31. Schmid, W.: Familial constitutional panmyelocytopathy. Fanconi's anemia (FA). II. A discussion of the cytogenetic findings in Fanconi's anemia. *Sem. Hemat.* **4**: 241–249, 1967.

32. Todaro, G.J., Green, H., and Swift, M.R.: Susceptibility of human diploid fibroblast strains to transformation by SV40 virus. *Science* **153**:1252–1254, 1966.

33. Poon, P.K., O'Brien, R.L., and Parker, J.W.: Defective DNA repair in Fanconi's anemia. *Nature* **250**:223–225, 1974.

34. Remsen, J., and Cerutti, P.: Deficiency of gamma ray excision repair in skin fibroblasts from patients with Fanconi's anemia. *Proc. Natl. Acad. Sci. USA* **73**:2419–2423, 1976.

35. Abels, D., and Reed, W.R.: Fanconi-like syndrome: immunologic deficiency, pancytopenia, and cutaneous malignancies. *Arch. Derm.* **107**:419–423, 1973.

36. Sirenavin, C., and Trowbridge, A.A.: Dyskeratosis congenita: clinical features and genetics aspects. *J. Med. Genet.* **12**:339–354, 1975.

37. Inoue, S., et al.: Dyskeratosis congenita with pancytopenia. *Am. J. Dis. Child* **126**:389–396, 1973.

38. Bryan, H.G., and Nixon, R.K.: Dyskeratosis congenita and familial pancytopenia. *JAMA* **192**:203–208, 1965.

39. Scoggins, R.B., et al.: Dyskeratosis congenita with Fanconi-type anemia: Investigations of immunologic and other defects. *Clin. Res.* **19**:409, 1971.

40. Ortega, J.A., et al.: Congenital dyskeratosis: Zinsser-Engman-Cole syndrome with thymic dysplasia and aplastic anemia. *Am. J. Dis. Child* **124**:701–704, 1972.

41. Steier, W., et al.: Dyskeratosis congenita: relationship to Fanconi's anemia. *Blood* **39**:510–520, 1972.

42. Carter, D.M., and Cohen, S.R.: Prenatal diagnosis of heritable skin diseases. In *Dermatology Update* (S.L. Moschella et al., Eds.). New York: Elsevier, 1979, pp. 23–44.

43. Mills, S.E., et al.: Intracranial calcifications and dyskeratosis congenita. *Arch. Derm.* **115**:1437–1439, 1979.

44. Sorrow, J.M., and Hitch, J.M.: Dyskeratosis congenita. *Arch. Derm.* **88**:156–163, 1963.

45. Addison, M., and Rich, M.S.: The association of dyskeratosis congenita and Fanconi's anemia. *Med. J. Aust.* **1**:797–799, 1965.

46. Srivastava, R.N.: Wiskott-Aldrich syndrome. *Arch. Dis. Child* **42**:604, 1967.

47. Cooper, M.D., et al.: Wiskott-Aldrich syndrome: an immunologic deficiency disease involving the afferent limb of immunity. *Am. J. Med.* **44**:499–513, 1968.

48. Parkman, R., et al.: Complete correction of the Wiskott-Aldrich syndrome by allogenic bone marrow transplantation. *N. Eng. J. Med.* **298**:921–927, 1978.

49. Shapiro, R.S., et al.: Wiskott-Aldrich syndrome: detection of carrier state by metabolic stress of platelets. *Lancet* **1**:121–123, 1978.

50. Blaese, R.M., et al.: Hypercatabolism of IgG, IgA, IgM and albumin in Wiskott-Aldrich syndrome: a unique disorder of serum protein metabolism. *J. Clin. Invest.* **50**:2231-2238, 1971.

51. Silver, H.K.: Rothmund's syndrome – Thomson's syndrome: an oculocutaneous disorder. *Am. J. Dis. Child* **111**:182–190, 1966.
52. Taylor, W.B.: Rothmund's syndrome – Thomson's syndrome. Congenital poikiloderma with or without juvenile cataracts: a review of the literature, report of a case, and discussion of the relationship of the two syndromes. *Arch. Derm.* **75**:236–244, 1957.
53. Kraus, B.S., et al.: The dentition in Rothmund's syndrome. *J. Am. Dent. Assoc.* **81**:895–915, 1970.
54. Reid, J.: Congenital poikiloderma with osteogenesis imperfecta. *Br. J. Derm.* **79**: 243–244, 1967.
55. Blinstrub, R.S., et al.: Poikiloderma congenitale: report of two cases. *Arch. Derm.* **89**:659–664, 1964.
56. Tritoch, H., and Liochka, G.: Zur histopatholgie der kongenitalen Poikilodermie Thomson. *Z. Haut. Geschl-Kr.* **43** (Suppl.):155–166, 1968.
57. Lowe, L.B.: Hereditary epidermolysis bullosa. *Arch. Derm.* **95**:587–595, 1967.
58. Wechsler, H.L., et al.: Polydysplastic epidermolysis bullosa and development of epidermal neoplasms. *Arch. Derm.* **102**:374–380, 1970.
59. Reed, W.B., et al.: Epidermolysis bullosa dystrophica with epidermal neoplasms. *Arch. Derm.* **110**:894–902, 1974.
60. Didolbar, M.S., et al.: Epidermolysis bullosa dystrophica and epithelioma of the skin. *Cancer* **33**:198–202, 1974.
61. Briggaman, R.A., and Wheeler, C.E.: Epidermolysis bullosa dystrophica-recessive: a possible role of anchoring fibrils in the pathogenesis. *J. Invest. Derm.* **65**:203–211, 1975.
62. Bauer, E.A.: Recessive dystrophic epidermolysis bullosa: evidence for an altered collagenase in fibroblast cultures. *Proc. Natl. Acad. Sci. USA* **74**:4646–4650, 1977.
63. Glinski, W., et al.: Cell mediated immunity in epidermodysplasia verruciformis. *Dermatologica* **153**:217–227, 1976.
64. Jablonska, S., et al.: On the viral etiology of epidermodysplasia verruciformis Lewandowsky-Lutz: electron microscope studies. *Dermatologica* **137**:113–125, 1968.
65. Jablonska, S., et al.: The ultrastructure of transitional states to Bowen's disease and invasive Bowen's carcinoma in epidermodysplasia verruciformis. *Dermatologica* **140**:186–194, 1970.
66. Rueda, L.A., and Rodriguez, G.: Verrugas humanas por Virus Papova. *Med. Cutan. Iber. Lat. Am.* **4**:113–136, 1976.
67. Prunieras, M.: Epidermodysplasia verruciformis. In: *Dermatology in General Medicine* (T.B. Fitzpatrick et al., Eds.; 2nd ed.). Ch. 166. New York: McGraw-Hill, 1979, pp. 1635–1637.
68. Prawer, S.E., et al.: Depressed immune function in epidermodysplasia verruciformis. *Arch. Derm.* **113**:495–499, 1977.
69. Jablonska, S., et al.: Twenty-one years of followup studies of familial epidermodysplasia verruciformis. *Dermatologica* **158**:309–327, 1979.
70. Jablonska, S., et al.: Epidermodysplasia verruciformis as a model in studies in the role of papovaviruses in oncogenesis. *Cancer Res.* **32**:583–589, 1972.
71. Mikhail, G.R., and Wertheimer, F.W.: Clinical variants of porokeratosis (Mibelli). *Arch. Derm.* **98**:124–131, 1968.
72. Caskey, R.J., and Mehregan, A.: Bowen disease associated with porokeratosis of Mibelli. *Arch. Derm.* **111**:1480–1481, 1975.
73. Guss, S.B., et al.: Porokeratosis plantaris et palmaris et disseminata. *Arch. Derm.* **104**:366–373, 1971.

74. Savage, J.: Porokeratosis (Mibelli) and carcinoma. *Br. J. Derm.* 76:489, 1964.
75. Bazex, A., and Dupre, A.: *Ann. Derm. Syph.* (Paris) 95:361-374, 1968.
76. Sarkany, I.: Porokeratosis Mibelli with basal cell epithelioma. *Proc. Roy. Soc. Med.* 66:435-436, 1973.
77. Girgla, H.S., and Bhattacharya, S.K.: Clinical study of porokeratosis: report of 10 cases. *Int. J. Derm.* 15:43-51, 1976.
78. Reed, R.J., and Leone, P.: Porokeratosis – a mutant clonal keratosis of the epidermis. *Arch. Derm.* 101:340-347, 1970.
79. Taylor, A.M.R., et al.: Chromosomal instability associated with susceptibility to malignant disease in patients with porokeratosis of Mibelli. *JNCI* 51:371-378, 1973.
80. Flegel, H.: Hyperkeratosis lenticularis perstans. *Hautarzt* 9:362, 1958.
81. Bean, S.F.: The genetics of hyperkeratosis lenticularis perstans. *Arch. Derm.* 106: 72, 1972.
82. Beveridge, G.W., and Langlands, A.O.: Familial hyperkeratosis lenticularis perstans associated with tumors of the skin. *Br. J. Derm.* 88:453-458, 1973.
83. Frenk, E., and Tapernoux, B.: Hyperkeratosis lenticularis perstans (Flegel): biologic model for keratinization occurring in the absence of Odland bodies. *Dermatologica* 153:253-263, 1976.
84. Burgess, G.H.: Keratoacanthoma. In: *Cancer Dermatology* (F. Helm, Ed.). Philadelphia, PA.: Lea and Febiger, 1979, pp. 133-139.
85. Tarnowski, W.M.: Multiple keratoacanthoma. *Arch. Derm.* 94:74-80, 1966.
86. Reed, R.J.: Keratocanthoma: entity or syndrome? *Bull. Tulane Univ. Med. Faculty* 26:117-130, 1967.
87. Epstein, N.N., Biskind, G.R., and Pollack, R.S.: Multiple primary self-healing squamous cell "epitheliomas" of the skin: generalized keratoacanthoma. *Arch. Derm.* 75:210-223, 1957.
88. Ereaux, L.P., and Schopflocher, P.: Familial primary self-healing squamous epithelioma of skin: Ferguson-Smith type. *Arch. Derm.* 91:589-594, 1965.
89. Sommerville, J., and Milne, J.A.: Familial primary self-healing squamous epithelioma of the skin (Ferguson-Smith type). *Br. J. Derm.* 62:485-490, 1950.
90. Jolly, H.W., and Carpenter, C.L.: Multiple keratoacanthoma. *Arch. Derm.* 93: 348-353, 1966.
91. Rook, A., and Chapion, R.H.: Keratoacanthoma. *NCI Monog.* 10:257-268, 1963.
92. Barr, R.J., Shneidman, D.W., and Graham, J.H.: Pseudomalignant and pseudobenignant lesions of the skin and subcutaneous tissues. In: *Dermatology Update* (S.L. Moschella, Ed.). New York: Elsevier, 1979, pp. 273-323.
93. Lever, W.F., and Schaumburg-Lever, G.: *Histopathology of the Skin* (5th ed.). Philadelphia, PA: Lippincott, 1972, 484 pp.
94. Gray, H.R., and Helwig, E.B.: Epithelioma adenoides cysticim and solitary trichoepithelioia. *Arch. Derm.* 87:102-114, 1963.
95. Gaul, L.E.: Heredity of multiple benign cystic epithelioma. *Arch. Derm.* 68:517-524, 1953.
96. Ziprkowski, K., and Schewach-Millet, M.: Multiple trichoepithelioma in a mother and two children. *Dermatologica* 132:248-256, 1966.
97. Welch, J.P., Wells, R.S., and Kerr, C.B.: Ancell-Spiegler cylindroma (turban tumors) and Brooke-Fordyce trichoepithelioma: evidence for a single genetic entity. *J. Med. Genet.* 5:29-35, 1968.
98. Korting, G.W., Hoede, N., and Gebharqt, R.: Kurzer Bericht uber einen maligne entarteten Spiegler-Tumor. *Derm. Monatsschr.* 156:141-147, 1970.

99. Lever, W.F., and Schaumburg-Lever, G.: Trichoepithelioma. In: *Tumors of the Epidermal Appendages* (5th ed.), Philadelphia PA: Lippincott, 1975, pp. 515-518.

100. Kechijian, P., Connors, R.C., and Ackerman, A.B.: Trichoepithelioma vs. basal cell cancer, criteria for histologic diagnosis. *J. Derm. Surg.* **1**:22-23, 1975.

101. Howell, J.B., and Anderson, D.E.: Transformation of epithelioma adenoides cysticum into multiple rodent ulcers: fact or fallacy. *Br. J. Derm.* **95**:233-242, 1976.

102. Greenbaum, S., and Shaffer, B.: Trichoepithelioma with basal cell epithelioma. *Arch. Derm.* **46**:564, 1942.

103. Howell, J.B., and Caro, M.R.: Basal cell nevus: its relationship to multiple cutaneous cancers and associated anomalies of development. *Arch. Derm.* **79**:67-80, 1959.

104. Southwick, G.J., and Schwartz, R.A.: The basal cell nevus syndrome. *Cancer* **44**: 2294-2305, 1979.

105. Clendenning, W.E., Bloch, J.B., and Radde, I.C.: Basal cell nevus syndrome. *Arch. Derm.* **90**:38-53, 1964.

106. Howell, J.B., and Mehregan, A.H.: Pursuit of the pits in the nevoid basal cell carcinoma syndrome. *Arch. Derm.* **102**:586-597, 1970.

107. Taylor, W.B., et al.: Nevoid basal cell carcinoma syndrome. *Arch. Derm.* **98**:612-614, 1968.

108. Berlin, N.I., et al.: Basal cell nevus syndrome. *Ann. Int. Med.* **64**:403-421, 1966.

109. Causon, R.A., and Kerr, G.A.: The syndrome of jaw cysts, basal cell tumours, and skeletal anomalies. *Proc. Roy. Soc. Med.* **57**:799-801, 1964.

110. Horland, A.A., Wolman, S.R., and Cox, R.P.: Cytogenetic studies in patients with basal cell nevus syndrome and their relatives. *Am. J. Hum. Genet.* **27**:47, 1975.

111. Jackson, R., and Gardere, S.: Nevoid basal cell carcinoma syndrome. *Cap. Med. Assoc. J.* **125**:850-860, 1971.

112. Doku, H.C., at al.: Chelitis glandularis. *Oral Surg.* **20**:563-571, 1965.

113. Schweich, L.: Chelitis glangularis simplex. *Arch. Derm.* **89**:301-302, 1964.

114. Rueleur-van Haeverbeck, A.: A propos de la cheilite glandulaire de puente. *Arch. Belg. Derm. Syph.* **25**:147-150, 1969.

115. Michalowski, R.: Chelitis glandularis, heterotopic salivary glands, and squamous cell carcinoma of the lips. *Br. J. Derm.* **74**:445-449, 1952.

116. Balus, L.: Ist die cheilitis glandularis eine pracancerose erkrankung? *Hautarzt.* **16**:364-367, 1965.

117. Kaloustian, V.M., and Kurban, A.K.: Hyperplasias, aplasias, dysplasias, and atrophies. Chapter 5. In: *Genetic Diseases of the Skin.* Berlin: Springer-Verlag, 1979, pp. 109-114.

118. Clouston, H.R.: Hereditary ectodermal distrophy. *Can. Med. Assoc. J.* **21**:18-31, 1929.

119. Williams, M., and Fraser, F.C.: Hidrotic ectodermal dysplasia – Cloustan's family revisited. *Can. Med. Assoc. J.* **96**:36-38, 1967.

120. Gold, R.J.M., and Scriver, C.R.: Properties of hair keratin in an autosomal dominant form of ectodermal dysplasia. *Am. J. Hum. Genet.* **24**:549-561, 1972.

121. Gold, R.J.M., and Kachra, Z.: Molecular defect in hidrotic ectodermal dysplasia. In: *First Human Hair Symposium* (A.C. Brown, Ed.). New York: Medcom Press, 1974, pp. 250-276.

122. Wilkinson, R.D., Schopflocher, P., and Rosenfeld, M.: Hidrotic ectodermal dysplasia with diffuse eccrine poromatosis. *Arch. Derm.* **113**:472-476, 1977.

123. Mauro, J.A., Maslyn, R., and Stein, A.A.: Squamous cell carcinoma of nail bed in hereditary ectodermal dysplasia. *NY State J. Med.* **1**:1065-1066, 1972.

124. Campbell, C., and KeoKam, T.: Squamous cell carcinoma of the nail bed in epidermal dysplasia. *J. Bone Joint Surg.* 48:92–99, 1966.
125. Bazex, A., Dupre, A., and Christol, B.: Genodermatose complexe de type indetermine associant une hypotrichose, un etat atrophodermique generalise et des degenerescences cutanees multiples (epitheliomas-baso cellulaires). *Bull. Soc. Fr. Derm. Syph.* 71:206, 1964.
126. Bazex, A., et al.: Atrophodermie folliculaire, proliferations baso-cellulaires et hypotrichose. *Ann. Derm. Syph.* 93:241–254, 1966.
127. Braum-Falco, O., and Marghescu, S.: Uber eine systematisierte follikulare atrophodermie mit keratosis palmoplantaris dissipata und keratosis follicularis. *Hautarzt* 18:13, 1967.
128. Curth, H.O.: The genetics of follicular atrophoderma. *Arch. Derm.* 114:1479–1483, 1978.
129. Viksnius, P., and Berlin, A.: Follicular atrophoderma and basal cell carcinomas. *Arch. Derm.* 113:948–951, 1977.
130. Gorlin, R.J., and Chaudhry, A.P.: Oral lesions accompanying pachyonychia congenita. *Oral Surg.* 11:541–544, 1958.
131. Colm, A.M., et al.: Pachyonychia congenita with involvement of the larynx. *Arch. Otolaryngol.* 102:233–235, 1976.
132. Jackson, A.D.M., and Lawler, S.D.: Pachyonychia congenita: a report of six cases in one family. *Ann. Eugen.* 16:142–146, 1951.
133. Anneroth, G., et al.: Pachyonychia congenila. *Acta Derm.* 55:387–394, 1975.
134. Maser, E.D.: Oral manifestations of pachyonychia congenita. *Oral Surg.* 43:373–378, 1977.
135. Witkop, C.J., and Gorlin, R.J.: Four hereditary mucosal syndromes. *Arch. Derm.* 84:762–771, 1961.
136. Joseph, H.L.: Pachyonychia congenita. *Arch. Derm.* 90:594–603, 1964.
137. McDonald, R.M., and Reed, W.B.: Natal teeth and steatocystoma multiplex complicated by hidradenitis suppurativa. *Arch. Derm.* 112:1132–1134, 1976.
138. Witkop, C.J.: Albinism. In: *Advances in Human Genetics* (H. Harris and K. Hirschborn, Eds.). Vol. 2. New York: Plenum, 1971, pp. 61–142.
139. King, R.A., and Witkop, C.J.J.: Hair bulb tyrosinase activity in oculocutaneous albinism. *Nature* 263:69–71, 1976.
140. Witkop, C.J., et. al.: Mutations in the melanin pigment system in man resulting in features of oculocutaneous albinism. In: *Pigmentation: Its Genesis and Biologic Control* (V. Riley, Ed.). New York: Appleton-Century-Crofts, 1972, pp. 359–377.
141. Witkop, C.J., et al.: Albinism. In: *The Metabolic Basis of Inherited Disease* (J.B. Stanbury, et al., Eds.); 4th ed. New York: McGraw-Hill, 1978, pp. 283–316.
142. Witkop, C.J., et al.: Ophthalmologic, biochemical, platelet, and ultrastructural defects in the various types of oculocutaneous albinism. *J. Invest. Derm.* 60:443–456, 1973.
143. Logan, L.J., et al.: Albinism and abnormal platelet function. *N. Eng. J. Med.* 284:1340, 1345, 1971.
144. Windhorst, D.B., et al.: A human pigmentary dilution band on a heritable subcellular structural defect – the Chediak-Higashi syndrome. *J. Invest. Derm.* 50:9–18, 1968.
145. White, J.G.: The Chediak-Higashi syndrome: a possible lysosomal disease. *Blood* 28:143–156, 1966.
146. Lockman, L.A., et al.: The Chediak-Higashi syndrome. Electrophysiologic and electron microscope observation in the peripheral neuropathy. *J. Ped.* 70:942–951, 1967.

147. Windhorst, D.B., et al.: The Chediak-Higashi anomaly and Aleutian trait in mink, homologous defects of lysosomal structure. *Ann. NY Acad. Sci.* **155**:818–846, 1968.

148. Zelickson, A.S., et al.: The Chediak-Higashi syndrome: formation of giant melanosomes and the basis of hypopigmentation. *J. Inves. Derm.* **49**:575–581, 1967.

149. Stossel, T.P., et al.: Phagocytosis in chronic granulomatous disease and the Chediak-Higashi syndrome. *N. Eng. J. Med.* **286**:120–123, 1972.

150. Mosher, D.B., et al.: Abnormalities of pigmentation. In: *Dermatology in General Medicine* (T.B. Fitzpatrick et al. Eds.). New York: McGraw-Hill, 1979, pp. 568–629.

151. Oettle, A.G.: Skin cancer in Africa. *NCI Monog.* **10**:197–214, 1963.

152. Keeler, C.E.: Albinism, xeroderma pigmentosum, and skin cancer. *NCI Monog.* **10**: 349–359, 1963.

153. Lassus, A., et al.: Vitiligo and neoplasms. *Acta Derm. Venereol.* **52**:229–232, 1972.

154. Johnson, B.E., et al.: Melanin and cellular reactions to ultraviolet radiation. *Nature* **235**:147–149, 1972.

155. Reed, W.B., et al.: Pigmentary disorders in association with congenital deafness. *Arch. Derm.* **95**:176–186, 1967.

156. Comings, D.E., and Odland, G.F.: Partial albinism. *JAMA* **195**:519–523, 1966.

157. Ziprkowski, L., et al.: Partial albinism and deaf mutism. *Arch. Derm.* **86**:530–539, 1962.

158. Goodman, R.M., et al.: Genetic considerations in giant pigmented hairy nevus. *Br. J. Derm.* **85**:100–157, 1971.

159. Voigtlander, V., and Jung, E.E.: Giant pigmented hairy nevus in two siblings. *Humangenetik.* **24**:79–84, 1974.

160. Greely, P.W., Middleton, A.G., and Curtin, J.W.: Incidence of malignancy in giant pigmented nevi. *Plas. Reconst. Surg.* **36**:26–36, 1965.

161. Reed, W.B., et al.: Giant pigmented nevi, melanoma, and leptomeningeal melanocytosis. *Arch. Derm.* **91**:100–119, 1965.

162. Pers, M.: Naevus pigmentosus giganticus. *Ugeskr. Laeg.* **125**:613–619, 1963.

163. Russell, J.L., and Reyes, R.G.: Giant pigmented nevi. *JAMA* **171**:2083–2086, 1959.

164. Lewis, M.G.: Melanoma and pigmentation of the leptomeninges in Ugandan Africans. *J. Clin. Path.* **22**:183–186, 1969.

165. Kaplan, E.N.: The risk of malignancy in large congenital nevi. *Plas. Reconst. Surg.* **53**:421–428, 1974.

166. Lorentzen, M., et al.: Incidence of malignant transformation in giant pigmented nevi. *Scan. J. Plas. Reconst. Surg.* **11**:163–167, 1977.

167. Sanderson, K.V., and Wilson, H.T.H.: Haber's syndrome. *Br. J. Derm.* **77**:1–8, 1965.

168. Robbins, J.H., et al.: Xeroderma pigmentosum: an inherited disease with sun sensitivity, multiple cutaneous neoplasms, and abnormal DNA repair. *Ann. Int. Med.* **80**:221–248, 1974.

169. Friedberg, E.C.: Xeroderma pigmentosum. *Arch. Path. Lab. Med.* **102**:3–7, 1978.

170. Cleaver, J.E.: Xeroderma pigmentosum: genetic and environmental influences in skin carcinogenesis. *Int. J. Derm.* **17**:435–444, 1978.

171. Sutherland, B.M., Rice, M., and Wanger, E.K.: Xeroderma pigmentosum cells contain low levels of photoreactivating enzyme. *Proc. Natl. Acad. Sci. USA* **72**:102–107, 1975.

172. Lehman, A.R., et al.: Xeroderma cells with normal levels of excision repair have a defect in DNA synthesis after UV irradiation. *Proc. Natl. Acad. Sci. USA* **72**:219–223, 1975.

173. Reed, W.B., et al.: Xeroderma pigmentosum: clinical and laboratory investigation of its basic defects. *JAMA* **207**:2073–2079, 1969.

174. Andrews, A.D., et al.: Relation of DNA repair processes to pathological aging of the nervous system in xeroderma pigmentosum. *Lancet* **1**:1318–1320, 1976.

175. Setlow, R.B., and Regan, J.D.: Defective repair of N-acetoxy-2-acetylaminofluorene-induced lesions in the DNA of xeroderma pigmentosum cells. *Biochem. Biophys. Res. Commun.* **46**:1019–1021, 1977.

176. Stich, H.F., and San, R.H.C.: Reduced DNA repair synthesis in xeroderma pigmentosom cells exposed to the oncogenic 4-nitroquinoline 1-oxide and 4-hydroxyaminoquinoline 1-oxide. *Mutat. Res.* **13**:279–282, 1971.

177. Epstein, J.H.: Systemic disease and light. In: *Dermatology Update* (S.L. Moschella, Ed.). New York: Elsevier, 1979, pp. 119–144.

178. Lynch, H.T., et al.: Spontaneous regression of metastatic malignant melanoma in two siblings with xeroderma pigmentosum. *J. Med. Genet.* **15**:357–367, 1978.

179. Hofman, H., Jung, E.G., and Schnyder, U.W.: Pigmented xerodermoid: first report of a family. *Bull. Cancer* (Paris) **65**:347–350, 1978.

180. McConnell, R.B.: Gastrointestinal cancer, genetics, and genetic markers. *Fron. Gastrointes. Res.* **4**:134–141, 1979.

181. Clarke, C.A.: Neoplasms of the gastrointestinal tract associated with inherited abnormalities of the skin. *Proc. Roy. Soc. Med.* **51**:326, 1958.

182. Howel-Evans, W., et al.: Carcinoma of the esophagus with keratosis palmaris et plantaris (tylosis). *Quar. J. Med.* **27**:413–429, 1958.

183. Shine, I., and Allison, P.R.: Carcinoma of the esophagus with tylosis. *Lancet* **1**: 951–953, 1966.

184. Clarke, C.A., and McConnell, R.B.: Six cases of carcinoma of oesophagus occurring in one family. *Br. Med. J.* **2**:1137–1138, 1954.

185. Harper, P.S., Harper, R.M.P., and Howel-Evans, A.W.: Carcinoma of the oesophagus with tylosis. *Quar. J. Med.* **39**:317–333, 1970.

186. Gentry, W.C., et al.: Multiple hamartoma syndrome (Cowden's disease). *Arch. Derm.* **109**:521–525, 1974.

187. Weary, P.E., et al.: Multiple hamartoma syndrome (Cowden's disease). *Arch. Derm.* **106**:682–690, 1972.

188. Nuss, D.D., et al.: Multiple hamartoma syndrome (Cowden's disease). *Arch. Derm.* **114**:743–746, 1978.

189. Burnett, J.W., et al.: Cowden disease: report of two additional cases. *Br. J. Derm.* **93**:329–336, 1975.

190. Brownstein, M.H., et al.: Cowden's disease: cutaneous marker of heart cancer. *Cancer* **41**:2393–2398, 1978.

191. Lloyd, K.M., and Dinnis, M.: Cowden's disease: a possible new symptom complex with multiple system involvement. *Ann. Int. Med.* **58**:136–142, 1963.

192. Wade, T.R., and Kopf, A.W.: Cowden's disease: a case report and review of the literature. *J. Derm. Surg. Oncol.* **4**:459–464, 1978.

193. Allen, B.S., Fitch, M.H., and Smith, J.G.: Multiple hamartoma syndrome. *J. Am. Acad. Derm.* **2**:303–308, 1980.

194. Reid, J.D.: Intestinal carcinoma in the Peutz-Jeghers syndrome. *JAMA* **229**:833–834, 1974.

195. Matuchansky, C., et al.: Peutz-Jeghers syndrome with metastasizing carcinoma arising from a jejunal hamartoma. *Gastroenterology* **77**:1311–1315, 1979.

196. Humphries, A.L., et al.: Peutz-Jeghers syndrome with colonic adenocarcinoma and ovarian tumors. *JAMA* **197**:296–298, 1966.

197. Utsunomiya, J., et al.: Peutz-Jeghers syndrome: its natural course and management. *Johns Hopkins Med. J.* **136**:71–82, 1975.

198. Christian, C.D.: Ovarian tumors: an extension of the Peutz-Jeghers syndrome. *Am. J. Obstet. Gyn.* **111**:529–534, 1971.

199. Gardner, E.J.: Followup study of a family group exhibiting dominant inheritance for a syndrome including intestinal polyps, osteomas, fibromas, and epidermal cysts. *Am. J. Hum. Genet.* **14**:376–390, 1962.

200. Weary, P.E., et al.: Gardner's syndrome: a family group study and review. *Arch. Derm.* **90**:20–30, 1964.

201. Watne, A.L., et al.: The diagnosis and surgical treatment of patients with Gardner's syndrome. *Surgery* **82**:327–333, 1977.

202. Gorlin, R.J., and Chaudhry, A.P.: Multiple osteomatosis, fibromas, lipomas, and fibrosarcomas of the skin, leiomyomas, and multiple intestinal polyposis. *N. Eng. J. Med.* **263**:1151–1158, 1960.

203. Binder, M.C., et al.: Colon polyps, sebaceous cysts, gastric polyps, and malignant brain tumors in a family. *Dig. Dis.* **23**:460–466, 1978.

204. Fraumeni, J.F., et al.: Sarcomas and multiple polyposis in a kindred: a genetic variety of hereditary polyposis? *Arch. Int. Med.* **121**:57–60, 1968.

205. Camiel, M.R., et al.: Association of thyroid carcinoma with Gardner's syndrome in siblings. *N. Eng. J. Med.* **278**:1056–1058, 1968.

206. MacDonald, J.M., et al: Gardner's syndrome and periampullary malignancy. *Am. J. Surg.* **113**:425–430, 1967.

207. Marshall, W.H., et al.: Gardner's syndrome with adrenal carcinoma. *Aus. Ann. Med.* **16**:242–244, 1967.

208. Naylor, E.W., and Libenthal, E.: Early detection of adenomatous polyposis coli in Gardner's syndrome. *Pediatrics* **63**:222–227, 1979.

209. Danes, B.S.: The Gardner syndrome: increased tetraploidy in cultured skin fibroblast. *J. Med. Genet.* **13**:52–56, 1976.

210. Yaffee, H.S.: Gastric polyposis and soft tissue tumors: a variant of Gardner's syndrome. *Arch. Derm.* **89**:806–808, 1969.

211. Turcot, J., et al.: Malignant tumors of the central nervous system associated with familial polyposis of the colon: report of two cases. *Dis. Colon Rect.* **2**:465, 1959.

212. Baughman, F.A., et al.: The glioma-polyposis syndrome. *N. Eng. J. Med.* **281**:1345, 1965.

213. Swenson, K.H., et al.: The glucagonoma syndrome. *Arch. Derm.* **114**:224–228, 1978.

214. Kahan, R.S., and Perez-Figaredo, R.A.: Necrolytic migratory erythema. *Arch. Derm.* **113**:792–797, 1977.

215. Goodenberger, D.M., et al.: Necrolytic migratory erythema without glucagonoma. *Arch. Derm.* **115**:1429–1432, 1979.

216. Binnick, A.N., et al.: Glucagonoma syndrome. *Arch. Derm.* **113**:749–754, 1977.

217. Kessingir, A., et al.: The glucagonoma syndrome and its management. *J. Surg. Oncol.* **9**:419–424, 1977.

218. Mallinson, C.N., et al.: Glucagonoma syndrome. *Lancet* **2**:1–5, 1974.

219. Boden, G., and Owen, O.E.: Familial hyperglucagonemia: an autosomal dominant disorder. *N. Eng. J. Med.* **296**:534–538, 1977.

220. Lambert, D., et al.: Genodermatose sclero-atrophiante et keratodermique des extremites. *J. Genet. Hum.* **26**:25–31, 1978.

221. Hureiz, C., et al.: Genodermatose sclero-atrophiante et keratodermique des extremites. *Ann. Derm. Syph.* (Paris) **96**:135–146, 1969.

222. Huriez, C., et al.: Apropos de 28 cas d'epidermolyse bulleuse dans 11 families dont une famile etudee du point de une genetique, sans mise en evidence de linkage. *Bull. Soc. Franc. Derm. Syph.* **75**:750–755, 1968.

223. Van der Hoeve, J.: Eye symptoms in tuberous sclerosis of the brain. *Trans. Ophthalmol. Soc. UK* **40**:329, 1920.
224. Nichel, W.R., and Reed, W.B.: Tuberous sclerosis. *Arch. Derm.* **85**:209–226, 1962.
225. Fitzpatrick, T.B., et al.: White leaf-shaped macules: earliest visible sign of tuberous sclerosis. *Arch. Derm.* **98**:1–6, 1968.
226. Tilger, W.: Ultrastructure of white leaf-shaped macules in tuberous scleros. *Arch. Derm. Forsch.* **248**:13–27, 1973.
227. Jimbow, K., et al.: Congenital circumscribed hypomelanosis: characterization based on electron microscopic study of tuberous sclerosis nevus depigmentosus and piebaldism. *J. Inves. Derm.* **64**:50–52, 1975.
228. Lagos, J.C., and Gomez, M.R.: Tuberous sclerosis: reappraisal of a clinical entity. *Mayo Clin. Prc. Med.* **64**:185–200, 1971.
229. Reed, W.B., Nichel, W.R., and Campion, G.: Internal manifestations of tuberous sclerosis. *Arch. Derm.* **87**:715–726, 1963.
230. Martin, G.I., et al.: Computer-assisted cranial tomography in early diagnosis of tuberous sclerosis. *JAMA* **235**:2323–2324, 1976.
231. Prompitak, A., et al.: An abortive case of tuberous sclerosis without mental deficiency or epilepsy in an adult. *Am. J. Ophthalmol.* **76**:255–259, 1973.
232. O'Callaghan, T.J., et al.: Tuberous sclerosis with striking renal involvement in a family. *Arch. Int. Med.* **135**:1082–1089, 1975.
233. Chonko. A.M., et al.: Renal involvement in tuberous sclerosis. *Am. J. Med.* **56**: 124–131, 1974.
234. Dwyer, J.M., et al.: Pulmonary tuberous sclerosis. *Quar. J. Med.* **40**:115–123, 1971.
235. Tod, P.A.: Radiological findings in tuberous sclerosis. *J. Coll. Radiol. Aus.* **6**:42–48, 1962.
236. Papnayotou, P., and Vezirtgie, E.: Tuberous sclerosis with gingival lesions. *Oral Surg.* **39**:577–581, 1975.
237. Cameron, S.J., and Dorg, A.: Cerebellar tumors presented with clinical features of pheochromocytoma. *Lancet* **1**:492–494, 1970.
238. Mendelow, A.D., et al.: Familial phaeochromocytoma with von Hippel's disease in one sister and ectopic adrenal cortex in the kidney in another. *Br. J. Surg.* **65**:138–140, 1978.
239. Tomita, T., et al.: Occult adenocarcinoma of the pancreas in a patient with Lindau's disease. *Dig. Dis.* **23**:80s–83s, 1978.
240. Knudson, A.G., and Strong, L.C.: Mutation and cancer: neuroblastoma and pheochromocytoma. *Am. J. Hum. Genet.* **24**:514–532, 1972.
241. Chatten, J., and Voorhees, M.L.. Familial neuroblastoma. report of a kindred with multiple disorders, including neuroblastoma in four siblings. *N. Eng. J. Med.* **277**: 1230–1236, 1967.
242. Griffin, M.E., and Bolande, R.P.: Familial neuroblastoma with regression and maturation to ganglioneurofibroma. *Pediatrics* **43**:377–382, 1969.
243. Adams, R.D.: Neurocutaneous diseases. In: *Dermatology in General Medicine* (T.B. Fitzpatrick et al. Eds.). New York: McGraw-Hill, 1979, pp. 1206–1246.
244. Crowe, F.W., et al.: *Clinical, Pathological, and Genetic Study of Multiple Neurofibromatosis.* Springfield, IL: Thomas, 1956.
245. Crowe, F.W.: Axillary freckling as a diagnostic aid in neurofibromatosis. *Ann. Int. Med.* **61**:1142–1143, 1964.
246. Johnson, B.L., and Charneco, D.R.: Cafe-au-lait spots in neurofibromatosis and in normal individuals. *Arch. Derm.* **102**:442–446, 1970.
247. Healey, F.H., and Mekelatos, C.J.: Pheochromocytoma and neurofibromatosis. *N. Eng. J. Med.* **258**:540–543, 1958.

248. Jimbo, K., et al.: Ultrastructure of giant pigmented granules (macromelanosomes) in the cutaneous pigmented macules of neurofibromatosis. *J. Inves. Derm.* **61**:300–309, 1973.

249. Glushien, A.S., et al.: Pheochromocytoma. *Am. J. Med.* **14**:317–327, 1953.

250. Fabricant, R.N., et al.: Increased levels of a nerve-growth-factor cross-reacting protein in "central" neurofibromatosis. *Lancet* **1**:4–7, 1979.

251. Fienman, N.L., and Yakovac, B.A.: Neurofibromatosis in childhood. *J. Ped.* **76**:339–346, 1970.

252. Riccardi, V.M., and Kleiner, B.: Neurofibromatosis: a neoplastic birth defect with two age-peaks of severe problems. *Birth Defects Orig. Art. Ser.* **23**(3c):131–138, 1977.

253. Brasfield, R.D., and Das Gupta, T.K.: Von Recklinghausen's disease: a clinicopathologic entity. *Arch. Surg.* **175**:86–104, 1972.

254. Lisch, K.: Uber beteilung der Augen, insbesondire das Vorkommen von Irisknotchen bei der Neurofibromatose (Rechlinghausen). *Z. Augenheilb.* **93**:137–143, 1937.

255. Riccardi, V.M., Kleiner, B., and Lubs, M.L.: Neurofibromatosis: variable expression is not intrinsic to the mutant gene. *Birth Defects Orig. Art. Ser.* **15**(56):283–289, 1979.

256. Riccardi, V.M.: Pathophysiology of neurofibromatosis. IV. Dermatologic insights into heterogencity and pathogenesis. *J. Am. Aca. Derm.* **3**:157–166, 1980.

257. Gorlin, R.J., and Vicars, R.A.: Multiple mucosal neuromas, pheochromocytoma, medullary carcinoma of the thyroid, and Marfanoid body build with muscular wasting: reexamination of a syndrome of neural crest malmigration. *Birth Defects* **7**:69–72, 1971.

258. Walker, D.M.: Oral mucosal neuroma – medullary thyroid carcinoma syndrome. *Br. J. Derm.* **88**:599–603, 1973.

259. Schimke, R.N.: Phenotype of malignancy: mucosal neuroma syndrome. *Pediatric* **52**:283–284, 1973.

260. Schimke, R.N., et al.: Syndrome of bilateral pheochromocytoma, medullary thyroid carcinoma, and multiple neuromas. *N. Eng. J. Med.* **279**:1–7, 1968.

261. Block, M.B., et al.: Multiple endocrine adenomatosis, Type IIb: diagnosis and treatment. *JAMA* **234**:710–714, 1975.

262. Samaan, H.A., et al.: Medullary carcinoma of the thyroid and astrocytoma. *Ann. Int. Med.* **56**:585–586, 1977.

263. Epstein, D.J., et al.: Werner's syndrome. *Medicine* **45**:177–221, 1966.

264. Bjornberg, A.: Werner's syndrome and malignancy. *Acta Derm. Venereol.* **56**:149–154, 1976.

265. Knotch, W., et al.: Uber das Verner-syndrom. *Hautarzt* **14**:145–152, 1963.

266. Fleischmajer, R., and Nedwich, A.: Werner's syndrome. *Am. J. Med.* **54**:111–116, 1973.

267. Goldstein, S., and Moerman, E.J.: Heat-labile enzymes in Werner's syndrome fibroblasts. *Nature* **255**:159, 1975.

268. Bolande, R.P.: Childhood tumors and their relationship to birth defects. In: *Genetics in Human Cancer: Progress in Cancer Research and Therapy* (J.J. Mulvihill et al., Eds.). Vol. 3. New York: Raven Press, 1977, pp. 43–75.

269. Mullins, J.F., et al.: The Kleppel-Trenaunay-Weber syndrome. *Arch. Derm.* **86**:202–206, 1962.

270. Owens, D.W., et al.: The Kleppel-Trenaunay-Weber syndrome with pulmonary vein varicosity. *Arch. Derm.* **108**:111–113, 1973.

271. Lamar, L.M., et al.: Kleppel-Trenaunay-Weber syndrome. *Arch. Derm.* **91**:58–59, 1965.

272. Goidanich, I.F., and Campanacci, M.: Vascular hemangiomata and infantile angioectatic osteohypoplasia of extremities. *J. Bone Joint Surg.* **44**:815–842, 1962.

273. Benedetto, A.V., et al.: Porphyria cutanea tarda in three generations of a single family. *N. Eng. J. Med.* **398**:458-362, 1978.
274. Grossman, M.E., et al.: Porphyria cutanea tarda. *Am. J. Med.* **67**:277-286, 1979.
275. Fromke, V.L., et al.: Porphyria variegata. *Am. J. Med.* **85**:80-88, 1978.
276. Topi, G., and D'Alessandro, G.L.: Inheritance of porphyria cutanea tarda. *Br. J. Derm.* **97**:617-627, 1977.
277. Perry, H.O.: Less common skin markers of visceral neoplasms. *Int. J. Derm.* **15**: 19-25, 1976.
278. Muhbauer, J.E., and Pathalc, M.A.: Porphyria cutanea tarda. *Int. J. Derm.* **18**: 767-780, 1979.
279. Buckman, K.J., et al.: Familial systemic lupus erythematosus. *Arch. Int. Med.* **138**:1674-1676, 1978.
280. Dubois, E.L.: *Lupus Erythematosus: a Review of the Current Status of Discoid and Systemic Lupus Erythematosus and Their Variants* (2nd ed.). Los Angeles, CA: USC Press, 1976.
281. Fessd, W.J.: Systemic lupus erythematosus in the community: incidence, prevalence, outcome, and first symptoms. *Arch. Int. Med.* **134**:1027-1035, 1974.
282. Kuehan, P.G., et al.: Familial occurrence of extramammary Paget's disease. *Cancer* **31**:145-148, 1973.
283. Oka, M., et al.: Simultaneous prostatic carcinoma and genital Paget's disease associated with subsequent adenocarcinoma. *Br. J. Urol.* **51**:49, 1974.
284. Gershwin, M.E., et al.: Increased frequency of HL-A8 in Sjogren's syndrome. *Tis. Ant.* **6**:342-346, 1975.
285. Whaley, K., et al.: Sjogren's syndrome. I. Sicca components. *Qtr. J. Med.* **166**: 297-302, 1973.
286. Henkin, R.I., et al.: Abnormalities of taste and smell in Sjogren's syndrome. *Ann. Int. Med.* **76**:375-383, 1972.
287. Bhoch, K.J., et al.: Sjogren's syndrome. *Medicine* **44**:187-231, 1965.
288. Stoltze, C.A., et al.: Keratoconjunctivitis sicca and Sjogren's syndrome. *Arch. Int. Med.* **106**:513-522, 1960.
289. Mason, A.M.S., et al.: Sjogren's syndrome – a clinical review. *Sem. Arthr. Rheum.* **2**:301-331, 1973.
290. Brouet, J.C., et al.: Biologic and clinical significance of cryoglobulins. *Am. J. Med.* **57**:775-788, 1974.
291. Ehrlich, E.I.: Oculocutaneous manifestations of rheumatic diseases. *Rhematology* **4**:1-2, 1973.
292. Chevrant-Bieton, J., et al.: Cutaneous manifestations of idiopathic hemochromatosis. *Arch. Derm.* **113**:161-165, 1973.
293. Kidd, K.K.: Genetic linkage and hemochromatosis. *N. Eng. J. Med.* **301**:209-210, 1979.
294. Cartwright, G.E., et al.: Hereditary hemochromatosis. *N. Eng. J. Med.* **301**:175-179, 1979.
295. Williams, R., et al.: The inheritance of idiopathic haemochromatosis: a clinical and liver biopsy study of 16 families. *Qtr. J. Med.* **31**:249-265, 1962.
296. Saddi, R., and Feingold, J.: Idiopathic hemochromatosis: an autosomal recessive disease. *Clin. Genet.* **5**:234-241, 1974.
297. Pollycove, M.: Hemochromatosis. In: *The Metabolic Basis of Inherited Disease* (J.B. Stanbury et al., Eds.; 4th ed.). New York: McGraw-Hill, 1978, pp. 1127-1164.
298. Simon, M., et al.: Idiopathic hemochromatosis. *N. Eng. J. Med.* **297**:1017-1021, 1977.

299. Carleton, A., et al.: Maffucci's syndrome (dyschondroplasia with haemangiomata). *Qtr. J. Med.* 11:203–228, 1942.
300. Sakurane, H.F., et al.: The association of blue rubber bleb nevus and Maffucci's syndrome. *Arch. Derm.* 95:28–36, 1967.
301. Berlin, R.: Maffucci's syndrome. *Acta Med. Scand.* 177:299–307, 1965.
302. Talbot, S., and Wyatt, E.H.: Blue rubber bleb naevi. *Br. J. Derm.* 82:37–39, 1970.
303. Walshe, M.M., et al.: Blue rubber bleb naevus. *Br. J. Med.* Vol. 2. 931–932, 1966.
304. Fretgin, D.F., and Potter, B.: Blue rubber bleb nevus. *Arch. Int. Med.* 116:924–929, 1965.
305. Rice, S.J., and Fischer, D.S.: Blue rubber bleb nevus syndrome. *Arch. Derm.* 86: 503–511, 1962.
306. Taylor, J.F., et al.: Kaposi's sarcoma in Uganda: a clinicopathological study. *Int. J. Cancer* 8:122–135, 1971.
307. Bluefarb, S.M.: *Kaposi's Sarcoma.* Springfield, IL: C.C. Thomas, 1957.
308. Beylot, C., et al.: Kaposi's sarcoma and malignant lymphoma. *Ann. Derm. Ven.* 104:817–823, 1977.
309. Gange, R.W., and Wilson-Jones, E.: Kaposi's sarcoma and immunosuppressive therapy: appraisal. *Clin. Exp. Derm.* 3:135–146, 1978.
310. Reynolds, W.A., et al.: Kaposi's sarcoma: a clinicopathologic study with particular reference to its relationship to the reticuloendothelial system. *Medicine* 44:419–443, 1965.
311. Olweny, C.L.M., et al.: Childhood Kaposi's sarcoma: clinical features and therapy. *Br. J. Cancer* 33:555–560, 1976.
312. McCarthy, W.D., and Pack, G.T.: Malignant blood vessel tumors: a report of 56 cases of angiosarcoma and Kaposi's sarcoma. *Surg. Gyn. Obstet.* 91:465–482, 1950.
313. Finlay, A.Y., and Marks, R.: Familial Kaposi's sarcoma. *Br. J. Derm.* 100:323–326, 1979.
314. Safai, B., et al.: Association of Kaposi's sarcoma with second primary malignancies. *Cancer* 45:1472–1479, 1980.
315. Schwartz, R.A., et al.: Squamous cell carcinoma in dominant type Epidermolysis Bullosa Dystrophica. *Cancer* 47:615–620, 1981.
316. Roberts, J.T., Byrne, E.H., and Rosenthal, D.: Familial variant of dermatofibroma with malignant in the proband. *Arch. Derm.* 117:12–15, 1981.
317. Carney, J.A., Hayles, A.B., Pearse, A.G.E., Perry, H.O., and Sizemore, G.W.: Abnormal cutaneous innervation in multiple endocrine neoplasia, type 2b. *Annals. Int. Med.* 94:362–363, 1981.

A recent article by Linus, et al., (*Arch Surg* 116: 1182-1184, Sept. 1981) has presented negative data for cancer association in the Peutz-Jegher's syndrome. This study was based upon 48 patients with Peutz-Jegher's syndrome seen at the Mayo Clinic, Rochester, MN, followed up for a median period of 33 years. Carcinoma of the small or large intestines did not develop in any patient with possibly one exception. Survival of patients with Peutz-Jegher's syndrome also was found to be similar to that of the general population. The authors therefore are skeptical about the premalignant potential of this rare syndrome, especially in the small intestine. They recommend surgical conservatism.

4
Dermatopathologic Aspects of
Cancer-associated Genodermatoses

Walter H. C. Burgdorf, M.D.

I will attempt to acquaint the non-dermatopathologist with the ways in which a skin biopsy may aid in diagnosing cancer-associated genodermatoses. Avoiding detailed discussions of microscopic features which can be found in the referenced articles as well as in standard textbooks, I will concentrate on interpreting skin biopsies and speculating on the relationship of microscopic features to the underlying disease process.

SYNDROMES WITH CUTANEOUS MARKERS
OF UNDERLYING MALIGNANCY

Acanthosis Nigricans

Acanthosis nigricans (AN) can clearly be inherited and it is definitely a marker of cutaneous malignancy. In general, however, only sporadic cases are associated with cancer. Even though AN may not be a true cancer-associated genodermatosis, we will consider it here because it is often biopsied.

AN is far more distinctive clinically than microscopically. The name is a misnomer to the pathologist as neither marked acanthosis nor increased pigment (nigricans) is a prominent feature. Instead, AN falls into the group of epidermal-papillary hyperplasias, featuring basketweave hyperkeratosis, as well as elongation of the rete ridges and dermal papillae. Lesions showing these features include seborrheic keratosis, actinic keratosis, verruca, several variants of ichthyosis, acrokeratosis verruciformis, and confluent and reticulated papillomatosis. This long list should make clear that the biopsy is rarely helpful in diagnosing AN.

The histological overlap also raises several interesting questions regarding possible epidermal-papillary growth factors. Seborrheic keratoses, when inherited, present at a relatively early age,[1] although they are usually seen only in elderly patients. When seborrheic keratoses occur suddenly in adults, it is often a sign of internal malignancy, known as the Leser-Trelat sign.[2]   There is considerable overlap between AN, Leser-Trelat, and other diffuse papillomatous eruptions which have been associated with underlying malignancies.   Some patients may have AN, multiple seborrheic keratosis, and other papillomas at the same time.[3,4]

Furthermore, AN has been associated with peripheral insulin resistance in some cases[5] and with vitamin A deficiency in others.[6]   Thus it is conceivable that several factors may lead to epithelial-papillary hyperplasia, manifesting itself in a number of clinical patterns, as well as being associated with internal malignancies.

Cowden's Syndrome

Brownstein has recently said that "the combination of multiple facial trichilemmomas, oral fibromas, and benign acral keratoses enables one to diagnose Cowden's syndrome at a stage before serious internal complications develop."[7]   Multiple facial trichilemmomas alone should suggest Cowden's syndrome, one genodermatosis which the dermatopathologist can be the first to diagnose.

Trichilemmomas appear as warty growths about the face which suggest a number of clinical diagnoses but appear distinct histologically as large pale tumors of the follicular infundibulum.   Brownstein[7] found a variable pattern ranging from classic trichilemmomas to inverted follicular keratoses.   Figure 4-1 shows a classic trichilemmoma from one of Brownstein's patients.

The oral fibromas and acral keratoses are similar to such lesions in patients without Cowden's syndrome, but their presence helps confirm the diagnosis. Thus these seemingly innocent skin findings serve as an early, reliable marker for both breast and thyroid carcinoma.

Ackerman[8] has suggested that trichilemmomas may be old human wart virus infections of the follicular infundibulum.   Brownstein[7] does not share this view; he found no wart virus in four trichilemmomas from Cowden's syndrome patients. Morphologically, I tend to agree with Brownstein, but in a speculative sense, a viral etiology with improper surveillance of a papovavirus as the underlying defect causing trichilemmomas, breast cancer, thyroid cancer, and many other defects would be a tidy explanation.

Gardner's Syndrome

About 65% of the patients with Gardner's syndrome have multiple cutaneous cysts.   These are erroneously called sebaceous cysts but are keratinous cysts, epidermoid type, because they contain keratin and have a cyst wall undergoing epidermal keratinization with a granular layer.   Epidermoid keratinous cysts are a common dermatopathologic finding, and it would be absurd to evaluate all patients with such lesions for intestinal disease.   Keratinous cysts of the trichilemmal type with the cyst wall undergoing trichilemmal keratinization without a

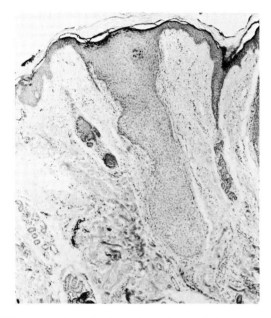

Figure 4-1. Trichilemmoma from the face of a patient with Cowden's syndrome. Tumor arises from hair through proliferation of trichilemmal cells which retain several characteristics: (a) clear cells, (b) tendency toward peripheral palisading best seen in middle third. Notice how much lighter and more bulbous the trichilemmoma is in comparison to the adjacent normal structures (H & E, 50X; reproduced from *British Journal of Dermatology* 100: 670, 1979, Figure 3). *(Courtesy of Martin H. Brownstein, M.D., Great Neck, NY, and Blackwell Scientific Publications)*

granular layer tend to be on the scalp, often calcify, and may develop proliferative changes in their walls. In a study of 60 families with hereditary trichilemmal keratinous cysts, no patient had intestinal polyps.[9]

Postsurgical desmoids in colectomy scars are more specific for Gardner's syndrome.[10] Desmoids do occur in women during or after pregnancy, but are very rare in males except in Gardner's syndrome. Thus a fibrous proliferation in such a scar should prompt a search for Gardner's syndrome. On the other hand, one should be reluctant to diagnosis fibrosarcoma in such desmoids, since they are benign clinically and rather bland histologically. Association with a cancer-associated genodermatosis does not always mean cancer.

Torre's Syndrome

Multiple cutaneous sebaceous gland tumors, and multiple keratoacanthomas have been associated with underlying malignancy, usually in a sporadic fashion and most often following the appearance of the visceral cancer.[11,12]   Lynch[13] and his coworkers have found multiple sebaceous adenomas in some of their familial cancer pedigrees.

Sebaceous adenomas and carcinomas are distinctly rare, and a single sebaceous tumor probably justifies a search for underlying malignancy. Several points of confusion arise. Most adults with any degree of sun exposure have senile sebaceous hyperplasia, consisting of tiny yellowish papules about hair follicle openings, especially on the forehead. These lesions show sebaceous proliferation about a simple follicle opening. Sebaceous tumors are usually dermal masses with varying degrees of organization and atypia, as Figures 4-2 through 4-4 illustrate.

Torre's syndrome should not be confused with Gardner's syndrome; the sebaceous tumors have nothing in common with the erroneously named sebaceous cysts of Gardner's syndrome.

Glucagonoma Syndrome

There are only two good clues to the glucagonoma syndrome – documenting elevated serum glucagon levels or finding necrolytic changes on a skin biopsy.

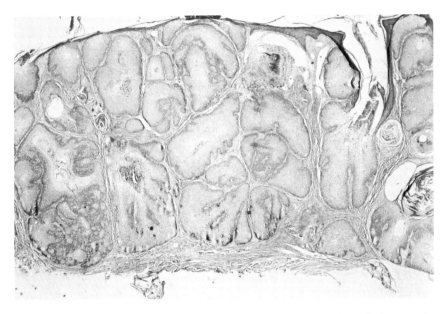

Figure 4-2. Papule from face of man with Torre's syndrome. Wide variety of sebaceous elements present, defying exact classification. On right hand one lobule is arising from follicle as in senile sebaceous hyperplasia (SSH), but overall complexity and atypia distinguish this from SSH (H & E, 125×). *(Histological material courtesy of Ali Fahmy, M.D., Ph.D., Oklahoma City, OK)*

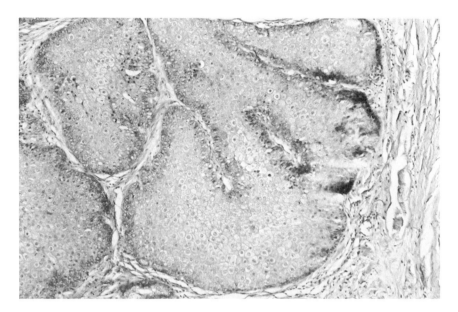

Figure 4-3. Lobule in the middle of Figure 4-2, showing a fairly typical sebaceous adenoma, which is somewhat more cellular than a normal sebaceous gland but lacks atypia (H & E, 500×). *(Histological material courtesy of Ali Fahmy, M.D., Ph.D., Oklahoma City, OK)*

While most reports of the glucagonoma syndrome have been sporadic, hyper-glucagonemia has been found in relatives of one patient with the glucagonoma syndrome.[14]

I have had the opportunity to study a number of biopsies from patients with glucagonoma syndrome and am most impressed with the marked variability. The key feature is the necrolytic epidermis. This may include epidermal blister formation, with or without acantholysis, and necrolytic or fusiform keratinocytes (Figures 4-5 through 4-7). There are other causes of a sick epidermis, including staphylococcal scalded skin syndrome, acute graft vs host disease, epidermal erythema multiforme, and toxic epidermal necrolysis, but such epidermal changes should at least suggest the glucagonoma syndrome.[15-17]

The role of glucagon in this fascinating picture is unclear. It has never been identified in the skin lesions, although it would seem useful to look for it with immunoperoxidase staining which so nicely identifies the hormone in the pancreas. Direct toxic effects from glucagon may be the explanation; alternatively, the epidermal well-being may be influenced by local alterations in carbohydrate metabolism.

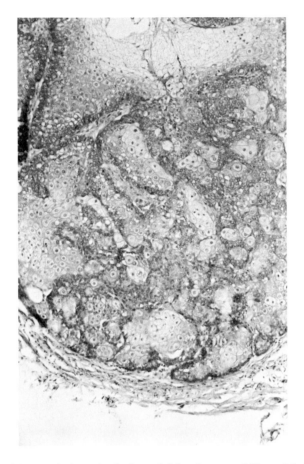

Figure 4-4. Highly atypical area in the lower left-hand corner of Figure 4-2. Taken alone, this pattern with wide variance in cell size and maturity might be interpreted as a sebaceous carcinoma (H & E, 500X). *(Histological material courtesy of Ali Fahmy, M.D., Ph.D., Oklahoma City, OK)*

Multiple Mucosal Neuroma Syndrome (MEN-III)

In MEN-III, a simple biopsy of a nodule on.the lip or tongue can provide a long head start toward the treatment of medullary carcinoma of thyroid. True neuromas of the skin and mucosal surface are quite rare.[18] Thus, if a patient has a well-encapsulated neuroma about the mouth (Figure 4-8), he has MEN-III and is at great risk for medullary carcinoma of the thyroid. These patients may also have pheochromocytomas. An association with neurofibromatosis has been sought, but MEN-III has true neuromas and far fewer café au lait spots.

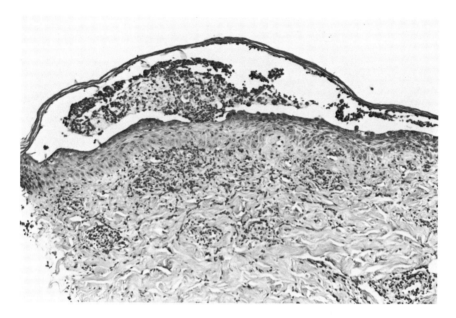

Figure 4-5. Pustule in glucagonoma syndrome. In this case, the 'sick' epidermis is manifested by high epidermal dissolution with acantholysis. The pustule contains inflammatory cells, which are also present diffusely throughout the dermis (H & E, 125×). *(Histological material courtesy of Troy Rollins, M.D., Eugene, OR)*

Neurofibromatosis

Neurofibromatosis (NF) provides a spectrum of challenges to the dermatopathologist. Initially, he may be asked to study a café au lait spot or confirm the presence of a neurofibroma. Later, he may have to evaluate malignant degeneration in a neurofibroma. The differential diagnosis of café au lait spots will be considered later in this chapter.

Isolated neurofibromas are puzzling both clinically and histologically. We often see adults with no stigmata of NF who have papillomas, similar to skin tags or degenerated nevi, which histologically show a neurofibroma, with a myxoid stroma, wavy cell nuclei, and numerous mast cells. It is hard to imagine that the patients have NF. When children and young adults have histologic neurofibromas, one must ask if they have NF.

Most superficial neurofibromas in patients with NF have a low malignant potential. The deep and plexiform neurofibromas, however, do undergo malignant degeneration: this will be discussed in Chapter 5. I would like to reemphasize the need to inform the surgical pathologist that the patient has NF when submitting such a tumor. Ackerman and Rosai[19] warn: "We know of only two circumstances in which the diagnosis of malignant schwannoma should be the primary consideration in the presence of a malignant tumor of soft tissues

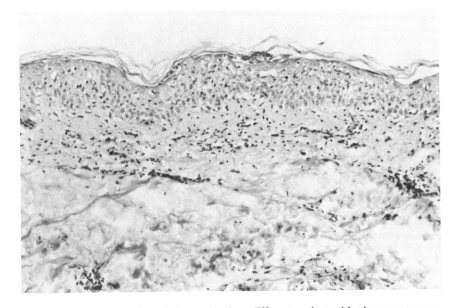

Figure 4-6. Marked epidermal destruction in a different patient with glucagonoma syndrome. Here, atypical shrunken keratinocytes are dispersed throughout an epidermis that looks almost spongiotic from the hydropic destruction. The degeneration is greater in the upper epidermis than along the basal layer, in contrast to the changes in lupus erythematosus. The dermal infiltrate is sparse (H & E, 125×). *(Histological material courtesy of Steven K. Spencer, Hanover, NH)*

composed of spindle cells: (1) when the tumor develops in a patient with Recklinghausen's disease and (2) when the tumor is obviously arising within the anatomic compartment of a major nerve or in continuity with an unquestionable neurofibroma."

The distinction between schwannomas and neurofibromas is needlessly confusing. In NF, there are two *types* of Schwann cell proliferation: the peripheral tumors are wavy, loose neurofibromas, while the more central schwannomas are usually well encapsulated, show palisading, and are in continuity with a nerve. The malignant degeneration occurs most often in the central tumors which are designated malignant schwannomas.

Another variant of the theme of NF is central NF.[20] Patients have bilateral acoustic neuromas; both cafe au lait spots and peripheral neurofibromas are present but unusual. It appears that studying serum nerve growth factors (NGF) may help distinguish between peripheral and central NF. In the former, NGF occurs in normal amount with increased functional activity, while in central NF there is an increased amount of NGF with normal to reduced function.[21]

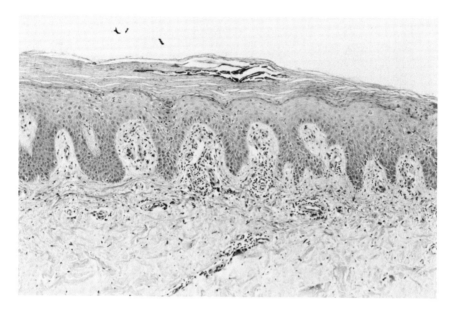

Figure 4-7. In this view, one can see how harmless glucagonoma syndrome may look. There is psoriasiform hyperplasia with elongation of the rete ridges and dermal papillary vessel proliferation and inflammation. The hydropic degeneration in the granular layer is the only clue that chronic dermatitis may not be the whole explanation (H & E, 125×). *(Histological material courtesy of Steven K. Spencer, Hanover, NH)*

Tuberous Sclerosis

All three of the cardinal skin findings in tuberous sclerosis (TS) can be identified through biopsy. The ash leaf or white hypopigmented macules will be considered under pigmentary disturbances. They are usually the first sign of TS and enable the diagnosis to be made early in life.

The shagreen patch is a connective tissue nevus. Isolated connective tissue nevi (CTN) exist, but if such a lesion is seen, a search for the other stigmata of TS is indicated. Histologically, CTN look surprisingly normal; special stains for elastin and collagen are often needed to make the correct diagnosis. Using these stains the dermis appears exceptionally "full," with increased amounts of one or both fibers. In questionable cases, comparison with a biopsy from clinically normal skin may help.

Finally, TS patients have a variety of angiofibromas. Those about the nose are best known; they were mistakably called adenoma sebaceum because the regional sebaceous hyperplasia was misinterpreted. The abnormality seems to be a proliferation of dense fibrous stroma about many small blood vessels. Fibromas

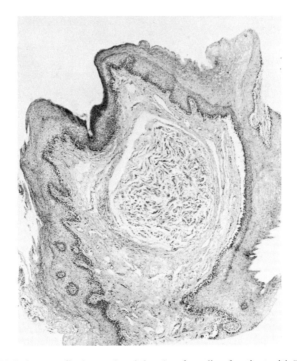

Figure 4-8. Well-circumscribed neural nodule taken from lip of patient with Type III multiple mucosal neuroma syndrome. The parakeratosis is normal for the area; the single proliferation of nervous tissue is not, which forces the correct diagnosis (H & E, 30×). *(Photomicrograph courtesy of Robert J. Gorlin, D.D.S., Minneapolis, MN)*

in other areas, including Koenen's periungual fibromas, tend to show fewer vessels and more fibrosis, often of a glial type (so designated because the giant fibroblasts are so large as to mimic glial cells).[22,23]

Tylosis

Tylosis or hyperkeratosis of the palms and soles is an overrated sign of cutaneous malignancy. In several pedigrees, including the family initially reported by Howel-Evans,[24] there is a perfect association between the presence of palmar-plantar keratoses and the later development of carcinoma of the esophagus. Cases of tylosis associated with sporadic internal malignancies have also been reported.[25,26]

The mechanism of disease in these two cases may be different. In Howel-Evans type tylosis, I imagine that a disturbance in keratinization leads to uncontrolled proliferation, producing both hyperkeratosis and squamous carcinoma.

In acquired tylosis, the associated tumors are often adenocarcinomas suggesting that perhaps the tumor secretes a compound interferring with keratinization.

Biopsy is an unsatisfactory way to evaluate keratodermas. All that is seen in a thickened stratum corneum overlyiing palmar or plantar skin. Some cases show epidermolytic hyperkeratosis, but this is not associated with malignancy. Thus, no information which could help interpret the possibility of a cancer-associated genodermatosis can be extracted from a biopsy. Perhaps someday ultrastructural studies of keratinization will allow us to subdivide different types of tylosis, making the morphologic identification of Howel-Evans tylosis and other cancer-associated keratodermas possible.

Fibrofolliculomas

Fibrofolliculomas are small flesh-colored nodules which histologically reveal an overproliferation of the normal perifollicular stroma compressing epithelial strands. While studying hereditary medullary carcinoma of the thyroid, Birt[27] identified a family in which some members had both fibrofolliculomas and thyroid cancer. There was not a perfect association. Hornstein and Knickenberg[28] describe two siblings with fibrofolliculomas, one of whom had intestinal polyps.

MULTIPLE CUTANEOUS MALIGNANCY SYNDROMES

In all these syndromes, the diagnosis becomes obvious as multiple tumors develop. The challenge to the dermatopathologist is to be suspicious of a multiple cancer syndrome based on early biopsies and beat the attending physician to the diagnosis. The age of the patient is usually the best clue.[29]

Basal Cell Nevus Syndrome

Basal cell carcinomas occupy a major part of every dermatopathology practice; it is hard to maintain a high index of suspicion when seeing common tumors. However, a basal cell carcinoma in a young patient or a calcified or ossified basal cell carcinoma should raise the question of basal cell nevus syndrome (BCNS). Many types of abnormal calcification occur in BCNS so it is not surprising that the skin tumors may also show this change. I have seen several unexpected features in biopsies from patients with BCNS (courtesy of Dr. Robert W. Goltz and Dr. Robert J. Gorlin). Occasionally, clinically normal skin will show nests of basal cell carcinoma. Also, in the BCNS patients with medulloblastoma, basal cell cancers will develop at an even earlier age in the radiation therapy portal used to treat the brain tumor. Finally, BCNS patients have tiny palmar pits whose pathogenesis is unclear. In some cases, basal cell carcinomas are adjacent to the pits.

Bazex Syndrome

Bazex described patients with multiple basal cell carcinomas, hypohidrosis, hypotrichosis, and follicular atrophoderma. I have seen histological material from only one pedigree with Bazex syndrome; the basal cell carcinomas had no features to distinguish them from ordinary tumors.

Follicular atrophoderma is another example of something clinically obvious becoming blurred histologically. There are perifollicular ice-pick marks over the hands, elbows, and face. Viksnins and Berlin[30] report no pathological findings in biopsies of pits; I have never seen step sections from such a biopsy but would hardly expect a hole or pit to disappear. Curth[31] shows one picture with some hyperkeratosis and dermal follicular atrophy but nothing to explain the ice-pick marks.

Multiple Self-healing Keratoacanthomas (Ferguson-Smith Syndrome)

Multiple keratoacanthomas (KA) or perhaps multiple self-healing squamous cell carcinomas represent a distinct clinical syndrome described in several generations of Scottish patients by several generations of Scottish doctors. The condition has been seen in families elsewhere. Some confusion exists over the term multiple KA which may refer to Ferguson-Smith patients, to patients with multiple "regular" KA, to those with eruptive KA of sudden onset, and to those with multiple pitch or tar induced KA.

The lesions described by Ferguson-Smith[32,33] studied histologically by Sommerville and Milne[34] are different from ordinary KA. In the usual KA, there is a cup-shaped proliferation of acanthotic epidermis with a ground glass appearance. The margin of the tumor is usually distinct with no evidence of invasion. In Ferguson-Smith tumors, the appearance is of an invasive squamous cell carcinoma with little organization, foci of invasion, and much inflammation. However, both regular and Ferguson-Smith KA usually heal spontaneously.

Viral-like particles were identified in KA almost 20 years ago but their presence has never been confirmed.[35] Chemical carcinogens can clearly cause KA, but familial susceptibility to them has not been established. We have seen multiple KA and squamous cell carcinomas develop on the hand of renal transplant patients. These individuals usually start out with multiple warts which change because of immunosuppression and excessive sunlight. Some biopsied lesions look like KA; others, like squamous cell carcinomas of Ferguson-Smith KA.

Multiple Hereditary Benign Cystic Epithelioma, Epithelioma Adenoides Cysticum of Brooke, Multiple Trichoepithelioma (MT)

MT about the nose is often misdiagnosed as tuberous sclerosis, basal cell nevus syndrome, or Cowden's syndrome, but the biopsy resolves all questions. Histologically, a hair follicle tumor is seen with varying patterns ranging from a well-developed hair follicle to a basaloid keratotic tumor, closely resembling a basal cell carcinoma. Cylindromas and syringomas may be seen in the same patient. Usually, multiple trichoepitheliomas are only a severe cosmetic problem, but some may behave clinically as basal cell carcinomas.

A solitary trichoepithelioma is trouble for two reasons: (1) it may be the first stigmata of MT, and (2) it may be a basal cell carcinoma. In adults, a single trichoepithelioma should be treated as a basal cell carcinoma.

Haber's Syndrome

Haber's syndrome includes familial rosacea-like dermatitis associated with a variety of epidermal changes including keratinous cysts — epidermoid type, dilated hair follicles, and basal layer proliferation from the epidermis and appendages.[36] Few cases have been seen and the malignant potential of these changes is uncertain.

Porokeratosis

Porokeratosis is a histological diagnosis, referring to epidermal disorders displaying a cornoid lamella or column of parakeratosis over a damaged granular layer. While most cases appear to be sporadic, McKusick[37] catalogues porokeratosis of Mibelli (isolated lesions, either annular or linear), disseminated superficial actinic porokeratosis (multiple annular plaques on sun-exposed skin), and guttate disseminated porokeratosis (multiple lesions everywhere including palms and soles) as genodermatoses, inherited in autosomal dominant fashion.

Porokeratosis seems to be a clonal disturbance in the epidermis, caused by light, trauma, or genetic factors. In many forms of porokeratosis, both in situ and invasive squamous cell carcinomas have been reported.[38] I have seen porokeratosis of Mibelli in renal transplant patients suggesting that immune suppression may reduce surveillance of abnormal epidermal clones, leading to their proliferation and expression.

Hyperkeratosis Lenticularis Perstans (HLP; Flegel's Disease)

Hyperkeratotic papules are found on the lower leg and dorsum of foot in HLP. Histologically, there is marked localized hyperkeratosis over an atrophic epidermis, often with a band-like dermal lymphocytic infiltrate. Many hyperkeratotic acral papules could fit this rather nonspecific description. HLP lesions lack Odland bodies, keratinocytic organelles which may release phospholipids to form the physiologic water barrier.[39] In one family with HLP, numerous skin cancers appeared, unrelated spatially or temporally to the hyperkeratotic plaques.[40]

PIGMENTARY CHANGES

Hyperpigmented Lesions

Skin acquires pigment because the melanocytes manufacture melanin, package it in melanosomes, and transfer it to keratinocytes.

Despite a number of confusing names and descriptions, there are basically three ways in which skin can be hyper-pigmented:

1. Increased amount of melanin
2. Increased number of melanocytes
3. Other cells (nevus cells, dermal nevus cells, melanoma cells) or materials (tattoos)

The melanin system can be studied histologically by:

1. Routine HE: melanocytes – clear cells in basal layer; melanin – fine brown granules in keratinocytes and macrophages
2. DOPA incubation of fresh skin: melanocytes with functioning enzyme system identified
3. Electron microscopy: melanosome morphology and location assessed

The foremost question in evaluating pigmented lesions concerns malignancy. Is this a malignant melanoma or is it likely to become one? Most malignant melanomas are sporadic and may be light induced; some pedigrees, however, show autosomal dominant inheritance of atypical moles (nevocytic nevi) which seem to have a high malignant potential. These familial melanoma pedigrees are discussed in Chapter 9. Xeroderma pigmentosa patients also develop multiple malignant melanomas. The dermatopathologist can help identify such patients by being alert to multiple atypical nevi and malignant melanomas in a single patient or given family.

Both congenital hairy nevi and cerebriform intradermal nevi associated with cutis verticis gyrata[41] may turn into malignant melanoma; evidence for a pattern of inheritance of either of these conditions is weak, and they will not be further considered.

The café au lait spot is a benign tan macule which has attracted the attention of dermatologists and geneticists for years. The challenge is to diagnose neurofibromatosis on the basis of café au lait spots. The number (greater than six), size (greater than 1.5 cm), and shape (relatively smooth border)[42] are used to separate the café au lait spots in NF from similar lesions in other conditions. In addition, multiple tiny tan macules in the axilla (axillary freckles) strongly suggest NF.

A café au lait or axillary freckle is far less specific histologically than clinically. Both may show increased amounts of melanin and/or increased number of melanocytes. Benedict et al.[43] used electron microscopy to identify giant melanosomes in both the café au lait spots and the normal skin of patients with NF.

Table 4-1 shows the other diseases where café au lait spots may be seen; it is only a partial list to demonstrate several points: (1) many conditions have café au lait spots, (2) all the conditions besides NF have other distinguishing features; (3) a normal person may have one or two café au lait spots. If he has several and appears otherwise normal, a lesion should be biopsied to look for giant melanosomes.

Table 4-2 lists a few of the conditions in which giant melanosomes have been found.[44,45] There is surprisingly little overlap between the two lists, but this most likely means that most cafe au lait spots associated with rare genodermatoses have not been studied for giant melanosomes. If a patient is clinically suspicious for NF and has giant melanosomes, he probably has NF. In Benedict's work,[43] 19 of 19 patients with NF had giant melanosomes while only one of 10 with Albright's showed them. However, some patients with NF do not have giant melanosomes.[46]

Another cause of confusion is nevus spilus; a single tan macule may be called nevus spilus even though it appears identical to a café au lait spot. Some consider nevus spilus a café au lait spot with tiny areas of more intense pigmentation.

Table 4-1. Clinical Conditions in which Café au Lait Spots May Be Seen.

Neurofibromatosis
Albright syndrome
Bloom syndrome
Xeroderma pigmentosum
Ataxia telangiectasia
Sturge-Weber syndrome
Basal cell nevus syndrome
Tuberous sclerosis
Dyskeratosis congenita
Fanconi anemia
Normal patients

Table 4-2. Pigmented Lesions Which May Have Giant Melanosomes on Electron Microscopy.

Neurofibromatosis
Albright syndrome
Chediak-Higashi syndrome
Tinea Versicolor
Nevocytic Nevi
Lentigo
Leopard syndrome
Nevus spilus
Normal skin

It is not important what one calls a single lesion; if multiple tan macules are present, NF should be suspected.

Café au lait spots may have an increased number of melanocytes but they usually show only an increased amount of melanin. The lentigo always has an increased number of melanocytes. Two genodermatoses with lentigines are Peutz-Jeghers[47] syndrome with perioral and acral lentigines and leopard[48] syndrome which as the name implies also has mulitple lentigines. Surprisingly, in both Peutz-Jeghers and leopard syndrome, nevocytic nevus cell nests have been seen in the larger lentigines.

Hypopigmented Lesions

Hypopigmented macules are another lesion intimately related to a common cancer-associated genodermatosis. The "ash leaf" macules (which are often not shaped like an ash leaf) are most often the earliest sign of tuberous sclerosis. Just as with cafe au lait spots, the clinical diagnosis is more helpful than a biopsy. Almost every person with TS, when examined carefully, with a Wood's light when needed, will have at least one hypopigmented macule. About 50% of TS patients will have more than five hypopigmented macules. More than one such lesion in an otherwise normal patient should still raise suspicion of TS.

In evaluating hypopigmented lesions histologically one must decide if melanocytes are absent or if melanin production is abnormal or nonexistent. Routine H & E sections may allow this distinction. In vitiligo and piebaldism, melanocytes are absent, but they are present in albinism and TS. Since melanocytes are present, one must check their ability to make melanin. In albinism, they lack a variety of enzymes essential to melanogenesis. A transfer block, preventing the transfer of melanosomes from melanocytes to keratinocytes, is the defect in nevus depigmentosus. The melanosomes may be too large, too small, abnormally grouped, or otherwise changed. In TS, the melanosomes are small and poorly pigmented.[49,50]

Diffuse Pigmentary Changes

Colors can range from pure white in albinism to very dark in hemachromatosis; they can be uniform or mottled and poikilodermatous (having hypo- and hyper-pigmentation) as in xeroderma pigmentosun, Fanconi anemia, and dyskeratosis congenita. Using the principles discussed under hyper- and hypopigmented lesions, one can evaluate these diffuse, varied changes. In most of the poikilodermas, the histopathology is not especially helpful. There is an atrophic actinically damaged epidermis, with epidermal-dermal junction damage disrupting melanocyte function and causing incontinence of pigment.

In Chediak-Higashi syndrome, which is an alleged variant of albinism, the skin is not truly white but more cream to light grey. Electron microscopy reveals giant melanosomes which apparently are not transferred properly into keratinocytes. Leukocytes also have azurophilic granules which interfere with their mobility and phagocytic ability. These granules may be found in other organ systems.[51] Thus, pathology can be most helpful in identifying this syndrome with its risk of recurrent infections and lymphoreticular cancer.

A final example of the use of pathology in studying hyperpigmentation can be drawn from hemochromatosis. These patients are identified by measuring serum iron, iron-binding capacity, and ferritin. The pigmentation of hemochromatosis is a "double whammy." Iron is clearly the main systemic problem: the entire dermis is full of iron which can be identified with special stains. Melanin appears in the upper dermis, as apparent postinflammatory hyperpigmentation. Yet melanin, not iron, causes the color. Patients with hemochromatosis and vitiligo have white spots even though the pale area is rich in iron.[52] Despite the fact that a biopsy is unnecessary in hemochromatosis, it surely opens a window on an unexplained interplay between iron and melanin.

Cutaneous Malignancies in Genodermatoses

Some cutaneous genodermatoses have lesions which are not intrinsically malignant, but tend to undergo malignant degeneration. I will attempt to group them in a speculative fashion.

Benign nongenetic hyperkeratotic lesions such as calluses, scars, and old draining sinuses have a tendency to develop squamous cell carcinomas (SqCCs). In several genodermatoses, this pattern is repeated. But there are also many hyperkeratotic conditions where malignant degeneration is rare. I suspect that the genetic makeup of the lesion has far more say about malignancy than does trauma. Patients with dyskeratosis congenita and Fanconi syndrome have marked leukokeratosis and may develop SqCCs. At least one unusual variant of ichthyosis also seems to be at risk for early development of SqCCs.[53] In hidrotic ectodermal dysplasia, pachyonychia congenita, and Rothmund-Thompson syndrome, the hyperkeratotic lesions may also evolve into SqCCs.

Sunlight is an important cocarcinogen in many genodermatoses. The countless photodermatoses show varying degrees of susceptibility to sunlight, ranging from xeroderma pigmentosum, where UV radiation leads to all types of skin cancers at an early age, to congenital lupus erythematosus where sun-induced lesions are at a small risk of milignant change. Another example is cheilitis glandularis where patients develop actinic damage and SqCCs on their protruding lips.[54]   The cheilitis in hereditary polymorphous light eruption of North American Indians is not premalignant, however.[55]

Another unusual condition is epidermolysis bullosa (EB), where the dystrophic variants are at considerable risk of developing squamous cell carcinoma (Figure 4-9).[56]   Since EB dystrophica (recessive) patients seem at far greater risk than EB dystrophica (dominant), it is valuable to pursue all procedures which may differentiate the two. Electron microscopy may help, as some authors feel the nature of the subepidermal anchoring fibril defect is different in the two forms. Why should a defect below the epidermal-dermal junction so predispose to epidermal (i.e., SqCC) cancer? Probably the scarring unifies EB with the hypertrophic premalignant diseases.

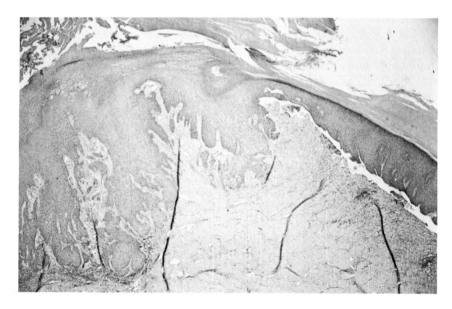

Figure 4-9. Squamous cell carcinoma (SCC) arising in recessive dystrophic epidermolysis bullosa (EB). On the left there is epidermal proliferation with atypical keratinocytes invading the dermis, representing a SCC. On the right, the acanthotic epidermis lies separate from the bulk of the dermis because of the EB (H & E, 30×). *(Histological material courtesy of Charles Palmer, M.D., Albuquerque, NM)*

A final group consists of those in which poor control of a virus seems to be the problem.[57]   Jablonska et al.[58] have recently subdivided epidermodysplasia verruciformis (EDV) into two groups, caused by two subvariants of the human wart virus.   One type tends to get cutaneous cancer in their warty lesions while the other does not.   Jablonska[59] has also shown that the papovavirus is easier to identify in the benign lesions than in those which have undergone malignant transformation.   The dermatopathologist can be of considerable help in diagnosing EDV and in assessing malignant change.   The original lesions are identical to plane warts, while a gradual progression can be seen to frankly invasive SqCC (Figure 4-10).

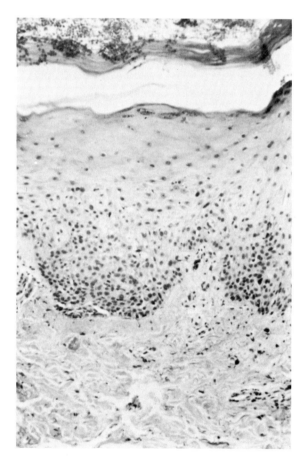

Figure 4-10 (A). This shows acanthosis and some epidermal disarray with insufficient granular layer changes to still suggest verruca plana.

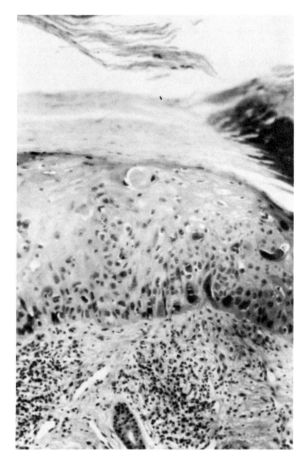

Figure 4-10 (B). This picture simply provides a transition to the highly malignant squamous cell carcinoma in situ.

EDV represents a defective response to a viral subtype; in other conditions, impaired immunity results in abnormal protection against many different organisms. Patients with DiGeorge's syndrome have reduced T-lymphocyte function; multiple SqCCs of the upper respiratory tract occurred in such a patient.[60] Abels and Reed described the Fanconi-like syndrome with pancytopenia, immunologic deficiencies, and multiple SqCCs.[61] Similarly oral and genital SCC in true Fanconi syndrome and the verrucous oral carcinomas in dyskeratosis congenita could represent unchecked human wart virus infection. It is unclear if such cancers truly represent impaired viral surveillance and malignant transformation or if they are simply another variation on trauma. In chronic mucocutaneous candidiasis, the hypertrophic oral infections may develop into cancers with no sug-

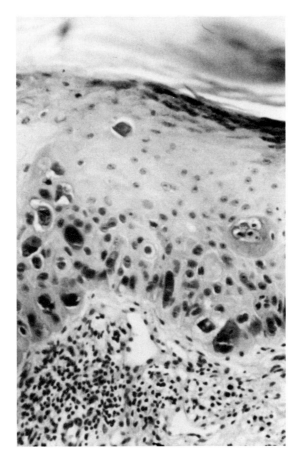

Figure 4-10 (C).   Many bizarre keratinocytes can be seen (H & E, 300X [A, B]. 500X [C]).
(Photomicrographs courtesy of Franklin Pass, M.D., Minneapolis, MN)

Figure 4-10.   These three views show the progression in epidermodysplasia verruciformis from a normal papule to a highly atypical intraepidermal carcinoma:

gestion that *Candida albicans* can transform cells.[62]   Finally, no matter what causes the tumors, reduced immunity may favor their spread.

Vascular Lesions

The categorization of cutaneous vascular lesions is no less confusing histologically than it is clinically.   However, several of the genodermatoses with vascular lesions are often biopsied and it behooves one to appreciate their features.

I consider three types of congenital hemangiomas:

1. Nevus flammeus — capillary dilation and/or hyperplasia associated with clinical port-wine stains, Sturge-Weber syndrome, and Klippel-Trenaunay syndrome
2. Capillary hemangioma — common strawberry hemangioma, consisting of many proliferative anastomosing vessels, often similar to a pyogenic granuloma, not associated with any genodermatoses
3. Cavernous hemangioma — large dermal and subcutaneous mass of mature vessels with endothelial lining and fibrous stroma; these hemangiomas are associated with two cancer-associated genodermatoses: blue rubber bleb nevus syndrome and Maffucci's syndrome

These can usually be separated clinically, but a biopsy should also help. There can be overlaps, with large thickened vessels occasionally seen with nevus flammeus or proliferative elements found near large vessels in cavernous hemangiomas, but the named feature should dominate.

There are two proliferative aspects of vascular tumors about which one must be warned. Any vascular lesion can show endothelial proliferation, with protrusion of cells into the lumen. These are seen in both Maffucci's syndrome and blue rubber bleb nevus syndrome. Although other malignancies are associated with these syndromes, the vascular lesions are not premalignant. The second proliferation is the pseudo-Kaposi sarcoma seen in the angiodermatitis of arteriovenous bypass.[63] Reddish nodules accumulate with vascular neogenesis and hemosiderin deposition, but no slits or atypical cells are seen.

Patients with congenital vascular or lymphatic disease of the extremities are at risk of developing the Stewart-Treves syndrome, or lymphangiosarcoma resulting from chronic edema. Nodules in such limbs should be biopsied promptly and a careful search made for anastomosing channels, Kaposi sarcoma-like areas, and atypical endothelial cells. The clinician should be aware of these possibilities and pursue all options until full clinicopathologic correlation has been obtained. Only in this way can the overdiagnosis of benign endothelial proliferations and the underdiagnosis of lymphangiosarcoma be prevented.

Another group of genodermatoses is associated with lymphomas rather than internal malignancy or skin cancer. These have been left for last because skin biopsy is least helpful in their diagnosis. They may also fit into the category of cancer caused by genetically impaired viral surveillance. Included in this group are Sjogren's syndrome, systemic lupus erythematosus, ataxia telangiectasia, Wiskott-Aldrich syndrome, Chediak-Higashi syndrome, and most of the other inherited immunodeficiencies. Systemic lupus erythematosus (LE) can be diagnosed by immunofluorescence examinations of normal skin for an LE band, while lip biopsy may show chronic lymphocytic inflammation about minor salivary glands in Sjogren's syndrome.

I would like to emphasize several points made in this chapter. First of all, dermatopathology can dramatically aid in diagnosing some important cancer-related genodermatoses, often long before the cancer itself becomes apparent. Two success stories of this decade are the diagnosis of Cowden's syndrome and glucagonoma syndrome on skin biopsies.

Secondly, an alert dermatopathologist can often use subtle clues, such as family association, age of patient, and multiplicity of lesions, to suggest multiple cancer syndromes like the basal cell nevus syndrome.

In addition, the dermatopathologist must be careful to not overinterpret single lesions. For example, a single innocent nevus spilus looks the same under the microscope as a café au lait spot from a neurofibromatosis patient and may even have giant melanosomes.

Finally, cancer markers are not always cancer markers. The best example is acanthosis nigricans which teaches several lessons. The clinical presentation is unique, while the histologic differential diagnosis may occupy several pages of a textbook. Acanthosis nigricans may be inherited and it may be a marker for malignancy, but it is almost never both inherited and a marker of malignancy in the same patient. Thus, as important as clinical correlation is in the daily practice of dermatopathology, it is even more important in the interpretation of rare, infrequently seen, and poorly understood genodermatoses associated with cancer.

REFERENCES

1. Bedi, T.R.: Familial congenital multiple seborrheic verrucae. *Arch. Dermatol.* **113**: 1441-1442, 1977.
2. Dantzig, P.I.: Sign of Leser-Trelat. *Arch. Dermatol.* **107**:902-905, 1973.
3. Schwartz, R.A., and Burgess, G.H.: Florid cutaneous papillomatosis. *Arch. Dermatol.* **114**:1803-1806, 1978.
4. Mikhail, G.R., Fachnie, D.M., Drukker, B.H., Farah, R., and Allen, H.M.: Generalized malignant acanthosis nigricans. *Arch. Dermatol.* **115**:201-202, 1979.
5. Kahn, C.R., Flier, J.S., Bar, R.S., Archer, J.A., Gorden, P., Martin, M.M., and Roth, J.: The syndromes of insulin resistance and acanthosis nigricans. Insulin-receptor disorders in man. *N. Eng. J. Med.* **294**:739-745, 1976.
6. Montes, L.F., Hirschowitz, B.I., and Krumdieck, C.: Acanthosis nigricans and hypovitaminosis A. Response to topical vitamin A acid. *J. Cutaneous Path.* **1**:88-94, 1974.
7. Brownstein, M.H., Mehregan, A.H., Bikowski, J.B., Lupulescu, A., and Patterson, J.C.: The dermatopathology of Cowden's syndrome. *Br. J. Dermatol.* **100**:667-673, 1979.
8. Ackerman, A.B.: Trichilemmoma. *Arch. Dermatol.* **114**:286, 1978.
9. Leppard, B.J., Sanderson, K.V., and Wells R.S.: Hereditary trichilemmal cysts: Hereditary pilar cysts. *Clin. Exp. Dermatol.* **2**:23-32, 1977.
10. Gardner's Syndrome. In: *Soft Tissue Tumors: Proceedings of the Thirty-ninth Annual Anatomic Pathology Slide Seminar* (discussed by F.M. Enzinger; W.H. Hartman, Ed.). ASCP, 1975, pp. 91-96.

11. Torre, D.: Multiple sebaceous tumors. *Arch Derm.* 98:549–550, 1968.
12. Houshoider, M.S., and Zeligman, I.: Sebaceous neoplasms associated with visceral carcinomas. *Arch. Dermatol.* 116:61–64, 1980.
13. Lynch, H.T., Lynch, P.M., Pester, J., and Fusaro, R.M.: The Cancer Family Syndrome. *Arch. Int. Med.* 141:607–611, 1981.
14. Boden, G., and Owen, O.E.: Familial hyperglucagonemia – an autosomal dominant disorder. *N. Engl. J. Med.* 296:534–538, 1977.
15. Binneck, A.N., Spencer, S.K., Dennison, W.L., Jr., and Horton, E.S.: Glucagonoma syndrome. Report of two cases and literature review. *Arch. Dermatol.* 113:749–754, 1977.
16. Kahan, R.S., Perez-Figaredo, R.A., and Neimanis, A.: Necrolytic migratory erythema. Distinctive dermatosis of the glucagonoma syndrome. *Arch. Dermatol.* 113: 792–797, 1977.
17. Swenson, K.H., Amon, R.B., and Hanifin, J.M.: The glucagonoma syndrome. A distinctive cutaneous marker of systemic disease. *Arch. Dermatol.* 114:224–228, 1978.
18. Holm, T.W., Prawer, S.E., Sahl, W.J., Jr., and Bart, B.J.: Multiple cutaneous neuromas. *Arch. Dermatol.* 107:608–610, 1973.
19. Ackerman, L.V., and Rosai, J.: *Surgical Pathology* (5th ed.). St. Louis, MO: C.V. Mosby, 1974, p. 1131.
20. Allen, J.C., Eldridge, R., and Young, D.: Early-onset acoustic neuroma: genetic, clinical and nosologic aspects. *Birth Defects: Original Article Series.* 10(10): 171–184, 1974.
21. Fabricant, R.N., Todaro, G.J., and Eldridge, R.: Increased levels of a nerve-growth-factor cross-reacting protein in "central" neurofibromatosis. *Lancet.* I:4–7, 1979.
22. Ackerman, A.B., and Kornberg, R.: Pearly penile papules. *Arch. Dermatol.* 108: 673–675, 1973.
23. Bhawan, J., and Edelstein, L.: Angiofibromas in tuberous sclerosis: a light and electron microscopic study. *J. Cut. Path.* 4:300–307, 1977.
24. Howel-Evans, W., McConnell, R.B., Clarke, C.A., and Sheppard, P.M.: Carcinoma of the oesophagus with keratosis palmaris et plantaris (tylosis): a study of two families. *Quart. J. Med.* 27:413–430, 1958.
25. Parnell, D.D., and Johnson, A.M.: Tylosis palmaris et plantaris. Its occurrence with internal malignancy. *Arch. Dermatol.* 100:7–9, 1979.
26. Millard, L.G., and Gould, D.J.: Hyperkeratosis of the palms and soles associated with internal malignancy and elevated levels of immunoreactive human growth hormone. *Clin. Exp. Dermatol.* 1:363–368, 1976.
27. Birt, A.R., Hogg, G.R., and Dube, W.J.: Hereditary multiple fibrofolliculomas with trichodiscomas and acrochordons. *Arch. Dermatol.* 113:1674–1677, 1977.
28. Hornstein, O.P., and Knickenberg, M.: Perifollicular fibromatosis cutis with polyps of the colon: a cutaneointestinal syndrome sui generis. *Arch. Dermatol. Res.* 253: 161–175, 1975.
29. Summerly, R.: Basal-cell carcinoma. An aetiological study of patients aged 45 and under with special reference to Gorlin's syndrome. *Brit. J. Dermatol.* 77:9–15, 1965.
30. Viksnins, P., and Berlin, A.: Follicular atrophoderma and basal cell carcinomas. The Bazex syndrome. *Arch. Dermatol.* 113:948–951, 1977.
31. Curth, H.O.: The genetics of follicular atrophoderma. *Arch. Dermatol.* 114:1479–1483, 1978.
32. Smith, J.F.: A case of multiple primary squamous-celled carcinomata of the skin in a young man, with spontaneous healing. *Brit. J. Dermatol.* 46:267–272, 1934.
33. Smith, J.F.: Multiple primary, self-healing squamous epithelioma of the skin. *Brit. J. Derm. Syph.* 60:315–318, 1948.

34. Sommerville, J., and Milne, J.A.: Familial primary self-healing squamous epithelioma of the skin. *Brit. J. Derm. Syph.* 62:485-490, 1950.
35. Zelickson, A.S., and Lynch, F.W.: Electron microscopy of virus-like particles in a keratoacanthoma. *J. Invest. Derm.* 37:79-83, 1961.
36. Sanderson, K.V., and Wilson, H.T.H.: Haber's syndrome. Familial rosacea-like eruption with intraepidermal epithelioma. *Brit. J. Dermatol.* 77:1-8, 1965.
37. McKusick, V.A.: *Mendelian inheritance in man.* Baltimore, MD: The Johns Hopkins University Press, 1978, pp. 326-327.
38. Coskey, R.J., and Mehregan, A.: Bowen disease associated with porokeratosis of Mibelli. *Arch. Dermatol.* 111:1480-1481, 1975.
39. Frenk, E., and Tapernoux, B.: Hyperkeratosis lenticularis perstans (Flegel): biologic model for keratinization occurring in the absence of Odland Bodies? *Dermatologica* 153:253-262, 1976.
40. Beveridge, G.W., and Langlands, A.O.: Familial hyperkeratosis lenticularis perstans associated with tumors of skin. *Brit. J. Dermatol.* 88:453-458, 1973.
41. Orkin, M., Frichot, B.C., III, Zelickson, A.S.: Cerebriform intradermal nevus. A cause of cutis vericis gyrata. *Arch. Dermatol.* 110:575-582, 1974.
42. Crowe, F.W., and Schull, W.J.: Diagnostic importance of café au lait spots in neurofibromatosis. *Arch. Int. Med.* 91:758-766, 1953.
43. Benedict, P.H., Szabo, G., Fitzpatrick, T.B., and Sinesi, S.J.: Melanotic macules in Albright's syndrome and in neurofibromatosis. *JAMA* 205:618-626, 1968.
44. Konrad, K., Wolff, K., and Honigsmann, H.: The giant melanosome: model of deranged melanosome morphogenesis. *J. Ultrastruct. Res.* 48:102-123, 1974.
45. Weiss, L.W., and Zelickson, A.S.: Giant melanosomes in multiple lentigines syndrome. *Arch. Dermatol.* 113:491-494, 1977.
46. Silvers, D.N., Greenwood, R.S., and Helwig, E.B.: Café au lait spots without giant pigment granules. *Arch. Dermatol.* 110:87-88, 1974.
47. Bartholomew, L.G., Moore, C.E., Dahlin, D.C., and Waugh, J.M.: Intestinal polyposis associated with mucocutaneous pigmentation. *Surgery, Gynecology & Obstetrics* 115:1-11, 1962.
48. Voron, D.A., Hatfield, H.H., and Kalkhoff, R.K.: Multiple lentigines syndrome: case report and review of the literature. *Am. J. Med.* 60:447-456, 1976.
49. Tilgen, W.: Ultrastructure of white leaf-shaped macules in tuberous sclerosis. *Arch. Dermatol. Forsch.* 248:13-27, 1973.
50. Jimbow, K., Fitzpatrick, T.B., Szabo, G., and Hori, Y.: Congenital circumscribed hypomelanosis: characterization based on electron microscopic study of tuberous sclerosis, nevus depigmentosus and piebaldism. *J. Invest. Dermatol.* 64:50-62, 1975.
51. Zelickson, A.S., Windhorst, D.B., White, J.G., and Good, R.A.: The Chediak-Higashi syndrome: formation of giant melanosomes and the basis of hypopigmentation. *J. Invest. Derm.* 49:575-581, 1967.
52. Perdrup, A., and Poulsen, H.: Hemochromatosis and vitiligo. *Arch. Dermatol.* 90:34-37, 1964.
53. Senter, T.P.: Carcinoma in atypical ichthyosiform dermatosis. *Arch. Dermatol.* 115:979-980, 1979.
54. Schweich, L.: Diagnosis: Cheilitis glandularis simplex (Puente and Acevedo). *Arch. Dermatol.* 89:301-302, 1964.
55. Birt, A.R., and Hogg, G.R.: The actinic cheilitis of hereditary polymorphic light eruption. *Arch. Dermatol.* 115:699-702, 1979.
56. Reed, W.B., College, J., Jr., Francis, M.J.O., Zachariae, H., Mohs, F., Sher, M.A., and Sneddon, I.B.: Epidermolysis bullosa dystrophica with epidermal neoplasms. *Arch. Dermatol.* 110:894-902, 1974.

57. Prawer, S.E., Pass, F., Vance, J.C., Greenberg, L.J., Yunis, E.J., and Zelickson, A.S.: Depressed immune function in epidermodysplasia verruciformis. *Arch. Dermatol.* 113:495–499, 1977.

58. Jablonska, S., Orth, G., Jarzqbek-Chorzelska, M., Glinski, W., Obalek, S., Rzesa, G., Croissant, O., and Favre, M.: Twenty-one years of follow-up studies of familial epidermodysplasia verruciformis. *Dermatologica* 158:309–327, 1979.

59. Jablonska, S., Dabrowski, J., and Jakubowicz, K.: Epidermodysplasia verruciformis as a model in studies on the role of papovaviruses in oncogenesis. *Cancer Res.* 32: 583–589, 1972.

60. Tewfik, H.H., Ptacek, J.J., Krause, O.J., and Latourette, H.B.: DiGeorge syndrome associated with multiple squamous cell carcinomas. *Arch. Otolaryngol.* 103:105–107, 1977.

61. Abels, D., and Reed, W.B.: Fanconi-like syndrome. Immunologic deficiency, pancytopenia, and cutaneous malignancies. *Arch. Dermatol.* 107:419–423, 1973.

62. Richman, R.A., Rosenthal, I.M., Solomon, L.M., and Karachorlu, K.: Candidiasis and multiple endocrinopathy with oral squamous cell carcinoma complications. *Arch. Dermatol.* 111:625–627, 1975.

63. Earhart, R.N., Aeling, J.A., Nuss, D.D., Mellette, J.R.: Pseudo-Kaposi sarcoma. A patient with arteriovenous malformation and skin lesions simulating Kaposi Sarcoma. *Arch. Dermatol.* 110:907–910, 1979.

5
The Neural Crest, Its Migrants, and Cutaneous Malignant Neoplasms Related to Neurocristic Derivatives

R.J. Reed, M.D.

Introduction

The neural crest is derived from the neuroectoderm and has a separate brief existence.[1,2]   As a provisional embryonic depot, it is progressively depleted by emigration of its cells. The migrants influence the development and organization of embryonic tissue.[1-3] In part they lose their identity in an interplay with the invaded tissue, but some persist as specialized cells.[3] The neural crest has been identified as the source of cranial mesenchyme, Schwann cells, at least some neurocrine cells, sympathetic ganglion cells, and melanocytes.[1-5]

The migration of neurocristic cells is anticipated by a peculiar isolation of individual cells in a widened interstitial space. In their migration and differentiation, neurocristic cells are influenced in part by the matrix they invade[6] and by transient encounters with other cells.[3] Glycosaminoglycans and collagens are requisites for differentiation in some areas.[6] Although the basic phenotype may be determined prior to migration,[7] the bulk of the evidence indicates that the specific function of neurocristic cells is not predetermined.[8] The pluripotency of neurocristic cells[2] is variously expressed in tumorous dysplasias.[9]

In the cranium, neurocristic mesectodermal cells contribute to the mesenchyme.[4,5] In sites other than the cranium, the influence of migratory neurocristic cells on mesenchymal differentiation is not well defined. A cell, whose role is comparable to that of the cranial mesectodermal cell, has not been defined for the late developing somites. Neurocristic derivatives influence developing embryonic, mesenchymal cells, and many malignant schwannomas have mesenchymal qualities.[9] The evidence indicates a close relationship between mesenchyme and specialized tissues, presumed to be derived from the neural crest. It also suggests that neurocristic cells function as organizers which influence differentiation, maturation, and stabilization of the target organs.[3]

Dysplasias of neurocristic origin are characterized by tumorous malformations.[9] If the neurocristic influence on the development and organization of tissue is defective, the affected tissue is distorted in form and often grows at an increased or disproportionate rate.[10-16]   The abnormal growth continues after birth and results in alterations of form and, often, function.[9]   In aggregate, the distorted tissue qualifies as a tumorous dysplasia. The melanocytic nevi, plexiform neurofibromas, ganglioneuromas, and neuroblastomas are examples of tumorous dysplasias.[9]

In tumorous dysplasias, differentiation acquires prognostic significance. The more closely the morphology of the tumor approaches mature or postnatal tissue, the better the prognosis.   Conversely those tumorous dysplasias whose morphologic characteristics mimic embryonic tissue are likely to be characterized by aggressive local growth and often by metastases. A distinction should be made between malignant embryonic tumorous dysplasias of childhood, and mature tumorous dysplasias of adults that transform into malignant neoplasms. Neuroblastoma as a tumorous dysplasia has persistent embryonic qualities (arrested differentiation).   In primary or metastatic sites, it may mature into a ganglioneuroma.   Rarely, a mature ganglioneuroma may dedifferentiate into a neuroblastoma.   There is, however, the potential in an adult for a ganglioneuroma to transform into a malignant schwannoma.   Plexiform neurofibroma, as a mature tumorous dysplasia, is characterized by persistent local growth of relatively mature cellular components.   Its related malignant schwannoma usually has mesenchymal qualities[9] and is characteristically a complication of adult life.[17]

Neurocristopathies, APUD Cells, and Apudomas

The neurocristic migrant may effect tumorous dysplasias in diverse organs and of diverse cell types.   Some of the bewildering clinical patterns are embraced in syndromes such as the mucosal neuroma syndrome and neurofibromatosis. Neurocristic tumorous dysplasias are conceptually grouped under the term *neurocristopathies*.[18]   Many of the cells in neurocristic tumorous dysplasias share biochemical and ultrastructural features (amine content and/or amine precursor uptake and decarboxylation; APUD).[19-23]   Conceptually, tumorous dysplasias with APUD features are grouped under the term, apudomas.[21]   At the ultrastructural level, tumors in the neurocristopathies and the apudomas are composed of cells with characteristic, cytoplasmic vesicles.[21]   These dense cored vesicles are markers for neurocristic and APUD cells. The melanosome may represent a special evolution of the dense cored vesicle.

The concepts of neurocristopathies, the APUD system, and apudomas may be overly broad.   The basis for the expanded concept of neurocristopathies has been in large part inference and speculation.[24,25] Many APUD cells are more likely to be of endodermal than of neurocristic origin.[26] Not all apudomas are accepted as neurocristic tumorous dysplasias. Accepted neural crest derivatives are the sympathetic ganglion cells, melanocytes, paraganglionic chief cells, C cells of the thyroid, and Schwann cells. There are questions regarding the origin of Schwann cells.[27]

For the enterochromaffin system and the pancreatic islets, an origin from the neural crest has not been established.[25,26,28] In tumorous dysplasias, the enterochromaffin and the melanocytic systems share features. The parent cells contain distinctive cytoplasmic organelles. They reside at an epithelial-stromal interface, in a site ideally suited to mediate reactions between two units. In their postnatal migrations, they emigrate from epithelium into mesenchyme. In the latter location they form tumorous dysplasias and are neurotropic. If the enterochromaffin system is not of neural crest origin, an embryologic process in which cells sequester from a primary germ layer (endoderm?), proliferate as a separate embryologic structure, and later emigrate from the depot to repopulate a specific epithelium (i.e., pancreas, intestinal epithelium) should be anticipated. By interaction with mesenchyme and epithelium, the migrants should acquire specific characteristics at the termination of their journey. Such a locus which is depleted by emigration of undifferentiated cells has not been identified.

In a model system of migratory cells, the interplay between migrants, mesenchyme, and epithelium influences the characteristics of the migratory cells and the invaded mesenchyme.[29] In the development of the gonads, germ cells migrate from the yolk sac entoderm to their site of residence (genital ridge). In the chick, the migration is accomplished through the blood stream. The migration is terminated in an area in which coelomic (mesodermal) epithelium and the adjacent mesenchyme are hyperplastic. In the female, the migrants concentrate in cords of cells (granulosa cells) in the cortex of the developing ovary. In the male, they concentrate in cords of cells (Sertoli cells) in the medulla. The site of residence (medulla or cortex) influences, and is influenced by, the germ cells. The Leydig or theca cells are mesodermal in origin. The origin of the sex cords is controversial, but sex cord tumors in the adult are occasionally teratomatous.[30]

In summary, the ectoderm and endoderm have their distinctive systems in which migrants serve as organizers of mesenchyme, and influence the differentiation and maturation of the invaded tissue. In this context, the neurocristic cells are the ectodermal homologue of the endodermally derived germ cells. Perhaps the teratomatous potential of neurocristic cells in some tumorous dysplasias[9] is partially explained by "germ cell" qualities.

Ectopic Hormone Production

Ectopic production of hormones has been observed with tumors of the neurocristic and the enterochromaffin systems. For these two systems, overlap in specific ectopic hormones (i.e., ACTH) has been cited as supportive evidence for the common neuroectodermal origin of the two systems.[31] Other syndromes of ectopic hormone production are related to antidiuretic hormone, parathormone, gastrin, thyrotrophins, or gonadotrophins.[32]

Derepression of Gene Function and Tumors with Ectopic Hormone Production

Derepression of gene function has been offered as an explanation for syndromes in which hormones are produced ectopically by tumors.[32] For proponents of the concept, all malignant cells are totipotent with the capability to occasionally express the gene functions of specific endocrine cells. The category of tumors with ectopic production of ACTH can be divided into a carcinoid-oat cell (enterochromaffin) group and a pheochromocytoma-neuroblastoma (neurocristic) group.[30] If derepression of gene function plays a role in the pheochromocytoma-neuroblastoma group, it influences neurocristic derivatives. Derepression of gene function may play a role in these peculiar syndromes, but anomalous or ectopic production of hormones probably expresses the embryologic potential of specific neurocristic or enterochromaffin cells. Ectopic ACTH production by both neurocristic and enterochromaffin tumorous dysplasias may express a basic role in the body's economy. Is the pituitary the only normal source of corticotrophins, or are minute amounts occasionally contributed by other endocrine systems?

Oat cell carcinomas are prominent in the list of tumors which produce ectopic hormones.[31] The plasma membranes of tumor cells in oat cell carcinoma share some surface antigens with certain endodermally derived epithelial cells of the digestive tract and some with neurocristic cells (Schwann cells) of the peripheral nervous system.[33] The shared antigens do not resolve the dilemma of the embryologic source of the malignant cells. They may provide an explanation for the sensory neuropathy associated with some carcinomas of the lung.

Amyloid as a Stromal Marker for Cells with APUD Qualities

Stromal deposits of amyloid characterize some of the visceral tumors in neurocristic syndromes.[9] The deposits apparently represent the extracellular accumulation of secretory products (peptides).[34] They are characteristic of medullary carcinoma of the thyroid (Figure 5-1) but have been identified in other dysplasias such as paragangliomas and intestinal gangliocytic paragangliomas.[35] The amyloid (APUD amyloid) in neurocristic tumorous dysplasias differs from immuno-amyloid.[34]

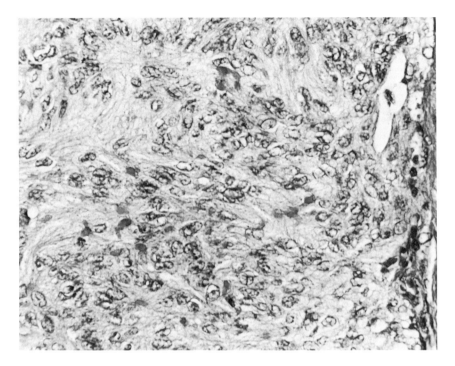

Figure 5-1. Spindle cells with intercellular deposits of amyloid characterize this medullary carcinoma of the thyroid (H & E).

Cutaneous Neurocristopathies: Inheritance and Potential for Malignant Transformation

Neurofibromatosis is an autosomal dominant trait[36] with a potential for malignant transformation of its tumorous dysplasias. Neurofibromas are multicellular in origin.[37]

The mucosal neuroma syndrome is an autosomal dominant trait.[36,38] A proclivity for malignant transformation of the true neuroma is not documented.

In the skin, neuroblastomas and ganglioneuromas are cutaneous metastases with rare exceptions.

If tuberous sclerosis has neurocristic qualities, its cutaneous manifestations are benign hamartomas with no tendency for malignant transformation.[9] With the exception of hamartomas of the central nervous system, its tumoral, visceral lesions show little or no proclivity for malignant transformation. It is an autosomal dominant trait.[10,36]

Melanocytic nevi express a neurocristic dysplasia: they have a potential for malignant transformation.[39] The frequency with which melanocytic nevi become melanomas has not been defined. Melanocytic nevi, at least in some families, are manifestations of a genodermatosis, but studies relating the distribution and number of nevi to familial traits are not available. If attention is given to melanomas rather than melanocytic nevi, familial cases are documented. The familial atypical multiple mole-melanoma (FAMMM) syndrome is an autosomal dominant trait.[36]

The melanosis neurocutaneous syndrome is characterized by multiple cutaneous nevi and lentigines, and by meningeal melanosis and melanocytosis.[40] Its cutaneous and meningeal lesions have a potential for malignant degeneration. The congenital nevus of the garment or giant hairy type is a premalignant lesion.[41] It shares features with, or is one of the cutaneous manifestations of, the neurocutaneous melanosis syndrome. The giant hairy nevus is an autosomal dominant trait.[36]

Xeroderma pigmentosum is manifested in part by melanocytic hyperplasias, dysplasias, and melanomas.[42] It is an autosomal recessive trait[36] in which a genetic, enzymatic defect hampers repair of UV-induced alterations in DNA.[43] The basic defect does not reside solely in cells of neural crest origin.

Blastomas: Nuclear and Cytoplasmic Phases, Maturation and Retrodifferentiation, Fetal Antigens and Isoenzymes; Neuroblastoma and Related Tumors as a Model

Histologically, the extremes of cellular differentiation qualify as nuclear and cytoplasmic phases. In the nuclear phase, the cytoplasm is subservient to the needs of the nucleus. The cytoplasm is likely to be scanty, basophilic, and occasionally metachromatic. Specialization is not characteristic of the nuclear phase: all of the cells in the nuclear phase are relatively indistinguishable. The connective tissue expression of the nuclear phase is a mucinous matrix. The nuclear phase is adapted to rapid growth, a property expressed histologically by a high mitotic rate. Embryonic tissue is basically an expression of the nuclear phase.

In the cytoplasmic phase, the nucleus is subservient to the cytoplasm. Its functions are directed to the formation of genetically coded metabolic units. The metabolic units are transferred to the cytoplasm and incorporated into organelles. They directly determine the metabolic functions in the cytoplasm. Morphologically distinctive cytoplasmic features express the influence of nuclear-derived metabolic units. The cytoplasmic phase is one of cytoplasmic specialization: it finds expression in distinctive extracellular products, either secretions or supporting matrix. Mitoses are infrequent.

An intermediate phase combines the properties of the cytoplasmic and nuclear phases, but does not permit the full expression of either. It finds its counterpart in fetal tissues, in which a compromise is established between the need for rapid growth and the need for the formation of specialized cytoplasmic products.

These three phases find expression in tumorous dysplasias. If a tumorous dysplasia has embryonic qualities, it is a blastoma. Its cells have prominent hyperchromatic nuclei, large nucleoli, and scanty basophilic cytoplasm. They are rather uniformly undifferentiated: each cell resembles its neighbor. Mitoses are numerous. Matrix is scanty or mucinous.

In a tumorous dysplasia that is a grotesque distortion of adult tissue, the component cells are in a cytoplasmic phase. Cytoplasmic structures are distinctive for each cell line in the dysplasia. Mitoses are infrequent. Intermediate expressions in a tumorous dysplasia are likely to resemble fetal tissue.

A neuroblastoma is composed of cells in the nuclear phase. This blastomatous dysplasia may disseminate and rapidly destroy the host. There is, however, the potential for spontaneous regression of the primary tumor, a peculiar necrotizing and lytic process. A second alternative finds expression in a conversion of cells to a cytoplasmic phase, and the acquisition of fetal or adult properties. In a neuroblastoma the conversion may be expressed in varying degrees. The primary lesion or the metastases may undergo partial or complete regression, or partial or complete maturation. Metastases often show a synchronous pattern of maturation: different metastatic lesions are likely to be histologically indistinguishable.

Neuroblastomas in which foci of maturation clearly define the direction of differentiation are classified as differentiating neuroblastomas (Figure 5-2). A differentiating neuroblastoma has a significant potential for metastasis. Some lesions progressively differentiate into relatively mature tissue with random, small blastomatous foci. The potential for continued local growth is significant, but metastases are unlikely. Lesions in this category are classified as ganglioneuroblastomas or immature ganglioneuromas. As the final expression of maturation, a tumor is composed of disorganized but relatively mature tissue and, in the category of neuroblastoma, qualifies as a ganglioneuroma.

Sampling errors inherent in biopsy specimens make it difficult to exclude immature foci in large lesions that otherwise qualify as ganglioneuromas. In an occasional ganglioneuroma, the occult foci may offer an explanation for a reversion to a blastoma after years of stable quiescence. A less common path of malignant transformation is expressed by proliferation of ganglion cells and neoplastic spindle cells or Schwann cells. A lesion of the latter type qualifies as a malignant ganglioschwannoma (Figure 5-3).

Most neuroblastomas are derived from cells that were embryologically destined for the adrenal medulla. Peculiarly, the differentiating blastoma acquires ganglioneuromatous rather than chromaffin qualities. If a neuroblastoma is truly a dysplasia of precursory chromaffin cells, the latter cells and ganglion cells

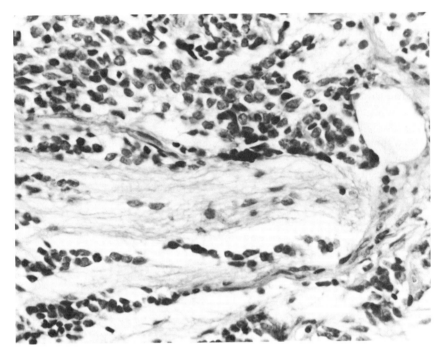

Figure 5-2. Three histologic features of a differentiating neuroblastoma are demonstrated: (1) septation, (2) a delicate mesh of fibrils, and (3) carrot-shaped nuclei with a cytoplasmic process from the pointed extremity (H & E).

must be close functional and embryologic relatives. The ganglion cell directs and limits its secretory product to its synapse. The adrenal medullary cell (chromaffin cell) liberates its secretory product into the blood stream. The blastoma and its relatives secrete amines that are metabolites of vasoactive amines.[44] Determinations of the metabolites are occasionally an aid in the diagnosis of neuroblastoma and in the anticipation of its clinical course.

The clinicopathologic concepts of nuclear and cytoplasmic phases find their counterparts in the G and S cycles of individual cells.[45] In a neoplastic system of cells, the nuclear phase corresponds to stem cells or retrodifferentiated cells, and the cytoplasmic phase to differentiated cells. The regressive steps in neoplastic retrodifferentiation are assumed to proceed in an orderly manner to recapitulate in reverse order the processes of embryonic and fetal differentiation.[44] In fact, most malignant tumors in adults do not acquire blastomatous qualities. They are composed of cells in which nuclear and cytoplasmic features are variously combined but disorganized. By the preservation of cytoplasmic proper-

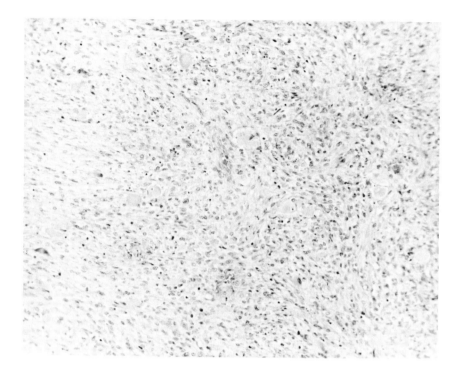

Figure 5-3. This mediastinal tumor is composed of spindle cells and irregularly distributed ganglion cells. It qualifies as a malignant ganglio-schwannoma. Intralesional transformation finds expression in neoplastic Schwann cells rather than retrodifferentiation to a neuroblastoma (H & E).

ties, we are able to classify tumors histologically as carcinomas or sarcomas and to qualify them as specific variants (i.e., adenocarcinoma, squamous cell carcinoma, rhabdomyosarcoma). In occasional cases, a distinctive pattern in a metastatic site provides a clue as to the site of the primary tumor. Invariably, histologic clues in the cytoplasm and in the extracellular matrix serve to distinguish a retrodifferentiated cancer cell from a malignant blast cell. A suppression or omission of cytoplasmic gene function does not adequately account for the histologic characteristics of most retrodifferentiated cancer cells. The simultaneous and disorderly expression of cytoplasmic and nuclear phases characterizes most patterns of malignant retrodifferentiation in the adult. Retrodifferentiation does account for the formation or release of embryonic or fetal antigens, isoenzymes, and cell coats from some malignant cells.[7,46,47]

The concepts of maturation and retrodifferentiation are intertwined with concepts of organizers whose evocators influence the development and maturation of tissue. The evocators have become morphogens. Cyclic AMP has been identified as a morphogen for neuroblastomas.[48]

Common Features of Immune-mediated Tumor Progression (Intralesional Malignant Transformation)

Many autosomal dominant disorders find clinical expression in tumorous dysplasias. In neurocristic tumorous dysplasias in the adult, a transformation to a malignant tumor characteristically is a slowly evolving phenomenon. Over a period of months and years, it is manifested by increasing cellularity, degrees of nuclear atypism, loss of overall symmetry, and mitotic activity. The malignant lesion may manifest fetal qualities, such as the mesenchymal properties of the malignant schwannoma, or may show anaplasia. A de novo malignant tumor is not characteristic of the malignant transformation of a neurocristic dysplasia.

The transformation to a malignant tumor is assumed to require at least two genetic "hits." In autosomal dominant dysplasias, the first hit is the expression of an inborn genetic defect. The second hit is an acquired alteration of the genome. A true blastoma may represent florid expression of the inborn hit: it is not comparable to a malignant tumor which evolves in an adult by intralesional transformation of a benign tumorous dysplasia. The two hit theory does not adequately account for the cytologic variability of melanocytic dysplasias and melanomas. The cytologic variability in the melanocytic neoplastic system suggests that multiple hits produce multiple clones of cells, some of which fail and regress, while others form the substrate for progressive intralesional transformations.

In our guidelines for malignant transformation of a neurocristic dysplasia, a role was developed for slowly progressive phenomena rather than de novo or spontaneous appearance of a malignancy in previously normal tissue. On this basis, three of the four accepted variants of cutaneous malignant melanoma show intralesional transformations[49] that may relate to processes in the transformation of familial melanocytic dysplasias. Clinicopathologic correlations form a basis for the classification of cutaneous melanomas,[50] but generally the malignant melanocyte expresses its embryologic heritage. The movement of the malignant melanocyte into connective tissue mimics the migration of its embryonic precursor from the neural crest into mesenchyme. The morphologic features of a malignant melanoma are an expression of the specific characteristics of the tumor cells and the host immune response.[51] Some melanomas have two distinct phases in their evolution. In the initial phase of growth, tumor cells are relatively protected in the epidermis. A population of dysplastic melanocytes in the epidermis is the source of the dysplastic dermal melanocytes. Migrants in the dermis are exposed to a hostile immune response. Many of the migratory cells succumb; those that survive are loosely aggregated and are isolated from neighboring nests by an inflamed fibrous matrix. In this initial phase, the host's immune response limits local growth in the dermis but allows tumor cells to proliferate and spread in the epidermis. This defines the radial growth phase[49] in biologic terms and expresses it in terms of host immune intolerance.[51] Tumor cells in the epidermis are relatively protected from the host immune response.

The altered relationship between the host and the tumor is manifested in the dermis by an active interplay between aggressive lymphocytes and target cells. The interplay is concerned with progressive-regressive phenomena and the emergence of immune tolerance. In the evolution of a melanoma, a change in the relationship between tumor cells and immune response finds expression in a significantly different pattern of growth. Tumor cells aggregate to form a nodule. The expanding nodule elevates the epidermis and deforms the interface between the papillary and reticular dermis. This pattern of growth defines the vertical growth phase in biologic terms: it qualifies as a phase of host immune tolerance.[51] Some melanomas bypass the phase of immune intolerance and from their inception form an expanding nodule. One additional feature relates to histologic patterns. Some melanomas, after a variable period of expansile growth in the papillary dermis, infiltrate the reticular dermis between collagen bundles. This infiltrating pattern relates in part to migratory habits of melanoma cells but, in some examples, correlates with a significant depression in host immune response, particularly cell-mediated immunity.[51]

Cutaneous Neurocristic Tumorous Dysplasias

In the skin, benign neurocristic tumorous dysplasias include:

1. Melanocytic nevi and lentigines
   a. Congenital
   b. Acquired
   c. Blue nevus
   d. Spindle cell nevus
   e. Neurocutaneous melanosis syndrome
2. Nerve sheath tumors
   a. Neurofibroma (solitary or plexiform)
   b. Schwannoma (rare in the skin)
3. True neuroma (composite nerve sheath and axonal tumor)

In tuberous sclerosis, the epidermal melanocyte seems to have a pivotal role in the evolution of the facial angiofibroma (adenoma sebaceum).[52] Although the evidence is indirect, the cutaneous lesions of tuberous sclerosis may qualify as neurocristic dysplasias. They include:

1. Angiofibroma
2. Connective tissue nevus (shagreen patch)

The malignant counterparts of the benign neurocristic tumorous dysplasias are:

1. Malignant melanoma (relationship of subvariants, with exception of giant hairy nevus, to reported cases of familial melanoma is not clearly defined)
   a. Superficial spreading melanoma
   b. Lentigo maligna melanoma
   c. Acral lentiginous melanoma
   d. Nodular melanoma
   e. Malignant cellular blue nevus (common expression of melanoma arising in giant hairy nevus)
   f. Malignant spindle cell nevus
   g. Melanoma of soft parts (clear cell sarcoma: neurocutaneous syndrome is not defined)
   h. Melanomas, not otherwise classified
2. Nerve sheath tumors
   a. Mesenchymal (fibroblastic, mixed mesenchymal, or teratoid), malignant schwannoma (usual expression of malignant transformation of plexiform neurofibroma)
   b. Protoplasmic malignant schwannoma
   c. Melanocytic malignant schwannoma (melanoma of soft parts: neurocutaneous syndrome is not defined)
   d. Neuroepithelioma (not related to neurocutaneous syndromes)
3. Composite nerve sheath and nerve cell tumors: neuroblastoma and its differentiated variants (cutaneous lesions are metastases)

The Melanogenic, Neurocristic Cell: Its Acquisition of Schwann Cell Qualities in Tumorous Dysplasias

Oncogenetic-ontogenetic speculations. Embryologically, dispersed neurocristic cells are likely to acquire melanocytic characteristics. Neurocristic cells in local aggregates are likely to show neuronal differentiation.[27] The melanocyte has APUD qualities.[23] In postnatal life in the skin, it resides in the basal portion of squamous epithelium. It may reside temporarily in the dermis. The mongolian spot is a clinical marker for a dermal population of melanocytes whose existence in the dermis is brief. The cellular blue nevus may represent a tumorous dysplasia of the transitory dermal melanocyte.[53] If the transitory dermal melanocyte has a role, it most likely is concerned with the differentiation and development of the dermis (i.e., the adventitial and reticular dermis as functioning units).

The melanocyte, in its benign, acquired tumorous dysplasias (nevi), recapitulates the functions of a migratory, neurocristic cell whose roles include the development of the dermis (transitory organizer) and pigmentation and metabolism of the epidermis (permanent resident). These capabilities are recapitulated in the differentiation of epithelioid nevus cells (postnatal, migratory melanocytes) and characterize the type A, B, and C nevus cells.[53] The type A melanocyte is gregarious and melanogenic. It clusters with its neighbors in rounded nests. The nests might be compared to the cellular aggregates in the neural crest. The type B cell is merely a transition phase between types A and C. The type C nevus cell shuns its neighbors and isolates itself in a fibrous matrix. It is dispersed, fibrogenic, and usually amelanotic. Generally, the epithelioid nevus cell is not both melanogenic and fibrogenic. Fibrogenesis is an expression of Schwann cell differentiation. The transformation of a melanogenic cell into a fibrogenic cell expresses the common embryonic heritage of the melanocyte and Schwann cell.[53] In embryonic development, the site of residence at the termination of the migration of the neurocristic, precursory cell determines the expression of one or the other of these potentials.[2] In postnatal migrations in the evolution of tumorous dysplasias, a specialized cell (melanocyte) reverts to a less differentiated state and acquires characteristics of its embryonic relative (Schwann cell).[53] The latter cells are generally not melanogenic, but are fibrogenic and have cholinesterase activity. The biphasic properties of the acquired nevus prompted Masson to propose a dual origin from melanocytes and Schwann cells.[54] In acquired nevi the migratory melanocyte moves into and expands the papillary dermis. A similar preference for the papillary dermis characterizes a long period in the evolution of superficial spreading malignant melanoma and in part expresses growth characteristics that are basic to the migratory, epithelioid melanocyte.[53] In the congenital nevus, melanocytes have a characteristic distribution in the reticular dermis.[55]

In the cellular blue nevus, a single cell line expresses melanocytic and schwannian characteristics.[56] The spindle, migratory melanocyte is commonly fibrogenic and melanogenic, and usually neuroid. In spindle cell nevi, the migratory cells commonly extend into the reticular dermis.[53] An understanding of the migrations of the spindle nevus cell is basic to an understanding of the evolution of spindle cell malignant melanomas. Many spindle cell melanomas induce relatively little stroma in the papillary dermis. Early in their evolution, tumor cells extend into the reticular dermis. Lentiginous patterns in radial growth components usually correlate with spindle cell patterns in vertical growth components. Spindle cell melanomas in a vertical growth phase are commonly neuroid. Their cells form elongated, neuroid fascicles, or they are desmoplastic. In the desmoplastic phase, individual cells are isolated in a stroma mediated in part by the tumor cells.[57] Neurotropism with invasion of nerve sheaths and endoneurial spaces is a common feature (Figure 5-4). Rarely does a desmoplastic melanoma

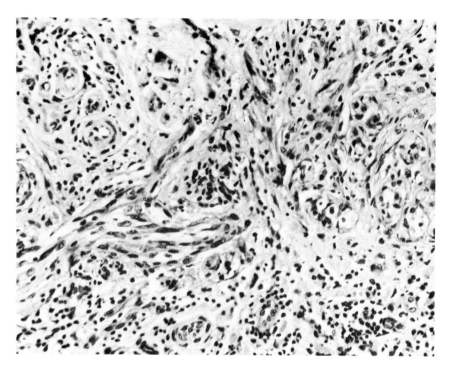

Figure 5-4. Fascicles of atypical spindle cells are cut in longitudinal and cross section. In this neurotropic melanoma, the tumor cells have acquired Schwann cell characteristics (H & E).

acquire distinctive neuroid features that simulate a traumatic neuroma.[58] In the latter type, rigid fascicles of spindle cells extend from involved nerves into adjacent soft tissue (Figure 5-5) and in some examples are accompanied by argyrophilic fibers that resemble axon cylinders. Lesions of this neuromatous type usually are preceded by a lentiginous melanocytic dysplasia, such as lentigo maligna (Figure 5-6). Minimal deviation melanomas[49] have been precursory lesions in a few examples. Rarely does the neuromatous pattern evolve de novo without a precursory melanocytic dysplasia. In the neurotropic or neuromatous melanoma,[58] the tumor cells have acquired Schwann cell characteristics, and some of the cells function as axon sheath cells (malignant neuroma or neuromatous melanoma).

The neurotropic melanoma is primarily a tumor of sun-exposed surfaces and fair-faced, elderly patients.[58] It has a distinctive clinical course characterized by local infiltrative growth and multiple local recurrences. There is a potential for dedifferentiation of tumor cells and progressive biologic aggression. Metastases to lymph nodes, or by way of the blood stream, are common late in the evolution

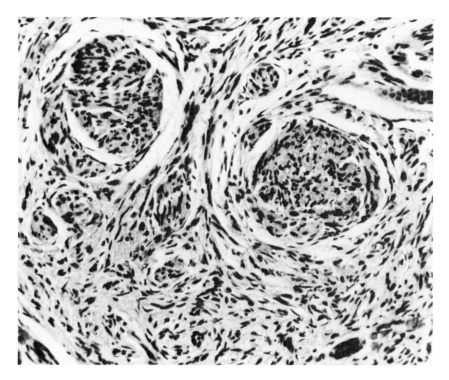

Figure 5-5. Tumor cells have infiltrated small peripheral nerves in this neurotropic melanoma (H & E).

of the tumor. The clinical course may also be determined by progressive local infiltration of soft tissues and extension into the cranial cavity.

Superficial Spreading Melanoma as a Model of Interactions between Target Cells and Host Immune Response

Superficial spreading melanoma[50] is the most common form of cutaneous malignant melanoma. Its vertical growth phase follows the radial growth phase by a period of months or years. Clinically, the radial growth phase is an irregular papule or plaque that is variegated brown or black, red, white, and blue. The vertical growth phase is a nodule within the papule or plaque.

Histologically, the radial phase (immune intolerance) is characterized by melanocytic dysplasia, epidermal hyperplasia, and host immune response.[49] The melanocytes are plump, often melanogenic, and actively migratory. They have round, hyperchromatic nuclei and prominent nucleoli. In their migrations in the epidermis, they are rounded and fill the space between neighboring keratinocytes.

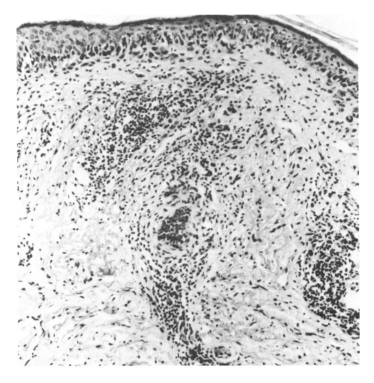

Figure 5-6. This precursory lesion of a neurotropic melanoma shows the pattern of lentigo maligna. A small infiltrated nerve is represented near the lower margin of the field (H & E).

In the basal portion of the epidermis, they form rounded nests that are irregularly distributed. Nests and individual tumor cells migrate into the papillary dermis. They are widely spaced and isolated in an inflamed, widened papillary dermis. The host immune response is cellular. It is composed of lymphocytes, histiocytes, and plasma cells. The inflammatory cells stimulate a fibrous matrix that resembles the stroma of the papillary dermis.

In the superficial spreading melanoma, the melanocytes often show regional variations in degrees of cytologic dysplasia.[49] Two phenomena determine the evolution of the radial component. The host immune response may succeed focally, or occasionally entirely, in the eradication of the offending population of melanocytes (regression).[49] Regression is seen histologically as a laminated fibrous scar in which the inflammatory infiltrate is variable and the dysplastic cells are reduced in number or destroyed (Figure 5-7). In the interplay between host immune response and dysplastic melanocytes, resistant clones of tumor cells may be selected. This change in tumor cells and in the effects of host immune response is manifested histologically by a significant change in growth patterns. Nests of tumor cells aggregate to form an expanding nodule in the pap-

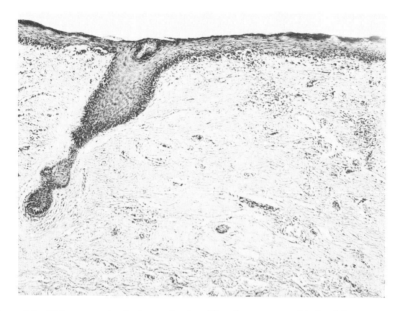

Figure 5-7. Melanocytes in the hyperplastic epidermis are arranged in lentiginous patterns. The papillary dermis is widened and fibrotic. There are patchy perivascular infiltrates of lymphocytes. The fibrous scar marks an area of regression in a superficial spreading malignant melanoma (H & E).

illary dermis (vertical growth phase, or initial immune tolerance). Within the expanding nodule, there are often two or more distinctive cytologic patterns, some of which may deviate minimally from a population of nevus cells.[49] In this initial phase of vertical growth or host immune tolerance, the cellular immune response is usually well developed. Focal or complete regression may occur.[49] If undisturbed by surgical intervention, superficial spreading malignant melanoma undergoes one additional biologic change. The growth pattern changes from an expansile nodule in the papillary dermis to diffuse infiltrates in the reticular dermis. This change in the biology of the tumor is accompanied by a significant depression of the cellular host immune response (final phase of host immune tolerance), and by cytologic uniformity in the infiltrating cells (selection of a single, aggressive clone). Spontaneous regression is uncommon in this phase.

Superficial Spreading Melanoma: Clinicopathologic Correlations

1. The radial growth phase is a melanocytic dysplasia rather than a malignant neoplasm: the tumor cells are susceptible to the host immune response. Metastases are unlikely in this evolutionary phase. If metastases

occur, they do not contradict the concept of melanocytic dysplasia. Carcinoma in situ of the uterine cervix is a severe dysplasia, and metastases are accepted as an occasional complication.

2. The clinical variation in surface colors relates to histologic patterns. The brown and black are related to viable, pigmented tumor cells. The red is related to inflammation and amelanotic tumor cells. The white and blue represent areas of partial or complete regression.

3. The three biologic stages relate directly to changes in the relationship between tumor cells and host immune response. They correlate with prognosis and are given recognition in Clark's levels of invasion. Level II invasion defines the phase of host immune intolerance. Level III invasion defines the initial phase of immune tolerance. Level IV invasion defines the final phase of immune tolerance. Level V invasion is simply an extension beyond an arbitrary anatomic boundary. It is a measure of increasing bulk rather than a change in the biology of the tumor.

4. The prognosis of a melanoma may be approached by a simple measurement of increasing bulk (Breslow[59]). A measurement of a lesion from the granular level of the epidermis to the deep margin of the tumor provides a guide to the prognosis. Increasing height correlates with a worsening prognosis. Therapeutically, a lesion measuring less than 0.75 mm in height is unlikely to metastasize. This measurement embraces most level II melanomas and a small percentage of level III melanomas. In the range of 0.75 to 1.50 mm, it is difficult to predict regional lymph node metastases. It has been recommended that prophylactic lymph node dissections are not indicated in this range.[59] For lesions greater than 1.50 mm there is a correlation between height and prognosis.

5. Nevus cell populations may provide a marker for a precursory tumorous dysplasia (nevus).[49]

Characterization of Radial Growth Component of Superficial Spreading Melanoma as a Melanocytic Dysplasia

In the radial growth phase of superficial spreading melanoma (phase of immune tolerance), metastases are unlikely. The radial growth phase qualifies as a premalignant dysplasia in which the epidermis and papillary dermis are the domain of the dysplastic cells. The premalignant dysplasia is defined by:

1. Variations in cytologic atypism
2. Occasional remnants of a nevus (nests of cells with nevus cell characteristics)
3. Infiltrates of lymphocytes and histiocytes
4. Intermingling of lymphoid cells (aggressor cells) and melanocytes (target cells)
5. Focal regression with laminated fibrosis of papillary dermis

6. Widely spaced nests of dysplastic cells and individual dysplastic cells in the papillary dermis

Definition of Premalignant Melanocytic Dysplasias

The six features that characterize the radial growth phase of superficial spreading melanoma define a premalignant melanocytic dysplasia. The halo nevus qualifies as a related process.[49]   The lesions in the B-K mole syndrome[60,61] and in the FAMMM syndrome[62] also qualify as premalignant melanocytic dysplasias. The latter two syndromes appear to be identical. For purposes of discussion they will be referred to as the *multiple nevi–familial melanoma* syndromes (MNFM). They embrace a group of familial cases with clinically abnormal moles.[60-62] With the passage of time, some of the moles show pigmentary changes and some are transformed into malignant melanomas. The peculiar moles, some of which are precursors of melanomas, show the histologic features of an atypical melanocytic dysplasia (Figures 5-8 through 5-10). They provide a link between nevi and melanomas, and a model for the evolutionary changes between the two. As a model, they offer guidelines for the interpretation of atypical dysplastic changes in acquired and congenital nevi. They also confirm the atypical, dysplastic qualities of the halo nevus[49] (Figures 5-10 and 5-11). They anticipate the occasional halo nevus that evolves into a melanoma (Figure 5-11).

The halo nevus generally is a symmetrical process, clinically and histologically. It has uniform, gradually sloping margins, and its halo is circumferentially symmetrical. The atypical nevus with significant degrees of melanocytic dysplasia is an asymmetrical process. The lesion is irregular in outline and pigmentation. Intraepidermal spread of dysplastic melanocytes away from the main portion of the lesion is a common histologic finding. A halo, if present, is irregular in outline at the periphery. Its outline is not uniformly related to the periphery of the atypical nevus. Symmetry characterizes the gross and histologic features of benign nevi and mild melanocytic dysplasias. Asymmetry characterizes moderate and marked melanocytic dysplasias.

Although basic reaction patterns are shared in the evolution of some familial melanomas and superficial spreading melanomas, fundamental questions remain unanswered. In the MNFM syndromes, are the nevus cells antigenically abnormal? Is the progression from genetically and antigenically abnormal nevus cells to melanoma cells the expression of genetically determined progressive changes, or do they reflect the clonal selection of precursory melanoma cells by the host's immune response?

Lentigo Maligna as a Model for the Influence of Environmental Factors on the Genetically Predisposed

Freckled skin qualifies as a defective covering with an unusual susceptibility to injury by sunlight. It is a racial defect, especially associated with Celtic descent.

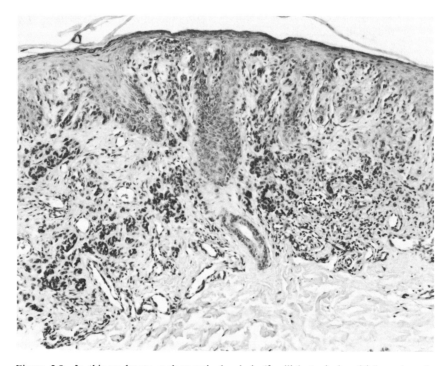

Figure 5-8. In this moderate, melanocytic dysplasia (familial atypical multiple mole-mela-noma syndrome), atypical melanocytes form rounded nests at the dermal-epidermal inter-face and in the widened papillary dermis. Some of the nests of cells are outlined by lami-nated fibrous tissue. The nests of cells are irregular in distribution (asymmetry). Melanocytes with nevus cell characteristics are clustered near the interface between the papillary and reticular dermis (H & E).

Actinically damaged, fair skin is afflicted by a variety of keratoses, carcinomas, and melanomas. One particular example, the lentigo maligna, is more or less peculiar to sun-damaged, fair skin. It qualifies as an actinic lentigo, and its inva-sive counterpart is lentigo maligna melanoma.[63] In history, Hutchinson's des-cription of the malignant freckle[64] anticipates much of the current information on the evolution of malignant melanoma. It clearly defines a premalignant lenti-go (radial growth phase) in which a melanoma (vertical growth phase) eventuates. Lentigo maligna shares with superficial spreading melanoma the features of progression-regression.[49] It has distinctive features in the radial growth phase and the vertical growth phase. In the epidermis, the dysplastic melanocytes are relatively confined to the basal portion (Figure 5-6). The epidermis is usually atrophic, rarely hyperplastic with elongated rete ridges. The dysplastic melano-

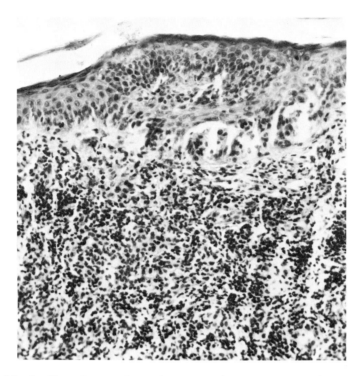

Figure 5-9. In this moderate melanocytic dysplasia (familial atypical multiple mole-melanoma syndrome), the changes simulate a halo nevus. Diffuse lymphoid infiltrates mask the melanocytic population in the dermis (H & E).

cytes show regional variations in atypism. Even neighboring melanocytes may show significant differences. The dysplastic melanocytes often have well-developed dendrites. They appear to lie within lacunae. If they form aggregates, the nests are oval with their long axis parallel to the surface of the skin. Host immune response in the papillary dermis is variable but often minimally developed. In the vertical growth phase, the melanocytes are commonly spindle cells. In the latter configuration, they rarely induce a significant amount of stroma in the papillary dermis to acquire the characteristics of polypoid level III invasion. The spindle cells usually extend into the reticular dermis (actinically damaged, elastotic dermis) early in the evolution of the vertical growth phase and may do so in the biologic radial phase (prior to the formation of an expansile nodule).

Lentigo maligna melanoma is a biologically indolent tumor. Metastases are infrequent[63] and do not relate closely to the prognostic indices of Clark or Breslow. The indolent behavior of lentigo maligna melanoma is not found in the lentiginous radial growth component or in the common spindle cell quality of

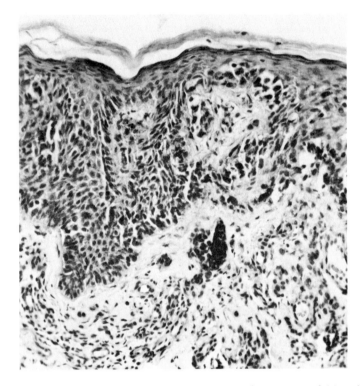

Figure 5-10. The laminated fibrous tissue which marks a focally successful host immune response outlines some of the elongated rete ridges (familial atypical multiple mole-melanoma syndrome). Dysplastic melanocytes are distributed in a lentiginous pattern in the epidermis (H & E).

the vertical growth component. Acral lentiginous melanomas share both features with lentigo maligna melanomas but at deep levels IV and V are fatal in 80% of the cases at five years.[65]

Nevus cell patterns are common in the dermis beneath lentigo maligna. They may provide a marker for the precursory melanocytic tumorous dysplasia.

Acral Lentiginous Melanoma as a Model for the Influence of Genetic Factors on the Distribution and Histologic Character of Cutaneous Melanoma

If lentigo maligna has special significance for the fair-complexioned patient, acral lentiginous melanoma has special significance for the black patient.[65] It is a paradox that melanomas in the Negro arise almost exclusively in nonpigmented atrichic areas such as the palms and soles, the subungual areas, and the mucous

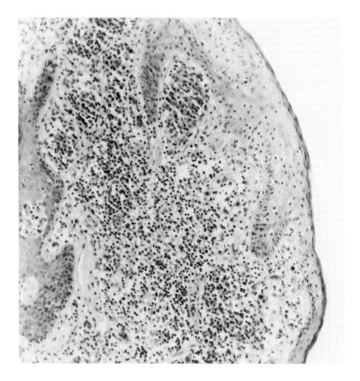

Figure 5-11. In this melanocytic lesion dysplastic melanocytes intermingle with lymphocytes. The tumor cells metastasized to regional lymph nodes. The lesion qualifies as a minimal deviation melanoma and is a histologic simulant of a halo nevus (H & E).

membranes.[65] The acral lentiginous melanoma may evolve for years in its radial growth phase (immune intolerance; Figures 5-12 and 5-13). In its vertical growth phase, it is usually a spindle cell tumor and commonly shows invasion to level IV or deeper. The suggestion that antimelanoma chalones are available in the pigmented skin but lacking in the amelanotic areas is interesting speculation.[66]

Xeroderma Pigmentosum as a Model for the Influence of the Environment and of a Genetic Defect on the Induction and Progression of Acquired Tumorous Dysplasias

Many autosomal recessive disorders are expressed at an enzymatic level. Xeroderma pigmentosum (XP) is an autosomal recessive, heritable disorder. It is manifested by defective, enzymatic repair of environmental damage to autosomal genes.[43] The damage is produced by exposure of the skin to UV light. The damaged, autosomal genes are not unique to XP; the defective repair of damaged

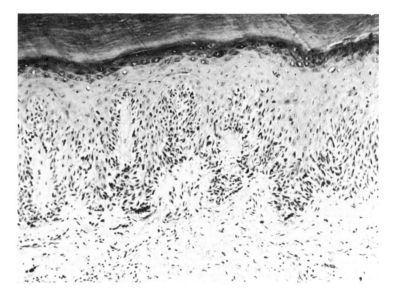

Figure 5-12. Lentiginous melanocytic dysplasia of the radial component of an acral lentiginous melanoma (H & E).

genes is unique. The genetic defects are mirrored in the formation of genetically determined, metabolic units. Histologically, the metabolic defects are correlated with acquired epithelial and melanocytic dysplasias and malignant neoplasms.[67] The cutaneous keratoses, carcinomas, lentigines, and melanomas, which involve the sun-damaged, fair skin of elderly Celts, also involve the skin in XP, but they do so with an alarming incidence, and at a disturbingly early age. In XP, as in the fair-complexioned, elderly Celt, the damage to exposed cells is indiscriminate: ectodermal as well as neural crest derivatives are affected. The genetic defect is clinically manifested by acquired, cellular dysplasias. Protection of the patient from UV irradiation will prevent the dysplasias and malignant neoplasms, but it does not correct the basic defect.

XP as a model for the effects of UV irradiation on the skin provides evidence that damage to the epidermis and melanocytes is the primary carcinogenic response. The connective tissue also is damaged, but its role as a primary determinant in cutaneous carcinogenesis is doubtful.

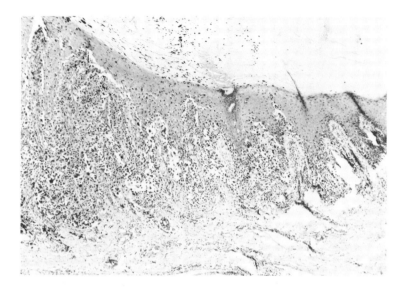

Figure 5-13. Progressive dysplasia from the periphery of a lesion (*right*) to the center of a lesion (*left*) characterizes the radial component of acral lentiginous melanoma (H & E).

The Congenital Nevus as a Model for Intralesional Transformation of a Congenital Tumorous Dysplasia

The congenital nevus is clinically evident at birth or shortly thereafter.[55] Its clinical features are variable; they are best displayed in the clinical setting of the giant hairy (garment, or bathing trunk) nevus. The latter lesion is a large, pigmented nevus that may also be hairy. It is commonly accompanied by multiple small nevi and lentigines. Histologically, the congenital nevus is characterized by periappendageal accumulations of epithelioid nevus cells and by thin rows of similar nevus cells between collagen bundles of the reticular dermis[55] (Figure 5-14). Other patterns include compound nevus (nests of nevus cells at the dermal-epidermal interface and in the papillary dermis) and blue nevus. The small epithelioid cells that are distributed in the reticular dermis are distinctive; they provide a marker for small congenital nevi that are otherwise difficult to distinguish clinically from acquired nevi.[55]

The characteristic histologic patterns of a congenital nevus are common beneath, and adjacent to, nodular melanomas and superficial spreading melanomas. In most melanocytic dysplasias (atypical hyperplasias), remnants of a benign nevus are a requisite for diagnosis. Their prevalence in melanocytic dysplasias

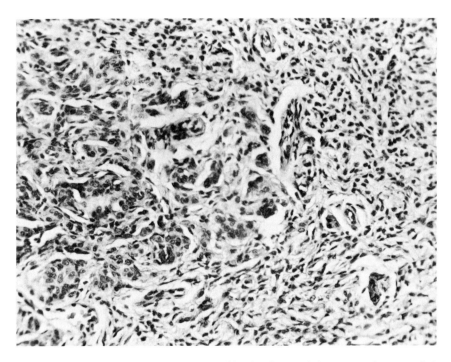

Figure 5-14. *right*: Nevus cells are arranged in the characteristic pattern of a congenital nevus in an infant. *left*: Moderately dysplastic melanocytes form nests and fascicles (H & E).

implicates congenital nevi of both the giant and the small varieties and acquired nevi as common precursory lesions of melanoma.

The incidence of melanoma in a giant hairy nevus is not defined. It has been estimated to be 13%.[68] The latter figure is derived from reported cases and is undoubtedly too high. On the basis of statistical predictions, the estimated incidence is 6%.[41] In the Negro, the melanoma arising in a giant hairy nevus is an exception to the preferential localization of melanomas to amelanotic areas.

The *neurocutaneous melanosis syndrome* is related to the congenital giant hairy nevus syndrome.[69] Its cutaneous manifestations have features of the giant hairy nevus. Rarely is the cutaneous lesion a peculiar blastoma containing primitive small cells, ganglion cells, and melanocytes[69] (Figures 5-15 and 5-16). In the central nervous system the lesions are confined to the pia-arachnoid and the perivascular spaces. They consist of melanocytes and clusters of melanophages. In infancy, hydrocephalus is a complication. Leptomeningeal and cutaneous melanomas are additional complications. The blastomas are conceptually, but not biologically, related to the melanotic neuroectodermal tumor of infancy.[70]

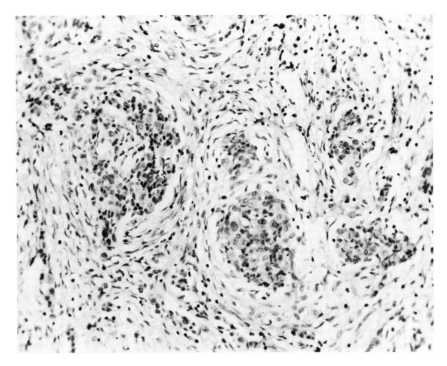

Figure 5-15. Neuroid fascicles with small dark and large pale cells are supported by a fibrous matrix (neurocutaneous differentiating melanoblastoma) (H & E).

The melanomas which complicate giant hairy nevi in infancy are peculiar. They have blastomatous qualities and deserve recognition as melanoblastomas.

In the adult, the melanomas arising in giant hairy nevi qualify as nodular or superficial spreading variants. They characteristically evolve through stages of progressive dysplasia in which the host's immune response plays a significant role.

Histologically, congenital nevi commonly show dysplastic changes. In the papillary dermis, a dysplasia is manifested by abnormal clusters of cells (abnormal in size and distribution) and by cytologic atypism. Within the abnormal aggregates, the cells show variations in nuclear size and staining. Mitoses may be occasional features. Often in an adult, the dysplastic changes are accompanied by a host immune response (lymphoid infiltrates and focal regression with lamellar fibrosis of the papillary dermis). This superficial form of melanocytic dysplasia produces widening of the papillary dermis (elevation of the skin surface) and irregularities in the contour at the surface (papillomatosis). The lesion may persist for months or years in this borderline phase and may manifest its potential by multiple local recurrences. If undisturbed, it may evolve into a malignant mela-

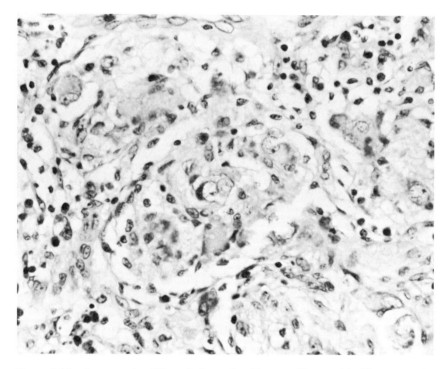

Figure 5-16. In areas, the differentiating melanoblastoma illustrated in Figure 5-15 has ganglioneuromatous qualities. Ganglion cells are supported by a vacuolated matrix (H & E).

noma. The changes are similar to those seen in the precursory lesions in the familial melanoma syndrome.

The second or blastomatous form of intralesional malignant transformation involves the melanocytic population in the reticular dermis. The blastomatous melanocytes commonly acquire spindle cell qualities but may be epithelioid. They may or may not be melanogenic. If the cells are spindle shaped, they demonstrate many of the qualities of a blue nevus but form disorganized patterns and are cytologically atypical. Mitoses are a common feature. The tumor cells have dense nuclear membranes and are supported by a mucinous matrix (Figure 5-17). They evolve from dysplastic cells without a significant interplay with the host's immune response. Lymphoid infiltrates are inconspicuous. In melanoblastomas of infancy, it is difficult to correlate the atypical changes with biologic aggression. Adequate local excision is recommended. Lymph node dissections in infants are of questionable value unless the lymph nodes are clinically involved.

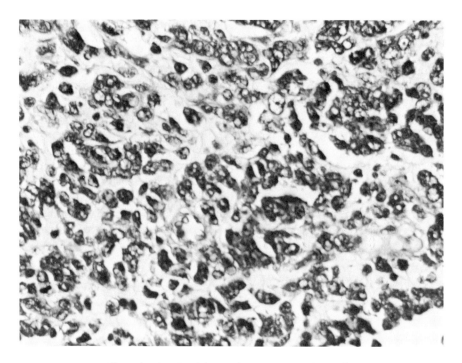

Figure 5-17. Undifferentiated cells with marginated nuclear chromatin are supported by a mucinous matrix in this melanoblastoma. The tumor arose in a giant hairy nevus in an infant and metastasized to regional lymph nodes and to the skin of the face and scalp (H & E).

Von Recklinghausen's Disease as a Model of Intralesional Transformation and Neoplastic Recapitulation of Fetal Properties

The cutaneous, tumorous manifestations of von Recklinghausen's disease include solitary cutaneous neurofibromas, solitary subcutaneous neurofibromas, plexiform neurofibromas, and occasional ganglioneuromas.[69] The cutaneous neurofibroma is a soft, sessile or pedunculated tumor. The subcutaneous, solitary neurofibroma is a circumscribed, encapsulated tumor whose nerve of origin is usually inconspicuous or not identified. The cutaneous plexiform neurofibroma is usually dermal as well as subcutaneous: a plexus of tortuous, irregularly enlarged nerves is supported by a distinctive, neuroid, fibrous matrix.[9] It is a diagnostic stigma of neurofibromatosis.[69]

In the skin, the dysplasia of von Recklinghausen's disease is tumorous but has distinctive relationships with the dermis. The tumors with rare exceptions accommodate the skin appendages in a regular pattern (Figure 5-18). The adjacent dermis is not compressed. In essence, the tumor accommodates to a fibrous defect in the dermis. It qualifies as a dysplasia of dermal fibrous tissue.[9] The implications of this observation are:

1. In the skin, the tumorous dysplasia of neurofibromatosis expresses defective maturation and formation of the reticular dermis (Figure 5-19).
2. The prominence of neural crest derivatives and neural tissues in these fibrous dysplasias of the dermis provides evidence that neural crest derivatives play a role in the formation and maturation of the dermis.
3. In this neural crest dysplasia in which the tumorous lesions are grotesque distortions of peripheral nerves and perineurial fibrous tissue, a defect in mesenchyme is inlaid with neuroid tissue.

The solitary cutaneous neurofibroma has little or no proclivity for malignant transformation. In neurofibromatosis, the plexiform neurofibroma and the large

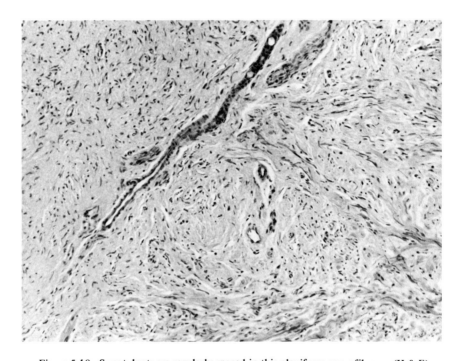

Figure 5-18. Sweat ducts are regularly spaced in this plexiform neurofibroma (H & E).

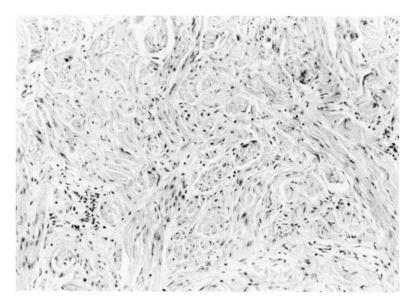

Figure 5-19. The dermal portion of this plexiform neurofibroma is indistinguishable from a connective tissue nevus of the dermis (H & E).

neurofibromas with subcutaneous components are potential sites for malignant transformation. The precursory phases between a neurofibroma and a malignant schwannoma have not been clearly defined. By implication, the transformation from a benign to a malignant process is abrupt and complete. De novo transformation of the latter type undoubtedly occurs, but a slow, progressive transformation through multiple stages of cellularity and cytologic atypism is a more likely sequence. If melanomas are selected as a comparable model, tumors that evolve by progressive dysplasia (radial growth patterns or immune intolerance) outnumber those that evolve de novo (nodular melanomas or spontaneous immune tolerance). If attention is paid to transition areas between frankly malignant portions of a malignant schwannoma and the adjacent neurofibroma, it is possible to identify the atypical, dysplastic precursor of the malignant lesion. In the transitional areas of atypism and hypercellularity, the cells are not uniformly arranged in tortuous fascicles. They are loosely aggregated in a fibrous or myxomatous matrix (Figure 5-20). Transitional patterns in either the endoneurial component or the perineurial component may be misdiagnosed as a fully evolved malignant schwannoma. The latter error in part accounts for the commonly reported experience that malignant schwannomas are rather indolent tumors with long periods of active local disease.[9]

In a malignant schwannoma, fascicles of fibroblastic spindle cells in a fibromyxomatous matrix form the common pattern. Regional variations include

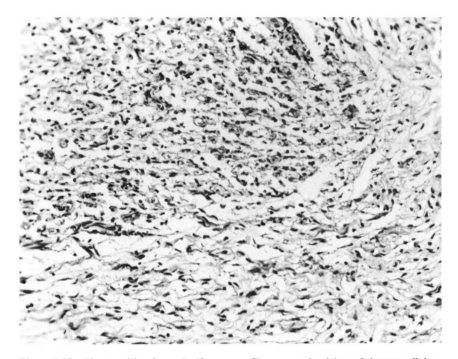

Figure 5-20. The transition from plexiform neurofibroma on the right to Schwann cell dysplasia on the left is abrupt (H & E).

chondroid and rhabdomyomatous patterns.[69] The patterns in the usual malignant schwannoma are histologic simulacra of fetal mesenchyme (Figure 5-21). The transformation of a neuroid tumorous dysplasia into a malignant mesenchymal tumor is a remarkable phenomenon. Either neural crest derivatives have mesenchymal potentials, or the neuroid dysplasias are peculiar expressions of altered mesenchyme. Mesenchymal malignant schwannoma is descriptive of neither the precursory tumor (a neurofibroma rather than a schwannoma) nor the histologic features.

In terms of histopathology, the common or mesenchymal malignant schwannoma is a fibroblastic, spindle cell tumor. The tumor cells have homogeneous cytoplasm and are arranged in rigid fascicles. Alternate fascicles (Figure 5-22) tend to be light (pale) or dark (basophilic). Often they are accompanied by a central, delicate blood vessel. Perithelial patterns are common. Foci of chondroid or rhabdomyomatous differentiation are occasional regional variations (Figures 5-23 and 5-24). Ideally, remnants of a plexiform neurofibroma should be found adjacent to the malignant tumor.

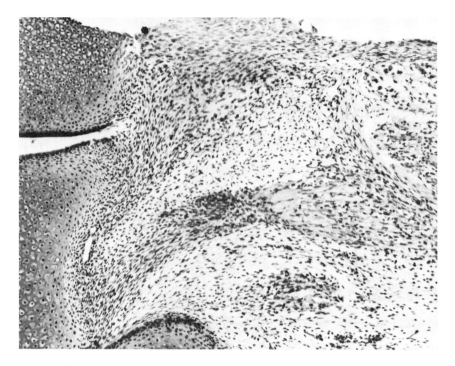

Figure 5-21. Fetal mesenchyme forms light and dark fascicles. In the center of the field, the dark fascicle blends with a fascicle of developing skeletal muscle. Fetal cartilage and a joint are represented on the left (H & E).

The protoplasmic, malignant schwannoma is also a fasciculated tumor (Figure 5-25). The tumor cells are plump and preponderantly either spindle or epithelioid (Figure 5-26). The fascicles are coarse and compactly aggregated. Minimal deviation patterns resemble a benign schwannoma (Figure 5-27). Bordering stellate areas of necrosis, the tumor cells form palisades (Figure 5-27). Starburst or storiform patterns are common in protoplasmic and fibroblastic malignant schwannomas (Figures 5-25 and 5-28). Some protoplasmic malignant schwannomas share features with the neurotropic melanoma (Figure 5-29).

In the teratoid malignant schwannoma,[71] islands of glandular epithelium are irregularly distributed in a tumor that otherwise qualifies as malignant schwannoma (Figure 5-30).

The teratoid, malignant schwannoma and the protoplasmic, or epithelioid malignant schwannoma are rare variants. The protoplasmic or epithelioid malignant schwannoma occurs in the clinical setting of von Recklinghausen's disease, but some examples are sporadic. Occasional examples may represent malignant

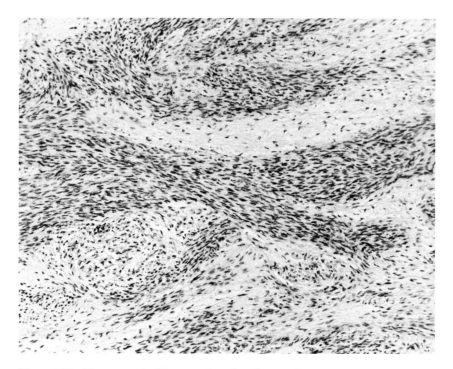

Figure 5-22. The pattern in this mesenchymal malignant schwannoma mimics the alternating light and dark fascicles in fetal mesenchyme shown in Figure 5-21 (H & E).

transformation of a benign schwannoma. Neuroepitheliomas of peripheral nerves (Figure 5-31) are not a manifestation of neurofibromatosis.

Other lesions occasionally associated with the tumorous dysplasias of peripheral nerves include meningiomas, pheochromocytomas, schwannosis of the central nervous system, and rarely gliomas.[69] Most of the associated lesions are of neuroectodermal origin, particularly of neural crest origin. These varied manifestations are related to the widely dispersed character of the neural crest derivatives. They clearly illustrate the bewildering clinical aspects of genodermatoses expressing neural crest dysplasias.

The Mucosal Neuroma Syndrome (Multiple Endocrine Neoplasia Type IIb or III): a Model of the Dispersed Nature of Neurocristic Dysplasias

The mucosal neuroma syndrome[38,72,74] is characterized by medullary carcinoma of the thyroid (a tumor of neurocristic C cells;[75] Figure 5-1), a high incidence of bilateral adrenal pheochromocytomas (tumors of neurocristic adrenal medullary

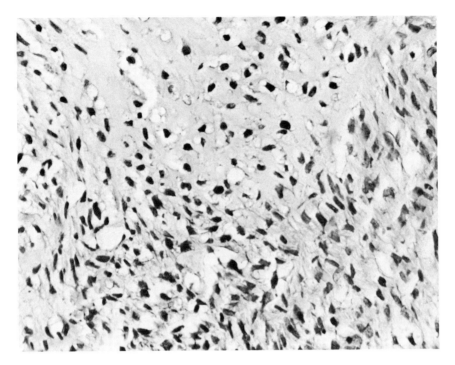

Figure 5-23.   This mesenchymal malignant schwannoma shows chondroid differentiation (H & E).

cells), mucosal neuromata (dysplasias of neurocristic Schwann cells and the peripheral extensions of neurocristic ganglion cells; Figures 5-32 through 5-34), a Marfanoid habitus, and abnormalities of intestinal neural plexuses.[76] The tumorous dysplasias and carcinomas in the mucosal neuroma syndrome clearly affect tissues of neurocristic derivation.

In multiple endocrine neoplasia (MEN) Type II (medullary thyroid carcinoma, pheochromocytoma, and parathyroid hyperplasia or adenoma), the tumors appear to be of clonal rather than multiclonal origin.[77]   In addition, a hormone-like nerve growth factor may be involved.[78]

If the pluripotency of neural crest cells is accepted, the parent cells of the adrenal medulla, the C cells of the thyroid, and the sympathetic ganglia are close embryonic relatives.   Involvement of multiple organ systems in MEN-IIb exemplifies the dispersed quality of the precursory neurocristic cell. The elevated level of nerve growth factor in a patient with medullary carcinoma of the thyroid may offer an alternate explanation for the mucosal neuromata in MEN-IIb. Perhaps the secretions of the medullary carcinoma have a specific stimulatory effect on mucosal (autonomic?) nerves.

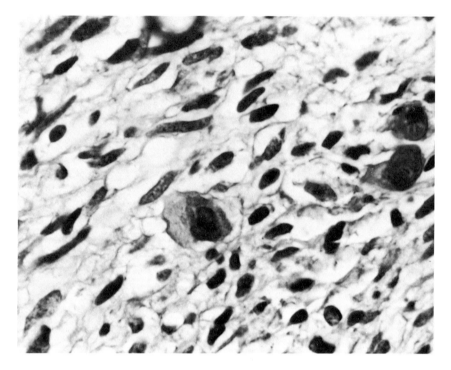

Figure 5-24. This mesenchymal malignant schwannoma contains foci of rhabdomyosarcoma (H & E).

Mesenchymal Dysplasias and the Neural Crest

Dermatofibrosarcoma protuberans (DFSP)[79] has features of a neurocristic tumorous dysplasia. Melanocytes have been identified in some examples[80] (Figure 5-35). The tumor characteristically has two distinct phases in its life history. An indurated, relatively stable plaque is often present from early childhood. After a rather stable period in which the plaque slowly enlarges, one or more nodules develop.

The histology of the plaque is often deceptively innocent. Uniform, elongated spindle cells are fibroblastic. They are supported by a delicate fibrous matrix and are arranged in interlacing fascicles (Figure 5-35). The interlacing fascicles produce starburst patterns. They extend from the plaque into the subcutaneous fat. They dissect the lobules of adipose tissue and blend with the deep fascia. At the ultrastructural level, some of the features suggest Schwann cell or perineurial cell differentiation.[79] The melanocytes and the ultrastructural features are compatible with a neurocristic tumorous dysplasia. The storiform patterns

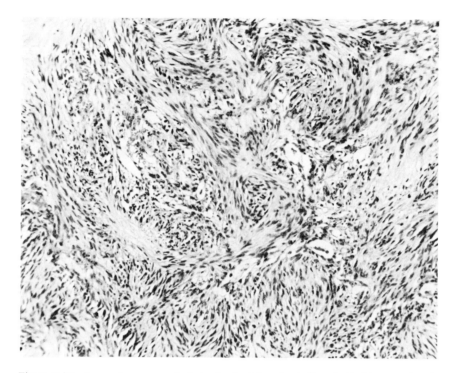

Figure 5-25. In a pulmonary metastasis, the fascicles of spindle cells in this protoplasmic malignant schwannoma form starburst patterns. The cells palisade around zones of necrosis (H & E).

as seen in DFSP are occasionally seen as regional variations in a plexiform neurofibroma.[69]

If the plaque stage of DFSP is a tumorous dysplasia, it is manifested in the organization and development of the reticular dermis and the subcutaneous fat. The evidence indirectly implicates a role for neurocristic cells in the formation of the skin, including the reticular dermis and the subcutaneous fat.

Cutaneous Pigmentation and Neurocristopathies

The neurocristic genodermatoses share the marker of cutaneous pigmentation. In neurocutaneous melanosis syndrome, giant congenital nevus syndrome, and multiple nevi-familial melanoma syndrome, the pigmented markers are nevi and lentigines. In neurofibromatosis and in occasional cases of multiple neuroma syndrome, the marker is the café au lait spot.[9,69] In tuberous sclerosis, the marker is the ash leaf spot.[81]

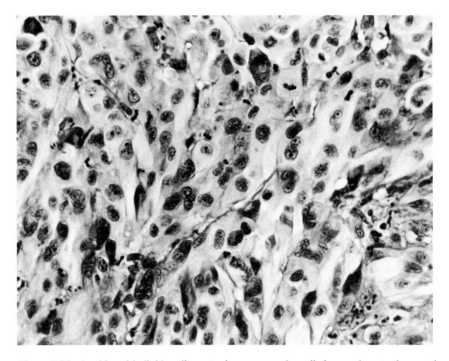

Figure 5-26. In this epithelioid malignant schwannoma, the cells have pale cytoplasm and are arranged in fascicles. The tumor shares cytologic features with some melanomas (H & E).

The café au lait spot has special significance. If it is a marker of neurocristic dysplasias, does its presence in polyostotic fibrous dysplasia of bone imply a role for a neurocristic dysplasia? Polyostotic fibrous dysplasia is an apparent mesenchymal dysplasia.[82] It shares features with neurocristic dysplasias:

1. Endocrine abnormalities
2. Systematized lesions in a selected organ system (bones in fibrous dysplasia as opposed to peripheral nerves in neurofibromatosis)
3. Disorganized growth at a rate greater than that of adjacent, uninvolved tissue
4. Defective maturation of involved tissue (woven bone)
5. Café au lait spots
6. Occasional malignant transformation of dysplastic lesions

Fibrous dysplasia of bone may be a peculiar skeletal manifestation of a neurocristic dysplasia.

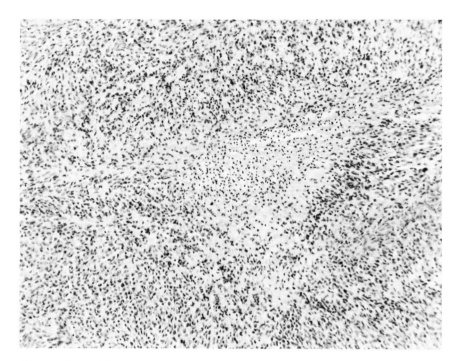

Figure 5-27. Minimal deviation patterns characterize some malignant schwannomas. Lesions of this type may represent malignant transformation of a schwannoma. The tumor cells form palisades around a stellate area of necrosis (H & E).

The mesenchymal property of the neural crest is expressed in some way in the fibrous tissue of the dermis. By location and function, the adventitial dermis is ideally suited to interact with epithelium. The melanocyte is situated in a pivotal position between the two. Hyperpigmentation is a feature of some conditions involving the epidermis and the adventitial dermis (acanthosis nigricans). The fibrous hamartomas of the butterfly area of the face in the tuberous sclerosis complex have significant melanocytic components.[52] Melanocytes drop from the epidermis into the papillary dermis. In the latter location they are fibrogenic. They stimulate the fibrosing process which eventuates in the clinical lesion classified as adenoma sebaceum (melanocytic angiofibroma). The lamina propria of the intestinal tract is in continuity with, and an extension of, the adventitial dermis. The juvenile retention polyp is a fibrous hamartoma of the lamina propria of the large intestine.[83] Familial cases of juvenile polyposis are recognized and occasionally are associated with a family history of familial polyposis or carcinoma.[83] Cases of familial juvenile polyposis have been associated with

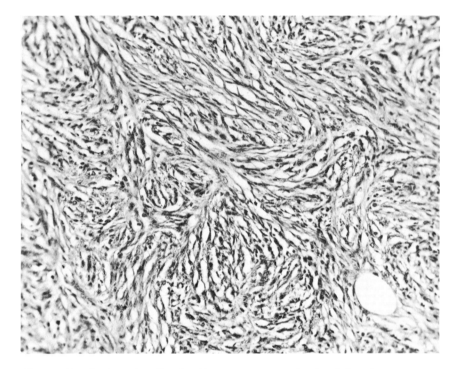

Figure 5-28. Starburst (storiform) patterns are seen as regional variations in some mesenchymal malignant schwannomas (H & E).

polypoid ganglioneurofibromatosis of the intestinal tract and with cutaneous neurofibromas.[83]   Familial juvenile polyposis may be a peculiar intestinal manifestation of a neural crest dysplasia and is occasionally associated with cutaneous lesions.

If pigmented cutaneous or mucosal lesions mark an acquired or cutaneous neural crest dysplasia, the Peutz-Jeghers syndrome deserves attention. In this syndrome, mucocutaneous lentigines are a marker,[84] and adenomatous polyps are widespread in the intestinal tract. The hyperplastic epithelium in the polyps has the differentiated features of the intestinal or gastric epithelium in the site of origin. The polyps have a peculiar mesenchymal component consisting of a branched stalk of hypertrophied smooth muscle. Perhaps Peutz-Jeghers syndrome is a peculiar expression of a neurocristopathy.

Cutaneous Neurocristic Genodermatoses and Related Visceral Tumors

The widely dispersed nature of the migratory neurocristic cell becomes evident in a study of visceral lesions associated with the neurocutaneous syndromes. With few exceptions, the related visceral tumors are also of neural crest origin.

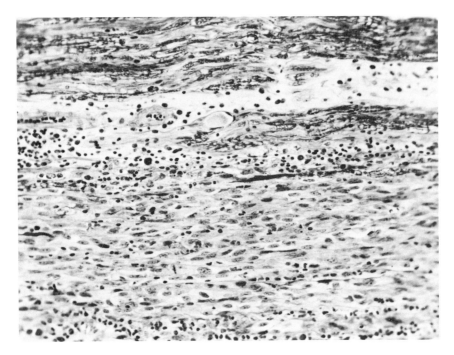

Figure 5-29. This protoplasmic malignant schwannoma is infiltrating a peripheral nerve. It is a histologic simulant of the neurotropic melanoma (H & E).

It is implied in these widespread disorders that the precursory cells in the neural crest begin their migration in concert and, genetically, are similarly dysplastic. In some syndromes, secretions derived from dysplastic cells may effect hyperplasias or tumors in genetically normal endocrine systems. In this manner, the parathyroid disease associated with multiple endocrine neoplasias may be unrelated to the basic genetic defect: it may merely reflect the influence of the secretory products of dysplastic cells on the parathyroid glands.[21]

In neurofibromatosis, the associated visceral lesions include pheochromocytoma, meningiomas and meningiomatosis, central nervous system schwannosis, gliomas, and muscular defects in the walls of arteries, particularly the renal artery.[85] The great vessels with the exception of endothelium are apparently derived from mesoectodermal (neurocristic) cells.[5] Dysplasias of the great vessels in neurofibromatosis are manifested by mural defects and by intimal hyperplasias. Stenosis of the renal artery is a complication. Muscular arteries in the renal parenchyma may be affected. There are peculiar plexiform neurofibromas which contain aneurysmally dilated blood vessels. They qualify as aneurysmal neurofibromas (Figure 5-36).

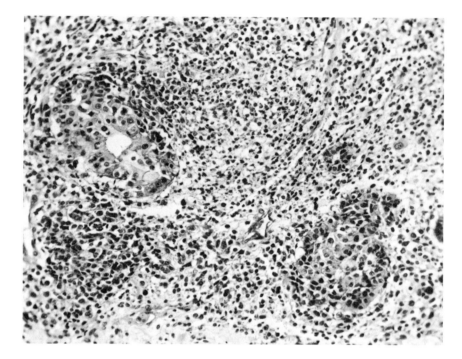

Figure 5-30. Epithelial (glandular) differentiation characterizes this teratoid malignant schwannoma (H & E).

In tuberous sclerosis, the associated visceral lesions include multiple endocrine adenomas, angiomyolipoma of the kidney, vascular and epithelial hamartomas of the lungs, polycystic disease of the kidney, liver, and pancreas, glial hamartomas, and rhabdomyoma of the heart.[86] Vascular lesions comparable to those in neurofibromatosis have been described. The mesenchymal quality of the visceral tumorous dysplasias in the tuberous sclerosis syndrome apparently contradicts a proposed role for a neuroectodermal or neurocristic dysplasia. On the other hand, the neural crest contributes to the media of great vessels[5] and to cranial mesenchyme.[4,5] In addition, mesenchymal dysplasias involving the dermis and blood vessels are occasional features of the neurocristic dysplasias of neurofibromatosis. Adipose tissue and smooth muscle may be significantly influenced by neural crest derivatives. Neurocristic dysplasias may find expression in tumors composed of smooth muscle cells and lipocytes[86] (Figure 5-37).

The mucosal neuroma syndrome is associated with pheochromocytoma and medullary carcinoma of the thyroid.[73]

The neurocutaneous melanosis syndrome is associated with melanosis and melanocytic tumors of the leptomeninges.[69]

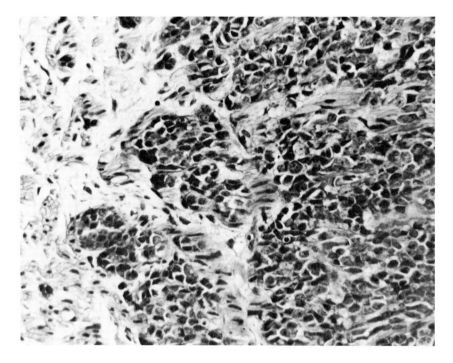

Figure 5-31. This neuroepithelioma is infiltrating a peripheral nerve. It has blastomatous qualities (H & E).

Conclusions

In the evolution of most acquired melanocytic tumorous dysplasias, the epidermal melanocyte clusters with its neighbors in nests and fascicles. The nondispersed character of melanocytes in the nests and fascicles turns off the melanogenic functions. The transformed cells become actively migratory and shun their neighbors as they move into the dermis. In their dispersed state in a new environment (the dermis), they acquire Schwann cell properties and are fibrogenic. Clearly, the melanocyte and Schwann cells are embryonic relatives. It is equally clear that the evolution of a nevus recapitulates a significant embryonic role of the neurocristic migrant, namely the development and maturation of the dermis.

If migratory melanocytes recapitulate the role of neurocristic migrants in the development of the dermis, the melanocytic activity (epidermal melanocytic hyperplasia and "dropping off" into the dermis) in the angiofibroma of the tuberous sclerosis complex assumes a major pathogenic role. The migratory melanocyte mediates the fibrogenesis which characterizes the angiofibroma. A role for neurocristic cells in the evolution of the mesenchymal hamartomas in

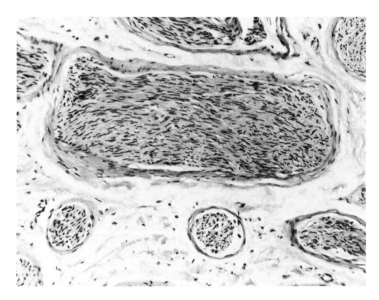

Figure 5-32. Peripheral nerves are increased in number and are hypercellular in this mucosal specimen from a patient with multiple mucosal neuromas (H & E).

the tuberous sclerosis complex is difficult to define, but may reflect the abnormal activities of organizers and evocators.

Two major variants of malignant neoplasms are exemplified in neurocristic dysplasias. In infants the tumors are usually blastomatous with a potential for spontaneous regression or maturation. The role of the host immune response in either process is neither defined nor discernible at a histologic level. The blastomas are in part the expressions of arrested development. They histologically and biochemically mimic fetal and embryonal tissues. Immature teratomas are blastomas in which two or more germ layers are represented.

In the second major category, the malignant neoplasms evolve by progressive changes in a system of dysplastic cells. The process characteristically evolves in an adult and is manifested by neoplastic retrodifferentiation of cells in a cytoplasmic phase. The cells generally express nuclear and cytoplasmic qualities in abnormal patterns. A role for the host immune response is defined and histologically discernible. Having acquired the characteristics of a malignant neoplasm, a tumor in this category is unlikely to revert to its former quiescent state or mature.

REFERENCES

1. Horstadius, S.: *The Neural Crest, Its Properties and Derivatives in the Light of Experimental Research.* London: Oxford University Press, 1950.

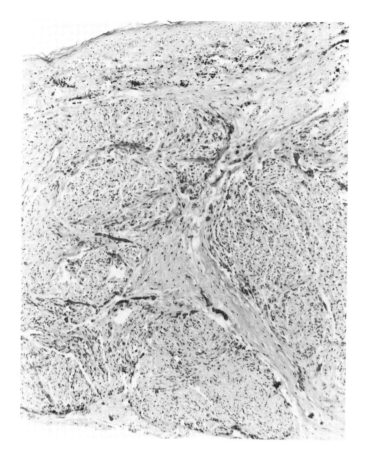

Figure 5-33. In this solitary true neuroma the altered nerve forms circumscribed, encapsulated aggregates in the dermis. In the aggregates, the spindle cells form interlacing fascicles (H & E).

2. Weston, R.P.: The migration and differentiation of neural crest cells. *Advan. Morphogenesis* 8:41, 1971.

3. Holtfreter, J.: Mesenchyme and epithelia in inductive and morphogenetic processes. In: *Epithelial-Mesenchymal Interactions* (R. Fleischmajer and R.E. Billingham, Eds.). Baltimore, MD: Williams and Wilkins, 1968, pp. 1–30.

4. LeLievre, C.S.: Participation of neural crest-derived cells in the genesis of the skull in birds. *J. Embryol. Exp. Morph.* 47:17–37, 1978.

5. LeLievre, C.S., and LeDouarin, N.M.: Mesenchymal derivatives of the neural crest: analysis of chimaeric quail and chick embryos. *J. Embryol. Exp. Morph.* 34:125–154, 1975.

6. Derby, M.A.: Analysis of glycosaminoglycans within the extracellular environments encountered by migrating neural crest cells. *Dev. Biol.* 66:321–336, 1978.

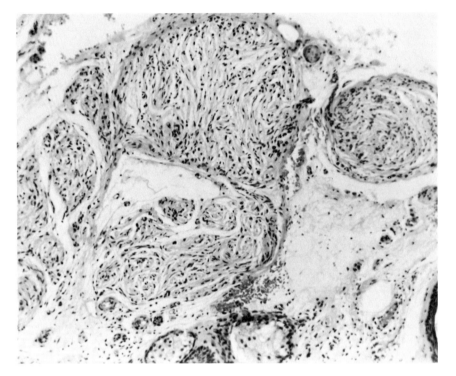

Figure 5-34. The nerve of origin for a solitary true neuroma is tortuous and hypercellular. The solitary neuroma is a histologic simulant of mucosal neuromas in the multiple neuroma syndrome (H & E).

7. Cohen, A.M.: Independent expression of the adrenergic phenotype by neural crest cells in vitro. *Proc. Natl. Acad. Sci. USA* **74**:2899–2903, 1977.

8. Noden, D.M.: An analysis of the migratory behavior of avian cephalic neural crest cells. *Dev. Biol.* **42**:106–130, 1975.

9. Reed, R.J.: Cutaneous manifestations of neural crest disorders (neurocristopathies). *J. Int. Dermatol.* **16**:807–826, 1977.

10. Willis, R.A.: The hamartomatous syndromes; their clinical, pathological and fundamental aspects. *Med. J. Aust,* **1**:827–833, 1965.

11. Williams, E.D., and Pollock, D.J.: Multiple mucosal neuromata with endocrine tumors. A syndrome allied to von Recklinghausen's disease. *J. Pathol. Bacteriol.* **91**: 71–80, 1966.

12. Brasfield, R.D., and Das Gupta, T.K.: von Recklinghausen's disease: a clinicopathologic study. *Ann. Surg.* **175**:86–104, 1972.

13. Lichtenstein, B.W.: Neurofibromatosis (von Recklinghausen's disease of the nervous system): analysis of the total pathologic picture. *Arch. Neurol. Psychiat.* **62**:822–839, 1949.

14. Venner, B.: Multiple neurofibromatosis. *Aust. NZ. J. Surg.* **25**:110–117, 1955.

15. Steiner, A.L., Goodman, A.D., and Powers, S.R.: Study of a kindred with pheochromocytoma, medullary thyroid carcinoma, hyperparathyroidism, and Cushing's disease. Multiple endocrine neoplasia, type 2. *Medicine* **47**:371–409, 1968.

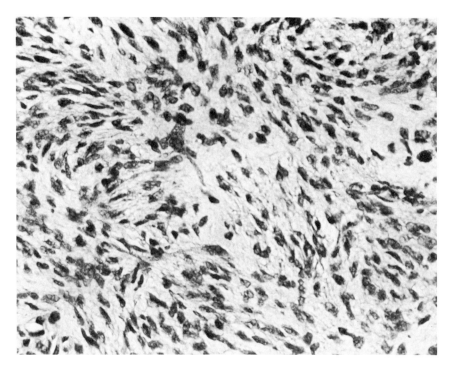

Figure 5-35. In this dermatofibrosarcoma protuberans, there are pigmented dendritic melanocytes (one is seen above the center of the field) (H & E).

16. Nickel, W.R., and Reed, W.B.: Tuberous sclerosis: special reference to the microscopic alterations in the cutaneous hamartomas. *Arch. Dermatol.* 85:209–224, 1962.

17. Riccardi, V.M., and Kleiner, B.: Neurofibromatosis: A neoplastic birth defect with two age peaks of severe problems. *Birth Defects* 13:131–138, 1977.

18. Bolande, R.P.: The neurocristopathies: a unifying concept of disease arising in neural maldevelopment. *Human Pathol.* 5:409–429, 1974.

19. Pearse, A.G.E., and Takor Takor, T.: Neuroendocrine embryology and the APUD concept. *Clin. Endocrinol.* 5:229$_s$–244$_s$, 1976.

20. Pearse, A.G.E.: The cytochemistry and ultrastructure of polypeptide hormone producing cells (the APUD series) and the embryologic, physiologic and pathologic implications of the concept. *J. Histochem. Cytochem.* 17:303–313, 1969.

21. Pearse, A.G.E.: The APUD cell concept and its implications in pathology. *Pathol. Annual* 9:27–41, 1974.

22. Pearse, A.G.E., and Polak, J.M.: Neural crest origin of the endocrine polypeptide (APUD) cells of the gastrointestinal tract and pancreas. *Gut* 12:783, 1971.

23. Rost, F.W.D., Polak, J.M., and Pearse, A.G.E.: The melanocyte. Its cytochemical and immunological relationship to cells of the endocrine polypeptide (APUD) series. *Virchows Arch.* 4:93–101, 1969.

24. Weichert, R.F.: The neural ectodermal origin of the peptide secreting endocrine glands. *Am. J. Med.* 49:232–241, 1970.

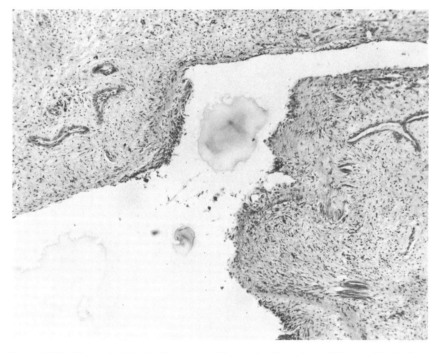

Figure 5-36. Vessels in this plexiform neurofibroma in the region of the parotid gland are aneurysmal. The media in the aneurysmal portion is deficient (H & E).

25. Andrews, Ann: APUD cells, apudomas, and the neural crest. *S. Afr. Med. J.* **50**: 890-898, 1976.

26. Pictet, R.L., Rall, L.B., Phelps, P., and Rutter, W.J.: The neural crest and the origin of the insulin-producing and other gastrointestinal hormone-producing cells. *Science* **191**:191-192, 1975.

27. Weston, J.A.: Neural crest cell migration and differentiation. In: *Cellular Aspects of Neural Growth and Differentiation,* UCLA Forum in Medical Sciences, #14. Los Angeles, CA: University of California Press, 1971, pp. 1-19.

28. Fontaine, J., LeLievre, C., and LeDouarin, N.M.: What is the developmental fate of the neural crest cells which migrate into the pancreas in the avian embryo? *Gen. Compar. Endocrinol.* **33**:394-404, 1977.

29. Karasanyi, H.L., and Nagele, R.G., Jr.: The role of the cell surface in the migration of primordial germ cells in early chick embryos: effects of concanavalin A. *J. Embryol. Exp. Morph.* **46**:5-20, 1978.

30. Scully, R.E.: Androgenic lesions of the ovary. In: *The Ovary* (International Academy of Pathology Monograph; H.G. Grady and D.E. Smith, Eds.). Baltimore, MD: Williams & Wilkins, 1963, pp. 143-174.

31. Skrabanek, P., Nat, D.R., and Powell, D.: Unifying concept of non-pituitary ACTH-secreting tumors. *Cancer* **42**:1263-1269, 1978.

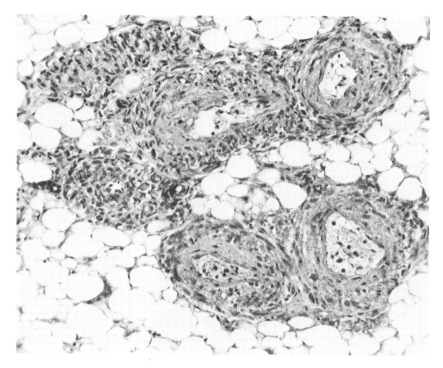

Figure 5-37. Abnormal vessels and aggregates of smooth muscle cells and lipocytes characterize this angiomyolipoma of the kidney in the tuberous sclerosis complex (H & E).

32. Omenn, G.S.: Recognition of ectopic hormone syndromes produced by tumors. *Birth Defects* 7:73–78, 1971.

33. Bell, C.E., and Seetharam, S.: Identification of the Schwann cell as a peripheral nervous system cell possessing a differentiation antigen expressed by a human lung tumor. *J. Immunol.* 118:826–831, 1977.

34. Pearse, A.G.E., Ewers, S.W.B., and Polak, J.M.: The genesis of apudamyloid in endocrine polypeptide tumors. Histochemical distinction from immunoamyloid. *Virchows Arch.* 10:93–107, 1972.

35. Reed, R.J., Daroca, P.J., Jr., and Harkin, J.C.: Gangliocytic paraganglioma. *Am. J. Surg. Pathol.* 1:207–216, 1977.

36. Lynch, H.T., and Frichot, B.C., III: Skin, heredity and cancer. *Sem. Oncol.* 5:67–84, 1978.

37. Fialkow, P.J., Sagebiel, R.W., Gartler, S.M., and Rimoin, D.: Multiple cell origin of hereditary neurofibromas. *N. Engl. J. Med.* 284:298–300, 1971.

38. Gorlin, R.J., and Vickers, R.A.: Multiple mucosal neuromas, pheochromocytoma, medullary carcinoma of the thyroid and marfanoid body build with muscle wasting: reexamination of a syndrome of neural crest malmigration. *Birth Defects* 7(6):69–72, 1971.

39. Cochran, A.J.: Histology and prognosis in malignant melanoma. *J. Pathol.* 97:459–468, 1969.
40. Slaughter, J.C., Hardman, J.M., Kempe, L.G., and Earle, K.M.: Neurocutaneous melanosis and leptomeningeal melanomatosis in children. *Arch. Pathol.* 88:298–304, 1969.
41. Lorentzen, M., Pers, M., and Bretteville-Jensen, G.: The incidence of malignant transformation in giant pigmented nevi. *Scand. J. Plast. Reconstr. Surg.* 11:163–167, 1977.
42. Bartholdson, L., Lilja, J., Mobacken, H., and Waldenstrom, J.: Xeroderma pigmentosum—biochemical and therapeutic aspects. *Scand. J. Plast. Reconstr. Surg.* 11:173-177, 1977.
43. Epstein, J.H., Fukuyama, K., Reed, W.B., and Epstein, W.L.: Defect in DNA synthesis in skin of patients with xeroderma pigmentosa demonstrated in vivo. *Science* 168:1477, 1970.
44. Uriel, J.: Cancer, retrodifferentiation, and the myth of Faust. *Cancer Res.* 36:4269–4275, 1976.
45. Gartler, S.M.: Patterns of cellular proliferation in normal and tumor cell populations. *Am. J. Pathol.* 86:685–692, 1977.
46. Fishman, W.H., and Singer, R.M.: Regulatory controls of oncotrophoblast proteins and developmental alkaline phosphatases in cancer cells. *Cancer Res.* 36:4256–4261, 1976.
47. Chiarugi, V.P.: Cell-coat glycosaminoglycans in cellular transformation and differentiation. *Exp. Cell Biol.* 44:251–259, 1976.
48. Chang, J.H.T., and Prasad, K.N.: Differentiation of mouse neuroblastoma cells in vitro and in vivo induced by cyclic adenosine monophosphaste (CAMP). *J. Ped. Surg.* 11:847–856, 1976.
49. Reed, R.J., Ichinose, H., Clark, W.H., Jr., and Mihm, M.C., Jr.: Common and uncommon melanocytic nevi and borderline melanomas. *Sem. Oncol.* 2:119–147, 1975.
50. Clark, W.H., Jr., From, L., Bernardino, E.A., and Mihm, M.C., Jr.: The histogenesis and biologic behavior of primary human malignant melanoma of the skin. *Cancer Res.* 29:705–727, 1969.
51. Reed, R.J.: Consultation case. *Am. J. Surg. Pathol.* 2:215–220, 1978.
52. Reed, R.J., Hairston, M.A., and Palomeque, F.E.: The histologic identity of adenoma sebaceum and solitary melanocytic angiofibroma. *Dermatol. Int.* 5:3-11, 1966.
53. Reed, R.J.: *Melanocytic Nevi and Related Tumors of the Skin: An Atlas of Dermatopathology.* Chicago, IL: American Society of Clinical Pathologists, 1975.
54. Masson, P.: My conception of cellular nevi. *Cancer* 4:9–38, 1951.
55. Mark, G.J., Mihm, M.C., Liteplo, M.G., Reed, R.J., and Clark, W.H.: Congenital melanocytic nevi of the small and garment type. *Human Pathol.* 4:395–418, 1973.
56. Masson, P.: Melanogenic system: nevi and melanomas. *Pathol. Ann.* 2:351–397, 1967.
57. Conley, J., Lattes, R., and Orr, W.: Desmoplastic malignant melanoma. *Cancer* 28:914–936, 1971.
58. Reed, R.J., and Leonard, D.: Neurotropic melanoma: a variant of desmoplastic melanoma. *Am. J. Surg. Pathol.* (in press).
59. Breslow, A.: Tumor thickness, level of invasion and node dissection in stage I cutaneous melanoma. *Ann. Surg.* 182:572-575, 1975.
60. Clark, W.H., Jr., Reimer, R.R., Greene, M., Ainsworth, A., and Mastrangelo, M.J.: Origin of familial malignant melanomas from heritable melanocytic lesions. *Arch. Dermatol.* 114:732-738, 1978.

61. Greene, M.H., Reimer, R.R., Clark, W.H., and Mastrangelo, M.J.: Precursor lesions in familial melanoma. *Sem. Oncol.* 5:85–87, 1978.
62. Lynch, H.T., Frichot, B.C., III, and Lynch, J.F.: Familial atypical multiple mole-melanoma syndrome. *J. Med. Genet.* 15(5):352–356, 1978.
63. Clark, W.H., Jr., and Mihm, M.C., Jr.: Lentigo maligna and lentigo-maligna melanoma. *Am. J. Pathol.* 55:39–67, 1969.
64. Hutchinson, J.: Lentigo-melanosis. A further report. *Arch. Surg. (London)* 5:253–256, 1894.
65. Arrington, J.H., III, Reed, R.J., Ichinose, H., and Krementz, E.T.: Plantar lentiginous melanoma: a distinctive variant of human cutaneous malignant melanoma. *Am. J. Surg. Pathol.* 1:131–143, 1977.
66. Copeman, P.W.M., Lewis, M.G., and Bleehan, S.S.: Biology and immunology of vitiligo and cutaneous malignant melanoma. In: *Recent Advances in Dermatology* (A. Rook, Ed.). Edinburgh: Churchill Livingstone, 1973, pp. 245–284.
67. Mascaro, J.M.: Xeroderma pigmentosa. In: *Cancer of the Skin* (R. Andrade et al., Eds.). Philadelphia: W.B. Saunders, 1976, pp. 573–595.
68. Reed, W.B., Becker, S.W., Sr., Becker, S.W., Jr., and Nickel, W.R.: Giant pigmented nevi, melanoma, and leptomeningeal melanocytosis. *Arch. Derm.* 91:100–119, 1965.
69. Harkin, J.C., and Reed, R.J.: Tumors of the peripheral nervous system. *Atlas of Tumor Pathology* (2nd series, fascicle 3). Washington, D.C.: Armed Forces Institute of Pathology, 1969.
70. Borello, E.D., and Gorlin, R.J.: Melanotic neuroectodermal tumor of infancy – a neoplasm of neural crest origin – report of a case associated with high urinary excretion of vanilmandelic acid. *Cancer* 19:196–206, 1966.
71. Woodruff, J.M., Chernik, N.L., Smith, M.C., Millette, W.B., and Foote, F.W., Jr.: Peripheral nerve tumors with rhabdomyosarcomatous differentiation (malignant "triton" tumors). *Cancer* 32:426–439, 1973.
72. Khairi, M.R.A., Dexter, R.N., Burzynski, N.J., and Johnston, C.C., Jr.: Mucosal neuroma, pheochromocytoma and medullary thyroid carcinoma: multiple endocrine neoplasia type 3. *Medicine* 54:89–112, 1975.
73. Gorlin, R.J., Sedano, H.O., Vickers, R.A., and Cervenka, J.: Multiple mucosal neuromas, pheochromocytoma and medullary carcinoma of the thyroid – a syndrome. *Cancer* 22:293–299, 1968.
74. Williams, E.D.: Medullary carcinoma of the thyroid. In: *Calcitonin, 1969 – Proceedings of the Second International Symposium.* (S. Taylor and G.V. Foster, Eds.). London: Heinemann, 1969, p. 483.
75. Chong, G.C., Beahrs, O.H., Sizemore, G.W., and Woolner, L.H.: Medullary carcinoma of the thyroid gland. *Cancer* 35:695–704, 1975.
76. Carney, J.A., Go, V.L.W., Sizemore, G.W., and Hayles, A.B.: Alimentary tract ganglioneuromatosis. A major component of the syndrome of multiple endocrine neoplasia, type 2b. *N. Engl. J. Med.* 295:1287–1291, 1976.
77. Baylin, S.B., Gann, D.S., and Hsu, S.: Clonal origin of inherited medullary thyroid carcinoma and pheochromocytoma. *Science* 193:321–323, 1976.
78. Bigazzi, M., Revoltella, R., Casciano, S., and Vigneti, E.: High level of nerve growth factor in the serum of a patient with medullary carcinoma of the thyroid gland. *Clin. Endocrinol.* 6:105–112, 1977.
79. Alguacil-Garcia, A., Unni, K.K., and Goellner, J.R.: Histogenesis of dermatofibrosarcoma protuberans: an ultrastructural study. *Am. J. Clin. Pathol.* 69:427–434, 1978.
80. Smith, J.L., Jr.: Tumors of the corium. In: *The Skin* (E.B. Helwig and F.K. Mostofi, Eds.). Baltimore, MD: Williams & Wilkins, 1971, pp. 533–557.

81. Fitzpatrick, T.B., Szabo, G., Hori, Y., Simone, A.A., Reed, W.B., and Greenburg, M.H.: White leaf-shaped macules: earliest visible sign of tuberous sclerosis. *Arch. Dermatol.* 98:1–6, 1968.

82. Reed, R.J.: Fibrous dysplasia of bone. *Arch. Pathol.* 75:480–495, 1963.

83. Reed, R.J.: Cystic stromal polyposis (juvenile polyposis). *Check Sample, Anatomic Pathology* #4D, Council on Anatomic Pathology, ASCP, 1977.

84. Morson, B.C., and Dawson, I.M.P.: *Gastrointestinal Pathology,* London: Blackwell Scientific, 1972, pp. 221–224.

85. Salyer, W.R., and Salyer, D.C.: The vascular lesion of neurofibromatosis. *Angiology* 25:510–519, 1974.

86. Inglis, K.: The relation of the renal lesions to the cerebral lesions in the tuberous sclerosis complex. *Am. J. Pathol.* 30:739–755, 1954.

6
Radiological Aspects of the Gastrointestinal Cancer-associated Genodermatoses

Roger K. Harned, M.D.

INTRODUCTION

A radiographic examination is often the primary diagnostic procedure in patients with one of the cancer-associated genodermatoses. Patients with genodermatoses such as Gardner's or Peutz-Jeghers syndromes are usually referred to the radiologist with symptoms related to the presence of gastrointestinal polyps. In such cases, the radiologist has a unique opportunity to confirm or establish the correct diagnosis. It is important for him to be familiar with the genodermatoses that are concurrent with internal malignancy. He may be the first to recognize that intestinal polyps in a young patient with associated skin lesions may represent a serious hereditary disease. Failure to recognize such disease may result in tragedy for the individual patient and for other members of his family that may be similarly afflicted.[1]

Diagnostic Methods for Evaluating the Gastrointestinal Tract

Since many of the cancer-associated genodermatoses involve small polyps of the gastrointestinal tract, precise radiographic methods of examination are necessary. Although the traditional, single contrast barium studies of the esophagus, stomach, small bowel, and colon are adequate for detecting large neoplasms, double contrast (air and barium) examinations are almost mandatory to diagnose small lesions. Investigators such as Gelfand, Laufer, Miller, and Rogers have stressed the improved accuracy of double contrast examinations over single contrast studies for early detection of gastrointestinal malignancy and small polyps.[2-16]

Improved methods for examining the small intestine, such as enteroclysis, have recently been introduced and will hopefully enhance the discovery of previously unrecognized small bowel pathology.[17-21] The modalities of com-' puted tomography, ultrasound, endoscopic retrograde cholangiographic pancreatography and percutaneous transhepatic cholangiography have almost revolutionized the diagnostic approach to pancreatic, biliary, and retroperitoneal lesions. Arteriography and radionuclide studies continue to be reliable methods for evaluating gastrointestinal pathology. Thus, the radiologist of today, in an average sized medical center, can utilize new and improved diagnostic approaches to the internal manifestations of the genodermatoses.

THE GASTROINTESTINAL POLYPOSIS SYNDROMES

Since the radiologist plays a dominant role in diagnosing lesions of the gastrointestinal tract, emphasis in this chapter will be placed on the genodermatoses associated with gastrointestinal polyposis. The major syndromes in this category include: Gardner's, Peutz-Jeghers, and multiple hamartoma. Other syndromes such as: Turcot, Cronkhite-Canada, Torre's and juvenile polyposis will be discussed briefly because they are important in the differential diagnostic considerations.

Gardner's Syndrome

Gardner's syndrome (GS) is a classic example of a genodermatosis associated with gastrointestinal cancer. The original features of this syndrome: autosomal dominant inheritance, multiple soft tissue tumors, skeletal osteomatosis, and polyposis coli were described by Gardner and coworkers from 1951 to 1962.[22-26] This disease is of particular clinical importance because of the high incidence of colon carcinoma and other malignancies in affected patients. GS is closely related to familial polyposis coli (FPC), and some investigators believe these entities are different expressions of the same disease. Table 6-1 lists the components of GS. The important radiographic manifestations will be considered separately in the subsequent paragraphs.

Gastrointestinal. *Colon Polyps.* The polyps involving the colon in GS have the same biological behavior, morphology, and location as the polyps found in FPC.[1] The majority of these polyps are adenomatous. Morphologically they may be either sessile or pedunculated with the sessile form predominating. The polyps are characteristically small varying from 2 to 3 mm up to 1.0 cm.[1] In the majority of cases, they are distributed throughout the entire colon in a carpet-like fashion (Figure 6-1). Occasionally, segmental distribution may occur with involvement more extensive on the left side of the colon, including the rectum. Early in the course of this disease, the polyps may be sparse and scattered, appearing as tiny nodules with apparent normal intervening mucosa. A double contrast examination is the radiographic procedure of choice to identify such

Table 6-1. Features of Gardner's Syndrome.

I. Autosomal dominant inheritance

II. Time of onset
   A. Symptoms related to gastrointestinal polyps present in 3rd–4th decade
   B. Skin and bone lesions may present earlier

III. Cutaneous and subcutaneous lesions
   A. Sebaceous cysts
   B. Fibromas
   C. Lipomas, neurofibromas

IV. Gastrointestinal lesions
   A. Colon
      1. Adenomatous polyps
      2. Diffuse distribution but may be sparse and segmental
      3. Colon involved in all patients
      4. Colon carcinoma will develop in 100% of untreated patients
   C. Stomach
      1. Hyperplastic or adenomatous polyps
      2. Fundus and body involved, antrum may be spared
      3. Involved in 60–90% of patients
      4. Cancer uncommon, but may occur
   D. Duodenum
      1. Polyps in 90% of patients
      2. High incidence of duodenal and periampullary carcinoma

V. Fibromatosis
   A. Tendency to fibrous tissue proliferation
   B. Desmoid tumors, keloid formation
   C. Mesenteric and retroperitoneal fibrosis

VI. Bone lesions
   A. Occur in 50% of patients
      1. May precede colon polyps
      2. May appear before or during puberty
   B. Skull and facial bones
      1. Osteomas – outer table of calvarium
      2. Osteomas – paranasal sinuses, mandible
   C. Long bones
      1. Localized cortical thickening
      2. Osteomas and exostosis
   D. Malignant bone tumors uncommon
      1. Fibrosarcomas
      2. Osteogenic sarcomas

VII. Dental abnormalities
   A. Odontomas
   B. Unerupted supernumerary teeth
   C. Hypercementosis
   D. Numerous caries

VIII. Other associated neoplasms
   A. Adrenal carcinomas and adenomas
   B. Thyroid carcinoma
   C. Leiomyomas
      1. Gastric
      2. Retroperitoneal

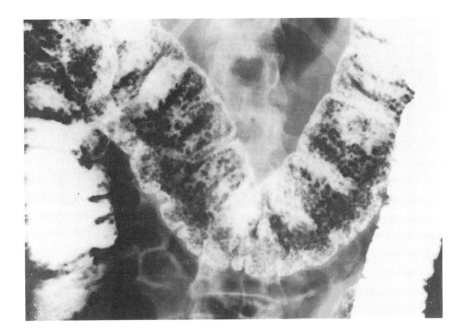

Figure 6-1. Double contrast colon examination. This is the classic appearance of multiple, small sessile polyps diffusely distributed throughout the colon in a patient with Gardner's syndrome. *(Courtesy of Wylie J. Dodds, M.D., Milwaukee, WI. Reprinted with permission from Gastrointestinal Radiology. Copyright Springer-Verlag, New York, Inc.)*

small, punctate lucencies (Figure 6-2). If a single contrast colon study is utilized, these minute polyps present as serrations along the lateral margin of the bowel wall (Figure 6-3A and B). Meticulous preparation of the colon is necessary to accurately evaluate the colon of these patients. It is not uncommon to have an associated lymphoid hyperplasia of the terminal ileum in GS.[27,28] Proctoscopic or colonoscopic examination, with biopsy, is mandatory to confirm the adenomatous character of the polyps before colectomy is considered.

The colonic polyps are not present at birth and usually develop during the second decade.[26] In the majority of cases, they are not evident radiographically until after puberty.[1] There have been reports of polyps occurring in children less than 10 years of age in families with FPC.[1,30,31] One report sites multiple colon polyps in a 4-month-old infant,[32] but such an occurrence is uncommon.

As in FPC, colon carcinoma will develop in 100% of untreated patients with GS by age 50 years.[33,34] Clinical symptoms referable to the gastrointestinal tract such as rectal bleeding, abdominal pain, and diarrhea commonly present in the third or fourth decades of life.[32] With GS, the average age of death in un-

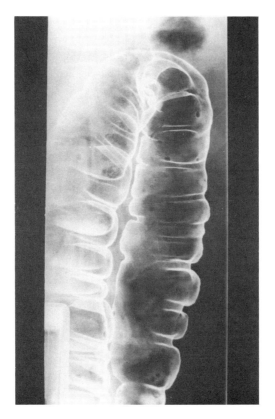

Figure 6-2. Double contrast examination. Tiny polyps in the splenic flexure area of the colon in a patient with familial polyposis coli. These small lesions are best seen with a double contrast study.

treated patients dying with colon carcinoma is 41 years.[35] The colon carcinomas have the typical radiographic appearance of adenocarcinoma. They may be annular, polypoid, or flat, or they may present as asymmetric or symmetric narrowing of the lumen (Figure 6-4). The colon cancers of GS are notoriously synchronous.

Gastric and Duodenal Polyps. Gastric polyps have been reported to occur in at least 5% of the patients with GS and uncommonly in FPC.[1,36] Recent reports, however, now indicate that gastric polyps as well as duodenal polyps occur in 65-90% of the patients with FPC and should be considered an integral part of the syndrome.[37-40] Gastric polyps are also as prevalent in GS.[38,41,42] The polyps are hyperplastic in most of the cases, but adenomatous polyps can also occur

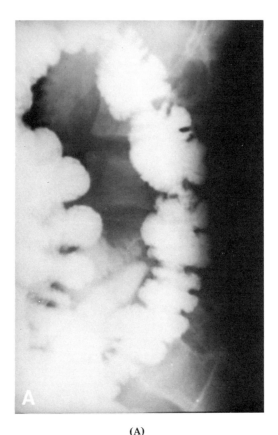

(A)

Figure 6-3. (A) Single contrast colon examination. These small polyps in a patient with familial polyposis coli present as serrations along the lateral and medial margins of the colon. They are not as well seen in comparison to a double contrast colon examination. (B) Single contrast colon examination in a patient with Gardner's syndrome showing multiple small polyps. *(Courtesy of David H. Stephens, M.D., Rochester, MN)*

and there are reports of gastric carcinoma developing in some cases.[43] These gastric polyps appear radiographically as small circumscribed lucencies seldom larger than 1.0 cm. (Figure 6-5A, B, and C). Distribution of the polyps may be throughout the entire stomach, but several cases have been described in which the antrum was not involved.[37,38] As previously discussed, a double contrast examination is the radiographic procedure of choice to detect these small polyps. Endoscopy may also be used as the initial diagnostic study or as a complementary procedure to the radiographic examination. Endoscopy, however, must eventually be utilized to establish the histology of the polyps by biopsy.

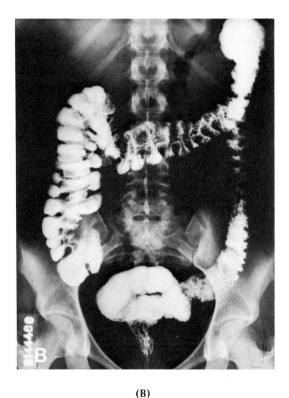

(B)

Figure 6-3. (Continued)

Other Associated Gastrointestinal Malignancies — Duodenal Carcinoma. Individuals with GS have a predilection to develop gastrointestinal neoplasms other than colon carcinomas. They have a particular tendency to develop duodenal, periampullary, and pancreatic carcinomas[44-46] (Figure 6-6). These findings, along with the recent knowledge that gastric polyps are prevalent in both FPC and GS, stress the possibility that these two polyposis syndromes are part of a spectrum of the same disease. McKusick considered the gene that determines GS as different from that of FPC.[41] This concept, however, has been questioned by other investigators who believe that FPC and GS are not separate genotypes.[38,47,48] Smith states that the two syndromes may represent opposite poles of a spectrum of genotypes produced by a single pleiotropic gene with varying expressivity.[1,47,48]

The occurrence of gastric and duodenal polyps in these patients raises the question of the frequency with which polyps may also be present in the jejunum and ileum (Figure 6-7). Perhaps the frequency of small bowel polyps is not

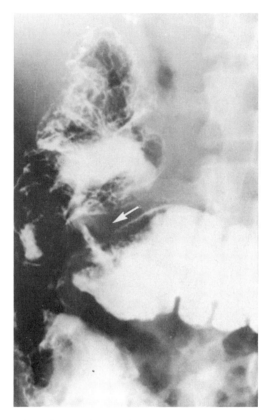

Figure 6-4. An annular adenocarcinoma of the proximal transverse colon (arrow) in a patient with Gardner's syndrome. *(Courtesy of Wylie J. Dodds, M.D., Milwaukee, WI. Reprinted with permission from Gastrointestinal Radiology. Copyright Springer-Verlag, New York, Inc.)*

appreciated since the specialized techniques of double contrast radiography and endoscopy have not been available for the small intestine. However, as noted in the introduction, the recently introduced enteroclysis method for examining the small bowel may enlighten us as to the occurrence of small bowel polyps in FPC and GS. Familial polyposis of the entire gastrointestinal tract, a separate entity from GS, has been described but has been considered extremely rare.[49] It now appears that extracolonic intestinal polyps are not uncommon and familial polyposis of the entire gastrointestinal tract may be more common than previously recognized.

Since there is potential for adenomatous polyps to occur in any area of the gastrointestinal tract in GS and FPC, the radiologist is obligated to thoroughly and conscientiously study the entire gastrointestinal tract including the small

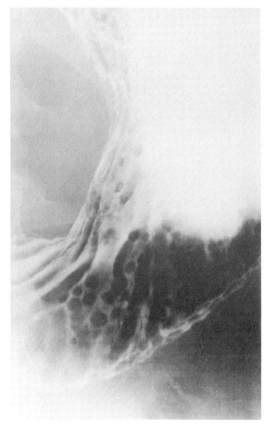

(A)

Figure 6-5. Double contrast examination of the stomach in a patient with familial polyposis coli showing distribution of hyperplastic polyps: (A) in the gastric body and (B) in the fundus. (C) Diffuse gastric polyposis in a patient with Gardner's syndrome. *(Reprinted with permission from Radiology, Oak Brook, IL).*

bowel. Particular attention should be paid to the descending and transverse duodenal segments in GS because of the predilection for neoplasms to occur in the pancreaticoduodenal area. A baseline examination of the pancreas with ultrasound or computed tomography may also be indicated in the initial evaluation of these patients.

Other Extraintestinal Lesions. *Associated Internal Neoplasms.* Adrenal carcinomas and adenomas have been described with GS.[46,50] The case reports are limited so this type of associated tumor is probably rare. If an adrenal neo-

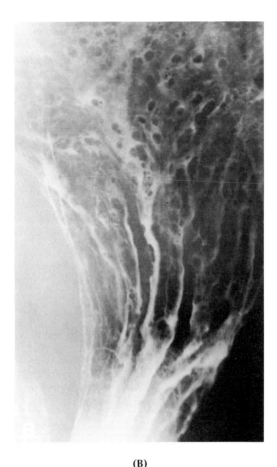

(B)

Figure 6-5. (Continued)

plasm is suspected, radiographic evaluation may be helpful. Plain film abdominal examination may show mottled calcium deposits in the adrenal gland, and the tumor may cause anterior displacement of a barium-filled stomach. Selective adrenal arteriography and venography, as well as computed tomography and ultrasound, will give information concerning the origin and extent of the tumor.[51]

Cases of thyroid carcinoma occurring with GS are documented in the literature.[52] Other internal neoplasms that have been described include gastric leiomyomas, retroperitoneal leiomyomas, and neurofibromas.[46,53] Although the incidence of these tumors is uncommon, most authors agree that their association with GS is more than coincidental and that they are representative of the broad spectrum of this disease. Physicians must be aware that patients with GS have the potential to develop unusual internal neoplasms.

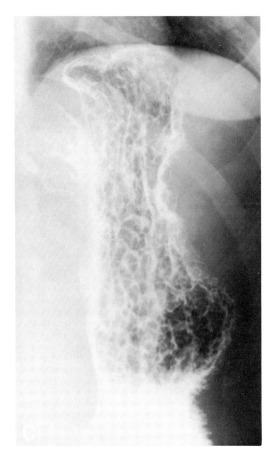

(C)

Figure 6-5. (Continued)

Cutaneous Lesions. The cutaneous manifestations of this syndrome have been discussed in Chapter 3. They generally consist of sebaceous cysts distributed most commonly over the face, scalp, and back and, occasionally, on the extremities (Figure 6-8). The subcutaneous tumors include fibromas, lipomas, leiomyomas, and neurofibromas. The cutaneous and subcutaneous lesions are usually multiple. Skin lesions may present before gastrointestinal symptoms manifest and, therefore, can serve as a signal to investigate the alimentary tract for polyps.[54]

Fibromatosis. There is a significant predisposition in GS for proliferation of fibrous tissue, resulting in the formation of mesenteric fibromatosis, desmoid tumors, retroperitoneal fibrosis, intraperitoneal adhesions, fibrosarcoma, and

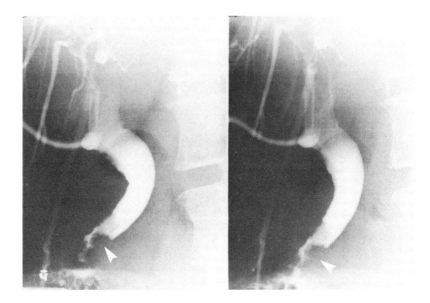

Figure 6-6. Ampullary carcinoma (arrow) in a patient with familial polyposis coli.

breast and parotid fibromatosis.[1,25,42,46,48,53,55-60] Fibromata in various forms have been reported to occur in at least 8% of the patients with GS and as much as 45%.[46,61] Although mesenteric fibromatosis may occur spontaneously, it is more common for this condition to develop following the trauma of abdominal surgery.[1,55,57,58] The desmoid tumors or fibromata may be large, discrete masses displacing adjacent organs (Figure 6-9). Resection is the treatment of choice and recurrence is not uncommon if the tumor is incompletely excised.[55] The mesenteric fibromatosis may also be diffuse and locally infiltrative. If the tumor is in intimate association with adjacent blood vessels, total resection may be impossible.[55] Most of the fibrous tumors in GS are benign; however, cases of fibrosarcoma have been documented in the literature.[25,46,56,58] Intraperitoneal adhesions causing small bowel obstruction following surgery in patients with GS occur frequently.[56,57]

Diagnostic imaging procedures aid in identifying and localizing the extent of the fibrous tumor masses. If intestinal obstruction is present, barium studies may show the exact site of obstruction and characterize whether it is the result of an adhesion or a neoplasm[62] Characteristic displacement of the stomach, small bowel, or colon may localize the intra-abdominal or retroperitoneal location of the fibromatosis. Arteriography may also localize the tumors and demonstrate their vascular pattern; however, most of these tumors are avascular.[63] The

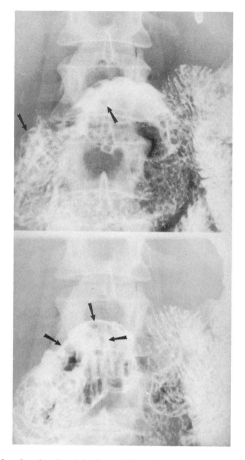

Figure 6-7. Polyps in the duodenal bulb and loop (arrows) in a patient with Gardner's syndrome.

newer imaging modalities, such as computed tomography and ultrasound, will probably prove to be the most accurate methods for identifying these fibrous neoplasms. It is well to keep in mind that an abdominal mass which develops, following colectomy, in a patient with GS may be a benign fibrous tumor and not a recurrent adenocarcinoma.

Bone Lesions. Bone abnormalities have been reported in approximately 50% of the patients with GS.[64] Both the bone and soft tissue lesions tend to appear before or during puberty and may precede the development of colonic polyposis.[1,54] The bone lesions of GS vary from localized cortical thickening, exostoses,

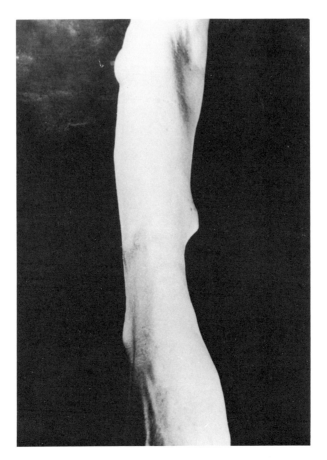

Figure 6-8. Inclusion cysts involving the forearm of a patient with Gardner's syndrome. *(Courtesy of Wylie J. Dodds, M.D., Milwaukee, WI. Reprinted with permission from Critical Reviews in Clinical Radiology and Nuclear Medicine. Copyright The Chemical Rubber Co., CRC Press Inc.)*

and osteomas to large protuberant bony masses.[65] The radiologist, depending on his knowledge of GS, should be able to select the proper radiographic views of the bony skeleton which will yield the greatest amount of information.

The osseous lesions of the skull in GS consist of two types according to Chang: dense osteomas arising from the outer table of the bony calvarium and osteomas arising near the paranasal sinuses and facial bones[65] (Figure 6-10). The ethmoid, sphenoid, and frontal sinuses, as well as the frontal and parietal bones and zygomas, are affected in order of decreasing frequency.[66] Anterior-posterior, laterals, Towne's, and submental-vertex radiographic views of the skull, as well as paranasal sinus projections, should be adequate to demonstrate these lesions.

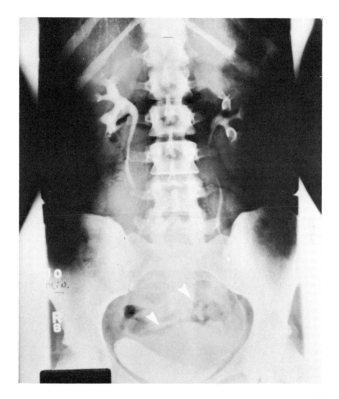

Figure 6-9. Pelvic fibromatosis (arrows) displacing left ureter in a patient with Gardner's syndrome. *(Courtesy of Carol B. Stelling, M.D., Charlottesville, VA)*

A dense osteoma originating at the angle of the mandible is one of the most characteristic bone changes in GS[65,66] (Figure 6-11). The cancellous portion of the mandible and maxilla may show small densities near the roots of the teeth, which are believed to be endosteal osteomas.[66] Dental abnormalities in GS include: hypercementosis, supernumerary and unerupted teeth, odontomas, and numerous caries.[1,25,65] Radiographic studies of the mandible should include anterior-posterior and both oblique views. However, Panorex studies of the mandible and maxilla are the most accurate and are preferred if this type of equipment is available (Figure 6-12).

Pedunculated osteomas, exostosis, and localized cortical thickening are the lesions most often seen in the long bones of patients with GS[1,65,66] (Figure 6-13A and B). These changes are characteristically limited to the diaphysis. Localized cortical thickening is probably the most common lesion involving the long bones, with the femoral and tibial shafts most frequently affected.[65] These lesions are bilateral in the majority of cases and occur most often in the radii,

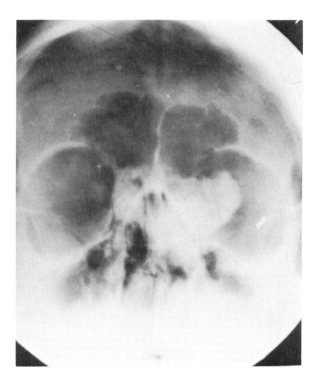

Figure 6-10. Dense osteomas involving the ethmoid sinuses in a patient with Gardner's syndrome. *(Courtesy of Wylie J. Dodds, M.D., Milwaukee, WI. Reprinted with permission from Critical Reviews in Clinical Radiology and Nuclear Medicine. Copyright The Chemical Rubber Co., CRC Press Inc.)*

ulnas, femurs, tibias, and fibulas.[66] Shortening and slight bowing of the long bones may also occur. The short tubular bones of the hands and feet may show similar changes of cortical thickening and exostosis.

The superior margins of the ribs, the inferior pubic rami, and the ilium below the anteroinferior iliac spine, all may have a wavy thickening of the cortex. The carpal and tarsal bones are rarely involved.[65]

Malignant tumors of bone, such as fibrosarcomas and osteogenic sarcomas, although infrequent, have been reported in association with GS.[61,67,68]

Management. Early diagnosis for the prevention of malignancy is the goal in the management of GS. As previously noted, the dermatologic and osseous manifestations may appear early in life with the gastrointestinal polyposis presenting

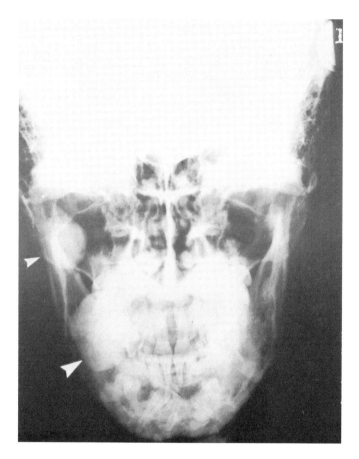

Figure 6-11. Osteomas (arrows) originating from the right mandibular ramus in a patient with Gardner's syndrome. *(Courtesy of Mervyn Thynne, M.D., Cleveland, OH)*

from 17 to 35 years of age.[54,69] Duncan suggests that all members of a family with a history of GS should be carefully evaluated for soft tissue tumors and should have roentgenograms of the skull, facial, and long bones as well as dental films to detect manifestations of the disease.[54] Proctosigmoidoscopy, as well as upper and lower gastrointestinal roentgenograms, should be performed. If no abnormalities are found, he recommends an annual examination for the appearance of external tumors and for occult blood in the stool. Roentgenograms of the skull and facial bones at 5-year intervals should be obtained.[54]

The initial therapy for patients with a diagnosis of FPC or GS is either total colectomy with ileoproctostomy or proctocolectomy with ileostomy and is usually deferred until the patients reach their late teens.[1,61] Total colectomy

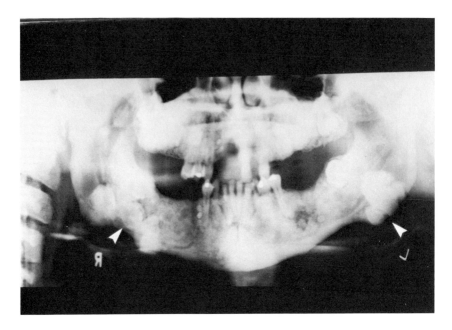

Figure 6-12. Panorex study of the mandible in a patient with Gardner's syndrome showing dense osteomata (arrows). *(Courtesy of Mervyn Thynne, M.D., Cleveland, OH)*

with ileoproctostotomy is the preferred surgical procedure — provided the patients are reliable and will return for annual proctoscopic follow-up examinations. Recurrent polyps can be fulgurated at that time and biopsies obtained for lesions suspicious for adenocarcinoma.[1] There are reports documenting spontaneous regression of rectal polyps following colectomy.[59,70-72] However, other reports state that there is a 4-22% incidence of carcinoma developing in the rectal stump.[73,74]

The recent evidence of extracolonic polyps occurring in significant numbers of patients with FPC and, particularly, GS raises questions about their long-term course and appropriate management. As previously noted, most of the gastric polyps associated with these syndromes have been hyperplastic, but adenomatous polyps also occur and cases of gastric carcinoma are documented.[43] The increased incidence of duodenal carcinoma in GS[44-46,75] suggests the same cancer-polyp relationship as in the colon. Boley recommended colectomy and partial gastrectomy when both colon and stomach polyps were present.[76] Cases have been reported of FPC in which gastric polyps did not involve the antrum which would allow for partial gastrectomy.[37,38] Boley also recommended termination of the procedure without resection when polyposis was found to involve the jejunum or ileum since total eradication of the disease would be im-

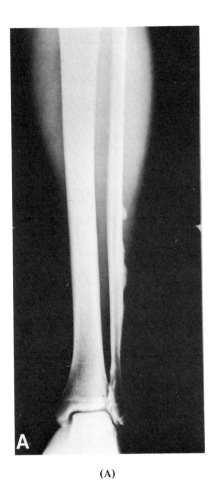

(A)

Figure 6-13. Gardner's syndrome patients showing: (A) osteomas involving the fibular diaphysis and (B) osteomas and periosteal thickening involving the femoral diaphysis (arrows). *(Courtesy of Mervyn Thynne, M.D., Cleveland, OH)*

possible.[76] It seems correct that in cases of FPC and GS with gastric polyposis, only colectomy should be performed since the malignant potential of gastric polyps is not definitely established. Conservative management of gastric polyps might also be supported by the observation that polypoid lesions of the stomach regressed in two cases reported in the literature.[38]

How to adequately follow these patients who have known polyps in the stomach and duodenum remains an unanswered question. Since the majority of these individuals are young, complete radiographic studies of the stomach and small intestine annually for the remainder of their lives do not seem feasible because

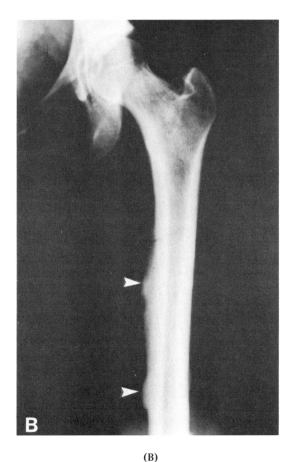

(B)

Figure 6-13. (Continued)

of the radiation exposure. A baseline upper gastrointestinal radiographic examination should be obtained, however, at the time of initial diagnosis for comparative purposes in the future. The flexible endoscopes now available allow for efficient and accurate examinations of the stomach and descending duodenum. Thus it would seem that endoscopy of the stomach and duodenum, as well as occult blood testing of the stool, at two-year intervals would be a more practical method for following asymptomatic patients. A detailed enteroclysis examination of the small intestine, perhaps, could be carried out at six-year intervals. Development of symptoms directed to the gastrointestinal tract should, of course, warrant immediate, thorough, radiographic examination followed by endoscopy if necessary.

The Problem of Heterogeneity of Polyp Expression. Bussey reports that the average number of colon polyps in a patient with FPC varies from 300 to 3,000.[77] The lowest number of polyps recorded in a case of polyposis from the St. Marks series was 150. Therefore, it has been suggested that 100 adenomatous polyps is the dividing line between the polyposis and nonpolyposis patients.[34,77]

Lynch, however, described two families with FPC which included patients with classic diffuse polyposis coli and patients with only solitary polyps but in whom the colon cancer predisposition was equally as high.[78] This variation in the phenotypic presentation of polyps in a kindred raises a question as to the minimal number of polyps necessary to establish the diagnosis of FPC. He suggests that variable penetrance of the dominant P gene could explain the variable patterns seen in the two kindreds. Lynch believes that these data indicate a need to reevaluate our criteria for diagnosing FPC, particularly regarding the site and number of colon polyps in high risk patients from families with a tendency to colon cancer and /or "classic FPC."

Oldfield's Syndrome

This entity was originally described by Oldfield as a distinct polyposis syndrome.[79] However, it is now recognized as a variant of Gardner's syndrome.

Oldfield described three members from one family with multiple sebaceous cysts, polyposis coli, and a tendency to develop colon carcinoma. The bone lesions and fibrous tumors characteristic of classic Gardner's syndrome were not present. The sebaceous cysts were typically located over the entire body including the face and neck. One patient in Oldfield's report presented with cysts on his scalp, back, and face at 6 years of age. The colon polyps did not manifest themselves or at least cause symptoms until puberty. The polyps were adenomatous, and adenocarcinoma of the rectosigmoid developed in two of the reported individuals.

Peutz-Jeghers Syndrome

Peutz-Jeghers syndrome (PJS) is an uncommon disease with the cardinal features of mucocutaneous melanotic pigmentation, gastrointestinal polyposis, and autosomal dominant inheritance. The original characteristics of the syndrome were described by Peutz in 1921, and the mode of inheritance was established by Jeghers in 1941.[80,81] Both sexes are equally affected and there is no racial distribution. A positive family history is present in half of the patients, and the remaining 50% represent sporadic mutations.[1,75,82,83] Over 300 cases of PJS have now been described showing that polyps involve not only the small intestine but also the stomach, duodenum, and colon and, in rare instances, the respiratory and urinary tracts as well.[1,75,82-86] Clinical recognition of this disease is important since there is a definite tendency for these patients to develop alimentary tract carcinoma[87-90] (see Table 6-2).

Distribution and Characteristics of the Gastrointestinal Polyps. The alimentary tract polyps in PJS are distributed from the esophagus to the rectum with small bowel polyps present in over 50% of the cases. Of the patients examined, 30% have polyps in the colon, while the stomach is involved in approximately 25%.[83,84,91] Polyps may rarely be present in the esophagus.[92] The polyps are usually multiple, either pedunculated or sessile, and vary in size

Table 6-2. Features of Peutz-Jeghers Syndrome.

I. Autosomal dominant inheritance

II. Mucocutaneous lesions
    A. Pigmented lesions usually evident in infancy or early childhood
    B. Mucosal pigmentation
        1. Mucosal surface of lower lip, buccal mucosa
        2. Bluish-gray blotches
        3. Do not fade with increasing age
    C. Skin pigmentation
        1. Face, palms of hands, soles of feet
        2. Brown or black macules
        3. May fade with increasing age

III. Gastrointestinal lesions
    A. Small bowel
        1. Involved in over 50% of patients
        2. Hamartomatous polyps
        3. Intussusception common, bleeding common
    B. Colon
        1. Involved in 30% of patients
        2. Polyps tend to be adenomas but may be hamartomas
    C. Stomach
        1. Involved in 25% of patients
        2. Polyps – adenomas or hamartomas
    D. Esophagus – polyps are rare
    E. Polyps in stomach, duodenum, and colon should be regarded as potentially malignant; increased tendency for carcinomas to develop in these areas
    F. Polyps of the alimentary tract appear in early childhood, gastrointestinal symptoms present in adolescence or young adult

IV. Associated neoplasms
    A. Ovarian
        1. Occur in 5% of female patients
        2. Usually theca cell granulosa type
    B. Polyps in other areas
        1. Ureters, urinary bladder
        2. Bronchi, maxillary sinuses, nasal choanae

from 0.1 to 3.0 cm.[1,82] Carpeting of the small intestine with tiny polyps has been described but does not occur in the stomach or colon.[93] Intussusception secondary to a polyp in the small intestine is quite common, while intussusception in the colon is unusual.[82]

Early investigators considered the small bowel polyps of PJS to be precancerous adenomas.[81,94] It is now accepted that these polyps are benign, nonproliferating hamartomas.[82-84,88,93,95] The question of whether these hamartomas undergo true malignant degeneration has not been completely resolved; however, if such degeneration does occur, it is exceedingly rare.[90,93,96-98] Gastric and duodenal polyps in the majority of patients with PJS show the histologic features of hamartomas, but adenomatous polyps with malignant potential may occur. Colonic polyps in this disease are usually proliferative lesions indistinguishable from adenomatous polyps.[1,84,99]

Most evidence indicates that patients with PJS have a greater risk of developing gastrointestinal tract carcinoma than individuals in the general population.[82,88] Of these patients, 2-3% will develop alimentary tract adenocarcinoma.[75,90] Although a few cases of ileal and jejunal carcinoma have been reported,[87,90,97] it is an uncommon occurrence[83] and the most common sites for carcinoma in PJS are the colon, stomach, and duodenum[87,88] (Figures 6-14 and 6-15).

Roentgen Features. Radiographic examination of these patients is necessary to confirm the diagnosis, determine the extent of gastrointestinal involvement, and determine the presence or absence of malignancy. Clinical symptoms are related to the gastrointestinal polyposis, and the most frequent presenting symptom is abdominal pain, secondary to small bowel intussusception.[88] Most of the intussusceptions are transient and the attacks remit spontaneously.[82,84] Occasionally, large intussusceptions may not reduce, resulting in a small bowel obstruction. In such cases, plain film examination of the abdomen utilizing supine, upright, and decubitus views, may show the obstruction or a soft tissue mass at the site of intussusception. Barium contrast studies will usually delineate the location and cause of the obstruction. It is not unusual while examining the small bowel during fluoroscopy to see the intussusceptions form and reduce spontaneously[1] (Figures 6-16 and 6-17).

Enteroclysis examination of the small bowel[17-21] with double contrast technique is the preferred method to demonstrate small polyps. Patients with PJS must be examined with meticulous technique. Tiny polyps may be overlooked unless the small bowel loops are systematically, manually compressed and separated during fluoroscopy[1,82] (Figures 6-18A and B). Hypotonic studies during enteroclysis may be helpful in studying a particular small bowel segment.

The double contrast method is also preferred to examine the stomach, duodenum, and colon. Gastric and duodenal polyps are usually multiple, but solitary

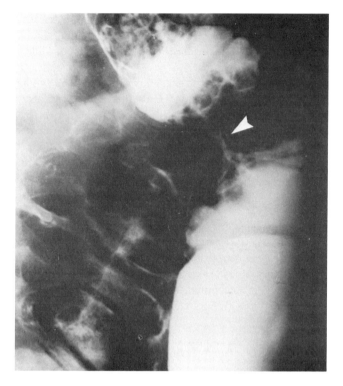

Figure 6-14. Adenocarcinoma of the proximal descending colon (arrow) in a patient with Peutz-Jeghers syndrome. *(Courtesy of Wylie J. Dodds, M.D., Milwaukee, WI. Reprinted with permission from Critical Reviews in Clinical Radiology and Nuclear Medicine. Copyright The Chemical Rubber Co., CRC Press Inc.)*

polyps have been found.[82] Colon polyps, when present, are multiple, varying in number from 2 to 12 with the pedunculated variety being the most common (Figure 6-19).

Rectal bleeding and melena are the second most common presenting symptoms of PJS occurring in approximately 30% of the patients.[82,83] Massive gastrointestinal bleeding is rare. Barium studies of the small bowel or stomach seldom show evidence of ulcerations involving the polyps. Arteriography, however, has demonstrated hypervascularity of the small bowel hamartomas and may also show evidence of intussusception by the stretching and distortion of mesenteric vessels.[100]

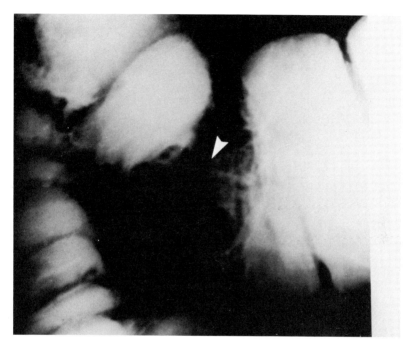

Figure 6-15. Adenocarcinoma of the proximal transverse colon (arrow) in a patient with Peutz-Jeghers syndrome. *(Courtesy of Wylie J. Dodds, M.D., Milwaukee, WI)*

Extra-Alimentary Lesions. Polyps occurring in the ureters, bladder, renal pelvis, bronchi, maxillary antra, and nasal choanae have been reported in patients with documented PJS.[85,86,93] It is not established whether these lesions are actually part of the syndrome or coincidental findings. If symptoms or history suggest respiratory or urinary tract involvement, chest, skull, and paranasal sinus radiographs, as well as intravenous urography, may be indicated.

Ovarian tumors, particularly granulosa cell tumors, occur with greater frequency in female patients with PJS than in the general population.[92,101-103] Humphries reports that the incidence of ovarian tumors in this syndrome is approximately 5%.[103] The age range for the occurrence of these neoplasms has been from 4 to 60 years, with more than half found in females 22 years or younger.[102] Some investigators believe that ovarian neoplasms should be included as part of the syndrome. It would seem that the incidence is high enough to warrant a thorough investigation of females with PJS to exclude the presence of coexisting ovarian tumors. Ultrasound or computed tomography of the pelvis would be helpful in such an evaluation.

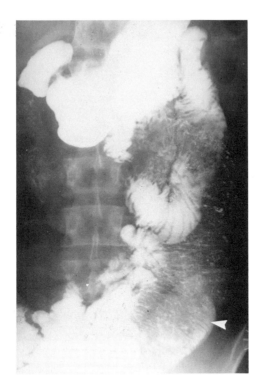

Figure 6-16. An adult patient with Peutz-Jeghers syndrome showing an area of intussusception (arrow) secondary to hamartomatous polyps of the jejunum.

Mucocutaneous Pigmentation. A detailed discussion of the skin changes in PJS has been presented in Chapter 3. The abnormal pigmentation appears in infancy or early childhood.[95] The cutaneous component consists of oval, brown, or black macules distributed around the mouth, eyes, nostrils, and less commonly on the volar aspects of the hands and feet[75,82,93] (Figure 6-20A and B). The mucosal pigmentation is almost pathognomonic for PJS and is composed of brown or black blotches on the lips, usually the lower lip, and buccal mucosa[75,82,93] (Figure 6-21). The cutaneous lesions may fade and disappear during the patient's adult life, while the mucosal pigmentation remains unchanged. Patients with the characteristic pigmentation of PJS without intestinal polyposis have been described but are rare.[93]

Management and Follow-up. Similar problems in management discussed for Gardner's syndrome patients also apply to patients with PJS. These individuals

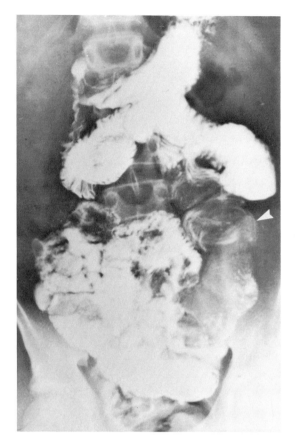

Figure 6-17. A 12-year-old boy with Peutz-Jeghers syndrome. Multiple polyps are present throughout the small bowel with an area of intussusception (arrow). *(Courtesy of Tom H. Smith, M.D., Kansas City, MO)*

are usually young, and radiation exposure for diagnostic purposes should be kept to a minimum. Cases are reported where the diagnosis was established as early as 8 and 11 months of age based on the typical mucocutaneous pigmentation.[104] However, symptoms related to polyps in the gastrointestinal tract apparently do not manifest until puberty, although Morens suggest that rectal polyposis may be more common in younger patients with PJS than previously recognized.[104] Gastrointestinal malignancy in the infant or child of early age with PJS is apparently rare. Thus, in an asymptomatic child, complete radiographic evaluation of the alimentary tract probably should be reserved until puberty. The purpose of an examination at that time would be to determine the extent of gastrointestinal involvement and to have a baseline for comparative purposes in the future. The

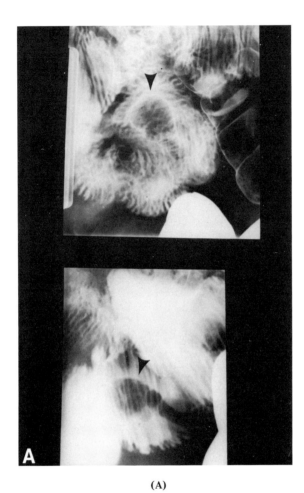

(A)

Figure 6-18. Small bowel examination of a 17-year-old female with Peutz-Jeghers syndrome showing: (A) a pedunculated hamartomatous polyp (arrow) and (B) a large sessile polyp in the jejunum (arrows).

patient of older age, puberty and beyond, should have a complete radiographic evaluation of the gastrointestinal tract at the time of initial diagnosis.

Evidence now indicates that polyps in the stomach, duodenum, and colon in PJS should be regarded as potentially malignant.[87] With the availability of flexible endoscopes, it would seem reasonable to prophylactically remove as many polyps in these areas as is safely possible in the asymptomatic patient. Of course, any polyps in the stomach, duodenum, or colon that are large (diameter of 2.0 cm or greater), show an increase in size, or change in contour should be

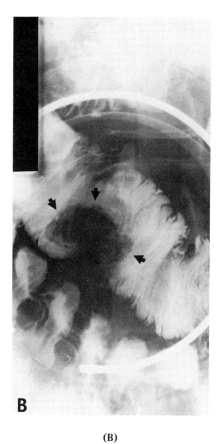

B

(B)

Figure 6-18. (Continued)

considered suspicious for malignancy and be resected. Dodds suggests a more conservative approach to the small bowel polyps in PJS and does not believe that prophylactic resection of small intestinal segments is necessary.[87] He is of the opinion that small bowel polyps, even if large but benign in appearance, can be safely watched in the asymptomatic patient. Small intestinal surgery should be performed in PJS only for significant small bowel obstruction, severe bleeding, or suspected malignancy.[1] Preservation of as much functional gastrointestinal tract tissue as possible should be the goal, since subsequent development of polyps may necessitate further surgery.[75]

Yearly evaluation of the stool for occult blood and endoscopic examination of the stomach, duodenum, and colon in patients with PJS at intervals of two years may be a satisfactory method of follow-up. Further radiographic examina-

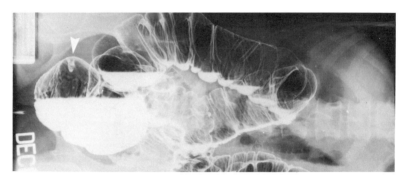

Figure 6-19. Double contrast colon examination in a 17-year-old female with Peutz-Jeghers syndrome demonstrating a pedunculated polyp in the rectum (arrow).

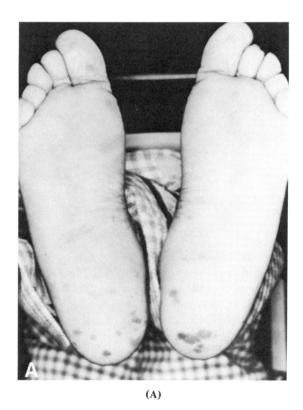

(A)

Figure 6-20. Pigmented macules in a patient with Peutz-Jeghers syndrome involving: (A) soles of the feet and (B) palms of the hands. *(Courtesy of Wylie J. Dodds, M.D., Milwaukee, WI. Reprinted with permission from Critical Reviews in Clinical Radiology and Nuclear Medicine. Copyright The Chemical Rubber Co., CRC Press Inc.)*

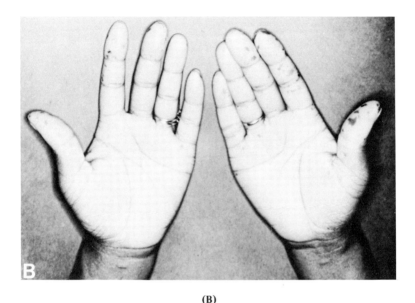

(B)

Figure 6-20. (Continued)

tion of the gastrointestinal tract, once the diagnosis has been made, would be reserved for those patients who develop symptoms.

Torre's Syndrome

Torre's syndrome (TS) has the salient features of multiple, benign sebaceous adenomas of the skin associated with visceral carcinomas, particularly of the gastrointestinal tract. At least ten cases have been described in the literature,[105-112] and a familial tendency has been suggested.[110,111] The age range has been from 36 to 65 years, with no racial or sex distribution.[108,112]

Cutaneous Manifestations. The skin lesions are sebaceous adenomas contrasting to the sebaceous cysts occurring in Oldfield's syndrome. There is an unusual discrepancy in location of single and multiple sebaceous tumors in TS. Isolated, single adenomas have a predilection for the head and neck, while multiple adenomas are more likely to have a truncal distribution.[108,112] In the majority of cases, the visceral carcinomas were diagnosed prior to the appearance of the sebaceous tumors, but in a few cases, the skin lesions preceded the internal malignancy.[106,108]

Visceral Carcinomas. The visceral carcinomas in TS are located primarily in the gastrointestinal tract, with colon carcinoma predominating. The colon neoplasms

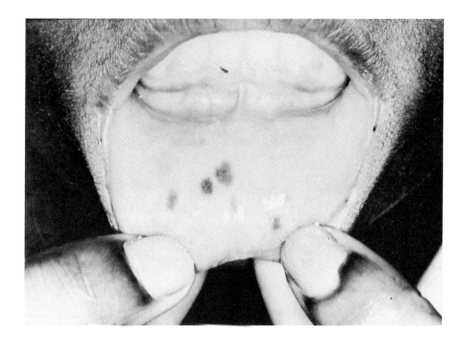

Figure 6-21. Bluish-black pigmented blotches of the lower lip mucosa in a patient with Peutz-Jeghers syndrome. *(Courtesy of Wylie J. Dodds, M.D., Milwaukee, WI)*

have a definite tendency to be synchronous and metachronous.[108,112] Although colon polyps have been reported in afflicted patients, there does not appear to be a polyposis predisposition.[108] Other gastrointestinal tract neoplasms that have been reported in TS include carcinoma of the duodenum, ampulla, and stomach.[105,106,108] Laryngeal carcinoma, transitional cell carcinoma of the ureter and urinary bladder, and endometrial carcinoma are other internal malignancies associated with this syndrome.[108,109] The visceral carcinomas tend to be low grade without any unique clinical or histologic characteristics.[112] Perhaps the hallmark of these tumors is their inclination to be multiple, arising in different segments of the alimentary tract throughout the course of the disease. The average reported survival time after the diagnosis of the original malignant neoplasm is 12 years, and the majority of patients have had at least 5-year survivals.[112] Metastases are uncommon.

Roentgen Manifestations and Management. The roentgen characteristics of the neoplasms in TS are no different from the usual carcinomas of the gastrointestinal tract. Radiologists should be aware of the synchronous disposition of the colon tumors and the possible development of carcinomas in the stomach or duodenum. The small intestine, thus far, has not been implicated. Any patient that develops a sebaceous adenoma following the diagnosis of a gastrointestinal carcinoma probably should be suspect for this syndrome. Once the diagnosis of TS has been established, thorough yearly radiographic or endoscopic evaluations of the stomach, duodenum, and colon may be necessary to detect occult malignancy. Unfortunately, the sebaceous adenomas appear before the onset of internal malignancies in only the minority of patients with TS. It has been recommended that any patient presenting with sebaceous adenomas, particularly on the eyelids, should have a careful evaluation of the gastrointestinal tract.[110,111]

Multiple Hamartoma Syndrome (Cowden's Disease)

Multiple hamartoma syndrome (MHS) is a disorder composed of a combination of verrucous, papular, and lichenoid mucocutaneous lesions, fibrocystic breast disease, carcinoma of the breast, benign and malignant thyroid tumors, gastrointestinal polyposis, and nervous system abnormalities.[113-116] There is an autosomal dominant pattern of inheritance. The age at onset of MHS varies from childhood (5 years) to age 45 years. Although gastrointestinal malignancies have not been described, it appears that the potential is present, and thus MHS is included in this chapter.

Mucocutaneous Lesions. All patients with MHS exhibit mucocutaneous lesions with variability in the degree to which each type of lesion is encountered.[114] Biologically, the skin lesions can be considered to be benign hamartomas.[115] Lichenoid papules are the most common cutaneous lesions and are located on the neck and pinnae, and clustered around the orifices of the eyes, nose, and mouth.[114] Other cutaneous manifestations include papillomatous lesions around the facial orifices, hyperkeratotic flat-topped papules on dorsa of the hands and wrists, translucent keratoses of palms and soles of the hands and feet, multiple lipomas, and occasionally cutaneous angiomas. The mucosal changes include papular, gingival, and palatal lesions, papillomatous lesions of the buccal mucosa, facial areas, and oropharynx, and a pebbly, scrotal appearance of the tongue.[114,115]

Gastrointestinal Lesions. Multiple alimentary tract polyps have been found in a significant number of these patients, most frequently in the colon, but also in the stomach.[114-116] Unfortunately, not all of the cases have been adequately studied to establish a definite pattern of occurrence or histologic identification of the polyps. Biopsies of the colon polyps have shown a variety of tumors varying from adenomatous, inflammatory, and lipomatous polyps to ganglioneuromas.[114] No malignant gastrointestinal neoplasms have been reported. Biopsies were apparently not obtained in the cases of gastric polyposis.[114,115] There are no reports of small intestinal polyps.

Other Neoplasms. Thyroid tumor formations, varying from goiters to adenomas and carcinomas, have been found in almost every patient with MHS.[114] Fibrocystic disease of the breast has been described in every female patient, and there is a very high incidence of breast carcinoma.[114-116] Brownstein reports that of the documented cases of Cowden's disease in females, at least 40% have developed breast carcinoma.[115] The central nervous system may be affected in this syndrome, as manifested by meningioma, mental dullness, and intention tremor.[116]

Radiographic Findings. The radiographic findings of the polyps involving the stomach and colon would not differ from those described in association with the other polyposis syndromes. In MHS the radiologist has the added responsibility of evaluating these patients for breast carcinoma, by use of mammography, and evaluating the thyroid for carcinoma, goiter, or adenoma with radionuclide studies and ultrasound.

Turcot Syndrome

Turcot syndrome (TS) is a rare affliction belonging to the gastrointestinal polyposis syndromes, but without a consistent dermatologic component. Its features include central nervous system tumors, polyposis coli with a probable predilection for colon adenocarcinoma, and an autosomal recessive mode of inheritance. Eight cases have been reported in the literature.[42,117-119] The majority of patients have been 12 to 24 years of age. One patient had an associated thyroid adenocarcinoma.[119]

Central Nervous System Tumors. The predominate CNS neoplasms were supratentorial glioblastomas. Medulloblastomas involving the fourth ventricle and spinal cord have also been described.[117,119] Most of the patients presented with signs and symptoms referable to the CNS such as seizures and headaches. A minority of the patients complained of diarrhea, rectal bleeding, or vague stomach distress.[42,117] Death as a result of CNS tumors occurred in almost all cases by age 25 years.

Skin Lesions. A definite association with skin disease has not yet been established for this syndrome. No skin lesions were characterized in Turcot's patients.[117] In three of Baughman's cases, however, café au lait spots and pigmented nevi were described.[118] Yaffe has suggested a possible relation between Gardner's syndrome and TS.[42]

Gastrointestinal Manifestations. The gastrointestinal polyps in Turcot syndrome are limited to the colon[42,117-119] and distributed primarily in the rectosigmoid. Three cases have demonstrated diffuse colon polyposis.[42,118] The polyps are probably benign adenomas, but the histopathology is not completely described in most of the reports. Malignant lesions of the colon developed in three of the patients.[117,118]

Cronkhite-Canada Syndrome

Cronkhite-Canada syndrome (CCS) is an unusual disorder characterized by diffuse gastrointestinal polyposis and ectodermal abnormalities consisting of alopecia, skin hyperpigmentation, and onychotrophia.[120-128] This disease usually presents in the sixth or seventh decade. There is no racial or sexual predisposition and no familial tendency. Although colon carcinoma has been described,[83,123] it is a rare occurrence and there is no definite predilection for gastrointestinal malignancy. Cronkhite-Canada syndrome, therefore, is not one of the genodermatoses but is included in this chapter for completeness in the differential diagnosis of gastrointestinal polyposis syndromes.

Polyps in CCS are always present in the stomach and colon and have been reported in the small bowel in over half of the patients.[83] Esophageal polyps may occur rarely.[128] Histologically, the polyps were originally thought to be adenomatous,[120] but they are now regarded as inflammatory polyps similar to the juvenile type.[83,126]

The most common presenting symptom is severe, watery diarrhea. The patients are seriously ill; many have hypoproteinemia, electrolyte imbalance, edema, and hypocalcemia.[83,128] There is a tendency for spontaneous remission in males, but females generally show a downhill course resulting in death within 6–18 months following the onset of diarrhea.

Juvenile Polyposis Syndromes

The combination of a genodermatoses and gastrointestinal cancer is not present in any of the juvenile polyposis syndromes. However, it is essential that the radiologist be familiar with these varied syndromes in children and infants. He should not mistake simple, juvenile polyps of the colon in a child for familial polyposis coli. He must understand the grave clinical implications of severe diarrhea in an infant with juvenile gastrointestinal polyposis and unusual ectodermal changes. He should be aware of recent reports suggesting an association between juvenile polyposis and malignancy of the gastrointestinal tract. For these reasons, this complicated group of syndromes is presented with this chapter.

Juvenile Polyps of the Colon. The solitary juvenile polyp is the most common polypoid lesion of the colon occurring in infants and children.[129] Juvenile polyps are often referred to as retention or inflammatory polyps and have certain histological features distinguishing them from adenomatous polyps. These features include an abundant connective tissue stroma, dilated cystic glands, and a single layer of columnar epithelium that is often ulcerated.[1,129-133] Morson considers the juvenile polyp a hamartoma.[99] The polyps are usually single, but approximately one-third are multiple. Eighty to ninety percent occur in the rectum and sigmoid.[131] Most are pedunculated (Figure 6-22). The peak age incidence in children is 4 to 6 years, and there is a slight male predominance. Rectal bleeding is the most common clinical presentation. The polyps tend to

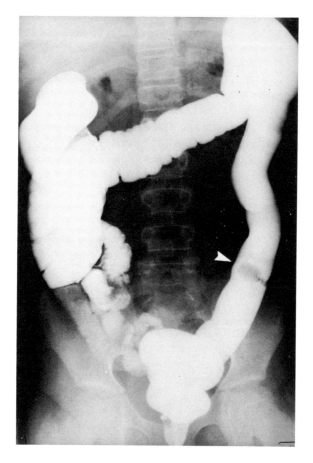

Figure 6-22. Pedunculated juvenile polyp of the descending colon (arrow) in a 10-year-old female.

decrease in frequency after the child reaches 12 years of age because of spontaneous regression or autoamputation. Surgical intervention is not usually necessary unless severe bleeding or intussusception develops. In the majority of cases, these solitary juvenile polyps have no malignant potential, no familial tendency, and no associated mucocutaneous lesions.

Generalized Juvenile Gastrointestinal Polyposis — Familial Type. Sachatello has reported generalized juvenile gastrointestinal polyposis in three members of a kindred.[134] He believes this is a hereditary syndrome characterized by juvenile polyps involving the stomach, small intestine, and colon in various combinations. The polyps may be present at birth or manifest at a later time in life and are responsible for symptoms related to chronic blood loss or bouts of intussusception. The ages of his patients ranged from 7 to 63 years. There was no evidence of gastrointestinal malignancy and no dermatologic lesions.

There have been recent reports indicating that juvenile polyposis, in at least some cases, is an inherited disease with an increased incidence of gastrointestinal cancer.[77,133,135,136] Although most of the cases consist of multiple juvenile polyps, solitary juvenile polyps have also been implicated and the distinction between these two groups is becoming less clear.[77,135] Stemper presented a kindred in which at least 10 members have had single or multiple juvenile polyps of the stomach and colon, and 11 members have had gastrointestinal neoplasms including gastric, duodenal, and colon carcinoma.[135] The question of whether there is a malignant potential to the juvenile polyps themselves or to the colonic mucosa from which they arise is not resolved.[77] A proportion of juvenile polyps in cases of juvenile polyposis have shown atypical epithelial changes indistinguishable from the atypia that may be seen in adenomas.[77,137] It is also known that adenomas and carcinomas can occur in association with juvenile polyposis.[77,137-139]

Therefore, we are now aware that associated gastrointestinal cancer has been found in some patients with juvenile polyposis and in their family members. It appears that the actual incidence of malignancy among juvenile polyposis cases is slightly higher than expected in the general population.[77] The exact genetics of juvenile polyposis associated with gastrointestinal malignancy awaits further long-range case studies.

Generalized Juvenile Gastrointestinal Polyposis — Nonfamilial Type. Reports of this type of juvenile polyposis are sparse in the medical literature.[131,140,141] The patients are infants, usually less than 12 months of age, presenting with bloody diarrhea, protein-losing enteropathy, and cachexia. Macrocephaly related to the presence of multiple arachnoid cysts may be present.[142] Ectodermal changes similar to those seen in adults with Cronkhite-Canada syndrome have been described.[140] The stomach, small bowel, and colon are invariably involved with multiple juvenile polyps. Esophageal polyps have not been reported.[142]

There is no familial predisposition. No gastrointestinal malignancies have been reported, but the disease is almost always fatal by 18 months of age because of uncontrolled malnutrition problems or complications of an unrecognized intussusception.

Generalized Gastrointestinal Adenomatous Polyps. Yonemoto described three cases with generalized polyposis (adenomatous) of the entire gastrointestinal tract.[49] An adenocarcinoma was found in one of these patients. The patients were children ranging in ages from 9 to 11 years. There were no other manifestations of the polyposis syndromes such as mucocutaneous or bone lesions. The relationship to familial polyposis coli is not clear except that the autosomal dominant mode of inheritance is the same. Gastric and small intestinal polyps are becoming an accepted part of Gardner's syndrome and of familial polyposis coli (as discussed earlier in this chapter), and the entity described by Yonemoto may yet be another variant of these diseases.

GASTROINTESTINAL NON-POLYPOSIS SYNDROMES

Other genodermatoses associated with alimentary tract malignancies but without dominant polyposis components will be discussed in this section. Familiar diseases of particular interest to the radiologist include hemochromatosis and celiac sprue as well as lesser known disorders such as tylosis palmaris et plantaris, ataxia telangiectasia, and familial hyperglucagonemia.

Tylosis Palmaris et Plantaris

The only genodermatosis known to be definitely associated with esophageal carcinoma is tylosis palmaris et plantaris (TPP).[143] This association was first described by Howel-Evans in 1958,[144] and only a few additional cases have been documented since.[145,146] The characteristic components of this uncommon disease include thickening of the skin of the palms and soles, esophageal carcinoma, and an autosomal dominant inheritance. Both sexes are equally affected and there is no racial preference.

Skin Manifestations. Tylosis is a form of dyskeratosis with the distinctive feature of pronounced thickening of the skin of the palms and soles.[144] Hyperhidrosis is also commonly present. Occasionally only the soles will manifest the dyskeratosis. There are two clinical types of inherited tylosis: early onset, presenting at age 3-12 months, and late onset, presenting at age 5-15 years.[144-146] The early onset type is more common in clinical dermatologic practice.[145] Esophageal carcinoma appears to be associated only with the late onset variety.[144]

Esophageal Cancer. After age 35, the risk of developing esophageal carcinoma for these patients steadily increases, and by 65 years of age, 95% of all tylotics will develop this cancer.[144,145] In the families described, there were no cases of esophageal cancer in patients who did not show tylosis. As in the general population, the dominant carcinoma is squamous cell and the most common locations for the tumor are in the middle and lower thirds of the esophagus. However, esophageal cancer in TPP occurs ten years earlier than expected in the general population.[143]

Diagnosis and Management. Roentgenologic evaluation in the form of an esophagram is usually the first diagnostic procedure for any patient with suspected esophageal carcinoma. Unfortunately, most patients do not present to the radiologist until symptoms of dysphagia are present, and by the time a radiographic diagnosis is established, the disease is often far advanced.

A more aggressive approach seems logical for patients with TPP who have a known high risk to develop esophageal carcinoma. After reaching the age of 30 years, any patient with TPP probably should have a baseline double contrast examination of the esophagus for comparative purposes in the future. This could be followed annually by a screening procedure such as exfoliative cytological analysis.[147] Any gastrointestinal symptom should be immediately investigated. The investigation should include both radiographic and endoscopic examinations of the esophagus. The roentgenologic description of esophageal cancer in TPP is not well documented. The tumor probably has the usual appearance of an ulcerative, fungating or infiltrative lesion (Figure 6-23).

Epidermolysis Bullosa

Epidermolysis bullosa (EB) is a rare hereditary skin disease in which bullae are formed on the skin and mucous membranes spontaneously or with minor trauma. Two major forms are recognized,[148] simplex and dystrophic. The simplex, milder form is characterized by nonscarring bullae of the skin after minimal trauma, occurs in infancy, and is transmitted by autosomal dominant inheritance. The dystrophic, severe type occurs at birth, is transmitted by an autosomal recessive gene, and is characterized by destructive bullae and vesicles involving the skin and mucous membranes. A majority of these patients develop contractures secondary to scar formation from infected bullae. Dystrophic changes also affect the nails and teeth.[148-150] Associated neoplasms, some including the gastrointestinal tract, have been described with this disease.

Associated Neoplasms. Bullous involvement of the mucous membranes of the eyes, nose, oropharynx, and genital tract are common in EB.[148] Esophageal involvement is not as prevalent but is also recognized in the recessive dystrophic

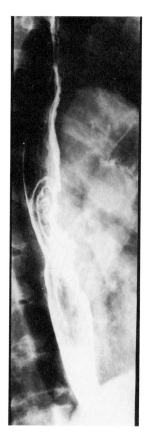

Figure 6-23. Double contrast esophagram showing a large squamous cell carcinoma of the mid-esophagus.

type.[148-150] Recurring esophageal bullae lead to scarring and stenosis. The stenotic areas are most frequently located in the proximal and distal thirds of the esophagus[149] (Figure 6-24). Dysphagia is the most common presenting symptom in these cases, usually occurring before the age of 14 years.[149] Postcricoid esophageal webs have been described.[149] The recurrent scarring and stenosis in EB suggests a potential for development of esophageal carcinoma; however, this relationship has not been definitely established. One case of carcinoma (cell type not designated), originating at the gastric cardia and extending into the esophagus, has been reported in a 38-year-old female with EB.[148,151] Squamous cell carcinoma of the oral mucosa has also been reported in this disease.[150,152] Squamous and basal cell carcinomas of the skin, most commonly of the lower extremities, are documented in patients with EB.[150]

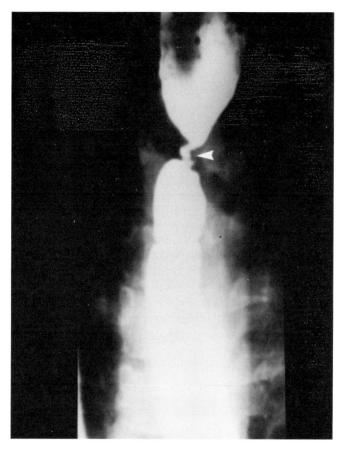

Figure 6-24. Esophagram showing a stricture (arrow) and esophageal web (immediately distal to the stricture) in a patient with epidermolysis bullosa. *(Courtesy of Tom H. Smith, M.D., Kansas City, MO)*

Dyskeratosis Congenita

Dyskeratosis congenita (DC) is a rare genodermatosis with multisystemic manifestations. The important features of this disease include: hyperpigmentation of the skin, nail dystrophy, leukoplakia of the mucous membranes, pancytopenia, and an increased incidence of solid malignant tumors.[153-165] Although the mode of inheritance is not definitely established, it is generally believed to be transmitted as a sex-linked recessive trait occurring predominantly in males.[153,159] The patients are usually of slight build with sparse hair and hypogonadism,[155] and approximately 40% will have subnormal intelligence.[153] Pancytopenia and malignancy are the major causes of death. Some investigators suggest that there are similarities between DC and Fanconi anemia.[154,166]

Skin Manifestations. The disease usually presents before puberty, at approximately 5–12 years of age, and in some cases is present at birth.[153,155] The most characteristic dermatologic manifestations are reticulated skin hyperpigmentation, nail dystrophy, and leukoplakia of the oral mucosa. Less frequent skin changes include hyperhidrosis and hyperkeratosis of palms and soles and bullous eruptions. The most common location for leukoplakia is the oral mucosa; less common locations are the urethra, glans penis, vagina, and rectoanal region.[155,158,160-164]

Associated Malignant Neoplasms. Sirinavin, in his review of 51 cases of DC, found a definite increased incidence of solid malignant tumors.[153] The neoplasms were usually diagnosed between 20 and 45 years of age, and involved the tongue, buccal and oral mucosa, nasopharynx, skin, cervix, and vagina. Most of these lesions were squamous cell carcinomas. Of particular interest are three documented cases of gastrointestinal tumors: two adenocarcinomas of the rectum and one squamous cell carcinoma of the esophagus.[155,156,165] This may indicate a tendency toward development of alimentary tract cancers in DC. No description of the radiographic appearance of these tumors was given.

Familial Hyperglucagonemia

Syndromes caused by functioning pancreatic islet cell neoplasms are well recognized: Zollinger-Ellison syndrome (gastrin-secreting tumor), watery diarrhea, hypokalemia, hypochlorhydria syndrome (non-beta islet cell tumor), and hyperglycemia (insulinoma). The least common of these tumors is the alpha-cell tumor which is associated with the rare, familial hyperglucagonemia syndrome (FH).[167] The FH syndrome consists of migratory necrotizing skin lesions, diabetes, anemia, autosomal dominant inheritance, and a glucagon-secreting pancreatic tumor.[167-172] The age range is from 40 to 69 years, and it is more common in females.[172]

Dermatological Features. The skin rash is distinctive and is described as a necrolytic, migratory erythema with certain features of pemphigus.[169] The erythematous rash progresses to bullous lesions with superficial necrolysis. As the original lesions heal, others develop. The eruption is most severe on the lower abdomen, groin, and perineum, and between the thighs and buttocks.[169] Anemia and diabetes are almost always present in these patients. The skin rash and diabetes may regress following resection of the glucagonoma.[172]

Radiographic Manifestations. The majority of glucagonomas are located in the tail of the pancreas and most are malignant.[172] Hepatic metastases are not uncommon. These tumors are usually diagnosed before the patient is seen by the radiologist. Therefore, his function is to confirm the clinical impression and localize the lesion.[167] Localization is important since the neoplasms often are small and cannot be palpated during surgery. Angiography utilizing selective and subselective catheterization techniques has been, up to now, the most reliable method of localizing these rare neoplasms.[167,172,173] The different functioning islet cell tumors usually cannot be distinguished radiographically.[167] They are characteristically well-circumscribed vascular tumors with a late capillary blush[167,172-174] (Figure 6-25). As the neoplasms enlarge, the supplying arteries may dilate, and typical tumor vascularity will become evident.[172] Displacement of vessels by the tumor mass is common. Hepatic metastases are almost always hypervascular (Figure 6-26). Selective catheterization of pancreatic veins to obtain blood samples for radioimmunoassay may be helpful in the diagnosis of a glucagon-secreting tumor.[175]

Barium contrast studies of the upper gastrointestinal tract are usually of no help in diagnosing these tumors because of their small size. However, if the tumor is large enough, the classic signs of a pancreatic mass such as displacement of the stomach and duodenal loop may be evident (Figure 6-27A and B). Ultra-

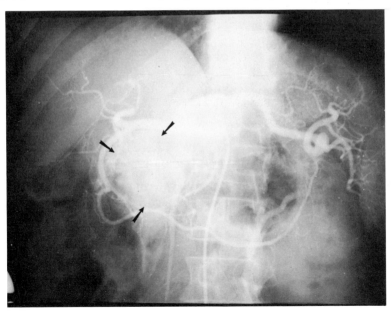

Figure 6-25. Selective arteriogram of the celiac artery in a patient with familial hyperglucagonemia. Note the large, vascular glucagonoma (arrows) in the head of the pancreas.

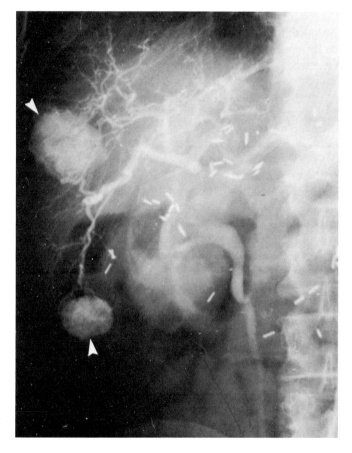

Figure 6-26. Selective arteriogram of the right hepatic artery showing vascular metastases (arrows) to the liver in a patient with familial hyperglucagonemia.

sound and particularly computed tomography with contrast enhancement may prove to be the diagnostic methods of choice for these tumors in the future.

Ataxia Telangiectasia (Louis-Bar Syndrome)

Ataxia telangiectasia (AT) is an autosomal recessive syndrome characterized by cerebellar ataxia, oculocutaneous telangiectasia, recurrent sinopulmonary infections, and an increased incidence of malignant neoplasms.[176-180]

Neuromuscular Manifestations. The cardinal symptom of this disease is cerebellar ataxia, usually appearing before the age of 5 years, and manifested by clumsiness

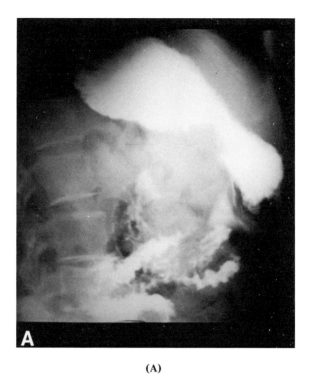

(A)

Figure 6-27. (A) Displacement of the stomach anteriorly and (B) effacement of the gastric antrum by a large glucagonoma in the head of the pancreas.

and unsteady gait.[176-178,181,182] The ataxia is progressive and incapacitating within 6-8 years.[178] Other features include choreoathetoid movements, hypotonia, dysarthria, and abnormalities of conjugate eye movements.[181,183,184] Retardation of growth is also a frequent feature.[176] The intelligence of these patients is usually normal.[176]

Oculocutaneous Changes. Oculocutaneous telangiectasia appears later than ataxia, becoming evident at about 5-6 years of age.[177,181,182] The telangiectasia characteristically begins in the bulbar conjunctiva, sparing the parietal portion.[177] Cutaneous telangiectasias are first noted in the ears, across the butterfly area of the face, across the bridge of the nose, and periorbitally.[177,179] As the patient's age increases, the neck, hands, feet, and antecubital and popliteal regions become involved. Telangiectasia has not been demonstrated in gastrointestinal viscera, and bleeding from mucous membranes is an inconspicuous feature of AT compared to hereditary hemorrhagic telangiectasia (Rendu-Osler-Weber syndrome).[181]

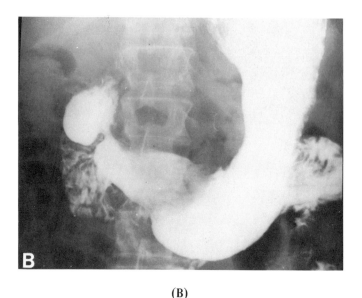

(B)

Figure 6-27. (Continued)

Sinopulmonary Involvement. Sinopulmonary infections occur in about 85% of cases.[176] These include sinusitis, bronchitis, and pneumonia.[177,182] The recurrent infections lead to bronchiectasis and pulmonary fibrosis. Chronic pulmonary disease is usually the cause of death, often occurring in adolescence.[177]

Immunologic Deficiencies. A common finding in AT is a marked deficiency in serum IgA.[178,183] There is also a concomitant decrease of IgA in the intestinal mucosal plasma cells.[183] In many of these patients the thymus has been abnormally small, and histological examination has shown thymic dysplasia and decrease in thymic lymphocytes.[178,180] Swift reports that increases in the serum α-fetoprotein in patients with AT are more consistent than the immunoglobulin deficiencies.[185]

Associated Malignancies. Peterson emphasized that patients with AT have a susceptibility to develop lymphoreticular malignancies.[178] Hodgkin's disease, reticulum cell sarcoma, lymphosarcoma, and lymphocytic leukemia have all been reported.[178,186] Other malignant tumors associated with AT include frontal lobe glioma, cerebellar medulloblastomas, and ovarian dysgerminomas.[178,182,184,187,188]

Mucinous adenocarcinoma of the stomach was described in two members of a large Negro sibship by Haerer.[180] Both patients were females, had a decrease in serum IgA levels, and succumbed to the adenocarcinoma in their early teens. The mother of these children also developed gastric cancer. Thus, she would have to be heterozygous for the AT gene. Since the mode of inheritance is autosomal recessive, her two affected children would be homozygous. The occurrence of gastric carcinoma in the mother suggests a heterozygote effect of the deleterious recessive gene.[143] This is an important concept. Swift suggests that over 5% of all persons dying from any malignancy before age 45 may carry the gene for AT. Therefore, according to Swift, each gene for an autosomal recessive syndrome which predisposes to tumor formation in heterozygotes may be associated with a small but important fraction of all genetic predisposition to malignancy.[185]

There is an apparent increased incidence of gastric and colonic carcinoma as well as lymphoma of the bowel in all enteropathic types of immunoglobulin deficiencies.[189]

Sholman has now reported an increased incidence of pancreatic neoplasm in patients with AT.[190] He believes that the risk of a patient with AT dying from pancreatic carcinoma is 15 times greater than that of the general population. These patients, in his opinion, are also at greater risk for developing diabetes mellitus.

Roentgen Findings. Discussions of the radiographic changes in AT are sparse. Upper gastrointestinal examinations were performed on the two patients with gastric adenocarcinoma, but the tumor was only described as "large." No detail of the roentgen appearance for the cases of pancreatic carcinoma are available. The only other reference to radiographic examinations occurs in the changes of chronic lung disease, such as peribronchial infiltration which resembles cystic fibrosis.[178] Marshak has reported on the roentgen features of small bowel immunoglobulin deficiency syndromes.[189] These features include a malabsorption pattern seen in IgA-deficient sprue consisting of small bowel dilatation and fragmentation of the barium column secondary to hypersecretion. Multiple nodular defects and thickening of the small intestinal folds are other manifestations of the immunoglobulin deficiency syndromes seen on barium examinations of the small bowel.[189] It is conceivable that some of these changes may be evident if small bowel studies are performed in the future on patients with AT.

Radiosensitivity. Studies have shown that patients with AT have an unusual radiosensitivity, not unlike the sensitivity of patients with xeroderma pigmentosum to ultraviolet.[191-193] AT patients who receive conventional radiotherapy for treatment of various malignant neoplasms have a tendency to develop severe complications often leading to a premature death.[192] The molecular basis for this clinical radiosensitivity is believed to be the result of a deficient DNA repair mechanism.[192-194]

Familial Malignant Melanoma

Familial malignant melanoma is characterized by an early age of onset, an excess frequency of multiple, primary melanomas, and an increased incidence of associated neoplasms.[195-198] In at least 3% of the families with melanoma, there is evidence to indicate an autosomal dominant mode of inheritance.[197-200] Melanoma has been found to be associated with other inherited disorders with cutaneous markers including xeroderma pigmentosum, von Recklinghausen's neurofibromatosis, and the congenital form of giant pigmented nevus.[197,201-203]

Lynch and Frichot have recently described malignant melanoma in association with a distinguishing cutaneous phenotype characterized by multiple, large, reddish-brown to pink moles, pigmentary leakage, and with an apparent autosomal dominant mode of inheritance. The authors believe that this may constitute a new familial melanoma syndrome and suggest that this disorder be named the familial atypical multiple mole-melanoma syndrome (FAMMM).[196,197,204]

Associated Neoplasms. Evidence compiled by Lynch and associates indicates that there is an excess of multiple, primary malignant tumors in certain melanoma-prone families.[195,203,205] These tumors include carcinoma of the breast, lung, gastrointestinal tract, lymphoreticular malignancies, and sarcoma. Fraser found a 20% incidence of coexisting neoplasms in his patients with malignant melanoma.[206] Of particular interest are the increased number of alimentary tract tumors, especially carcinomas involving the stomach and colon. In Lynch's study of five families with malignant melanoma, the associated gastrointestinal malignancies included six cases each of stomach and colon cancer, one each of pancreas and gallbladder, and two involving the liver.[195] Physicians therefore, should search for familial occurrences in patients with malignant melanoma and be aware of the possibility of coexisting neoplasms.[195]

Roentgen Manifestations. Malignant melanoma (melanosarcoma) is a common metastatic tumor to the gastrointestinal tract.[21] In McNeer's series,[207] necropsy of patients dying from melanoma showed a frequency of metastasis of 58% to the small intestine, 26% to the stomach, 22% to the colon, and 53% to the pancreas; 70% had metastasis to the lungs and 60% to the liver. Primary melanoma of the alimentary tract is rare since melanoblasts are usually not found in the entodermal epithelium.[21,208] Metastatic melanoma is a cellular tumor producing minimal desmoplastic response and, therefore, has a roentgen appearance similar to lymphosarcoma.[208]

The lesions of melanosarcoma commonly present on contrast examination of the gastrointestinal tract as submucosal or intraluminal nodules.[21,208] They have a tendency to central ulceration which gives the characteristic "bulls-eye" or "target" appearance (Figures 6-28A and B). The neoplastic nodules may become large enough to cause obstruction or intussusception of the small intestine. Aneurysmal dilatation of the bowel, not unlike lymphosarcoma, can also occur. If necrosis of the tumors is extensive, fistula or sinus tracts may develop.[208] Melanoma of the large bowel is usually located in the rectum, and the tumors are often large with ulceration and necrosis.[209] The differential diagnosis of melanoma involving the alimentary tract includes leiomyoma, leiomyosarcoma, lymphosarcoma, and Kaposi sarcoma.[21]

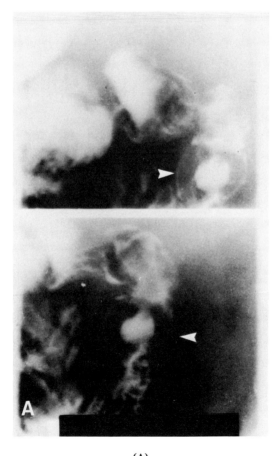

(A)

Figure 6-28. Metastatic melanosarcoma: (A) to the duodenum (arrow) and (B) to the gastric fundus (arrow), representing the classic "target" sign.

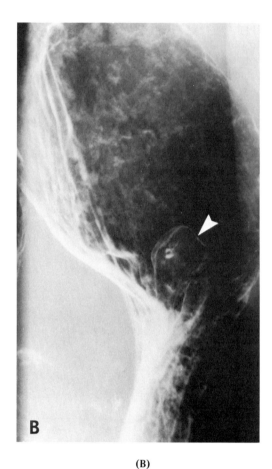

(B)

Figure 6-28. (Continued)

Wiskott-Aldrich Syndrome (Aldrich Syndrome)

The Aldrich syndrome (AS) is a sex-linked recessive, immunodeficiency disorder characterized by thrombocytopenia, chronic eczema, and an extreme susceptibility to bacterial infections.[210-213] The disease occurs only in males, with onset in early infancy and death usually before the age of puberty.[212-213] Immunologic IgM levels are very low, and IgA and IgG levels usually normal.[213] There is an approximate 10% incidence of malignancy developing in these children.[213] Purpura and melena are prominent clinical manifestations. Superficial infections such as impetigo, furunculosis, and conjuctivitis are the most common recurrent infections.[212] However, bronchopneumonia, otitis media, and sinusitis also commonly occur.

The majority of malignancies seen in AS are of lymphoreticular origin and include malignant lymphoma and leukemia.[211,213-215] The gastrointestinal tract, particularly the small intestine, was involved with reticulum cell sarcoma in several reported cases. No roentgen studies were apparently attempted on these young patients, and the neoplasms of the gastrointestinal tract were found on postmortem examination.

Sclero-Atrophic and Keratotic Dermatosis of Limbs (Sclerotylosis)

This little known genodermatosis has the characteristics of atrophic fibrosis of the skin and extremities, hypoplasia of the nails, and keratoderma of the palms and soles. It is associated with skin and bowel cancer, and has an autosomal dominant mode of inheritance.[191,204]

Neurofibromatosis (von Recklinghausen's Disease)

Neurofibromatosis (NF) is a hereditary, hamartomatous disorder characterized by multiple pedunculated or sessile skin nodules, café au lait spots, osseous abnormalities, and neurogenic tumors involving the central and peripheral nervous systems.[216,217] The disease involves the neuroectoderm, mesoderm, and endoderm, and has the potential of occurring in any organ system of the body.[216] Two forms of the disease, peripheral NF and central NF, related to circulating levels of serum nerve growth factor are now suggested.[218] Peripheral NF (von Recklinghausen's disease) is the most common form. Central NF is the less common variety and is characterized by a later age of onset and a clinical picture in which the central nervous system is predominately affected. The serum levels of nerve growth factor may be increased in the central form.[218] Both forms are inherited as an autosomal dominant trait. Associated malignant neoplasms, including sarcomas of peripheral nerves and somatic soft tissues, are not uncommon. Sarcomatous degeneration of gastrointestinal neurofibromas is of particular interest for this chapter.

Skin Lesions as Diagnostic Criteria. Café au lait spots (small areas of cutaneous pigmentation) are important in establishing the diagnosis of NF.[219,220] Less than 1% of normal children have more than two café au lait spots.[220] A child or adult with five or more such pigmented areas, 0.5 cm or more in diameter, most probably has NF.[219,220] The typical cutaneous neurofibromas are multiple, soft, sessile or pedunculated, vary in size, and are predominately located on the trunk. Lisch spots (multiple, dark pigmented nodules of the iris) are an important ocular sign of this disease. They are usually bilateral, and may be easily recognized or may only be identifiable with a slit lamp.[216]

Bone Changes. Bone abnormalities occur in approximately 30-50% of the cases.[217] Holt and Hunt discuss these lesions in detail.[216,221-223] Kyphoscoliosis of the spine, particularly cervical kyphosis with anterior and posterior scalloping of the vertebral bodies, is the most common lesion in NF.[216] Dysplastic changes of the skull and facial bones, most commonly distortion of the orbit, petrous, and sphenoid bones, are often present. Focal gigantism involving any bone, congenital bowing, and pseudoarthrosis of the tibia and fibula are all characteristic osseous manifestations of this syndrome.[216]

Associated Malignant Neoplasms. Secondary malignant neoplasms with sarcomatous degeneration are commonly reported in association with NF and include neurofibrosarcoma, liposarcoma, rhabdomyosarcoma, and sarcomas of peripheral nerves and somatic soft tissues.[224-226] This incidence of sarcomatous degeneration is variously reported to be from 2 to 4%.[224,227] Pheochromocytomas in adults also occur frequently in this disease.[216,227,228] Other tumors with a significantly high occurrence rate in NF are central nervous system neoplasms such as optic nerve gliomas, cerebral and cerebellar astrocytomas, meningiomas, acoustic neuromas, and intramedullary gliomas of the spinal cord.[216,224] Cutaneous malignant tumors described in association with NF are squamous and basal cell carcinomas and malignant melanoma.[227] Reich and Wiernik have suggested that patients with this disease are also at greater risk for developing leukemia.[229]

Gastrointestinal. The gastrointestinal tract is involved in 25% of patients with multiple NF.[217] The tumors may be single or multiple and have been reported in all segments of the alimentary tract, including the ampulla of Vater and the appendix.[216,217,230-233] They most frequently occur in the small intestine, especially the ileum.[230]

Small intestinal neurofibromas, with or without von Recklinghausen's disease, are rare.[217,234] All ages may be affected, but the highest incidence is in the 40--60 year age group.[230] The majority of the lesions are benign, but sarcomatous degeneration occurs in 15% of patients, usually those over 40 years of age.[235] The tumors may be asymptomatic, but if ulceration develops, bleeding will result leading to anemia.[231] As the neoplasms enlarge, palpable masses may develop as well as intestinal obstruction and perforation.[217,230] The tumors originate in the submucosa, are usually encapsulated, and may be pedunculated.[230] Preoperative demonstration of intestinal neurofibromas depends upon barium contrast studies, preferably enteroclysis. Radiographically, they usually present as multiple, sharply demarcated, intraluminal or submucosal defects.[230] Intussusception occurs not infrequently. Ulcerations commonly occur and in a benign lesion will appear small and well defined (Figure 6-29). However, ulcerations in a malignant tumor may be large and irregular.[230] A less common roentgen finding is compression and displacement of the small bowel by a large extraluminal tumor.[208] The neoplasms are hypervascular, and intestinal angiography may identify the exact number and location of the tumors as well as their blood

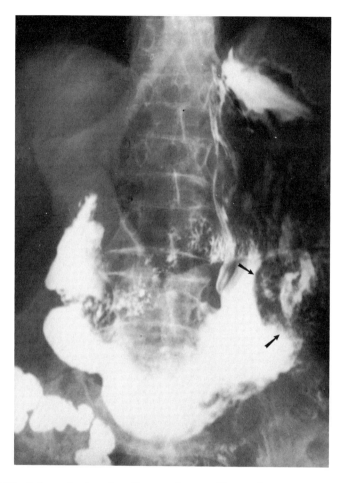

Figure 6-29. A large, benign ulcerating gastric neurofibroma (arrows) in a patient with neurofibromatosis.

supply.[217,236] Radiographically, and even by histologic examination, it may be impossible to differentiate between a benign tumor and a sarcoma.[230]

Neurofibromas involving the rectum and colon are not as common as in the small intestine, but several cases have been documented.[232] Patients with neurofibromas located in the rectosigmoid may present with the classic signs of any rectal neoplasm, such as diarrhea or constipation, bleeding, and pain. Radiographically, by use of barium studies, the colon lesions may be single or multiple and, as in the small bowel, may appear as intraluminal or intramural defects. The colonic segments may be distorted or displaced by extra-alimentary neurofibromas originating in retroperitoneal or intra-abdominal locations (Figure 6-30A, B, and C). Neurofibromas arising in the presacral or rectovaginal areas are not uncommon, and they often will produce extrinsic contour defects of the rectum. Actual bony erosions of the sacrum or coccyx may occur in such cases.[232] A case of neurofibroma of the colon simulating Hirschsprung's disease has been described.[233] Ultrasound and computed tomography are excellent diagnostic modalities to identify the intra-abdominal and retroperitoneal tumors that occur in this disease.

Management. When the diagnosis of multiple NF is first suspected or established, baseline barium studies of the entire gastrointestinal tract should be performed in the adult patient. Individuals with known NF, who consequently develop abdominal symptoms, anemia, or an abdominal mass, should have immediate

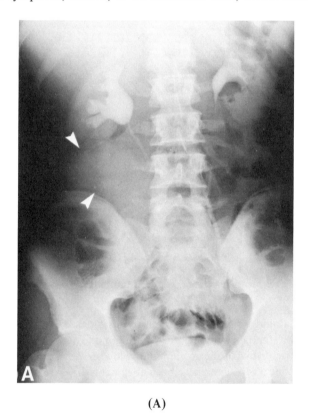

(A)

Figure 6-30. A retroperitoneal malignant schwannoma in a patient with neurofibromatosis: (A) displacing the right ureter medially (arrows) and (B) displacing the proximal transverse colon inferiorly (arrows). (C) Ultrasonic examination delineates the large neoplasm (arrows).

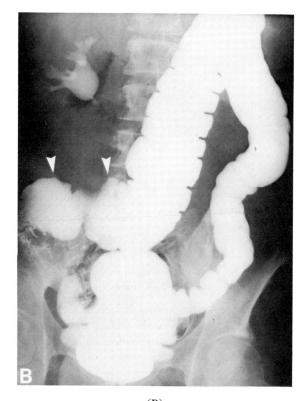

(B)

Figure 6-30. (Continued)

roentgen evaluation, particularly of the small intestine. Since there is a definite risk of sarcoma developing in these tumors after the age of 40 years, patients with known disease should be followed regularly with occult blood testing of the stool. If neoplasms develop, even in the asymptomatic patient, local excision or segmental resection should be performed when possible because of the danger of obstruction, intussusception, bleeding, and malignant degeneration.[217,231,235]

Celiac Sprue (Nontropical Sprue, Gluten Enteropathy)

Celiac sprue (CS) is a disease in which there is (1) intestinal malabsorption of carbohydrates, proteins, and fats; (2) a characteristic lesion of the intestinal mucosa; (3) clinical improvement on a gluten-free diet; and (4) an increased incidence of malignancy.[208,237,238] CS appears to be a hereditary disease, but the exact mode of inheritance is not completely established.[238,239]

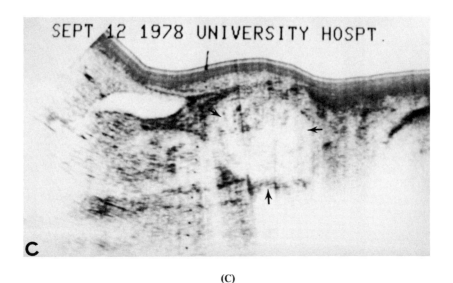

(C)

Figure 6-30. (Continued)

The disease is more common in females with an incidence of almost 2:1 over males.[238] The skin manifestations include glossitis, stomatitis, petechiae, and eczema.[240-242] Histologic changes of the small intestinal mucosa show flattening and loss of villi, and infiltration of the lamina propria with lymphocytes and plasma cells.[208,238]

Roentgen Manifestations. The classic changes noted on contrast examination of the small intestine are: dilatation, segmentation, and fragmentation of the barium column and thickening or thinning of the valvulae conniventes (Figures 6-31 and 6-32).[21,208] These changes are usually most evident in the jejunum but may also be seen in the ileum with extensive disease. The segmentation and fragmentation of the barium is secondary to increased intraluminal intestinal fluid.[208] Thickening of the valvulae conniventes (mucosal folds) is probably related to submucosal edema from the protein-losing enteropathy and to the amount of fluid within the bowel lumen.[21,208] Dilatation of the lumen is an important and constant finding of CS. The degree of dilatation is variable and is related to the severity of the disease.[208] Nonobstructive intussusception of the small intestine, probably related to the flaccid bowel, is occasionally present.[208]

Associated Malignancies. There is a definite increased incidence of lymphoma and esophageal carcinoma in patients with CS, and males are more susceptible to develop these malignancies than females.[21,208,238,243,244] Jejunal adenocarcinoma may also have an increased occurrence rate.[238] The overall incidence of malignancy in CS is approximately 15%.[243]

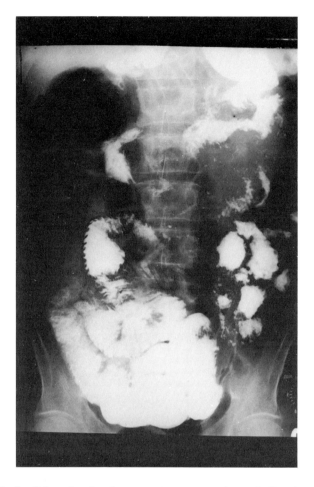

Figure 6-31. Small bowel series demonstrating segmentation and dilatation of intestinal loops in a patient with celiac sprue.

Lymphoma associated with CS occurs predominately in the jejunum with a high incidence of reticulum cell sarcoma. This complication presents in the fourth to seventh decades, after symptoms of CS have been present for an average of 20 years.[238] Lymphosarcoma in a patient with CS should be considered if fever develops, bowel hemorrhage or perforation presents, improvement does not result on a gluten-free diet, or an exacerbation of symptoms occurs while on maintenance therapy.[21,208] The roentgen features of lymphosarcoma as described by Marshak are listed in Table 6-3.[208] Primary or secondary lymphosarcoma of the small intestine may also occur with malabsorption and other manifestations of CS.[245] Differentiation from CS in these cases may be difficult.

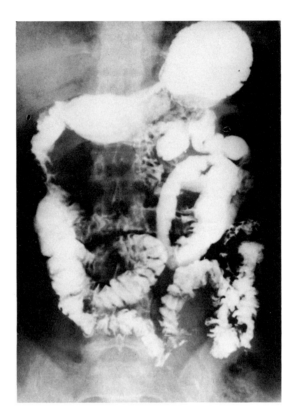

Figure 6-32. Effacement of the mucosa (moulage sign), dilatation, and fluid-filled loops of the small bowel in a patient with celiac sprue.

Esophageal carcinoma is also markedly increased in patients with CS.[243] The age of onset is in the sixth to seventh decade, with symptoms of CS present for approximately 50 years.[238]

Primary Hemochromatosis

Primary hemochromatosis (PH) is caused by a disorder of iron metabolism in which excess deposits of iron result in toxicity to the liver, pancreas, and heart.[246,247] The cardinal features of PH are: hepatic cirrhosis, diabetes mellitus, pigmentation of the skin, and cardiac failure.[246-249] Although there is controversy,[250,251] most investigators consider PH to be an inherited disorder, but the exact mode of inheritance has not been established.[247,252-256] It is usually an insidious, progressive disorder with clinical manifestations appearing between the ages of 40 and 60 years.[246-248] Males are afflicted more commonly than females, which

Table 6-3. Roentgen Features of Lymphosarcoma of the Small Intestine.*

I. Nodular form
  A. Intramural nodules
  B. Intraluminal nodules

II. Infiltrative form
  A. Thickened bowel wall
  B. Mucosal folds coarse and irregular or flattened and effaced
  C. Marked localized dilatation

III. Polypoid form
  A. Discrete polypoid mass
  B. May be large, bulky, pseudopedicle

IV. Endo-exoenteric form
  A. Large ulcer
  B. Fistulas communicating with adjacent bowel

V. Invasive form of mesentery
  A. Large extraluminal masses
  B. Displacement of adjacent organs

*From R. H. Marshak and A. E. Lindner, *Radiology of the Small Intestine.* Philadelphia, PA: W. B. Saunders, 1976.

is probably a reflection of the protective mechanism of menstruation for iron loss.[247] The disease is included in this section because of an increased incidence of hepatoma.

Skin Changes. Of patients with PH, 90% have skin hyperpigmentation and 10–15% have pigmentation on the oral mucous membranes.[248] The pigmentation ranges from a bronze or brown color to a bluish tinge and is most prominent on the face. Dermatological manifestations related to liver disease, such as spider angiomas, palmar erythema, and sparse body hair, are not uncommon.[247,248]

Radiographic Changes. Hepatomegaly is present in over 90% of patients with PH and results primarily from increased deposition of iron.[247] Splenomegaly may also occur but is apparently more common in the exogenous type of hemochromatosis.[257] Hepatomegaly and increased liver density will be evident on plain film studies of the abdomen. Perhaps the most accurate method for demonstrating these changes is computed tomography[258,259] (Figure 6-33).

There is an increased incidence of hepatoma in patients with PH ranging from 7 to 14%.[247,260] Hepatic angiography continues to be a reliable method for establishing the diagnosis of hepatoma; it is of particular value to the surgeon preoperatively in demonstrating the extent of the tumor and its vascular supply.[261,262] The classic angiographic appearance of a hypervascular hepatocellular carcinoma is that of dilated hepatic arteries, irregular tumor vessels throughout the lesion, and accumulation of contrast material (vascular lakes) in the

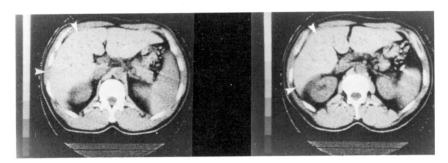

Figure 6-33. Computed tomography of the liver in a patient with hemochromatosis showing an increase in density of the hepatic parenchyma (arrows). *(Courtesy of David H. Stephens, M.D., Rochester, MN)*

capillary phase[262] (Figure 6-34A and B). Arteriovenous shunting may occasionally be present. The majority of hepatomas are highly vascular, but hypovascularity of these neoplasms, although uncommon, has been described.[261] Differential diagnostic problems for the hypervascular hepatomas include regenerating liver, liver cell adenoma, cavernous hemangiomas, and hypervascular liver metastases.[262] Computed tomography, ultrasound, liver scans, and radionuclide uptake studies are helpful in establishing the presence of a liver mass, but as discussed above, angiography should be performed prior to surgery. Other liver tumors found in PH include hemangioendothelial sarcoma,[263] osteogenic sarcoma,[264] and cholangiocarcinoma.[265]

A characteristic type of arthropathy has been described and occurs in approximately 50% of the patients with PH.[266-269] The patients present with pain and swelling of the hands, particularly of the second and third metacarpophalangeal joints. In most cases, the arthropathy is limited to the hands and wrists, but it may also involve the hips and knees. The roentgen findings include subchondral cysts of the second and third metacarpophalangeal joints, usually on the proximal side of the joint, but both sides may be involved as well. Often the cysts will have sclerotic margins.[266-269] Cysts and erosions may also be present in the carpal bones and inferior radioulnar joints. Joint space narrowing, with typical degenerative changes but without cyst formation, can be seen in the hips and knees. Chondrocalcinosis may also be present in these larger joints.[267] Calcification in the intervertebral disks of the lumbar spine has been reported to occur in 15% of the patients with PH and calcification of the ligamentum flavum in 8%.[270]

Pernicious Anemia

Pernicious anemia (PA) is included in this discussion because of its association with gastric carcinoma. There is a familial tendency to develop PA, and it is

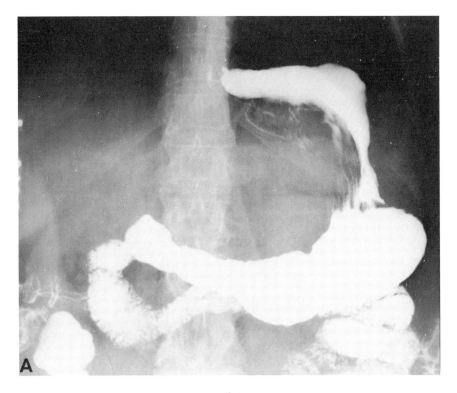

(A)

Figure 6-34. (A) Hepatoma in the left lobe of the liver causing a mass effect on the lesser curvature of the stomach and displacing the entire stomach to the left. (B) Arteriogram of the left lobe hepatoma demonstrating dilated hepatic arteries supplying the neoplasm and irregular tumor vessels throughout the lesion.

generally accepted as a genetic disease.[271-273] Dermatologic manifestations include glossitis, yellow coloration of the skin and sclerae, vitiligo, and premature graying of the hair.[274]

The increased incidence of gastric carcinoma occurring in patients with PA varies in the literature from 10 to 15%.[272,275-277] Some investigators believe that such figures are inaccurate because of limited and selected case material. They suggest that the actual incidence may be only two times higher than in the average population.[278] Thus, an association between PA and gastric carcinoma exists, but an exact pathogenetic relationship has not been definitely established.[279]

The radiologist should be aware of potential differences in the roentgen appearance of gastric carcinoma with PA in comparison to non-PA patients. Gastric carcinoma in PA tends to be located in the fundus or cardia and is more likely to be polypoid, and multicentric lesions are frequent.[276,278]

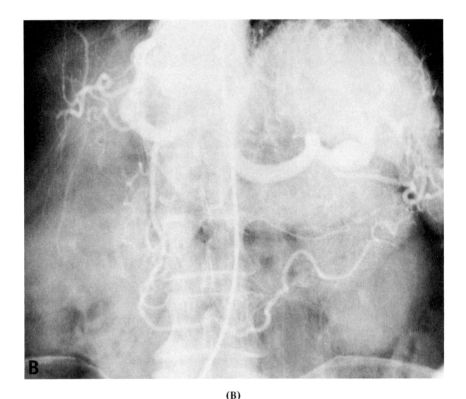

(B)

Figure 6-34. (Continued)

Kaposi Syndrome

Kaposi sarcoma (KS) is a multifocal neoplastic disease characterized by cutaneous, subcutaneous, and visceral tumors.[274,280,281] There is an increased incidence of the disease among South Africans, northern Italians, and eastern Europeans.[274,280,283] Males are affected more commonly than females, and the peak age incidence is between 50 and 70 years except in South Africa where a younger age group is affected.[274,280,282] It is a disease of unknown etiology although there are rare reports of KS affecting several members of a family, suggesting the possibility of autosomal dominant inheritance.[204,282-287] There is a high occurrence rate of associated primary malignancies including Hodgkin's disease and non-Hodgkin's lymphoma.[204,280,288]

Cutaneous Manifestations. The skin lesions are nodules and macules of a blue or purplish color.[274,280] The eruption is usually bilateral appearing first on the legs and feet, but it can involve any part of the body surface.[274] There is a tendency to develop edema which may be related to dermal lymph stasis.[280] Histologic studies of the skin lesions show them to be composed of freely anastomotic capillaries, with space between the blood vessels composed of tissue resembling well-differentiated fibrosarcoma.[281] The tumor has been classified by some as a hemangiosarcoma.[289] KS may present with skin lesions alone or with generalized lymphadenopathy.[280,290,291]

Gastrointestinal Manifestations. Internal organs, including the gastrointestinal tract, are affected in a high number of patients with KS.[274,281] Any portion of the alimentary tract may be involved, but radiological demonstration of the lesions is uncommon.[281] The tumors arise in the submucosa and appear as intramural nodules on contrast examinations.[208,281,292] Central ulceration of the nodules giving the classic "target" or "bulls-eye" configuration is not uncommon. The roentgenographic appearance of the small bowel in KS is similar to lymphosarcoma.[208,281] Gastrointestinal bleeding occurs frequently and results from ulceration of the larger lesions or sloughing of the intestinal mucosa, secondary to pressure from the submucosal masses.[208,281] As already mentioned, lymphomas may be associated with KS as a second primary malignancy. Clinical, laboratory, and roentgenographic evidence of malabsorption with KS has also been documented.[281]

Other Roentgen Manifestations.[280,293] Soft tissue roentgenograms of involved areas such as extremities may show single or multiple nodular densities. Cortical erosions and cysts may be present in bones adjacent to the soft tissue tumors. Chest films are usually without abnormalities in adults; however, enlarged hilar and mediastinal lymph nodes may be evident in children.

The material presented in this chapter is summarized in Table 6-4.

Table 6-4.

SYNDROME OR DISEASE	ASSOCIATED NEOPLASMS	DIAGNOSTIC ROENTGEN STUDIES
Gardner's	Colon polyps and carcinoma	Double contrast colon
	Stomach polyps and carcinoma	Double contrast stomach
	Duodenal polyps and carcinoma	Hypotonic duodenography
	Small bowel polyps	Enteroclysis
	Periampullary carcinoma	Hypotonic duodenography, US,* CT,†ERCP,‡PCTH8
	Desmoids, retroperitoneal and mesenteric fibromatosis	IVU,‖ US, CT
	Osteomas	Skull, facial bones, long bones
	Odontonomas	Panorex of mandible
	Adrenal adenomas and carcinomas	US, CT, IVU, adrenal arteriography and venography
	Thyroid carcinomas	Radionuclide scan, US
Peutz-Jeghers	Small bowel hamartomas	Enteroclysis
	Duodenal polyps and carcinoma	Hypotonic duodenography
	Stomach polyps and carcinoma	Double contrast stomach

Table 6-4. (Con't.)

SYNDROME OR DISEASE	ASSOCIATED NEOPLASMS	DIAGNOSTIC ROENTGEN STUDIES
Peutz-Jeghers (continued)	Colon polyps and carcinoma	Double contrast colon
	Ovarian	US, CT
	Ureteral, urinary bladder polyps	IVU, retrograde urography
	Bronchial, paranasal sinus polyps	PA, lateral chest, paranasal sinuses, bronchography
Torre's	Colon carcinoma	Double contrast colon
	Stomach carcinoma	Double contrast stomach
	Duodenal carcinoma	Hypotonic duodenography
	Ampullary carcinoma	Hypotonic duodenography, PCTH, ERCP, US
Multiple hamartoma	Breast carcinoma	Mammography
	Thyroid adenoma and carcinoma	Radionuclide scan, US
	Stomach polyps	Double contrast stomach
	Colon polyps	Double contrast colon
Turcot	CNS glioblastomas and and medulloblastomas	CT, radionuclide brain scan, cerebral antiography
	Colon polyps and adenocarcinoma	Double contrast colon
Tylosis palmaris et plantaris	Esophageal carcinoma	Double contrast esophagram
Epidermolysis bullosa	Esophageal carcinoma	Double contrast esophagram
Dyskeratosis congenita	Esophageal carcinoma	Double contrast esophagram
	Colon carcinoma	Double contrast colon
Wiskott-Aldrich	Lymphosarcoma small bowel	Enteroclysis
Familial hyperclucagonemia	Glucagonoma	Double contrast stomach, pancreatic arteriography, US, CT
Ataxia telangiectasia	Stomach carcinoma	Double contrast stomach
	Pancreatic carcinoma	Double contrast stomach, US, CT, pancreatic arteriography
	CNS gliomas	CT
	Ovarian dysgerminomas	US, CT
	Lymphosarcoma small bowel	Enteroclysis
Familial malignant melanoma	Breast carcinoma	Mammography
	Metastases to GI tract	Double contrast stomach, colon enteroclysis
	Lungs	PA and lateral chest
	Liver	US, CT, radionuclide scan

Table 6-4. (Con't.)

SYNDROME OR DISEASE	ASSOCIATED NEOPLASMS	DIAGNOSTIC ROENTGEN STUDIES
Neurofibromatosis	Sarcomas of peripheral nerves, somatic soft tissues	Soft tissue films of extremities and abdomen, CT, US
	CNS tumors	Myelography, CT, arteriography, tomography of petrous bone
	Pheochromocytoma	US, CT, arteriography
	Neurofibromas of GI tract	Double contrast stomach, colon, enteroclysis
Celiac sprue	Esophageal carcinoma	Double contrast esophagram
	Lymphosarcoma small bowel	Enteroclysis
Primary hemochromatosis	Hepatoma	CT, US, radionuclide scan, arteriography
Pernicious anemia	Stomach carcinoma	Double contrast stomach
Kaposi syndrome	Hemangiosarcomas of GI tract	Double contrast stomach, colon and enteroclysis

*US = ultrasound.

†CT = computed tomography.

‡ERCP = endoscopic retrograde cholangiopancreatography.

§PCTH = percutaneous transhepatic cholangiography.

‖IVU = intravenous urography.

REFERENCES

1. Dodds, W.J., and Lydon, S.B.: Intestinal polyposis syndromes. *CRC Rad. Nuc. Med.* 5:295, 1974.
2. Gelfand, D.W.: The Japanese-style double contrast examination of the stomach. *Gastrointest. Radiol.* 1:7, 1976.
3. Laufer, I., Mullens, J.E., and Hamilton, J.: The diagnostic accuracy of barium studies of the stomach and duodenum — correlation with endoscopy. *Radiology* 115:569, 1975.
4. Laufer, I.: A single method for routine double contrast study of the upper gastrointestinal tract. *Radiology* 117:513, 1975.
5. Laufer, I.: Assessment of the accuracy of double contrast gastroduodenal radiology. *Gastroenterology* 71:874, 1976.
6. Laufer, I.: *Double Contrast Gastrointestinal Radiology*, Philadelphia, PA: W.B. Saunders, 1979.
7. Montagne, J.P., Moss, A.A., and Margulis, A.R.: Double blind study of single and double contrast upper gastrointestinal examinations using endoscopy as a control. *AJR* 130:1041, 1978.
8. Skucas, J., and Schrank, W.W.: The routine air-contrast examination of the esophagus. *Radiology* 115:482, 1975.

9. Itai, Y., Kogune, T., Okuyama, Y., and Akiyama, H.: Superficial esophageal carcinoma, radiological findings in double contrast studies. *Radiology* **125**:597, 1978.

10. Goldstein, H.M., and Dodd, G.D.: Double-contrast examination of the esophagus. *Gastrointest. Radiol.* **1**:3, 1976.

11. Welin, S.: Modern trends in diagnostic roentgenology of the colon. *Br. J. Radiol.* **31**:453, 1958.

12. Miller, R.E.: Detection of colon carcinoma and the barium enema. *JAMA* **230**:1195, 1974.

13. Miller, R.E.: Examination of the colon. *Curr. Prob. Radiol.* **5**:1, 1975.

14. Rogers, C.W.: Method for double contrast study of the colon. *Med. Radiogr. Photgr.* **51**:30, 1975.

15. Laufer, I.: The double-contrast enema: myths and misconceptions. *Gastrointest. Radiol.* **1**:9, 1976.

16. Miller, R.E.: Cancer and the clean colon. *Appl. Radiol.* May/June:109, 1976.

17. Miller, R.E.: Personal communication, 1978.

18. Herlinger, H.: A modified technique for the double-contrast small bowel enema. *Gastrointest. Radiol.* **3**:201, 1978.

19. Ekberg, O.: Double-contrast examination of the small bowel. *Gastrointest. Radiol.* **1**:349, 1977.

20. Sellink, J.L.: Radiologic examination of the small intestine by duodenal intubation. *Acta. Radiol. "Diag" (Stock.)* **15**:318, 1974.

21. Sellink, J.L.: *Radiological Atlas of Common Diseases of the Small Bowel.* Leiden: Stenfert Kroese, 1976.

22. Gardner, E.J.: A genetic and clinical study of intestinal polyposis, a predisposing factor for carcinoma of the colon and rectum. *Am. J. Human. Genet.* **3**:167, 1951.

23. Gardner, E.J., and Plenk, H.P.: Hereditary pattern for multiple osteomas in a family group. *Am. J. Human Genet.* **4**:31, 1952.

24. Gardner, E.J., and Richards, R.C.: Multiple cutaneous and subcutaneous lesions occurring simultaneously with hereditary polyposis and osteomatosis. *Am. J. Human Genet.* **5**:139, 1953.

25. Gardner, E.J.: Follow-up study of a family group exhibiting dominant inheritance for a syndrome including intestinal polyps, osteomas, fibromas and epidermal cysts. *Am. J. Human Genet.* **14**:376, 1962.

26. Lynch, H.T.: Hereditary and colon cancer. *Nebr. Med. J.* **60**:222, 1975.

27. Dorazio, R.A., and Whelan, T.J., Jr.: Lymphoid hyperplasia of the terminal ileum associated with familial polyposis coli. *Ann. Surg.* **171**:300, 1970.

28. Vanhoutte, J.J.: Polypoid lymphoid hyperplasia of the terminal ileum in patients with familial polyposis coli and gardner's syndrome. *AJR* **110**:340, 1979.

29. Jones, E., and Cornell, W.P.: Gardner's syndrome, review of the literature and report on a family. *Arch. Surg.* **92**:287, 1966.

30. Peck, D.A., Watanabe, K.S., and Trueblood, H.W.: Familial polyposis in children. *Dis. Colon Rectum* **15**:23, 1972.

31. Sachatello, C.R.: Familial polyposis of the colon, a four-decade follow-up. *Cancer* **18**:581, 1971.

32. LeFevre, H.W., Jr., Jacques, T.F.: Multiple polyposis in an infant of four months. *Am. J. Surg.* **81**:90, 1951.

33. Hoffman, D.C., and Goligher, J.C.: Polyposis of the stomach and small intestine in association with familial polyposis coli. *Br. J. Surg.* **58**:126, 1971.

34. Bussey, H.J.R.: *Familial Polyposis Coli.* Baltimore, MD: John Hopkins University Press, 1975.

35. Watne, A.L., Johnson, J.G., and Chang, C.H.: The challenge of Gardner's syndrome. *Cancer* 19:266, 1969.
36. Lynch, H.T.: Hereditary and colon cancer. *Nebr. Med. J.* 60:268, 1975.
37. Denzler, T.B., Harned, R.K., and Pergam, C.J.: Gastric polyps in familial polyposis coli. *Radiology* 130:63, 1979.
38. Ushio, K., Sasagawa, M., Doi, H., et al.: Lesions associated with familial polyposis coli: studies of lesions of the stomach, duodenum, bones and teeth. *Gastrointest. Radiol.* 1:67, 1967.
39. Itai, Y., Kogure, T., Okuyama, Y., et al.: Radiographic features of gastric polyps in familial adenomatosis coli. *AJR* 128:73, 1977.
40. Utsunomiya, J., Maki, T., Iwama, T., et al.: Gastric lesions of familial polyposis coli. *Cancer* 34:745, 1974.
41. McKusick, V.A.: Genetic factors in intestinal polyposis. *JAMA* 182:271, 1962.
42. Yaffee, H.S.: Gastric polyposis and soft tissue tumors. A variant of Gardner's syndrome. *Arch. Dermatol.* 89:806, 1964.
43. Murphy, E.S., Mireles, M., and Beltran, A.: Familial polyposis of the colon and gastric carcinoma. *JAMA* 179:1026, 1962.
44. Melmed, R.N., and Bouchier, I.A.D.: Duodenal involvement in Gardner's syndrome. *Gut* 13:524, 1972.
45. Schnur, P.L., David, E., Brown, P.W., Jr., et al.: Adenocarcinoma of the duodenum and the Gardner syndrome. *JAMA* 223:1229, 1973.
46. Macdonald, J.M., Davis, W.C., Crago, H.R., and Berk, A.D.: Gardner's syndrome and periampullarly malignancy. *Am. J. Surg.* 113:425, 1967.
47. Smith, W.G.: Familial multiple polyposis: research tool for investigating the etiology of carcinoma of the colon. *Dis. Colon Rectum* 11:17, 1968.
48. Smith, W.G.: Multiple polyposis, Gardner's syndrome and desmoid tumors. *Dis. Colon Rectum* 1:323, 1958.
49. Yonemoto, R.H., Slayback, J.B., Byron, R.L. et al.: Familial polyposis of the entire gastrointestinal tract. *Arch. Surg.* 99:427, 1969.
50. Marshall, W.H., Martin, R.F., and Magkay, I.R.: Gardner's syndrome with adrenal carcinoma. *Aust. Ann. Med.* 16:242, 1967.
51. Kahn, P.C.: The radiologic identification of functioning adrenal tumors. *RCNA* 5: 221, 1967.
52. Camiel, M.R., Mule, J.E., Alexander, L.L., et al.: Association of thyroid carcinoma with Gardner's syndrome in siblings. *New Engl. J. Med.* 278:1056, 1968.
53. Collins, D.C.: The frequent association of other body tumors with familial polyposis. *Am. J. Gastro.* 31:376, 1959.
54. Duncan, B.R., Dohner, V.A., and Priest, J.H.: The Gardner syndrome: need for early diagnosis. *J. Pediat.* 72:497, 1968.
55. Chanco, A.G., and Rose, E.F.: Mesenteric fibromatosis following colectomy for familial polyposis. *Arch. Surg.* 104:851, 1972.
56. Parks, T.G., Bussey, H.R., and Lock-Hart Mummery, H.E.: Familial polyposis coli associated with extracolonic abnormalities. *Gut* 11:323, 1970.
57. Penn, D., Federman, Q., and Finkel, M.: Fibromatosis in Gardner's syndrome. *Am. J. Gastro.* 59:174, 1973.
58. Simpson, R.D., Harrison, E.G., Jr., and Mayo, C.W.: Mesenteric fibromatosis in familial polyposis. A variant of Gardner's syndrome. *Cancer* 17:526, 1964.
59. Johnson, J.G., Gilbert, E., Zimmerman, B., et al.: Gardner's syndrome, colon cancer and sarcoma. *J. Surg. Oncol.* 4:354, 1972.
60. Haggitt, R.C., and Booth, J.I.: Bilateral fibromatosis of the breast in Gardner's syndrome. *Cancer* 25:161, 1970.

61. Watne, A.L., Lai, H., Carrier, J., et al.: The diagnosis and surgical treatment of patients with gardner's syndrome. *Surgery* **82**:327, 1977.

62. Harned, R.K.: Barium sulphate is the contrast agent of choice in diagnosing obstruction of the small intestine. *Nebr. Med. J.* **60**:232, 1975.

63. Carillo, F.J., Ruzicka, F.F., and Clemett, A.R.: Value of angiography in the diagnosis of retractile mesenteritis. *AJR* **115**:396, 1972.

64. Dukes, C.E.: The control of precancerous conditions of the colon and rectum. *Canad. M.A.J.* **90**:630, 1964.

65. Chang, C.H., Piatt, E.D., Thomas, K.E., et al.: Bone abnormalities in Gardner's syndrome. *AJR* **103**:645, 1968.

66. Ziter, F.M.: Roentgenographic Findings in Gardner's syndrome. *JAMA* **192**:158, 1965.

67. Hoffmann, D.C., Bryan, M.B., and Brooke, N.: Familial sarcoma of bone in a polyposis coli family. *Dis. Colon Rectum* **13**:119, 1970.

68. Cabot, R.C.: Case records of the Massachusetts General Hospital, case #21061. *N. Engl. J. Med.* **212**:263, 1935.

69. Sanchez, M.A., Zali, M.R., Khalil, A.A., et al.: Be aware of Gardner's syndrome: a review of the literature. *Am. J. Gastro.* **71**:68, 1979.

70. Cole, J.W., McKalen, A., and Powell, J.: The role of ileal contents in the spontaneous regression of rectal adenomas. *Dis. Colon Rectum* **4**:413, 1961.

71. Hubbard, T.B., Jr.: Familial polyposis of the colon: the fate of retained rectum after colectomy in children. *Am. Surg.* **23**:577, 1957.

72. Localio, S.A.: Spontaneous disappearance of rectal polyps following subtotal colectomy and ileoproctostomy for polyposis of the colon. *Am. J. Surg.* **103**:81, 1962.

73. Bussey, H.R.: Progress report, gastrointestinal polyposis. *Gut* **11**:970, 1970.

74. Moertel, C.G., Hill, J.R., and Martin, A.A.: Surgical management of multiple polyposis. The problem of cancer in the retained bowel segment. *Arch. Surg.* **100**:521, 1970.

75. Erbe, R.W.: Inherited gastrointestinal-polyposis syndromes. *N. Engl. J. Med.* **294**: 1101, 1976.

76. Boley, S.J., McKinnon, W.M., and Marzulli, V.F.: The management of familial gastrointestinal polyposis involving stomach and colon. *Ped. Surg.* **50**:691, 1961.

77. Bussey, H.J.R., Veale, A.M.O., and Morson, B.C.: Genetics of gastrointestinal polyposis. *Gastroenterology* **74**:1325, 1978.

78. Lynch, H.T., Lynch, P.M., Follett, K.L., et al.: Familial polyposis coli: heterogeneous polyp expression in two kindreds. *J. Med. Genet.* **16**:1, 1979.

79. Oldfield, M.C.: The association of familial polyposis of the colon with multiple sebaceous cysts. *Br. J. Surg.* **41**:534, 1954.

80. Peutz, J.L.A.: Ober een zeer merkwaardige, geocombineerde familaire Polyposis van de Slijmvliezen van den Tractus intestinalis met die van de Neuskeelholte en Gepaard met eigen aardige Pigmentaties van Huiden Slijmvliezen. *Ned. Tijdschr. Geneeskd.* **10**:134, 1972.

81. Jeghers, H., Mckusick, V.A., and Katz, K.H.: Generalized intestinal polyposis and melanin spots of the oral mucosa, lips and digits: a syndrome of diagnostic significance. *N. Engl. J. Med.* **241**:933, 1949.

82. Godard, J.E., Dodds, W.J., Phillips, J.C., et al.: Peutz-Jeghers syndrome: clinical and roentgenographic features. *AJR* **113**:316, 1971.

83. Dodds, W.J.: Clinical and roentgen features of the intestinal polyposis syndromes. *Gastrointest. Radiol.* **1**:127, 1976.

84. Bartholomew, L.G., Moore, C.E., Dahlin, D.C. et al.: Intestinal polyposis associated with mucocutaneous pigmentation. *Surg. Gyn. Ob.* **115**:1, 1962.

85. Jancu, J.: Peutz-Jeghers syndrome involvement of the gastrointestinal and upper respiratory tracts. *Am. J. Gastro.* **56**:545, 1971.

86. Sommerhaug, R.G., and Mason, T.: Peutz-Jeghers syndrome and ureteral polyposis. *JAMA* **211**:120, 1970.

87. Dodds, W.J., Schulte, W.J., Hensley, G.T., et al.: Peutz-Jeghers syndrome and gastrointestinal malignancy. *AJR* **115**:374, 1972.

88. Dozois, R.R., Judd, E.S., Dahlin, D.C., et al.: The Peutz-Jeghers syndrome, is there a predisposition to the development of intestinal malignancy? *Arch. Surg.* **98**:509, 1969.

89. Reid, J.D.: Duodenal carcinoma in the Peutz-Jeghers syndrome. *Cancer* **18**(2): 970, 1965.

90. Reid, J.D.: Intestinal carcinoma in the Peutz-Jeghers syndrome. *JAMA* **229**:833, 1974.

91. McKittrick, J.E., Lewis, W.M., Doane, W.A., et al.: The Peutz-Jeghers syndrome. *Arch. Surg.* **103**:57, 1971.

92. André, R., Duhmael, G., and Bruaire, M.; Syndrome de Peutz-Jeghers avec polypose oesophagienne. *Bull. Soc. Med. Hop Paris* **117**:505, 1966.

93. Dormandy, T.L.: Gastrointestinal polyposis with mucocutaneous pigmentation (Peutz-Jeghers syndrome). *N. Engl. J. Med.* **256**:1093, 1957.

94. Berkowitz, S.B., Pearl, M.J., and Shapiro, N.H.: Syndrome of intestinal polyposis with melanosis of lips and buccal mucosa: study of incidence and location of malignancy. *Ann. Surg.* **141**:129, 1955.

95. Burdick, D., Prior, J.T., and Scanlon, G.T.: Peutz-Jeghers syndrome: a clinical pathologic study of a large family with a ten year follow-up. *Cancer* **16**(2):854, 1963.

96. Yun Ryo, R., M.D., Roh, S.K., Balkin, R.B., et al.: Extensive metastases in Peutz-Jeghers syndrome. *JAMA* **239**:2268, 1978.

97. Major, P.: Malignant neoplasms in Peutz-Jeghers syndrome. *JAMA* **240**:2155, 1978.

98. Utsunomiya, J., Gocho, H., Miyanaga, T., et al.: Peutz-Jeghers syndrome: its natural course and management. *Johns Hopkins Med. J.* **136**:71, 1975.

99. Morson, B.C.: Some peculiarities in the histology of intestinal polyps. *Dis. Colon Rectum* **5**:337, 1962.

100. Fenlon, J.W., and Schaekelford, G.D.: Peutz-Jeghers syndrome: case report with angiographic evaluation. *Radiology* **103**:595, 1972.

101. Christian, C.D.: Ovarian tumors: an extension of the Peutz-Jeghers syndrome. *Am. J. Ob. Gyn.* **3**;529, 1971.

102. Dozois, R.R., Kempers, R.D., Dahlin, D.C., et al.: Ovarian tumors associated with Peutz-Jeghers syndrome. *Ann. Surg.* **172**:233, 1970.

103. Humphries, A.L., and Peters, H.J.: Peutz-Jeghers syndrome with colonic adenocarcinoma and ovarian tumor. *JAMA* **197**:296, 1966.

104. Morens, D.M., and Garrey, S.P.: An unusual case of Peutz-Jeghers syndrome in an infant. *Am. J. Dis. Child.* **129**:973, 1975.

105. Torre, D.: Multiple sebaceous tumors. *Arch. Dermatol.* **98**:549, 1968.

106. Muir, E.G., Bell, A.J.Y., and Barlow, K.A.: Multiple primary carcinomas of the colon, duodenum, and larynx associated with kerato-acanthomata of the face. *Br. J. Surg.* **54**:191, 1967.

107. Bakker, P.M., and Tjon A Joe, S.S.: Multiple sebaceous gland tumors with multiple tumours of internal organs: a new syndrome? *Dermatologica* **142**:50, 1971.

108. Rulon, D.B., and Helwig, E.B.: Multiple sebaceous neoplasms of the skin: an association with multiple visceral carcinomas, especially of the colon. *Am. J. Clin. Pathol.* **60**:745, 1973.

109. Bitran, J., and Pellettiere, E.V.: Multiple sebaceous gland tumors and internal carcinoma: Torre's syndrome. *Cancer* **33**:835, 1974.

110. Jakobiec, F.A.: Sebaceous adenoma of the eyelid and visceral malignancy. *Am. J. Opth.* **78**:952, 1974.

111. Sciallis, G.F., and Winkelmann, R.K.: Multiple sebaceous adenomas and gastrointestinal carcinoma. *Arch. Dermatol.* **110**:913, 1974.

112. Leonard, D.D., and Deaton, R.W.: Multiple sebaceous gland tumors and visceral carcinomas. *Arch. Dermatol.* **110**:917, 1974.

113. Lloyd, K.M., and Dennis, M.: Cowden's disease: a possible new symptom complex with multiple system involvement. *Ann. Intern. Med.* **58**:136, 1963.

114. Weary, P.E., Gorlin, R.J., Gentry, W.C., et al.: Multiple hamartoma syndrome (Cowden's disease). *Arch. Dermatol.* **106**:682, 1972.

115. Brownstein, M.H., Wolf, M., and Bikowski, J.B.: Cowden's disease a cutaneous marker of breast cancer. *Cancer* **41**:2393, 1978.

116. Gentry, W.C., Eskritt, N.R., and Gorlin, R.J.: Multiple hamartoma syndrome (Cowden's disease). *Arch. Dermatol.* **109**:521, 1974.

117. Turcot, J., Depres, J., and St. Pierre, F.: Malignant tumors of the central nervous system associated with familial polyposis of the colon: report of two cases. *Dis. Colon Rectum* **2**:465, 1959.

118. Baughman, F.A., Jr., List, C.F., Williams, J.R., et al.: The glioma-polyposis syndrome. *N. Engl. J. Med.* **281**:1345, 1969.

119. Crail, H.W.: Multiple primary malignancies arising in the rectum, brain and thyroid. *US Nav. Med. Bull.* **49**:123, 1949.

120. Cronkhite, L.W., Jr., and Canada, W.J.: Generalized gastrointestinal polyposis: an unusual syndrome of polyposis, pigmentation, alopecia and onychotrophia. *New Engl. J. Med.* **252**:1011, 1955.

121. Johnston, M.M., Vosburgh, J.W., Wiens, A.T., et al.: Gastrointestinal polyposis associated with alopecia. Pigmentation and atrophy of the fingernails and toenails. *Ann. Intern. Med.* **56**:935, 1962.

122. Jarnum, S., and Jensen, H.: Diffuse gastrointestinal polyposis with ectodermal changes. *Gastroenterology* **50**:107, 1966.

123. DaCruz, G.M.G.: Generalized gastrointestinal polyposis. An unusual syndrome of adenomatous polyposis, alopecia, onychotrophia. *Am. J. Gastro.* **47**:504, 1967.

124. Orimo, H., Fujita, T., Yoshikawa, M., et al.: Gastrointestinal polyposis with protein-losing enteropathy, abnormal skin pigmentation and loss of hair and nails (Cronkhite-Canada syndrome). *Am. J. Med.* **47**:445, 1969.

125. Takahata, J., Okubo, K., Komeda, T., et al.: Generalized gastrointestinal polyposis associated with ectodermal changes and protein-losing enteropathy with a dramatic response to prednisolone. *Digestion* **5**:153, 1972.

126. Diner, W.J.: The Cronkhite-Canada syndrome. *Radiology* **105**:715, 1972.

127. Johnson, K., Soergel, K.H., Hensley, G.T., et al.: Cronkhite-Canada syndrome: gastrointestinal pathophysiology and morphology. *Gastroenterology* **63**:140, 1972.

128. Koehler, P.R., Kyaw, M.M., and Fenlon, J.W.: Diffuse gastrointestinal polyposis with ectodermal changes, Cronkhite-Canada syndrome. *Radiology* **103**:589, 1972.

129. Holgersen, L.O., Miller, R.E., and Zintel, H.A.: Juvenile polyps of the colon. *Surgery* **69**:288, 1971.

130. Ray, J.E., Heald, R.J., and Chir, M.: Growing up with juvenile gastrointestinal polyposis: report of a case. *Dis. Colon Rectum* **14**:375, 1971.

131. Soper, R.T., and Kent, T.: Fatal juvenile polyposis in infancy. *Surgery* **69**:692, 1971.

132. Silverberg, S.G.: "Juvenile" retention polyps of the colon and rectum. *Am. J. Dig. Dis.* **15**:617, 1970.

133. Veale, A.M., McColl, I., Bussey, H.R., et al.: Juvenile polyposis coli. *J. Med. Genet.* 3:5, 1966.
134. Sachatello, C.R., Pickeren, J.W., and Grace, J.T.: Generalized juvenile gastrointestinal polyposis. A hereditary syndrome. *Gastroenterology* 58:699, 1970.
135. Stemper, T.J., Kent, T.H., and Summers, R.W.: Juvenile polyposis and gastrointestinal carcinoma: a study of a kindred. *Ann. Intern. Med.* 83:639, 1975.
136. Haggitt, R.C., and Pitcock, J.A.: Familial juvenile polyposis of the colon. *Cancer* 26:1231, 1970.
137. Beacham, C.H., Shields, H.M., Raffensperger, E.C., et al.: Juvenile and adenomatous gastrointestinal polyposis. *Digestive Dis.* 23:1137, 1978.
138. Smilow, P.C., Pryor, C.A., and Swinton, N.W.: Juvenile polyposis coli. *Dis. Colon Rectum* 9:248, 1966.
139. Kaschula, R.O.: Mixed juvenile adenomatous and intermediate polyposis coli: report of a case. *Dis. Colon Rectum* 14:368, 1971.
140. Ruymann, F.B.: Juvenile polyps with cachexia. Report of an infant and comparison with Cronkhite-Canada syndrome in adults. *Gastroenterology* 57:431, 1969.
141. Berk, R.N., Rush, J.L., and Elson, E.C.: Multiple inflammatory polyps of the small intestine with cachexia and protein-losing enteropathy. *Radiology* 95:611, 1970.
142. Schwartz, A.M., and McCauley, R.G.: Juvenile gastrointestinal polyposis. *Radiology* 121:441, 1976.
143. Lynch, H.T., and Lynch, P.M.: Heredity and gastrointestinal tract cancer. In: *Gastrointestinal Tract Cancer* (M. Lipkin and R.A. Good, Eds.). New York: Plenum, 1978, pp. 241–274.
144. Howel-Evans, W., McConnell, R.B., Clarke, C.A., et al.: Carcinoma of the esophagus with keratosis palmaris et plantaris (tylosis). A study of two families. *Quart. J. Med.* 27:413, 1958.
145. Harper, P.S., Harper, R.J., and Howel-Evans, A.W.: Carcinoma of the esophagus with tylosis. *Quart. J. Med.* 39:317, 1970.
146. Shine, I., and Allison, P.R.: Carcinoma of the esophagus with tylosis (keratosis palmaris et plantaris). *Lancet* 1:951, 1966.
147. Nelson, R.S.: Tumors of the esophagus. In: *Gastroenterology* (Henry L. Bockus, Ed., 3rd ed.). Vol. 1. Philadelphia, PA: W.B. Saunders, 1974, p. 301.
148. Nix, T.E., and Christianson, H.B.: Epidermolysis bullosa of the esophagus: report of two cases and review of the literature. *South. Med. J.* 58:612, 1965.
149. Marsden, R.A., Gowar Sambrook, F.J., MacDonald, A.F., et al.: Epidermolysis bullosa of the oesophagus with oesophageal web formation. *Thorax* 29:287, 1974.
150. Didolkar, M.S., Gerner, R F., and Moore, G.E.: Epidermolysis bullosa dystrophica and epithelioma of the skin. Review of published cases and report of an additional patient. *Cancer* 33:198, 1974.
151. Sonneck, H.J., and Hantzschel, K.: Uler einen Fall von Epidermolysis Bullosa Dystrophica mit Oesophagusstenose und Kardiocarcinoma. *Hautarzt* 12:124, 1961.
152. Rockl, H.: Carcinoma Bei Epidermolysis Bullosa Dystrophica. *Hautarzt* 7:463, 1956.
153. Sirinavin, C., and Trowbridge, A.Z.: Dyskeratosis congenita: clinical features and genetic aspects. Report of a family and review of the literature. *J. Med. Genet.* 12:339, 1975.
154. Addison, M., and Rice, M.S.: The association of dyskeratosis congenital and Fanconi's anemia. *Med. J. Aust.* 1:797, 1965.
155. Cole, N.H., Cole, H.N., Jr., and Lascheid, W.P.: Dyskeratosis congenita. *Arch. Dermatol.* 76:712, 1957.
156. Garb, J.: Dyskeratosis congenita with pigmentation, dystrophia unguium and leukoplakia oris. *Arch. Dermatol.* 77:704, 1958.

157. Milgrom, H., Stoll, H.L., Jr., and Crissey, J.T.: Dyskeratosis congenita. *Arch. Dermatol.* 89:345, 1964.
158. Bryan, H.G., and Nixon, R.K.: Dyskeratosis congenita and familial pancytopenia. *JAMA* 192:203, 1965.
159. Garb, J.: Dyskeratosis congenita with pigmentation, dystrophia, unguium and leukoplakia oris: patient with evidence suggestive of Addison's disease. *Arch. Dermat. Syph.* 55:242, 1947.
160. Engman, M.F., Jr.: Congenital atrophy of the skin with reticular pigmentation: report of two cases. *JAMA* 105:1252, 1935.
161. Pastinszky, I., Vankos, J., and Racz, I.: Ein Beitrag zur Pathologie der Dyskeratosis Congenita Cole-Rauschkolb-Toomey. *Derm. Wschr.* 135:587, 1957.
162. Costello, M.J.: Dyskeratosis congenita with superimposed prickle-cell epithelioma on the dorsal aspects of the left hand. *Arch. Dermatol.* 75:451, 1957.
163. Costello, M.J., and Buncke, C.M.: Dyskeratosis congenita. *Arch. Dermatol.* 72:123, 1956.
164. Sorrow, J.M., Jr., and Hitch, J.M.: Dyskeratosis congenita: first report of its occurrence in a female and a review of the literature. *Arch. Dermatol.* 88:340, 1963.
165. Schamberg, I.L.: Dyskeratosis congenita with pigmentation, dystrophia unguius and leukokeratosis oris. *Arch. Dermatol.* 81:266, 1960.
166. Koszewski, B.G., and Hubbard, T.E.: Congenital anemia in hereditary ectodermal dysplasia. *Arch. Dermatol.* 74:159, 1956.
167. Auerbach, R.C., and Koehler, P.R.: The many faces of islet cell tumors. *AJR* 119:133, 1973.
168. Croughs, R.J., Hulsmans, H.A., Israel, D.E., et al.: Glucagonomas as part of the polyglandular adenoma syndrome. *Am. J. Med.* 52:690, 1972.
169. Mallinson, C.N., Bloom, S.R., Warin, A.P., et al.: A glucagonoma syndrome. *Lancet* 2:1, 1974.
170. McGavran, M.H., Unger, R.H., ReCant, L., et al.: A glucagon-secreting alpha-cell carcinoma of the pancreas. *N. Engl. J. Med.* 274:1408, 1966.
171. Boden, G., and Owen, O.E.: Familial hyperglucagonemia – an autosomal dominant disorder. *N. Engl. J. Med.* 296:534, 1977.
172. Cho, K.J., Wilcox, C.W., and Reuter, S.R.: Glucagon-producing islet cell tumor of the pancreas. *AJR* 129:159, 1977.
173. Deutsch, V., Adar, R., Jacob, E.T., et al.: Angiographic diagnosis and differential diagnosis of islet cell tumors. *AJR* 119:121, 1973.
174. Gray, R.K., Rosch, J., and Grollman, J.H., Jr.: Arteriography in the diagnosis of islet cell tumors. *Radiology* 97:39, 1970.
175. Ingemansson, S., Lunderquist, A., and Holst, J.: Selective catheterization of the pancreatic vein for radioimmunoassay of a glucagon secreting carcinoma of the pancreas. *Radiology* 119:555, 1976.
176. Boder, E., and Sedgwick, R.P.: Ataxia-telangiectasia. A familial syndrome of progressive cerebellar ataxia, oculocutaneous telangiectasia and frequent pulmonary infection. *Pediatrics* 21:526, 1958.
177. Karpati, G., Eisen, A.H., Andermann, F., et al.: Ataxia-telangiectasia. Further observations and report of eight cases. *Am. J. Dis. Child.* 110:51, 1965.
178. Peterson, R.D., Cooper, M.D., and Good, R.A.: Lymphoid tissue abnormalities associated with ataxia-telangiectasia. *Am. J. Med.* 41:342, 1966.
179. Reed, W.B., Epstein, W.L., Boder, E., et al.: Cutaneous manifestations of ataxia-telangiectasia. *JAMA* 195:126, 1966.
180. Haerer, A.F., Jackson, J.F., and Evers, C.G.: Ataxia-telangiectasia with gastric adenocarcinoma. *JAMA* 210:1884, 1969.

181. McKusick, V.A., and Cross, H.E.: Ataxia-telangiectasia and Swiss type agammaglobulinemia, two genetic disorders of the immune mechanism in related Amish sibships. *JAMA* 195:119, 1966.

182. Warkany, J.: *Congenital Malformations, Notes and Comments,* Chicago, IL: Year Book Publ., 1971, p. 270.

183. Eidelman, A., and Davis, S.D.: Immunoglobulin content of intestinal mucosal plasma-cells in ataxia-telangiectasia. *Lancet* 1:884, 1968.

184. Young, R.R., Austen, K.F., and Moser, H.W.: Ataxia-telangiectasia and the thymus. *Tr. Am. Neurol. A.* 89:28, 1964.

185. Swift, M.: Malignant disease in heterozygous carriers. *Birth Defects* 12:133, 1976.

186. Hecht, F., Koler, R.D., Rigas, D.A., et al.: Leukemia and lymphocytes in ataxia-telangiectasia. *Lancet* 2:1193, 1966.

187. Shuster, J., Hart, Z., Stimson, C., et al.: Ataxia-telangiectasia with cerebellar tumor. *Pediatrics* 37:776, 1966.

188. Dunn, H.G., Menwissen, H., Livingstone, C.S., et al.: Ataxia-telangiectasia. *Canad. MAJ.* 91:1106, 1964.

189. Marshak, R.H., Hazzie, C., Linder, A.E., et al.: Small bowel in immunoglobulin deficiency syndromes. *AJR* 122:227, 1974.

190. Sholman, L., and Swift, M.: Pancreatic carcinoma and diabetes mellitus in families of ataxia-telangiectasia probands. *Am. J. Hum. Genet.* 24:48a, 1972.

191. McKusick, V.A.: *Mendelian Inheritance in Man.* Baltimore, MD: Johns Hopkins University Press, 1978.

192. Paterson, M.C., Smith, B.P., Lohman, P.H.M., et al.: Defective excision repair of gamma ray damaged DNA in human (ataxia-telangiectasia) fibroblasts. *Nature* 260:444, 1976.

193. Taylor, A.M.R., Metcalfe, J.A., Oxford, J.M., et al.: Is chromatid-type damage in ataxia-telangiectasis after irradiation a GoA consequence of defective repair? *Nature* 260:441, 1976.

194. Arlett, C.F., and Lehmann, A.R.: Human disorders showing increased sensitivity to the induction of genetic damage. *Ann. Rev. Genet.* 12:95, 1978.

195. Lynch, H.T., Frichot, B.C., Lynch, J.D., et al.: Family studies of malignant melanoma and associated cancer. *Surg. Gynecol. Obstet.* 141:517, 1975.

196. Frichot, B.C.: New cutaneous phenotype in familial malignant melanoma. *Lancet* 1:864, 1977.

197. Lynch, H.T., Frichot, B.C., and Lynch, J.F.: Familial atypical multiple mole-melanoma syndrome. *J. Med. Genet.* 15:352, 1978.

198. Lynch, H.T., and Krush, A.J.: Hereditary and malignant melanoma: implications for early cancer detection. *Canad. Med. Assoc. J.* 99:17, 1968.

199. Cawley, E.P.: Genetic aspects of malignant melanoma. *Arch. Dermatol.* 65:440, 1951.

200. Anderson, D.E.: Clinical characteristics of the genetic variety of cutaneous melanoma in man. *Cancer* 28:721, 1971.

201. Lynch, H.T., Anderson, D.E., Smith, J.L., et al.: Xeroderma pigmentosum, malignant melanoma and congenital ichthyosis: a family study. *Arch. Dermatol.* 96:625, 1967.

202. Gartner, S.: Malignant melanoma of the choroid and von Recklinghausen's disease. *Am. J. Ophthalmol.* 23:73, 1940.

203. Lynch, H.T.: *Cancer Genetics.* Springfield, IL: C. Thomas, 1976, p. 639.

204. Lynch, H.T., and Frichot, B.C.: Skin, heredity and cancer. *Sem. Oncol.* 5:67, 1978.

205. Lynch, H.T.: *Skin, Heredity and Malignant Neoplasms.* Flushing, NY: Medical Examination Publ. Co., 1972, p. 239.

206. Fraser, D.G., Bull, J.G., Jr., and Dunphy, J.E.: Malignant melanoma and coexisting malignant neoplasms. *Am. J. Surg.* **122**:169, 1971.
207. Meneer, G., and DasGupta, T.: Life history of melanoma. *AJR* **93**:686, 1965.
208. Marshak, R.H., and Lindner, A.E.: *Radiology of the Small Intestine.* Philadelphia, PA: W.B. Saunders, 1976.
209. Templeton, F.E.: In: *Colonic Malignancy in Alimentary Tract Roentgenology* (A.R. Margulis and H.J. Burhenne, Eds.). Ch. 40. St. Louis, MO: C.V. Mosby Co., 1973,
210. Pearson, H.A., Shulman, R.N., Oski, F.A., et al.: Platelet survival in Wiskott-Aldrich syndrome. *J. Pediat.* **68**:754, 1966.
211. Ten Bensel, R.W., Stadlan, E.M., and Krivit, W.: The development of malignancy in the course of the Aldrich syndrome. *J. Pediat.* **68**:761, 1966.
212. Srivastava, R.N.: Wiskott-Aldrich syndrome. *Arch. Dis. Child* **42**:604, 1967.
213. Gatti, R.A., and Good, R.A.: Occurrence of malignancy in immunodeficiency diseases. *Cancer* **28**:89, 1971.
214. Kildeberg, P.: A case of Aldrich's syndrome. *Acta Paediat. (Suppl.)* **140**:120, 1963.
215. Coleman, A., Leikin, S., and Guin, G.H.: Aldrich's syndrome. *Clin. Proc. Child Hosp. (Wash.)* **17**:362, 1961.
216. Holt, J.F.: Neurofibromatosis in children. *AJR* **130**:615, 1978.
217. Davis, G.B., and Berk, R.N.: Intestinal neurofibromatosis in von Recklinghausen's disease. *Am. J. Gastroenterol.* **60**:410, 1973.
218. Fabricant, R.N., Todaro, G.J., and Eldridge, R.: Increased levels of a nerve-growth-factor cross-reacting protein in central neurofibromatosis. *Lancet* **1**:4, 1979.
219. Crowe, F.W., and Schull, W.J.: Diagnostic importance of café au lait spot in neurofibromatosis. *Arch. Inter. Med.* **91**:758, 1953.
220. WhiteHouse, D.: Diagnostic value of the café au lait spot in children. *Arch. Dis. Child* **41**:316, 1966.
221. Holt, J.F., and Wright, E.M.: The radiologic features of neurofibromatosis. *Radiology* **51**:647, 1948.
222. Holt, J.F.: Osscous manifestations of neurofibromatosis. *Proc. N. Engl. Roentgen Ray Soc.* **6**:57, 1950.
223. Hunt, J.C., and Pugh, D.G.: Skeletal lesions in neurofibromatosis. *Radiology* **76**:1, 1961.
224. D'Agostino, A.N., Soule, E.H., and Miller, R.H.: Sarcomas of the peripheral nerves and somatic soft tissues associated with multiple neurofibromatosis (von Recklinghausen's disease). *Cancer* **16**:1015, 1963.
225. Rodriquez, H.A., and Berthrong, M.: Multiple primary intracranial tumors in von Recklinghausen's neurofibromatosis. *Arch. Neurol.* **14**:467, 1966.
226. Gardner, W.J., and Turner, O.: Bilateral acoustic neurofibromas: further clinical and pathologic data on hereditary deafness and Recklinghausen's disease. *Arch. Neurol. Psychiatry* **44**:76, 1940.
227. Knight, W.A., Murphy, W.K., and Gottlieb, J.A.: Neurofibromatosis associated with malignant neurofibromas. *Arch. Dermatol.* **107**:747, 1973.
228. Schonebeck, J., and Lujngberg, O.: Recklinghausen's disease: a multifaceted syndrome. *Acta Path. Microbiol. Scand.* **78A**:437, 1970.
229. Reich, S.D., and Wiernik, P.H.: von Recklinghausen neurofibromatosis and acute leukemia. *Am. J. Dis. Child* **130**:888, 1976.
230. Marshak, R.H., Freund, S., and Maklansky, D.: Neurofibromatosis of the small bowel. *Am. J. Dig. Dis.* **8**:478, 1963.
231. Buntin, P.T., and Fitzgerald, J.F.: Gastrointestinal neurofibromatosis: a rare cause of anemia. *Am. J. Dis. Child* **119**:521, 1970.

232. Weston, S.C., Marren, M., Dohan, M.H., et al.: Neurofibroma of the rectum and colon. *ICS* **40**:285, 1963.

233. Staple, T.W., McAlister, W.H., and Anderson, M.S.: Plexiform neurofibromatosis of the colon simulating Hirschsprung's disease. *AJR* **91**:840, 1964.

234. River, L., Silverstein, J., and Topel, W.: Benign neoplasms of the small intestine. *Int. Abst. Surg.* **102**:1, 1956.

235. Levy, D., and Khatib, R.: Intestinal neurofibromatosis with malignant degeneration. *Dis. Colon Rectum* **3**:140, 1960.

236. Reuter, S.R., and Redman, H.C.: *Gastrointestinal Angiography.* Philadelphia, PA: W.B. Saunders, 1972, p. 100.

237. Trier, J.S.: Celiac sprue disease. *Gastrointestinal Disease* (M.H. Sleisenger and J.S. Fordtran, Eds.). Ch. 60. Philadelphia, PA: W.B. Saunders, 1978.

238. Kalser, M.H.: Celiac sprue. *Gastroenterology* (H.L. Bockus, Ed.). Ch. 59. Philadelphia, PA: W.B. Saunders, 1976.

239. MacDonald, W.C., Dobbins, W.O., and Rubin, C.E.: Studies of the familial nature of celiac sprue using biopsy of the small intestine. *N. Engl. J. Med.* **272**:448, 1965.

240. Marks, J., and Shuster, S.: Dermatogenic enteropathy. *Gut* **11**:292, 1970.

241. Bossak, E.T., Wang, C.T., and Adlersberg, D.: Clinical aspects of the malabsorption syndrome. *J. Mt. Sinai. Hosp.* **24**:286, 1957.

242. Friedman, M., and Hare, P.J.: Gluten-sensitive enteropathy and eczema. *Lancet* **1**: 521, 1965.

243. Harris, O.D., Cooke, W.T., Thompson, H., et al.: Malignancy in adult celiac disease and idiopathis steatorrhea. *Am. J. Med.* **42**:899, 1967.

244. Barry, R.E., and Read, A.E.: Celiac disease and malignancy. *Q. J. Med.* **42**:665, 1973.

245. Sleisenger, M.D., Almy, T.A., and Barr, D.P.: The sprue syndrome secondary to lymphoma of the small bowel. *Am. J. Med.* **15**:666, 1953.

246. Scheinberg, I.H.: The genetics of hemochromatosis. *Arch. In. Med.* **132**:126, 1973.

247. Finch, S.C., and Finch, C.A.: Idiopathic hemochromatosis, an iron storage disease. *Medicine* **34**:381, 1955.

248. Cawley, E.P., Hsu, Y.T., Wood, B.T., et al.: Hemochromatosis and the skin. *Arch. Dermatol.* **100**:1, 1969.

249. Dymock, I.W., Cassar, J., Pyke, D.A., et al.: Observations on the pathogenesis, complications and treatment of diabetes in 115 cases of hemochromatosis. *Am. J. Med.* **52**:203, 1972.

250. MacDonald, R.A.: Idiopathic hemochromatosis. A variant of portal cirrhosis and idiopathic hemosiderosis. *Arch. In. Med.* **107**:606, 1961.

251. MacDonald, R.A.: Idiopathic hemochromatosis. Genetic or acquired? *Arch. In. Med.* **112**:184, 1963.

252. Williams, R., Scheuer, P.J., and Sherlock, S.: The inheritance of idiopathic hemochromatosis. A clinical and liver biopsy study of 16 families. *Q. J. Med.* **31**:249, 1962.

253. Powel, L.W.: Iron storage in relatives of patients with hemochromatosis and in relatives of patients with alcoholic cirrhosis and hemosiderosis. *Q. J. Med.* **34**:427, 1965.

254. Morgan, E.H.: Idiopathic hemochromatosis: a family study. *Aust. Ann. Med.* **10**: 114, 1961.

255. Johnson, G.B., Jr., and Frey, W.G., III: Familial aspects of idiopathic hemochromatosis. *JAMA* **179**:747, 1962.

256. Balcerzak, S.P., Westerman, M.P., Lee, R.E., et al.: Idiopathic hemochromatosis: a study of three families. *Am. J. Med.* **40**:857, 1966.

257. Shanbrom, E., and Zheutlin, N.: Radiologic sign in hemosiderosis. *JAMA* **168**, 1958.

258. Stanley, R.J., Sagel, S.S., and Levitt, R.G.: Computed tomography of the liver. *RCNA* 15:331, 1977.
259. Mills, S.R., Doppman, J.L., and Nienhuis, A.W.: Computed tomography in the diagnosis of disorders of excessive iron storage of the liver. *J. Comp. Asst. Tomography* 1:101, 1977.
260. Berk, J.E., and Lieber, M.M.: Primary carcinoma of the liver in hemochromatosis. *Am. J. Med. Sci.* 202:708, 1941.
261. Nebesar, R.A., Pollard, J.J., and Stone, D.L.: Angiographic diagnosis of malignant disease of the liver. *Radiology* 86:284, 1966.
262. Reuter, S.R., Redman, H.C., and Siders, D.B.: The spectrum of angiographic findings in hepatoma. *Radiology* 94:89, 1970.
263. Sussman, E.B., Nydick, I., and Gray, G.F.: Hemangioendothelial sarcoma of the liver and hemochromatosis. *Arch. Path.* 97:39, 1974.
264. Maynard, J.H., and Fone, D.J.: Hemochromatosis with osteogenic sarcoma in the liver. *Med. J. Aust.* 2:1260, 1969.
265. McLoughlin, M.J., and Hill, M.Q.: Angiography in cholangiocarcinoma complicating hemochromatosis. *J. Can. Assoc. Radiol.* 21:238, 1970.
266. Schumacher, H.R., Jr.: Hemochromatosis and arthritis. *Arthritis Rheum.* 7:41, 1964.
267. Wardle, E.N., and Patton, J.T.: Bone and joint changes in hemochromatosis. *Ann. Rheum. Dis.* 28:15, 1969.
268. Dymock, I.W., Hamilton, E.B.D., Laws, J.W., et al.: Arthropathy of hemochromatosis. Clinical and radiological analysis of 63 patients with iron overload. *Ann. Rheum. Dis.* 29:469, 1970.
269. Hirsch, J.H., Killien, F.C., and Troupin, R.H.: The arthropathy of hemochromatosis. *Radiology* 118:591, 1976.
270. ByWaters, E.G.L., Hamilton, E.B.D., and Williams, R.: The spine in idiopathic hemochromatosis. *Ann. Rheum. Dis.* 30:453, 1971.
271. Hawkins, C.F., and Kendall, M.J.: Anemia in digestive tract disorders. In: *Gastroenterology*, (H.L. Bockus, Ed.). Ch. 169. Philadelphia, PA: W.B. Saunders, 1976.
272. Brandborg, L.L.: Polyps, tumors and cancer of the stomach. *Gastrointestinal Disease* (M.H. Sleisenger and J.S. Fordtran, Eds.). Ch. 42. Philadelphia, PA: W.B. Saunders, 1978.
273. McConnell, R.B.: Genetics in gastroenterology. *Gastroenterology* (H.L. Bockus, Ed.). Ch. 177, 1976.
274. Samitz, M.H.: Dermatologic gastrointestinal relationships. In: *Gastroenterology* (H.L. Bockus, Ed.). Ch. 166. Philadelphia, PA: W.B. Saunders, 1976.
275. Kaplan, H.S., and Rigler, L.G.: Pernicious anemia and carcinoma of the stomach — autopsy studies concerning their inter-relationship. *Am. J. Med. Sciences* 209:339, 1945.
276. Schell, R.G., Dockerty, M.B., and Comfort, M.W.: Carcinoma of the stomach associated with pernicious anemia: a clinical and pathologic study. *Surg. Gyneo. Obstet.* 98:710, 1954.
277. Zamcheck, N., Grable, E., Ley, A., et al.: Occurrence of gastric cancer with pernicious anemia at the Boston City Hospital. *N. Engl. J. Med.* 252:1103, 1955.
278. Frik, W.: Neoplastic diseases of the stomach. In: *Alimentary Tract Roentgenology* (A.R. Margulis and H.J. Burhenne, Eds.). Ch. 26. St. Louis, MO: C.V. Mosby, 1973.
279. Vilardell, F.: Chronic gastric disease and suction biopsy. In: *Gastroenterology* (H.L. Bockus, Ed.). Ch. 26. Philadelphia, PA: W.B. Saunders, 1976.
280. Mann, S.G.: Kaposi's sarcoma. Experience with ten cases. *AJR* 121:793, 1974.

281. Byrk, D., Farman, J., Dallemand, S., et al.: Kaposi's sarcoma of the intestinal tract: roentgen manifestations. *Gastrointes. Radiol.* 3:425, 1978.

282. Bluefarb, S.M.: *Kaposi's Sarcoma.* Springfield, IL: C.C. Thomas, 1957.

283. McGinn, J.T., Ricca, J.J., and Currin, J.F.: Kaposi's sarcoma following allergic angiitis. *Ann. Inter. Med.* 42:921, 1955.

284. Zeligman, I.: Kaposi's sarcoma in a father and son. *Bull. Johns Hopkins Hosp.* 107:208, 1960.

285. Epstein, E.: Kaposi's sarcoma and parapsoriasis en plaque in brothers. *JAMA* 219: 1477, 1972.

286. Templeton, A.C., and Dhru, D.: Kaposi's sarcoma in half-brothers. *Trop. Geogr. Med.* 27:324, 1975.

287. Finlay, A.Y., and Marks, R.: Familial Kaposi's sarcoma. *Br. J. Dermatol.* 100: 323, 1979.

288. Brasfield, R., and O'Brien, P.: Kaposi's sarcoma. *Cancer* 19:1497, 1966.

289. Palmer, P.E.S.: Hemangiosarcoma of Kaposi. *Acta Radiol. (Suppl.)* 316:5, 1972.

290. Bhana, D.: Kaposi's sarcoma of lymph nodes. *Brit. J. Cancer* 24:464, 1970.

291. Rylwin, A.M., Recher, L., and Hoffman, E.: Lymphoma-like presentation of Kaposi's sarcoma. *Arch. Derm.* 93:554, 1966.

292. Calenoff, L.: Gastrointestinal Kaposi's sarcoma: roentgen manifestations. *AJR* 114: 525, 1972.

293. Palmer, P.E.S.: Radiological changes of Kaposi's sarcoma. *Acta Unio. Internat. Contra Cancrum* 18:87, 1962.

7
Immune System Evaluation in Genetic Immunodeficiency Diseases Associated with Malignancies

J. Corwin Vance, M.D.

BACKGROUND

The role of the immune system in the etiology of human neoplasia has been widely studied but remains uncertain. It has been established that antigens are present on many tumors and that immune responses are active against those antigens. The effectiveness of such responses in preventing the emergence of neoplasia or in destroying a tumor once it has become established constitutes an active area of research. Many hypotheses of the etiology of human neoplasia have been proposed.[1] This discussion will focus on the role of the immune system in the development of cancer, with special reference to genetic diseases of immunodeficiency.

Some of the strongest evidence for the role of the immune system in neoplasia is the increased incidence of malignancies in the genetically determined immunodeficiency diseases (GDID) and acquired immunodeficiencies, such as patients undergoing immunosuppressive therapy for organ transplantation.[2-6] Only the GDID will be discussed here. In all genetic diseases with associated neoplasia, the possibility of involvement by the immune system should be considered. Among GDID, associated genetic but nonimmune defects also may play a role in the occurrence of neoplasia.

Three general hypotheses have been proposed for the involvement of the immune system in the etiology of neoplasia:

1. The immune system conducts an overall *surveillance* of the host for possible malignant cells. A defective surveillance mechanism permits the emergence or growth of malignancies.
2. *Immunostimulation,* possibly resulting from chronic infection or autoimmunity, might result in the occurrence of malignant diseases.

3. An immunodeficiency specific for a particular tumor antigen or an imbalance of regulatory influences may result in *tolerance* for a tumor and permit its growth.

The *surveillance* hypothesis was already contained in an early form in the work of Paul Ehrlich[7] and it has been widely accepted. The mounting evidence which fails to support the theory has been reviewed by Drew[8] who found the data on both sides to be inconclusive. The *immunostimulation* hypothesis is particularly strong in lymphomas, such as Burkitt's lymphoma.[9] It is of interest that lymphomas are the predominant malignancies in immunodeficiency patients.[4-6] Specific immune *tolerance* is a well-studied phenomenon, and tumor antigen tolerance may result in neoplasia. The specific deficiency in response to polysaccharide antigens in Wiskott-Aldrich patients may represent such a defect.[10]

The existence of antigens on the surface of tumors, such as leukemic cells, has been abundantly proved.[11] The host may respond with antibody or cell-mediated immunity, or both.[12-13] The presence of an active antitumor response sometimes correlates with a favorable clinical course, but in other cases no such association can be found. Correlations also occur between a favorable clinical response and the adequacy of the patient's responsiveness to less specific but more widely available tests of immune function, such as the delayed hypersensitivity skin tests and in vitro lymphocyte responsiveness to mitogens.[14] It is very difficult to generalize about the significance of specific test results, but patterns of abnormalities do emerge. For instance, Jones et al.[15] studied the total lymphocyte count, quantitative serum immunoglobulins, and delayed hypersensitivity skin tests in patients with non-Hodgkin's lymphomas. A severe degree of immunodeficiency was found in patients with a diffuse histologic type of tumor, whereas patients with a nodular histologic type had a lesser degree of immunodeficiency. A distinctive constellation of malignances is often associated with particular immunodeficiency diseases, which suggests that specific immune defects are associated with certain tumors. Gatti and Good[4] drew attention to the unusual constellation of malignancies in a number of primary immunodeficiency diseases. They also pointed out the increased incidence of malignancies, estimating that GDID patients have a risk 10,000 times that of an age-matched control group. More recently,[16] the estimated increased risk was reduced to about 100-fold; GDID patients had about 0.8 malignancy per 100 patients per year, whereas age-matched patients in the general population had an incidence of about 0.007 per 100 patients per year. Spector et al.[17] also noted that specific tumors, especially lymphomas and leukemias, were related to various GDID and thus indirectly to specific immune defects.

EVALUATION OF LYMPHOCYTE-ASSOCIATED IMMUNOCOMPETENCE

The complexity of both the immune system and immunological diseases requires an organized evaluation of immunocompetence. The most widely used laboratory tests for the evaluation of lymphocyte-associated immunocompetence are given in Table 7-1. It does not include any evaluation of the monocyte-macrophage-histiocyte series of cells, the granulocyte series, the complement system, or other local or systemic manifestations of immunity. Table 7-1 reflects the division of the lymphocyte-associated immune system into two parts, the thymus-dependent

Table 7-1. Evaluation of Lymphocyte-Associated Immunocompetence.

	T CELL (CELL-MEDIATED IMMUNITY)	B CELL (HUMORAL IMMUNITY)
Quantitative hematologic	1. Peripheral blood total lymphocyte count	1. Peripheral blood B-cell quantitation (e.g., immunofluorescent detection of surface immunoglobulin)
	2. Peripheral blood T-cell quantitation (e.g., by sheep red blood cell rosettes)	2. Serum (or secretory) immunoglobulin levels
Functional in vitro	3. Lymphocyte stimulation by mitogens (e.g., PHA or con-A)	3. Lymphocyte stimulation by mitogens (e.g., pokeweed)
	4. Lymphocyte stimulation by antigens (e.g., PPD, SK/SD, Candida)	
	5. Lymphocyte response to allogenic cells (e.g., mixed leukocyte reaction)	
	6. Lymphocyte mediator production (e.g., MIF)	
Functional in vivo	7. Induction of delayed-type hypersensivity (e.g., DNCB)	4. Serum antibody titers (e.g., isohemagglutinins, Schick test)
	8. Elicitation of delayed-type hypersensitivity (e.g., recall skin tests)	5. Induction of a primary antibody response (e.g., KLH, flagellin, etc.)
	9. Allograft rejection (e.g., skin grafts)	6. Elicitation of a secondary antibody response (e.g., diphtheria, tetanus, polio)
Anatomical	10. Lymphoid tissue biopsies (e.g., lymph nodes, thymus)	7. Lymphoid tissue biopsies (e.g., lymph nodes, intestine, spleen, bone marrow, tonsils)

or T-cell branch subserving cell-mediated immune functions, and the bone marrow or bursal-dependent B-cell branch subserving humoral immune functions. Not indicated are the innumerable interactions between the two divisions. It was designed in order to provide an overview of immune disturbances in the various GDID and to supply a framework in which to work when evaluating other diseases — in particular, diseases characterized by the development of malignancies. Patterns of abnormalities are easier to recognize when using such a system, thus aiding one in making diagnoses. Each test will be briefly discussed and then in the following section their use in several primary immunodeficiency diseases will be given.

T Cell (Cell-mediated Immunity)

Peripheral Blood Total Lymphocyte Count.[18] Most evaluations of cell-mediated immunity (CMI) should begin with a peripheral blood white cell count and an examination of a peripheral smear. Quantitation of the lymphocytes, and particularly the small lymphocytes which normally predominate, gives a rough evaluation of CMI, since a high proportion of the small lymphocytes in the peripheral blood are T cells. In general, if the total lymphocyte count is below 2,000 cells per cubic millimeter, lymphopenia is present. A single quantitation is not reliable because the number of lymphocytes normally varies. A transient lymphopenia or lymphocytosis may also be caused by a viral or other infection. Such infections are common occurrences in immunodeficient patients, and so may cause some confusion. Many GDID are characterized by a striking lymphopenia.

Peripheral Blood T-lymphocyte Quantitation.[19-21] T-lymphocytes are most often identified and quantitated in the peripheral blood by their ability to form rosettes with sheep erythrocytes. This is called the E rosette test and has been in use since the early 1970s when it was found that up to 80% of human peripheral blood lymphocytes spontaneously bind sheep erythrocytes. The latter gather in a group around T-lymphocytes, giving the appearance of a rosette, a rose-shaped cluster. Generally any lymphocyte having contact with three or more erythrocytes is counted as a rosette, abbreviated E^+. Figure 7-1 shows a Wright-stained smear of such a preparation. Both lymphocytes are T cells, but are abnormally large since the smear was prepared from a patient with Sezary syndrome, a T-cell leukemia. The exact nature of the receptor responsible for binding sheep erythrocytes is unknown. Thus while it is clear that E^+ cells are derived from the thymus, a certain degree of caution should be observed in interpreting their exact nature.

Differences in normal values are observed among laboratories. One cause is that the number of E^+ lymphocytes changes because of small variations in cell

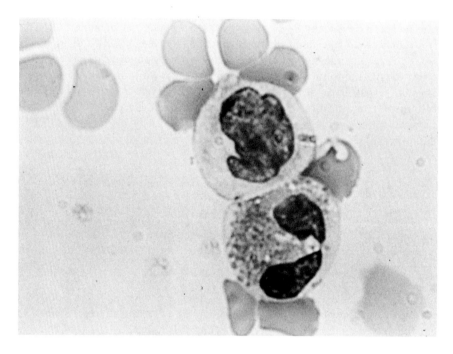

Figure 7-1. A rosette formation.

handling techniques and reagents. Thus a standard must be established in each laboratory. The E rosette test determines only the percentage of viable lymphocytes which are T cells. It is important to simultaneously perform a total lymphocyte count so that the absolute number of circulating T cells in a known volume of blood may be calculated. The absolute value is important since changes in the E^- B cells will also affect the relative proportion of E^+ cells. A second method by which T cells may be quantitated is by the use of antisera specific for human T cells.[21] More recently, monoclonal antibodies against T cells have been developed, and fluorescein-labelled anti-T cell antibodies conveniently distinguish T cells from B cells.

T-lymphocytes are known to be a functionally heterogeneous population, which may be subdivided by examination of cell surface receptors and antigens.[21-25] Some examples are given in Table 7-2. The subset of T cells expressing a surface membrane receptor for the Fc portion of IgG ($Fc\gamma R$) has been found to be associated with suppressor cell activity when analysis of their effect on B-cell responses is made, whereas T cells expressing a receptor for the Fc portion of IgM ($Fc\mu R$) are associated with helper cell activity.[22] Differentiation antigens are also present on T-cell surface membranes. The TH_1 antigen has been found

Table 7-2. Surface Markers on Human T-cell Subpopulations.

RECEPTORS	ASSOCIATED WITH
IgG-Fc (FcγR)	Supressor activity
IgM-Fc (FcμR)	Helper activity
ANTIGENS	
TH_1	Helper activity
TH_2	Supressor activity
Ia antigens	Expressed after activation

to be associated with helper cell activity, whereas TH_2 is associated with suppressor cell function.[23-25] The expression of Ia antigens on human lymphocytes was previously thought to be limited to B cells. However, such antigens have recently been found on T-lymphocytes having either helper or suppressor cell activity, but only after activation such as by mitogen stimulation.[25] In clinical diseases with immunodeficiency, it has become clear that changes in T-cell subsets are important,[26] but their determination has not yet become a widely available diagnostic tool and so was not included in Table 7-1.

T-lymphocyte Stimulation by Mitogens.[27-28] Stimulation of T-lymphocytes by mitogens is one of the most widely used and clinically important tests for the in vitro functional evaluation of the cell-mediated immune system. The plant extracts phytohemagglutinin (PHA) and concanavalin-A (con-A) are the most commonly used human lymphocyte mitogens, and while both stimulate B cells as well as T cells for practical purposes they may be considered T-cell mitogens. The method involves adding the mitogen to suspensions of peripheral blood lymphocytes, incubating them for about three days at $37°C$, and then adding radioactively labeled thymidine to the cultures. The quantity of thymidine incorporated into the cells, determined by liquid scintillation counting, is a measurement of DNA synthesis. Examination of the cells microscopically reveals that many have become transformed into large primitive appearing cells with a high degree of mitoses (blast transformation), and the proportion of such cells may also be counted as a measure of mitogen stimulation. The activation or stimulation of lymphocytes is an exceedingly complex process. The mitogenic plant extract first binds to the surface of the cells by a specific receptor. After binding occurs, many changes take place in the lymphocytes, a partial list of which includes: increased glucose uptake, increased potassium influx, increased calcium uptake, increased amino acid uptake, increased cyclic GMP levels, decreased cyclic AMP levels, increased endocytosis, increased acetylation of histones, increased RNA synthesis, increased protein synthesis, increased cell division, and increased size of lymphocytes. Mitogen stimulation, as a test of immunologic competence, measures only the efferent arm of the immune response. The antigen capture, processing, and recognition functions are not involved, and so are not evaluated. Mitogens are polyclonal stimulators, inducing proliferation in numerous clones of lymphocytes. A general or overall deficiency in lymphocyte function or numbers can be detected using this test, but the absence of a single clone cannot be detected and so mitogens are of little value in detecting more specific deficiencies.

The use of T-lymphocyte mitogens in the evaluation of patients with primary immune deficiencies has been well demonstrated.[28] In patients with DiGeorge's syndrome, there is a deficiency of T-lymphocytes and they are thus unable to respond to PHA or con-A. Patients with classical severe combined immune deficiency (SCID) lack both T cells and B cells, and so also fail to respond to mitogens. On the other hand, in patients with a deficiency limited to the B-cell system, such as Bruton's X-linked agammaglobulinemia, T-lymphocyte mitogenic responses are usually preserved. The mitogen response test is also important clinically in following the effects of therapy in immunodeficiency states. Mitogen responsiveness may return to normal coincident with successful treatment with such agents as transfer factor or bone marrow transplantation.[28]

Lymphocyte Stimulation by Antigens.[27,29,30] Stimulation of T cells by antigens is analogous to that by mitogens and is performed in a similar manner.[27] Instead of inducing a broad polyclonal activation as mitogens do, antigens activate the specific clones of lymphocytes committed to the particular antigen being tested. As a consequence, DNA synthesis and blast transformation, which are measured after five days in culture instead of three, are of a lower magnitude and are slower in reaching a peak. The afferent functions of recognition and processing of the specific antigens are required for an intact response, and so defects in those functions will be reflected by a reduced or absent response. Absence of previous exposure to the specific antigen will also result in a reduced response; thus, in order to confirm the significance of a negative result, either antigen exposure must be documented or a number of ubiquitous antigens must be studied. Bacterial and fungal antigens have been most widely used and include, among others, extracts from *Mycobacterium tuberculosis* (PPD), *Streptococcus* (SK/SD), *Candida albicans, Escherichia coli,* and *Staphylococcus aureus.* Antigens derived from viruses such as herpes, vaccinia, and mumps, and also tumor- or tissue-specific antigens have been used, particularly where disease-specific or disease-related antigen defects are suspected. In diseases in which the efferent arm of T-cell immune response is diffusely abnormal, the mitogen and antigen stimulation tests will usually be similarly reduced.

The ability of a patient's lymphocytes to respond in vitro to antigens generally corresponds with in vivo immune responses to the same antigens. A positive correlation has been established, for example, between the intensity of the recall skin test response to a particular antigen and the degree of in vitro lymphocyte responsiveness to the same antigen.[29] An example of the usefulness of the antigen stimulation test is in the evaluation of patients with chronic mucocutaneous candidiasis who have deficient lymphocyte transformation in vitro to candidal antigens and have frequent and severe infections with *Candida albicans.*[30] The recall skin test to *Candida* antigen is likewise usually negative, whereas anticandidal antibodies can frequently be detected in the serum.

Lymphocyte Response to Allogeneic Cells.[31-34] The one-way mixed leukocyte culture (MLC) is an in vitro model of allograft rejection developed for use in organ or tissue transplantation.[33] Blast transformation and proliferation of T cells results from their exposure to histocompatibility antigens present on the leukocytes of another individual. The MLC primarily detects antigenic differences at the lymphocyte-defined (LD) locus of the major histocompatibility complex (MHC). The method involves separating leukocytes (lymphocytes and monocytes) from the peripheral blood of two individuals. The cells of one person (the stimulator) provide the antigenic stimulus, and are treated with mitomycin C or x-irradiation to prevent DNA synthesis and cell division. These cells are mixed with the cells of the other person (the responder) whose immune response is to be tested. Radioactively labeled thymidine is added to the mixture after four to seven days, and the amount of thymidine taken up by the responding lymphocytes is counted by liquid scintillation.[31,33] When there is a histocompatibility antigen difference, 1-3% of the responder's lymphocytes become activated, which is higher than that seen in the antigen stimulation assay but less than in the mitogen stimulation assay.[34] Only those clones of T cells reactive to the LD transplantation antigens become activated. Previous exposure of the patient (i.e., the responder) to those specific antigens is not necessary. The MLC is a primary antigenic reaction during which the initial recognition process takes place, and in which macrophages are known to play a role.

Reduced MLC responsiveness has been observed in various primary immune deficiency disease, including SCID, Wiskott-Aldrich syndrome, and DiGeorge's syndrome.[28] If either the efferent of afferent arms of the immune system are diffusely abnormal, resulting in low antigen and mitogen stimulation assays, the MLC will usually likewise be depressed. Cases of dissociation of the PHA and MLC responses have been recorded in SCID.[28] The PHA response was absent while the MLC response was normal. There was no evidence, however, that the residual MLC responsiveness was of significant clinical benefit in those patients in whom it was preserved. In addition to its use as a diagnostic test, the MLC is used as a criterion for the selection of compatible donors in bone marrow transplantation.[31,33]

Lymphocyte Mediator Production.[35-38] Many biologically active compounds are secreted by lymphocytes after their activation by mitogens, antigens, or allogeneic cells. These lymphocyte mediators provide communication between cell types and also serve as a biological amplification mechanism. Migration inhibitory factor (MIF) has received the most detailed study and is generally the most useful test clinically.[35] MIF is a protein molecule which is released by either T- or B-lymphocytes after in vitro exposure to an antigen such as PPD, *Candida,* or SK/SD[36,37] Guinea pig peritoneal macrophages or human monocytes are generally used as indicator cells, and the inhibition of their migration by MIF is measured. Two separate assays are used, the *direct* and *indirect* methods.[35] In the direct (one-step) assay, the lymphocytes to be tested, the antigen, and the indicator monocytes are all cultured together and so the MIF released by the lymphocytes acts directly on the monocytes. It is impossible in this test to determine if a failure to inhibit migration is the result of a lymphocytic defect (no MIF produced) or a monocytic defect (unable to respond to MIF). In the indirect (two-step) assay, the lymphocytes are first cultured with the antigen and the MIF collected, and then the MIF is added to the indicator monocytes. Although the two-step system is more time consuming and requires larger numbers of cells, a defect can be more accurately determined since release of MIF and response to it are independently measured.[35]

This in vitro test generally correlates well with in vivo demonstrations of delayed-type hypersensitivity (DTH) such as recall skin test reactivity to the same antigens.[38] In some situations, however, the results of skin tests, lymphocyte blast transformation to mitogens and antigens, and MIF production do not correspond with each other. An immunodeficiency disease may have a comprehensive defect involving all of the assays, or it may be partial, affecting only one or two. The MIF test result has also been shown to change during the course of a disease and may be important prognostically or therapeutically.[35]

Induction of Delayed-type Hypersensitivity.[39,40] In order to test the afferent limb of the T-cell system in vivo, the patient must be exposed to an allergen with which he has had no previous contact. Several such allergens are available. Bacillus Calmette-Guerin (BCG) immunization has been used for patients with no previous exposure to tuberculosis; however, this assay involves the use of a live microorganism which might be injurious to an immunologically deficient patient. It is therefore contraindicated in most primary immune deficiency diseases. Kehole-limpet hemocyanin (KLH) has been used, but it may induce sensitization to shellfish antigens, thereby posing a danger to the patient. Dinitrochlorobenzene (DNCB) is the preferred allergen, and the method of Catalone et al.[39,40] is the one most widely used. Two preparations of DNCB (2,000 μg and 50 μg) are needed, and both are applied to the skin of one arm. After 24 hours, most normal individuals develop an irritant reaction at the site of highest DNCB concentration. On the fourteenth day after application, the two sites are checked for erythema and induration. If both sites show a reaction, the response is graded 4+, and if only the 2,000 μg site reacts it is graded 3+. If both sites are negative, an additional 50 μg challenge is applied to the opposite forearm and checked in 24-48 hours. If a response appears at the challenge site, sensitization is graded 2+. Over 96% of normal subjects will be sensitized and respond.[39] A much lower rate of sensitization has been demonstrated in patients with malignancies[40] and those with primary immune deficiency diseases affecting the T-cell arm, such as Wiskott-Aldrich syndrome[41] and ataxia telangiectasia.[42]

Elicitation of Delayed-type Hypersensitivity.[43-47] A battery of intradermal skin tests to selected antigens constitutes the easiest, safest, least expensive, and most informative screening assay for in vivo evaluation of T-lymphocyte function. The skin tests examine a patient's ability to recognize specific antigens with which he has had previous contact and his ability to mount a DTH cutaneous response to them. A negative skin test signifies either a lack of previous exposure or an inability to recognize or respond to a particular antigen. Thus, antigens to which the patient has had previous exposure are necessary, which is a drawback when testing very young children who have had little exposure to most antigens. To circumvent the problem of lack of exposure, a battery of skin tests is generally used. Almost 100% of apparently healthy adults will have a positive reaction to one or more skin tests if at least four antigens are applied simultaneously. Mumps antigen, candidin, trichophytin, streptokinase/streptodornase, and tuberculin are used.[43-45] The method involves the careful intradermal injection of 0.1 ml of each antigen separately on the forearms. After 48 hours, the diameter of erythema and induration are recorded. Generally 5 mm or more of induration is considered positive when the tests are used to evaluate immune function.

It is well known that anergy to a specific antigen occurs during an active infection in which the same antigen is released systemically. The PPD skin test is often negative during active tuberculosis.[46] Conditions such as age, leukocytosis, anemia, fever, and various bacterial and viral infections may also temporarily result in anergy.[45,47] Such complicating factors are unfortunately frequently present in patients being evaluated for immune deficiency states or malignancies.

Allograft Rejection.[48,49] The use of skin allografts is a time-honored method for evaluating cell-mediated immunocompetence. Because of its invasive nature, however, the use of this procedure must be limited. Skin grafts are technically easy to perform, rejection is simple to detect, and the time required to complete rejection provides a quantitative measurement. First an area of skin is excised from the recipient in order to provide a bed for the allograft. A slightly smaller area of skin is excised from a donor, placed on the bed, and observed. When a syngeneic graft (autograft) is performed, vascularization of the graft takes place within two or three days, and it is entirely normal histologically after four or five days. When an allograft is performed, the vascularization takes place in an identical manner, but then infiltration of the graft with inflammatory cells occurs. Inflammation, thickening, and necrosis appear in about seven days. Total cessation of blood flow to the graft and its sloughing off occur in about ten days. A second graft from the same donor is sloughed off in an accelerated manner (second set phenomenon), being complete in about seven days.

Rejection of a skin allograft is predominantly mediated by T-lymphocytes. Passively transferred cells but not serum are able to mediate the rejection. However, antibodies do play a role, as is particularly evident in hyperacute rejection reactions.[48] In patients with T-lymphocyte immunodeficiencies, graft rejection is often delayed and occasionally even absent.[49]

Lymphoid Tissue Biopsies.[50-53] The biopsy of lymphoid tissues is another invasive procedure which must be carried out cautiously. The indication for biopsy is often immunodeficiency with chronic and recurrent infections, so the incidence of infection is predictably high. Further, since there is often little lymphoid tissue to biopsy, the procedure may be more difficult than usual. In spite of such reservations, a biopsy is frequently indicated, primarily for diagnostic purposes. Characteristic histologic abnormalities are very useful in the diagnosis of many immune deficiency states.[51,52]

Two sites are often biopsied for information on cell-mediated defects: the peripheral lymph nodes and the thymus. A stimulated node is more informative than a nonstimulated one, so an immunization is usually first carried out. An antigen such as diphtheria-tetanus (DT) toxin may be given subcutaneously in the thigh, or a contact sensitizer such as oxazalone can be applied to the skin. After five to seven days, the effects of stimulation will be evident in the nodes, so an ipsilateral node draining the immunization site is excised surgically. Special attention is paid to the areas that contain predominantly T cells, such as the paracortical region.[50]

Thymic biopsy can also be carried out without prohibitive complications if done carefully.[53] It is less useful during an acute infectious episode, during antimetabolic therapy, or when the patient is under unusual stress, since those all affect thymic morphology and make the diagnosis of an immune deficiency state difficult. While a thymic biopsy may not be diagnostic for a particular disease, it does help delineate the syndromes and may prove helpful in planning therapy. For example, if the thymus is absent in a patient, transplantation of allogeneic thymic epithelium may be beneficial.

The following seven types of thymic abnormalities were delineated by Borzy et al.:[52] (1) total dysplasia, (2) partial dysplasia, (3) heterogenous cell population, (4) partial dysplasia with phagocytosis, (5) late fetal pattern, (6) normal pattern, and (7) ataxia telangiectasia pattern. The first five patterns were identified in persons with SCID, and the thymic histology helped to separate the subgroups of that disease. The ataxia telangiectasia (AT) pattern was specifically associated with AT, and the normal biopsies were found in patients with immunodeficiency with hyper-IgM and in those with secondary immunodeficiency. The severity of the thymic defect did not necessarily reflect the severity of the disease.[52]

B Cell (Humoral Immunity)

Peripheral Blood B-cell Quantitation.[54-59] A partial list of the surface markers of human B-lymphocytes is presented in Table 7-3. Immunofluorescent detection of surface immunoglobulin is the method most commonly used to identify B cells. Antisera are available which are directed against all classes of human immunoglobulin (polyvalent), individual immunoglobulin classes (IgG, IgM, IgA, IgE, and IgD), and the light chain types (kappa and lambda). The antisera are conjugated with a fluorochrome (fluorescein or rhodamine) for immunofluorescent detection. After incubation of peripheral blood lymphocytes with the appropriate antisera, the proportion of cells fluorescing is counted. Then the absolute B-lymphocyte count can be calculated if the total lymphocyte count is also known. By this method, between 15 and 30% of peripheral blood lymphocytes are identified as B cells in a normal population. Because of technical details there is a high degree of variability. For example, lymphocytes lacking surface immunoglobulin may have Fc receptors and so may passively absorb immunoglobulin present in the patient's serum, thereby giving a falsely elevated result.[58] Incubating the lymphocytes overnight gives the cells time to shed absorbed serum immunoglobulin and thus gives a more accurate measurement. The test serum itself may also absorb onto Fc receptors of other cell types. In order to prevent that complication, the Fc portion of the test serum is either removed enzymatically or blocked by the use of staphylococcal protein A which binds to the Fc portion of immunoglobulin molecules.

The other surface markers may be used to quantitate B cells, but they are less valuable. A rosette method detecting Fc receptors has been used, but it is now

Table 7-3. Surface Markers on Human B Cells.

Surface immunoglobulins

Histocompatibility antigens (HL-A)

Immune associated-like antigens (Ia)

B-cell differentiation antigen (BDA-1)

Receptors for Fc (IgM, IgG, IgE)

Receptors for complement (CR_1, CR_2)

Receptors for Epstein-Barr virus

Receptors for mouse erythrocytes

Receptors for monkey erythrocytes

recognized that certain T- and "null" lymphocyte subpopulations are also counted. A similar problem is encountered when complement receptors are used to quantitate B cells.

Peripheral blood B-cell quantitation is particularly valuable for characterizing the primary immune deficiency states.[54] For example, patients with Bruton's infantile X-linked hypogammaglobulinemia have a marked reduction of circulating B cells. Hypogammaglobulinemic patients having normal B-cell numbers generally have an acquired disease.

Identification of the various surface markers other than surface Ig is at times necessary diagnostically. For example, the B-cell subpopulation forming spontaneous rosettes with mouse erythrocytes is thought to be an early maturation phase, and such cells are absent in Bruton's disease and in immunodeficiency with thymoma.[54]

Serum (or Secretory) Immunoglobulin Levels.[60-72] Quantitation of serum immunoglobulins is generally the initial step in an evaluation of humoral immunity because of the usefulness of the test and its wide availability.[60-64] Protein electrophoresis is useful only as a rough screening procedure since it is highly imprecise and will fail to detect many selective immunoglobulin deficiencies. Immunoelectrophoresis is a commonly used screening procedure to uncover immunoglobulin deficiencies, but again, it is not accurate. A single radial immunodiffusion assay is generally used for precise measurement of the immunoglobulin classes IgG, IgA, IgM, and IgD.[65] A more sensitive radioimmunoassay is used for IgE quantitation.[69] Several technical difficulties must be kept in mind. First, serum immunoglobulin levels change with age, so normal values corrected for age variability must be consulted. Also, some patients with ataxia telangiectasia have monomeric IgM in their serum which diffuses more rapidly in agar than the pentameric form, thereby giving a falsely elevated value for IgM in the immunodiffusion test.

The importance of quantitation of individual immunoglobulin classes is underscored by the fact that selective deficiencies of IgA and IgM are two of the most common immunodeficiency diseases. Even IgG subclass quantitation is sometimes necessary since selective subclass deficiency occurs.[64] Serum IgD measurement is not routinely performed because it has not been shown to be necessary for the diagnosis of any GDID. Serum IgD may be abnormally low in patients deficient in all of the other major immunoglobulins, and also in some patients with selective IgA deficiency and Wiskott-Aldrich syndrome.[69] The serum IgD concentration is very low, representing only about 0.25% of the total serum immunoglobulin and is quite variable.[66,69] However membrane-bound IgD is found on the surface of a high proportion of peripheral blood B cells (usually in association with IgM) and may play an important role in B-cell maturation.[66-69] Some patients with SCID have an excess of IgD-bearing B cells relative to IgG- or IgA-bearing B cells. The suggestion has been made that in such cases a defect is present in the normal conversion from IgD- to IgG- or IgA-bearing B cells.[67,68] The functional importance of serum IgE is also ill defined, but its measurement is important in the diagnosis of several GDID.[69] The elevated levels of IgE found in a number of those diseases may reflect a deficiency of T-lymphocyte suppressor activity which normally regulates IgE synthesis.[70,71]

Measurement of secretory immunoglobulins may also be important. Patients with selective IgA deficiency may have abnormally low levels of IgA in their serum, their secretions, or both.[72] Total saliva or parotid saliva are the usual secretions measured, but others have also been studied. An absence of IgA in the respiratory secretions may be one factor responsible for the frequent infections seen at that site in selective IgA deficiency.

Lymphocyte Stimulation by Mitogens.[73-75] The mitogenic compound isolated from the plant pokeweed (*Phytolacca americana*) has been widely used as an in vitro test of B-cell function. A proliferation response, which is analogous to that produced by PHA and con-A, is stimulated by pokeweed mitogen (PWM), but both T and B cells are involved in approximately equal numbers, whereas with PHA and con-A, T cells are the predominant cell type activated.[73,74] The method of assay is analogous. In addition to inducing blast transformation of lymphocytes, PWM also stimulates the terminal differentiation of B-lymphocytes into immunoglobulin-synthesizing cells.[75] This response is quantitated by measurement of the immunoglobulins which are secreted into the medium by the stimulated cells. It is a more difficult assay to perform but is more specific for B-cell function than the mitogenic assay. In both pokeweed tests, antigen recognition and processing steps (afferent arm) of the immune response are bypassed; the effector arm alone is measured.

Serum Antibody Titers.[51,76] In vivo functional assays are usually indicated since severe defects in antibody formation can be present in the face of normal values in the in vitro tests. Isohemagglutinin titers and the Schick test are readily available and widely used. Early in life there is generally exposure to a number of ubiquitous antigens such as *E. coli*, streptococci (ASO titer), and heterologous erythrocyte antigens (heterophile titer). Antibodies to such antigens are sometimes called natural antibodies, and their titers demonstrate the ability of the patient to recognize and respond to specific antigens.

The isohemagglutinin titers measure the IgM antibody response to blood group antigens, and so they are a useful test of IgM functional integrity in all patients except those with blood type AB. Isohemagglutinin titers can be detected by 6 months of age, making the test valuable in all but very young children. Depressed titers are frequently seen in patients with severe B-cell abnormalities and are strikingly low in ataxia telangiectasia.[51]

The Schick test evaluates the IgG antibody response to diphtheria toxin. It is useful only in patients who have been exposed to the antigen either naturally or by receiving their routine diphtheria immunization. The test antigen is injected intradermally and the site examined after 96 hours. Erythema or edema of 10 mm or greater in diameter is a positive reaction, which indicates deficient anti-toxin antibody. The erythema and edema result from the effects of the toxin on the skin and are not to be confused with a delayed hypersensitivity response. Antibodies to the toxin make the test negative by neutralizing the effects of the toxin. Some patients having B-cell deficiency diseases nevertheless have a negative test, so a negative Schick test does not exclude the possibility of such a disease.[51]

Induction of a Primary Antibody Response.[77-81] The induction of a primary antibody response is an excellent measure of a patient's humoral immune capacity and is analogous to the use of DNCB to test cell-mediated immunity. The entire humoral immune process is evaluated, beginning with antigen processing and recognition, and including B-cell differentiation and proliferation, and finally immunoglobulin synthesis and secretion. It is a sensitive screening method for many B-cell immune deficiencies, but an abnormally low response gives no information concerning the exact site of the defect. A large number of antigens are available, and several should be used so that a failure to respond to a particular class of antigens will not be missed. Polysaccharide antigens, such as those from pneumococci, meningococci, or hemophilus, should be included since some patients have a selective deficiency to them. In young children the routine immunizations are convenient. The primary responses to typhoid, diphtheria, pertussis, or tetanus toxoid may be quantitated if there was no previous exposure. Killed polio virus vaccine may also be used. Living viral or bacterial vaccines should never be used since a progressive and possibly fatal infection might result in a severely immunoincompetent patient. In studying adult patients, it is necessary to select antigens to which they have had no previous exposure. KLH is such an antigen, but restricted usage has been recommended. Because of its origin in marine organisms, it might sensitize patients to sea foods. Bacteriophage ϕX174 has been used with good results.[80]

The method of inducing a primary antibody response requires that a baseline serum sample be drawn to detect any preexisting immunity to the antigen being tested. If antibodies are present, the immunization simply becomes a test of the secondary antibody response. Titers should then be drawn weekly for at least three weeks after antigen administration.

If a deficiency in secretory immunity is suspected, antibody responses in the secretions instead of the serum can be tested. Antigens which elicit secretory immunity under normal circumstances are selected, such as polio or influenza virus.

Elicitation of a Secondary Antibody Response.[77-81] This test is essentially the same as the foregoing, including use of the same method and many of the same antigens, but here antigens are selected to which the patient has had previous exposure. Only the primary sensitization phase is not tested. The assay is analogous to the recall skin tests used in cell-mediated immune evaluation, but is has the advantage of being more quantitative.

Lymphoid Tissue Biopsies.[50,51,82] Since biopsies are by nature a relatively invasive procedure, the expected benefits must be weighed against the risk of complications. Many tissues are very useful, including bone marrow, lymph nodes, spleen, tonsils, and intestine. The bone marrow is the most innocuous and provides information particularly about the early maturation stages of lymphoid cells. Lymph node biopsy, after a local immunization, is of particular benefit in evaluating the anatomy of B-cell response to antigens. Attention is paid especially to the development of germinal centers, where B cells predominate, and to the plasma cell response. The germinal centers are associated with the production of IgG antibody and the development of immunological memory. The lymph node plasma cell reaction occurs within a few days of antigen exposure, with large numbers of B cells proliferating in the cortex and then migrating to the medullary cords where plasma cells accumulate. This reaction occurs independently from the germinal center reaction and is associated with IgM antibody production.[50,51,82]

GENETICALLY DETERMINED IMMUNODEFICIENCY DISEASES

This section briefly reviews the clinical features of many of the GDID and includes a short summary of immunologic findings and the occurrence of malignancies in each. The significant immunological changes are demonstrated in an abbreviated form in Tables 7-4 through 7-19. In most cases, the exact nature of the underlying immunological defect remains unknown. The results of the immunological tests are primarily of diagnostic importance, and the emphasis is on the patterns of deficiency. The GDID have been divided into three major groups, those with combined T- and B-cell defects, those with predominantly B-cell defects, and those with predominantly T-cell defects. Examples have been selected from each group. There are large numbers of other genetic disease associated with malignancies, which are discussed extensively in other chapters of this book. They often have an associated immunodeficiency which would be revealed by the work-up suggested above, but the defect in the immune system is not felt to be

Table 7-4.   Immunologic Findings In Reticular Dysgenesis.

T CELL		B CELL	
Lymphocytes	Markedly reduced or absent	B cells	Markedly reduced or absent
T cells	Markedly reduced or absent	Ig's	All markedly reduced or absent
Mitogens	———	Mitogen	———
Antigens	———	Ab titers	———
MLC	———	1° Ab response	———
Mediators	———	2° Ab response	———
Induction	———	Lymphoid tissue biopsies	
Elicitation	———		
Allografts	———	Spleen	Lacks lymphocytes, plasma cells, and granulocytes
Lymphoid tissue biopsies		Bone marrow	Lacks myeloblasts, pro-myelocytes, myelocytes, metamyelocytes, band cells, granulocytes, lymphocytes, and plasma cells; reticular cells abundant; erythroid and megakaryocytic elements normal
Thymus	Lacks lymphocytes; Hassall's corpuscles, large reticular cells and reticular fibers present		
Nodes	Only rare lymphocytes; resemble a 10-week-old human embryo		
		GI tract	Lacks lymphocytes; reticular cells present

the primary event.   They will not be discussed here, but that is not to minimize the importance of the immune defects in the development of such cancers.

Reticular Dysgenesis[83-85]

Only four cases of this disease have been recorded, and all died in the first few weeks or months of life.   Sepsis was present, and there was little or no host defense detected.   Profound lymphocytopenia and granulocytopenia were characteristic findings.   Erythrocyte and platelet development were not affected.

Immunological evaluations have been limited.   There was a marked reduction or absence of serum immunoglobulins.   Circulating lymphocytes were either absent or markedly reduced.   Biopsies of all lymphoid tissues revealed the absence or reduction of lymphocytes, plasma cells, and granulocytes, but the presence of large reticular cells in abundance.   In the bone marrow, no precursors of either lymphocytes or granulocytes were present (Table 7-4). No patients have survived to develop cancer.

Severe Combined Immunodeficiency[86-91]

There are two forms of "classical" SCID, the *Swiss type* which is autosomal recessive in inheritance, and the *Gitlin type* which is X-linked recessive. Sporadic cases are also reported. Clinically they are all indistinguishable, coming to medical attention in the first weeks or months of life with severe infections. They often present earlier in life than patients with infantile X-linked agammaglobulinemia since the latter are better protected by passively transferred maternal IgG. The infections have been divided into four predominant sites of involvement: skin, respiratory, gastrointestinal, and septic. Chronic infections of the skin may be the first sign of the disease; they can be caused by *Candida* as well as various bacteria. The respiratory infections include bronchopneumonia, which may be a terminal event, and *Pneumocystis carinii* pneumonia, which can be treated successfully if the diagnosis is made early enough. Diarrhea is the predominant gastrointestinal symptom, and may result from either graft vs. host (GVH) or various bacterial or viral pathogens. Sepsis is a frequent cause of death. Vaccination with living agents must be strictly avoided since fatal BCG and vaccinia infections have also been recorded. Immunization with measles, polio, or other live viruses may also result in severe complications. Prompt diagnosis of SCID is essential so that treatment (bone marrow or fetal lymphoid tissue transplantation) may be instituted before serious complications have taken place. GVH disease is a frequent complication if any blood products containing viable lymphocytes are administered, and even in utero transfer of maternal lymphocytes to the fetus has been reported as a cause of GVH disease.

Classical SCID is characterized by the absence or profound reduction of almost all measurable immunological parameters (Table 7-5). There is a profound lymphopenia involving both T and B cells. Low levels of immunoglobulins are present. If high levels are found, the diagnosis of Nezelof's syndrome should be considered. It has been reported that the Swiss and Gitlin types may be separated on the basis of a positive MLC response in the latter, but it has not been consistently present. Lymphoid tissue biopsies are helpful diagnostically, but the incidence of infectious complications is very high.

Despite the early onset of the disease and rapid demise of its victims, a large number of malignancies have been recorded in SCID. The percentage of cancer observed in cases of SCID was between 1 and 1.5% in the Immunodeficiency-Cancer Registry (ICR) survey.[135] Lymphoreticular malignancies were predominant. The median age at the time of the diagnosis of cancer was 0.9 year (including all the different types of SCID). That was the youngest onset of malignancy in all of the primary immune deficiency diseases, as might be expected because of the early onset of immune deficiency.

Table 7-5. Immunological Findings in Classical SCID.

	T CELL		B CELL
Lymphocytes	Reduced – large lymphyo-cytes may be increased	B cells	Reduced or absent
T cells	Reduced or absent	Ig's	Variable but usually reduced or absent
Mitogens	Reduced or absent	Mitogens	Reduced or absent
Antigens	Reduced or absent	Ab titers	Hemagglutinins: reduced or absent; Schick test: positive
MLC	Reduced or absent		
Mediators	Reduced or absent	1° Ab response	Absent or poor response
Induction	Cannot be sensitized	2° Ab response	Absent or poor response
Elicitation	Absent	Lymphoid tissue biopsies	
Allograft rejection	No rejection takes place		
Lymphoid tissue biopsies		Bone marrow	Reduced numbers of lymphoblasts, lymphocytes, and plasma cells
Thymus	Embryonal or dysplastic, but usually present	GI	Lacks lymphocytes and plasma cells
Nodes	Reduced in number and size; lymphocytes and plasma cells are rarely present and germinal centers are reduced or absent	Tonsils	Lymphocyte numbers reduced

Nezelof's Syndrome.[92-94] Nezelof's syndrome is a sporadic or autosomal recessively inherited primary immunodeficiency disease which is often classified as a variant of SCID. Like classical SCID, it probably consists of a group of diseases. It is characterized by a combined immunodeficiency of severe degree, but it can be differentiated from SCID by the presence of normal or near normal levels of B cells and/or immunoglobulins. The term "SCID with B cells" is often used, which is then subdivided depending on the presence or absence of serum immunoglobulins. In some cases there is selective loss of individual serum immunoglobulin classes, whereas in others all immunoglobulins are absent.

Clinically, the disease is often somewhat milder and of later onset than classical SCID, but it generally begins within the first years of life. Untreated, patients rarely survive more than a year after its onset. They succumb to various infections, particularly those associated with T-cell deficiency. Gram-negative bacterial sepsis and generalized viral infections are particularly dangerous. *Candida albicans* and *Pneumocystis carinii* are common.

The characteristic immunologic findings include a lymphopenia resulting from the absence of T cells (see Table 7-6). All parameters of T-cell function are reduced or absent. Although the lymph nodes may be clinically hyperplastic, there is lymphocyte depletion in the T-cell dependent areas. Plasma cells may be normal. The thymus may be embryonal or dysplastic. On the humoral side, B cells are usually present and may even be elevated in number. Serum immunoglobulin defects are variable, being often normal, but specific immunoglobulin classes or all of them are sometimes reduced. Antibody responsiveness to antigens is usually abnormal. In those cases in which serum immunoglobulins are absent, even in the face of normal B-cell numbers, the functional tests are severely reduced or absent.

It has been found in some cases of Nezelof's syndrome that the absence of immunoglobulins resulted from a deficiency in the T cells necessary to help the B cells produce immunoglobulin. When T-lymphocytes from normal individuals were added to cultures of B cells from affected patients, the defect in immunoglobulin synthesis was overcome, and immunoglobulins were secreted into the medium.

Table 7-6. Immunologic Findings in Nezelof's Syndrome.

T CELL		B CELL	
Lymphocytes	Reduced	B cells	Normal or elevated
T cells	Reduced or absent	Ig's	Normal or deficiency in one or more classes of Ig's
Mitogens	Reduced or absent		
Antigens	Reduced or absent	Mitogen	Normal or reduced
MLC	Reduced or absent	Ab titers	Isohemagglutinins present or reduced
Mediators	Reduced or absent		
Induction	Reduced or absent	1° Ab response	Reduced, but some responses persist
Elicitation	Reduced or absent		
Allografts	Reduced or absent	2° Ab response	Reduced, but some responses persist
Lymphoid tissue biopsies		Lymphoid tissue biopsies	
Thymus	Dysplastic or embryonal		
Nodes	Lymphocyte depleteion in thymus-dependent areas; plasma cells may be normal	Spleen	Lymphocyte depletion in T-cell dependent areas; plasma cells abundant
		Intestine	Lymphocyte depletion; plasma cells abundant

The occurrence of malignancies in this syndrome has not been differentiated from classical SCID.

SCID with Adenosine Deaminase Deficiency.[95-103] The deficiency of adenosine deaminase (ADA) in some cases of SCID was the first enzymatic defect discovered to be associated with a primary immunodeficiency disease. The metabolic pathway for adenine nucleosides is shown in Figure 7-2. The enzyme ADA catalyzes the conversion of adenosine to inosine by hydrolytic deamination. Inosine is converted to hypoxanthine by purine nucleoside phosphorylase. Xanthine oxidase then catalyzes the conversion of hypoxanthine to xanthine and finally to uric acid. ADA is detectable in most tissues, including lymphoid cells and red blood cells where it is conveniently measured. It is now clear that about one-half of the recessively inherited cases of SCID have ADA deficiency. The enzyme system is quite heterogeneous, and the immunological defects produced by its deficiency are likewise variable. In most cases a structural gene mutation is the cause of the disease, resulting in an abnormal, inactive enzyme. In a few families, an ADA inhibitor has been found. In some cases, deficient red blood cell ADA has been found in patients with normal immune function. Preservation of ADA activity in the lymphoid cells apparently occurs, allowing for normal development of the immune system. Heterozygote carriers of ADA deficiency have about 50% of the normal enzyme levels. Individuals with a variant enzyme having about 10% of normal ADA activity have been found, who have normal immune function. The mechanism by which this enzyme deficiency causes such a profound immune deficiency is a matter for current debate. Adenosine and a number of

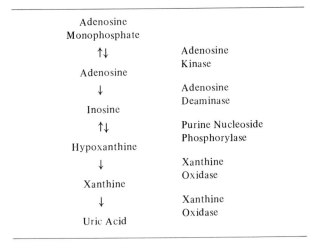

Figure 7-2. Metabolic pathway of adenosine deaminase.

its metabolites have been shown to be toxic for lymphocytes under certain circumstances.

The clinical course of SCID patients with and without ADA deficiency is identical. Distinctive skeletal abnormalities including cupping and flaring of the costochondral rib junction have been seen in many cases with ADA deficiency.

The immunological findings are likewise similar, so the table of immunologic findings will not be repeated. In some cases, a delay in the onset of the immune deficiency is seen. It is hypothesized that the transfer of maternal ADA to the fetus across the placenta allows for normal lymphoid differentiation. After birth, the ADA levels decline, and the immune system progressively involutes. This hypothesis is supported by differences in the thymus. In classical SCID, the thymus contains no Hassall's corpuscles or differentiated epithelium, whereas in ADA deficient SCID, Hassall's corpuscles and differentiated epithelium may be present, but involution of the lymphoid component is evident. The histological picture of the thymus in classical SCID is more embryonic, whereas in ADA deficiency it is largely dysplastic. It is evident that such differences may have profound implications where treatment is concerned. In the ICR survey, no instances of cancer associated with ADA deficiency were recorded.

Ataxia Telangiectasia[104-147]

Definition. Ataxia telangiectasia is an autosomal recessive syndrome characterized clinically by a progressive cerebellar ataxia and oculocutaneous telangiectases. A variety of endocrine abnormalities may be present. Progressive deficiency of immune function is an integral part of the clinical picture but is quite variable, involving both the humoral and cell-mediated arms of the immune response. Frequent infections, particularly of the sinopulmonary tract, and a high rate of malignancy are thought to be related to the immunological abnormalities. Defective DNA repair mechanisms may be etiologically important.

Historical Review. The term ataxia telangiectasia was introduced by Elena Boder and Robert Sedgwick in 1954.[104] Their detailed clinical report of eight patients firmly established the entity. It has since carried their proposed title, which incorporates the two most striking clinical findings: the severe, progressive cerebellar ataxia and the likewise progressive telangiectases. A previous report by Louis-Bar[105] of a single patient also included the characteristic findings, and some authors use her name in the title of the disease. The original description was probably that by Syllaba and Henner[106] in 1926 in which three siblings with familial choreoathetosis, ataxia, telangiectases, strabismus, muscle weakness, skin pigmentary changes, and endocrine abnormalties (goiter and hypoplastic genitalia) were reported. Boder and Sedgwick also directed attention to the 1957 clinical report by Wells and Shy,[107] in which two siblings with AT were described. Boder and Sedgwick were the first to emphasize the repeated sinopulmonary infections (sinusitis, bronchitis, pneumonia, otitis, and mastoiditis). They hypothesized that the complete syndrome had not been recognized earlier, since prior to the antibiotic era most of the patients probably died of infections at an early age. Furthermore, they were the first to observe the absence of the thymus at autopsy. One of their patients died at age 9 of a lymphosarcoma. The development of malignancies, particularly of the lymphoid system, has since been established as an important aspect of AT.

Clinical Characteristics. There is marked variability in AT with respect to its age of onset, clinical symptoms, and disease severity. Its clinical recognition usually depends on the presence of cerebellar ataxia in a young child who develops ocular and cutaneous telangiectases and who experiences an unusual number of sinopulmonary infections. It is a progressive disease with relentless deterioration in most of the clinical manifestations. It is probable that AT is inherited as an autosomal recessive trait.[108] Both sexes are equally affected. Vertical transmission has not been recorded, but siblings are frequently affected. Only in a few cases has parental consanguinity been found.[108] The infrequency of consanguinity implies either that there must be a high rate of spontaneous mutation or that the number of heterozygote carriers in the population must be great. Heterozygotes for AT may have an increased cancer risk. There is good evidence for an increased incidence of malignancy in family members of AT patients.[109]

Neurological Findings. The ataxia usually becomes evident in infancy or early childhood at about the time the child attempts to walk.[104,110,111] It begins as truncal ataxia, with swaying during sitting and standing, and an ataxic gait. Both usually progress to the point that patients become confined to a wheelchair. Athetoid movements and posturing have frequently been described and may become so prominent that the other ataxic manifestations are masked. An intention tremor and myoclonic jerks also develop. Drooling is frequent, and the speech becomes progressively slurred, slow, and scanning as the voice becomes slowly weaker. Nystagmus is often an early manifestation. Strabismus and ocular dyspraxia develop later. The motor milestones are delayed. A result of these neurological symptoms is a severe disability in visual-motor coordination. A further consequence is that learning, particularly in school, becomes increasingly difficult. Many children have been found to have normal intelligence when tested early, but show progressive deterioration. It is not clear if this is a direct result of the neurological disease or if it results from their learning disabilities and the physical difficulty they experience in taking tests. Late in the course of the disease, the deep tendon reflexes are reduced, and an extensor plantar response sometimes appears. The patients develop severe weakness and muscle wasting. The preception of vibration and position may be lost while pain and temperature sensations remain undiminished. All of these later, progressive neurological symptoms may be related to demyelination in the spinal cord which is detected tected in older patients.

Despite these multiple neurological symptoms, it has been noted by many authors that the patients have a remarkably equable disposition, making them relatively pleasant to care for.[110]

Some patients (about 5% in the series by McFarlin et al.[111]) have an unusually mild form of the disease in which the neurological symptoms are of later onset, milder in degree of severity, and more slowly progressive. It is possible that the few patients described before the use of antibiotics represented these mild cases.[110,111]

Cutaneous Findings. Telangiectases are an integral part of the syndrome.[109,112] The bulbar conjunctiva is the first site affected. The onset of the telangiectases is usually between the ages of 2 and 8 years, although one case has been recorded of their presence at birth and another with their onset at age 14.[111] They start as pink areas, often mistaken for conjunctivitis, on the temporal and nasal areas with sparing superior and inferior to the limbus.[112] They next appear on the face, particularly in the butterfly area, on the bridge of the nose, in the ears, and on the eyelids. Later the neck, posterior auricular areas, antecubital and popliteal fossae, and dorsa of the hands and feet become involved.[104,109,112] In some cases telangiectases of the oral mucous membranes have been found[104] and nasal bleeding has been a complication.[104] The cutaneous telangiectases were originally felt to be of arterial origin,[104] but capillary microscopy demonstrated that they branch from the subpapillary venous plexus.[112] It has been suggested that sunlight plays a partial role in their distribution[109] which would be consistent with the evidence indicating that there is a DNA repair defect in AT. It has been noted that activity may play a role since patients confined to a wheelchair early in their lives have been observed to have fewer telangiectases.[109] A reduced exposure to sunlight in those more severely affected patients might be a more likely explanation. It has been suggested that the telangiectases on the mucous membranes might be secondary to repeated trauma or therapeutic x-irradiation.[109] The telangiectases of the eyes and face are often striking and thus are frequently helpful in making the diagnosis. In the other sites they are often inconspicuous, and so must be specifically sought. Their presence in the central nervous system has been reported[104,113] but only in rare cases. Tortuosity of the vessels in the pulmonary vasculature has also been recorded.[114] This disease is not primarily a vascular disease such as Osler-Weber-Rendu, however. The neurological symptoms cannot be attributed to the vascular malfunctions even when abnormal vessels are present in the central nervous system.

There are many minor skin manifestations in AT.[109-113] Actinic keratoses are frequently encountered. Skin cancers, both basal cell and squamous cell carcinomas, have been found in relatively young individuals and in non-sun-exposed areas.[109] Their presence emphasizes both the aspect of premature aging which seems to be a part of the syndrome and the heightened susceptibility to cancer formation. Gray hair has been found to be prematurely present,[104,109] although it is not progressive. Poikiloderma is a common finding, with hyper- and hypopigmentation, atrophy, and telangiectasia. Other pigmentary changes include the occasional presence of café au lait spots, partial albinism, and vitiligo. Dry skin with follicular hyperkeratosis has been emphasized, as also has sclerodermatous texture which gives rise to "hidebound" skin and a "mask-like facies," in some patients.[109] These changes, together with the muscular atrophy often seen late in the disease, produce a strikingly aged appearance. As in many other immunodeficiency states, dermatitis is a frequent finding. It has been described as resembling atopic, seborrheic, or nummular dermatitis, but it responds poorly to the usual treatments for those conditions. When the pulmonary disease has progressed to a severe state, cyanosis and clubbing appear, a very poor sign prognostically.

Skin infections are frequent in AT and are those one expects to see with a depression in the T-cell-mediated immune functions. Viral infections seem to be of normal severity in early childhood. Vaccinia, measles, mumps, and chickenpox are usually well tolerated. The childhood immunizations are generally effective and not dangerous to the patient. As the disease progresses, however, viral infections are less well tolerated. Warts become a frequent problem. Impetigo commonly becomes recurrent and is difficult to eradicate from AT patients. Fungal infections have rarely been reported.[109]

Hirsutism is occassionally present in young and adult female patients.[109] This finding should alert the physician to evaluate the endocrinologic status of his patient since multiple endocrine abnormalities can be found in AT.

Skin biopsies from AT patients exhibit epidermal thinning, vascular dilation, dermal fibrosis, and clumping of the elastic tissue.[109] This resembles actinic elastosis and is suggestive evidence for the hypothesis that there is increased susceptibility to the adverse effects of solar irradiation in AT.

Respiratory Findings. An increased incidence of infections is one of the cardinal findings in AT.[104,110,111] Infections of the respiratory tract are characteristic, and their onset usually occurs early in the course of the disease. They may begin in the first year of life, but more typically have their onset between ages 3 and 8 years. Rhinitis, otitis, sinusitis, bronchitis, and pneumonia are frequently observed. As they progress, bronchiectasis may result, which then can further progress to respiratory insufficiency and death. The pathogens do not differ significantly from those usually observed in chronic bronchitis and bronchiectasis occurring in immunologically normal patients, and include both bacteria and viruses. The most frequent cause of death in AT is from such infections.

Endocrine Findings. The endocrine manifestations of the disease are generally of little diagnostic or prognostic value. They are not a constant feature and thus are probably not of primary etiologic significance, but such abnormalities are frequently encountered.[110,111]

Abnormal glucose metabolism was first reported by Schalch, McFarlin, and Barlow[115] who found an unusual form of insulin resistance. Others have confirmed their findings.[111] There is a glucose intolerance with glucosuria but no ketosis. The fasting plasma insulin level is elevated, excessive insulin is released in response to glucose, and the insulin fails to lower the blood glucose. Anti-insulin antibodies have not been detected, and other known causes of insulin resistance have been excluded. The underlying cause and significance of this metabolic abnormality remain unknown.

While accelerated aging of the skin and graying of the hair may give the patient a mature appearance, their sexual maturation is often retarded. Those patients who survive to the usual age of puberty often fail to develop secondary sexual characteristics. Sexual abnormalities can be seen at a very early stage of AT. Boder and Sedgwick[104] reported a case with small genitalia, hypospadias, and cryptorchism. Testicular or ovarian atrophy have been frequent findings, and hypospermatogenesis has been recorded.[116,117] The excretion of urinary 17-ketosteroids has been found to be reduced in some cases and probably reflects impaired gonadal function, although some patients with reduced 17-ketosteroid excretion have been found to have normal sexual development.[111,116] Gonadotropin levels have generally been normal.[111] Abnormalities have frequently been detected in the pituitary gland, including degenerative changes and abnormal appearing cells,[117-120] but those changes do not appear to be related to functional abnormalities. Adrenal function, as assayed by the excretion of 17-hydroxysteroids, has been normal in the majority of cases.[111]

There is also a constitutional deficiency with growth failure. Many patients fall below the third percentile for height and weight. This is not the result of a growth hormone deficiency since in most cases growth hormone levels are normal.[111]

Immunological Characteristics. While the immune deficiency is a very important aspect of AT, there is no specific diagnostic finding. The clinical picture, combined with the variable immune deficiency, are necessary to make the diagnosis. Prognostically, there is likewise no single immunological test which may be relied upon. The overall degree of immune dysfunction does correlate with the prognosis, however. In a study of 18 patients with AT, McFarlin, Strober, and

Waldman[111] divided AT into three groups on the basis of clinical criteria. They were:

  I.   Continuous, chronic sinopulmonary infection
 II.   Repeated infections in excess of normal
III.   No greater infectious complications than normal

There was an approximately equal distribution of patients among the three groups. The greatest degree of immunological impairment was present in group I, the least in group III. No specific immunological criteria could differentiate among the groups.

A gradually worsening reduction of cell-mediated immunity occurs in many AT cases. A defect in thymic differentiation has been suggested as its etiology.[121,122] A mild to moderate lymphocytopenia, usually resulting from a reduction of circulating T-lymphocytes, is a common finding[123,124] and is a valuable early sign of the disease. The immune deficiency cannot be explained simply by a lack of T cells since the degree of lymphocytopenia does not correlate with the other immune deficiencies. It has been suggested that the lymphocytopenia might be the result of an infectious episode, but that is unlikely since it has been seen in patients free of any infection. In fact, the paucity of peripheral lymphoid tissue in spite of frequent infections is a sign suggestive of AT.[123] Granulocytopenia and eosinophilia have been encountered, the significance of which remains obscure.[125]

The in vitro functional tests are commonly abnormal. The mitogen and antigen stimulation assays are frequently reduced. McFarlin and Oppenheim[126] demonstrated a plasma factor in AT patients which inhibited antigen stimulation. It has not been found in all patients having deficient antigen stimulation, and so it is probably not of primary etiological importance. Mitogenic responses have been found to change during the clinical course. Generally a depression of responsiveness signifies a poor prognosis, but the return of a previously abnormal response may also be a poor sign. Saxon and coworkers[127] reported a case in which a lymphocytic leukemia developed. The malignant cells responded normally to the mitogens PHA and con-A. Thus the return of mitogenic responsiveness signified the emergence of a T-cell malignancy. The results for mixed leukocyte cultures have been less frequently reported.[111,128] In some cases the MLC has been found to be preserved in the face of abnormal responses in most of the other in vitro and in vivo functional assays.

The in vivo T-cell functional assays are likewise severely impaired.[111,121,122,129] DNCB sensitization is frequently impossible, and the recall skin tests are usually all negative. The rejection of allografts by AT patients is often abnormal. In most cases graft rejection is delayed, but in some rejection never takes place. The use of allografts in AT should be limited. There is a danger of sensitizing patients to histocompatibility antigens present on the skin cells and passenger lymphocytes in the graft.

Lymphoid tissue anatomy is particularly important in the diagnosis of AT and is also useful in the evaluation for possible lymphoid malignancy.[111,114,118,122,129] Thymus biopsies may be technically difficult since the gland is usually either hypoplastic or absent. Normal thymus biopsies have been recorded in AT, however. The usual finding is severe lymphocyte depletion and a lack of corticmedullary differentiation, together with a lack of Hassall's corpuscles. Lymph node abnormalities include lymphocyte depletion from the cortical and paracortical areas, and hyperplasia of the reticular cells.

The humoral arm of the immune system is even more frequently impaired in AT than the cell-mediated arm. Quantitation of peripheral blood B cells may reveal normal or reduced numbers, and B cells having membrane-bound IgA may be normal even in the face of absent serum IgA.[128] Characteristically, there is a quite heterogeneous dysgammaglobulinemia. A reduction or absence of the immunoglobulin IgA in the peripheral blood has been estimated to occur in about 72% of the cases,[111,123,128-131] but normal or even elevated levels have also been reported. A gradual reduction of serum IgA levels may take place during the course of the disease. That is consistent with the hypothesis of immunologic attrition.[124,131] In some cases, however, elevation of IgA levels has been observed during the time in which the disease progressed clinically. A reduction of salivary IgA has been detected in some patients, but the serum and salivary levels were not necessarily dependent on each other and also did not correlate with the severity of the infections.[130] The transport piece for the immunoglobulin was found even in the absence of salivary IgA.[130] Metabolic studies of IgA have revealed that the reduced levels of serum IgA are in most cases the result of reduced synthesis.[129] Development of an anti-IgA antibody may result from the administration of blood products containing IgA. Its presence will cause hypercatabolism of endogenous IgA.[129] A reduction in the serum IgE levels has also been detected in many cases. It was suggested that the combination of deficiencies of IgA and IgE results in a more severe clinical course.[124] That suggestion has not been confirmed.[132] Serum levels of IgG, IgM, and IgD are also variable, but most commonly normal. Their turnover rates are likewise variable.[152]

Pokeweed mitogen responsiveness is usually reduced.[111,133,134] The isohemagglutinin titers are frequently normal, but may be reduced, as also are other "natural" antibody titers.[111] The antibody responses to both primary and secondary immunizations are highly variable. In a single patient, antibody responses to some antigens may be normal while there is no response to other antigens. The antibody responsiveness to immunization with blood group antigens may be sluggish as well.[106]

The bone marrow examination is often normal,[111,123] but a reduction of lymphocytes, IgA-containing cells, or plasma cells may be noted.[111,122] Lymph nodes often lack plasma cells and have rudimentary germinal centers.[111,122] Tonsils have deficient follicular development[52,111,122] or may be entirely absent.[123] Table 7-7 summarizes the immunologic data.

Table 7-7. Immunologic Findings in Ataxia Telangiectasia.

T CELL		B CELL	
Lymphocytes	Lymphocytopenia common; small lymphocytes predominantly affected	B cells	Usually normal, sometimes reduced
		Ig's	
T cells	Reduced, but may be normal or elevated (leukemia!)	IgG	Normal or may be elevated (chronic infection)
Mitogens	Usually reduced	IgA	Reduced or absent; rarely normal or elevated
Antigens	Usually reduced	IgM	Variable; may be normal, elevated, or reduced; low molecular weight IgM seen
MLC	Often normal		
Mediators	———		
Induction	Negative		
Elicitation	Usually all are negative	IgE	Reduced or absent
Allograft	Usually delayed and may get graft acceptance	IgD	Normal or rarely reduced or elevated
		Mitogen	Frequently reduced
Lymphoid tissue biopsies		Serum Ab titers	Usually normal, but may be reduced
Lymph nodes	Lymphocyte depletion with reticulum cell proliferation; may be normal	1° Ab response	Some antigens reduced while others simultaneously normal
Thymus	Consistently abnormal, sometimes absent; usually small with lymphocyte depletion, lack cortico-medullary differentiation, and Hassall's corpuscles absent; rarely normal	2° Ab response	Variably normal or reduced
		Lymphoid tissue biopsies	
		Bone marrow	Usually normal; may have reduced lymphocytes, IgA-containing cells, or plasma cells
		Lymph nodes	Germinal centers often rudimentary; plasma cells sometimes lacking
		Tonsils	Deficient follicular development

Malignancies in AT. In 1971 Gatti and Good[4] reviewed the occurrence of malignancies in primary immunodeficiency diseases. They found that the incidence in those patients was roughly 10,000 times that of the general age-matched population. Fully 10% of AT patients were found to develop malignancies. That was

confirmed by the ICR survey of patients with genetically determined immunodeficiency diseases with or without a malignancy.[135] Of 284 reported cases, 11.7%
had a malignancy. The registry collected 90 cases of malignancy in AT, the most
in any immunodeficiency disease. A few other diseases had a higher incidence of
malignancy, such as Wiskott-Aldrich with 15.4%, but AT is more common and
so accounted for more overall.

The histologic types of malignancies recorded by the ICR in AT were as follows:

1. Lymphoreticular   60 cases
2. Other mesenchymal, including Hodgkins   14 cases
3. Epithelial, including nervous system   16 cases

The age of onset of malignancies was early (median age, 9 years), and multiple
primary lesions were found in some patients. Interestingly, in some sibships, the
development of identical malignancies was recorded.[135]

Chromosome Abnormalities. The fascinating finding of chromosomal abnormalities in AT has drawn attention to the DNA repair mechanism, whose defects
could be etiologically important. In 1966, Hecht et al.[136] first reported chromosomal abnormalities in AT, a high degree (20-30%) of chromosomal breakage in
vitro. They drew an analogy with Fanconi anemia and Bloom's syndrome, both
of which also have chromosomal breakage and an increased incidence of malignancies. Pfeiffer[137] studied six cases of AT in 1970, finding abnormal chromosomes in two of them. In one case it appeared that clonal evolution was taking
place in the abnormal lymphocytes. The great variability noted among the abnormal cells was suggested as a possible origin for neoplastic evolution. Since
not all patients were found to have chromosomal abnormalities, he speculated
that exogenous factors might play a role. No link could be established between
the chromosomal abnormalities and the immunological defects.

Hecht et al.[138] followed a single case of AT over a period of 52 months. They
demonstrated that abnormal clones of lymphocytes arise, survive, and proliferate
in AT. Initially 1 or 2% of the lymphocytes carried a translocation involving
both number 14 chromosomes. The abnormal clone expanded to 56-78% of the
total. The fact that the chromosomal abnormality was quite specific became
very evident in 1975 after the reports of Oxford et al.[139] and McCaw et al.[140]
The former workers studied seven cases in which the D group and particularly
the 14q arm seemed to be affected. The latter investigators reported eight cases
in which 14q structural rearrangements were present. In one case, the abnormal
lymphocyte clone was observed to evolve into chronic lymphocytic leukemia.[140]

Recently Saxon, Stevens, and Golde[127] studied the functional characteristics
of the chronic lymphocytic leukemia T cells in an AT patient. A 14q+ tandem

translocation had been detected 11 years before the onset of the leukemia, and the leukemia evolved with that chromosomal abnormality. Receptors for both the Fc portion of IgM and the Fc portion of IgG were detected among the leukemic cells which were also capable of providing both helper and suppressor T-lymphocyte activity. They suggested that the malignancy occurred in an uncommitted T-lymphocyte capable of further differentiation into either helper or suppressor cells. It is of interest that an abnormality in differentiation in AT had been hypothesized earlier when it was discovered that there were markedly elevated levels of a-fetoprotein in the serum,[141] and also an undifferentiated thymus morphology.

An etiological role for the defective DNA repair mechanism had been suggested as early as 1967 when it was noticed by Gotoff that a patient with AT had a markedly enhanced clinical sensitivity to x-irradiation.[142] More recently Taylor et al.[143] studied the in vitro radiosensitivity of the chromosomes in patients with AT. They observed both chromatid-type damage (sister chromatid exchanges and chromatid breaks) and chromosome damage. They hypothesized that single-strand defects in the double helix of DNA would result in chromatid-type damage in mitoses if the damage were not repaired before mitosis. Double-strand defects could result in chromosomal abnormalities. They thus postulated that the observed defects in AT were a result of defective DNA repair mechanisms. No comment on the malignant potential of such a defect was made, but a comparison was made with xeroderma pigmentosum (XP) in which defective DNA repair has been well worked out and in which a very high incidence of malignancy is known. The effects of potentially lethal radiation damage were studied by Weichselbaum, Nove, and Little in 1978 in both XP and AT.[144] Their study suggested that it was excision repair which was defective. This was hypothesized to result in the accumulation of mutational damage which would in turn ultimately lead to malignancy. Chemical mutagens have been studied as well. Hoar and Sargent[145] found hypersensitivity of AT cells to such agents as mitomycin C (MC), actinomycin D, and methyl methanesulfonate (MMS). They felt that either excision be adequate to allow surgery to be done in emergencies.[153,160] By light microscopy, platelets are markedly reduced in size and highly variable in shape.[162] On the electron microscopic level, reduced organelles and increased numbers of tubules are present.[162] On bone marrow examination, a normal number of mega-karyocytes is found. The survival of normal homologous platelets in a WA patient has been shown to be normal.[162 164] However, the reduced survival of autologous platelets[162] and the finding of phagocytosed platelets in reticuloendothelial cells led Groettum et al.[162] to the hypothesis that autologous platelets are recognized as foreign and removed from the circulation. Splenectomy to increase platelet survival was a failure and resulted in enhanced susceptibility to infection.[154] Metabolic and functional defects have also been found in AT platelets.[162,165-167] Shapiro and his coworkers[167] reported the detection of WA carriers by applying a metabolic stress to the platelets (blockage of glycolysis by the inhibitor 2-deoxy-D-glucose) and observing their function (aggregation in response to adrenaline). Platelets from carriers of the WA syndrome trait failed to aggregate normally.

Infectious complications in WA syndrome usually begin later in the course of the disease but become progressively more frequent[159,168] and are a severe problem in many patients.[161] Practically every body surface and organ may become involved. Skin infections such as impetigo, furunculosis, abscesses, and cellulitis are very common, but chronic recurrent otitis media is probably more characteristic, being present in almost all patients.[169] Other infections include pneumonia, meningitis, sepsis, enteritis, peritonitis, osteomyelitis, blepharitis, sinusitis, etc.[151,156,162,168-170] A great variety of bacterial pathogens have been isolated, including both gram-positive and gram-negative organisms. Bacteria having polysaccharide capsules are often involved, but not exclusively. BCG has been safely given to some patients, probably because they received it before their enhanced susceptibility to infections developed. Viral pathogens are often tolerated better by younger patients. Varicella has been said to be well tolerated,[168] but cases rapidly followed by herpes zoster which sometimes becomes gangrenous have been reported.[151,158] Some cases have been complicated by viral pneumonia.[171] Herpes simplex often becomes recurrent in older children and may affect the eye.[162] It may disseminate and lead to a fatal outcome.[172] Warts may become a nuisance.[172,173] The immunity to hepatitis B appears to be relatively normal, however.[174] Other infectious problems include systemic or local candidiasis[168] and *Pneumocystis carinii* pneumonia.[158,168]

The characteristic skin eruption has been described as eczematous dermatitis, and is usually indistinguishable by distribution or morphology from common, chronic eczema of childhood. It is not present at birth but often appears days[154,162] or months[149,161,163] afterwards. Most commonly it begins on the face or scalp[154,177-179] and then spreads. The distribution includes the face and scalp, extremities (particularly the antecubital and popliteal fossae), buttocks,[154] and then the trunk and generalized skin.[155,176] Flares of the eruption are often associated with infections[177] or vaccinations.[168] The eruption frequently becomes secondarily infected and then develops hemorrhagic crusts.[148,154,185] repair or postreplication repair, or both, could result in the observed changes. Bleomycin, a radiomimetic drug which causes DNA strand scission has also been studied in AT.[146] Hypersensitivity to its effects was found, and the suggestion was made that the DNA repair defect would thus probably be in the rejoining of DNA strand breaks.

Viral oncogenesis has also been hypothesized to occur in AT. Joncas[147] noticed the persistence of Epstein-Barr virus (EBV) antibodies in about 50% of AT patients. Normally about 10% of individuals have such antibodies, which correlate with persistence of the virus. Similar levels (about 50%) are seen in Burkitt's lymphoma and nasopharyngeal carcinoma, two cancers possibly related to EBV. It was suggested that the genetic defect in the target cell, or perhaps the secondary immunological defect, allowed for viral persistence and transformation.

Wiskott-Aldrich Syndrome[148-192]

The Wiskott-Aldrich (WA) syndrome characteristically consists of these major features:

1. Thrombocytopenia with a bleeding diathesis
2. Increased susceptibility to infections of various types
3. An eczematous skin eruption

Any of them may dominate the clinical course, but all are usually present. A characteristic constellation of immunologic deficiencies and an increased incidence of lymphoreticular malignancies are also important features. It is usually inherited as a sex-linked recessive trait.[148-149]

The onset is generally in the first few months of life, and manifestations of the bleeding diathesis are usually the initial symptoms. Petechiae are frequently noted in the first few days of life, usually associated with thrombocytopenia, and they are useful in predicting if a newborn from a known kindred will be affected.[150-152] The Rumpel-Leede sign is often positive.[153] Blood in the stool, usually associated with diarrhea, is a sign which is present early in the course of the disease in many cases.[148,149,154-157] Bleeding from the circumcision site is common.[155] Epistaxis, hematuria, and hemorrhage from minimal trauma are also are also frequent complications.[153,158,159] In the initial stages of the disease, bleeding episodes are the most common cause of death, and gastrointestinal, adrenal, or intracerebral hemorrhages may be the terminal event.[154,160] Anemia secondary to the hemorrhagic diathesis is often observed and may require repeated transfusions. Thrombocytopenia of a variable degree and a prolonged bleeding time are uniformly present in WA syndrome. There is a report which suggests that the hemorrhagic complications do not necessarily correlate with the platelet count,[161] but platelet transfusions usually give temporary benefit and may even In rare cases it is mild or absent.[180] Topical treatment with steroid creams, antibiotics, coal tar, and soaks has had variable success, with some patients showing clearing of cutaneous lesions while others are resistant to any treatment. An allergic component has been frequently incriminated, but elimination diets and hyposensitization injections have only occasionally been of benefit,[153,154,161,176,181] and the injection sites carry a high risk of hemorrhagic or infectious complications. The skin is usually described as dry, scaling, and erythematous, and the pruritis is often severe. Seborrheic dermatitis, especially of the scalp is common. Petechiae and ecchymoses because of the bleeding tendency are also seen commonly, with showers of petechiae occurring at intervals throughout the course of the disease.[148]   A maculopapular rash resembling heat rash[154] and urticaria[153] have also been described.

Other reported findings include hepatomegaly, splenomegaly, failure to thrive, a variable eosinophilia, and even a case of alopecia totalis.[150,153,154,177,178]

A number of diseases have been described as variants of WA syndrome. A female case which lacked thrombocytopenia was described by Evans and Holzel.[172] Incomplete forms have been described in boys who lacked platelet defect or who lacked other of the signs and symptoms.[182]   An adult with WA syndrome has also been described.[183]   Judgement on the relationship of such cases to WA syndrome should be reserved until after the pathogenesis is better understood.

Immunological Characteristics. There are no immunological abnormalities which are specific for WA syndrome, the diagnosis depending primarily on the distinctive clinical features.   Defective immune function is uniformly present, but its nature is variable.   This has led to the speculation that there may be a group of related disorders contained within the diagnosis of WA syndrome having similar clinical features but different immune defects.[169]   Adding to the variability of immunological findings is the fact that some of the immune deficiencies are progressive,[168] while others may improve with time.[153]

It has been hypothesized that the seat of the immune deficiency in WA syndrome lies in the afferent limb, probably in antigen recognition or processing.[168,184]   The afferent limb of an immune response involves localization of antigens, antigen capture and processing by accessory cells, and antigen recognition by lymphocytes.   The effector limb, in contrast, involves lymphocyte proliferation, mediator production, antibody synthesis, and effector lymphocyte functions,

Krivit and Good[155] first reported that the isohemagglutinins were absent in their patients.   That defect has been confirmed and extended to include a failure of antibody synthesis to many other polysaccharide antigens.[150,155,161,168,169,176,185] Antibody responses to other classes of antigens were often, but not uniformly, normal.   The defective response to polysaccharide antigens is a striking and consistent abnormality, but it is by no means the sole defect.   The key observation was that nonspecific antigen-independent processes, such as lymphocyte proliferation in response to mitogens, were preserved whereas responses requiring the processing and recognition of specific antigens were deficient.   This led to the hypothesis that the defect was localized to the afferent limb of the immune response.[168,184]   In essence then, the defect in AT is an inability to initiate an immune response.   Once the response has begun, the effector elements are present and proceed normally.

Cooper et al.[168] hypothesized that the progressive decline in cellular immunity and the depletion of lymphocytes from the peripheral lymphoid tissues were secondary to the *defective antibody response* to polysaccharide antigens resulting in persistent antigenemia and chronic antigen stimulation of the T-cell system. In contrast, Blease et al.[184] felt that those changes were the result of an analogous defect of antigen processing and recognition by the *cell-mediated* arm of the immune response.

Since monocytes are active in the afferent limb of the immune response, they were studied by Spitler et al.[169] who uncovered a deficiency of Fc receptors for IgG on monocytes from some patients with WA. The same patients were found to respond favorably to transfer therapy. Functionally, the WA syndrome monocytes responded normally to chemotactic stimuli in Boyden chambers. Using the lymphocyte antigen stimulation assay, Blease et al.[186] found that WA syndrome macrophages functioned normally in vitro in antigen recognition and processing. They did not quantitate Fc-IgG receptors on the monocytes, and so one cannot be certain that their patients were not part of a subgroup having normal monocytic Fc receptors. Spitler et al.[169] found defective Fc-IgG receptors on only four of nine patients. Thus the functional significance of the monocyte Fc-IgG receptors in this disease remains unknown.

B cells in the peripheral blood of WA patients are quantitatively normal.[187] There is great variation in the quantitative immunoglobulin levels, and indeed, even in a single patient there may be marked variability in immunoglobulin levels.[188]

The most common pattern of immunoglobulin level is: IgG normal, IgM reduced, IgA elevated, IgE elevated, IgD elevated.[189] While the IgG is usually normal.[169] it may also be reduced[189] or elevated.[188] The subclasses of IgG are quite variable over time in WA syndrome, a finding not seen in normal serum.[188] The serum level of IgM is consistently reduced and its variability is even greater than IgG.[169,187,188] Hypercatabolism of IgG, IgA, and IgM has been documented, but it is usually balanced by an increased synthetic rate. Paraproteins of a benign nature have been detected in these patients, and they probably account for the elevated synthesis and much of the variability in immunoglobulin levels.[188] Pokeweed mitogen stimulation may be normal[185,187] or reduced.[153] The deficiency of isohemagglutinin titers was an early finding[155] and one which has been repeatedly confirmed, but some patients have normal levels[169] which shows that a failure to respond to polysaccharide antigens is not a sine qua non of the disease. The Schick test is often negative, thus demonstrating normal immunity to diphtheria. In one case, which paradoxically improved over time, the Schick test converted to negative at the age of 9 years.[153] The inability of WA syndrome patients to respond with a primary or secondary antibody response to polysaccharide antigens is a consistent defect,[155,168,184,185,187] although a few patients do respond normally.[169] The B-cell dependent areas of lymph nodes are generally well preserved, with germinal centers and the plasma cell reaction usually intact unless reticuloendothelial hyperplasia of a severe degree destroys the anatomy of the nodes.[155,168] Similar changes are noted in the spleen where, in addition, focal areas of hemorrhage are often noted.[155]

The T-cell side of immunity is usually normal when tested early in childhood, but it becomes progressively impaired with age. Lymphopenia is a frequent finding,[150,168,169] and it has been noticed that the lymphocytes which remain are larger, are more heterogeneous, and have lobulated nuclei.[185] The missing small lymphocytes are primarily T cells, which are often low in number.[187] The responsiveness of AT patients to T-cell mitogens such as PHA has usually been normal, which led to the hypothesis that the defect in AT is isolated in the afferent area.[168,169] Abnormally low responsiveness to PHA has also been noted in some patients, however.[153,169,170,185] The in vitro lymphocyte response to antigens is usually markedly reduced, in contrast to the response to mitogens.[169,189] The MLC response is likewise usually impaired.[153,169,185] The production of lymphocyte mediators in response to antigens is usually reduced.[169] Mitogens, on the other hand, have been reported to induce normal mediator release.[187] The impairment of cell-mediated immune function is clearly demonstrated in the tests for induction or elicitation in vivo. Sensitization to DNCB is usually reduced.[168,189] KLH[187] and BCG[161] sensitization are also impaired. The recall skin tests show anergy to most antigens.[169,187] Skin allografts done in WA syndrome have shown delayed rejection,[187] while one patient failed to reject the graft.[153] Lymphocyte depletion from T-cell dependent areas is a characteristic of WA syndrome. Early in the course of the disease lymph nodes may be normal,[189] but with time the lymphocyte depletion from the paracortical areas takes place.[150,168,189] The thymus may be normal[155] but is generally hypoplastic or atrophic,[189] and gradual lymphocyte depletion and focal areas of hemorrhage may be seen.[168] Table 7-8 summarizes the immunologic findings.

Malignancies in WA. The occurrence of malignancies in WA syndrome was noted by ten Bensel et al.[157] who reported two brothers with WA syndrome who developed cancers. They also noticed the unusual histologic patterns of malignancies. In the literature up to that time, three cases of malignant reticuloendotheliosis, two cases of myelogenous leukemia, two cases of malignant lymphoma, and a single astrocytoma of the brain had been reported. The preponderance of such unusual tumors suggested an etiological relationship. The histologic types of malignancy in WA reported by the ICR also showed a different pattern from other immunodeficiency disorders. Out of 45 malignancies, 34 were lymphoreticular, and of those, 12 were histiocytic lymphoma and nine were malignant reticuloendotheliosis.[17] Treatment may be associated with the unusual distribution of tumors to a limited extent. For example, five cases of lymphoreticular lymphomas have been reported in WA syndrome patients undergoing treatment with transfer factor.[153]

Among the genetically determined immunodeficiency diseases, WA syndrome is second only to immunodeficiency with thymoma for the incidence of cancer. In their review of malignancies in immunodeficiency diseases published in 1971, Gatti, and Good[4] recorded 13 malignancies and an estimated incidence of neo-

Table 7-8. Immunologic Findings in Wiskott-Aldrich Syndrome.

T CELL		B CELL	
Lymphocytes	Small lymphocytes consistently reduced, progressive	B cells	Normal
		Ig's	
T cells	Usually reduced, depletion sometimes progressive	IgG	Normal or elevated; subclasses may show variability
Mitogens	Usually normal	IgM	Reduced
Antigens	Markedly reduced	IgA	Elevated, sometimes normal or reduced
MLC	Reduced or normal	IgE	Elevated or normal
Mediators	Normal (if mitogen stimulated) or reduced (if antigen stimulated)	IgD	Elevated or normal
		Mitogen	Usually normal
		Serum Ab titers	
Induction		Isohemagglutinins	Absent or reduced, rarely normal
DNCB	Reduced or absent		
BCG	Tuberculin reaction often negative after BCG innoculation	Schick test	Sometimes remains positive
		1° Ab response	Specific inability to respond to polysaccharide antigens in most cases; other antigens reduced or normal
Elicitation	Reduced or absent		
Allografts	Delayed or absent rejection		
Lymphoid tissue biopsies		2° Ab response	Same as 1° response
		Lymphoid tissue biopsies	
Lymph nodes	Progressive depletion of lymphocytes from the thymus-dependent areas; thymus independent areas usually not affected	Lymph nodes	Germinal centers and plasma cell reaction normal; may have reticular cell hyperplasia
Intestine	Lymphoid tissue depletion	Spleen	May have reticular cell hyperplasia and areas of hemorrhage
Thymus	Hypoplastic or atrophic; differentiation normal; may have areas of hemorrhage	Bone marrow	Usually normal

plasia of 10% in WA syndrome. In the cumulative record of the ICR survey,[17] 15.4% of WA patients have developed a malignancy. They occurred at a very early age, the median age at the diagnosis of cancer being 6 years. That is second only to SCID in which the median age was 0.9 year. Familial malignancies have also been reported. In two brothers with WA, one had malignant reticulo-endotheliosis and the other myelogenous leukemia.[157] Overall, 10.4% of all WA cases reported by the ICR had a malignancy in a family member.[17]

In general, there have been three etiologies hypothesized for the increased incidence of malignancies in WA syndrome:

1. Chronic antigen stimulation of the reticuloendothelial system
2. Viral oncogenesis by any one of a number of possible viruses
3. Abnormal immune responses, either to tumors or to oncogenic agents

The concept of *chronic antigen stimulation* was discussed by Bruce and Blease[190] in their report of the presence of benign paraprotein in many WA syndrome patients. They drew attention to the fact that many patients have chronic lymphadenopathy showing reticuloendothelial hyperplasia, a characteristic of chronic antigen stimulation. The markedly elevated synthetic rate of the immunoglobulins in WA syndrome is also suggestive evidence for chronic antigen stimulation. The paraproteins were thought to represent overstimulation of a clone of plasma cells, perhaps resulting from a lack of specific antibody to the offending antigen. It is known that specific antibody responses are more often abnormal than nonspecific proliferative ones in WA, and that specific antibody inhibits further production of antibody in a feedback inhibition loop. Thus the paraprotein might represent the result of chronic stimulation by an antigen to which a specific antibody was not being produced. The concept has also received support from animal studies. Kreuger et al.[191] tested mice by immunosuppression combined with chronic antigen stimulation and demonstrated the development of malignant lymphomas.

Viral oncogenesis was discussed by Brand and Marinkovich[152] in their report of a case of WA syndrome with a malignant reticulosis limited to the brain. They emphasized that in a number of animals, including mice, cattle, cats, and fowl, malignant reticulosis may be induced by viral infection.

Abnormal immune responses might result in reduced resistance to viral infections and thus indirectly lead to viral oncogenesis. Support for this hypothesis was provided by Takemoto et al.[192] who also isolated a papovavirus from the brain and urine of a WA syndrome patient having a reticulum cell sarcoma of the brain. Decreased resistance to infections might also lead to chronic antigen stimulation by the persisting organisms. An immune surveillance hypothesis has also been discussed. The occurrence of malignancy in WA syndrome might result from a failure on the part of the immune system to recognize tumor antigens or tumor cells. Evidence against that hypothesis is the highly unusual nature of the malignancies which develop. Reticulum cell sarcoma localized to the CNS[158,171] and to the skin[153] are rare events. The more common malignancies of childhood such as neuroblastoma, Wilms' tumor, retinoblastoma, and rhabdomyosarcoma would be expected to escape from the immune surveillance as well, but are not a problem in WA syndrome.[158]

The prominent chromosomal abnormalities detected in ataxia telangiectasia are not seen in WA syndrome.[22]

Common Variable Immunodeficiency[193-202]

Among the primary immunodeficiency diseases, common variable immunodeficiency (CVI) is second only to selective IgA deficiency in its frequency of occurrence.[135]   A number of disorders are grouped under this diagnosis, making its precise definition difficult.[193]

The onset of clinical disease is usually delayed until adulthood, although children may also develop the disease.[194-196]   Males and females are equally affected. Pyogenic sinus and pulmonary infections of a chronic and recurrent nature are the usual heralds of this syndrome.   Progression of the pulmonary infections to bronchiectasis ultimately occurs.   Autoimmune disorders commonly accompany the disease, and include lupus erythematosus, rheumatoid arthritis, dermatomyositis, autoimmune thrombocytopenic purpura, hemolytic anemia, and pernicious anemia.   Similar diseases have been found in the families of CVI patients.[195] Gastrointestinal disorders are common, being present in up to 50% of the cases. They include diarrhea, steatorrhea, sprue, atrophic gastritis, pernicious anemia, nodular lymphoid hyperplasia, and protein-losing enteropathy.[197,198]   There is an increased incidence of *Giardia lamblia* infection,[197] and gastric carcinomas have been recorded as late consequences of the disease.[199,200]   Hepatosplenomegaly and lymphadenopathy are common − findings which would be encountered rarely in infantile X-linked agammaglobulinemia, the most likely disease with which CVI might be confused during childhood.

The characteristic immunologic finding is marked panhypoimmunoglobulinemia in the face of normal or reduced numbers of circulating B cells.[195]   A unifying factor in CVI is that there is a defect in some step in the pathway of maturation of B cells into functional immunoglobulin-secreting cells.[193]   The B-cell defects, however, are various.   In some cases, patients also lack circulating B cells, but in such cases B cells may be found in the tissues of the gut.   Some patients have B cells which are unable to respond at all to mitogenic or antigenic signals. In others, the B cells do respond and synthesize immunoglobulin, but are unable to secrete it because of a defect in glucosylation of the heavy chain of the immunoglobulins.[201]   Still other patients with CVI have a circulating inhibitor or suppressor T-cell population inhibiting their otherwise normal B cells.   Functional measurements of B cells, including existing antibody titers and primary and secondary antibody responses to immunization, are usually reduced or absent. In lymphoid tissue biopsies there may be a lack of plasma cells, whereas in other cases a nodular lymphoid hyperplasia is found.[197]   T-cell function is normal in the majority of cases, but it may be defective, and progressive deterioration of T-cell function over time occurs.[194]   Table 7-9 summarizes the above immunologic data.

Various malignancies have been reported in association with CVI. Many thymomas have been found.[202]   Epithelial malignancies are quite common, almost as frequent as lymphoreticular neoplasms — a situation which is similar to selective IgA deficiency.[135]   The cause of the increased epithelial cancers remains unknown, but it is interesting to note that both CVI and selective IgA deficiency have a high median age of onset of malignancy, 46 and 30 years, respectively, which is much higher than that seen in the other primary immunodeficiency

Table 7-9. Immunologic Findings in Common Variable Immunodeficiency.

T CELL		B CELL	
Lymphocytes	Sometimes reduced	B cells	May be normal, reduced, or absent
T cells	Sometimes reduced		
Mitogens	Sometimes reduced or absent	Ig's	
		IgG	Usually markedly reduced
Antigens	Sometimes reduced or absent	IgA	Usually reduced or absent
MLC	Sometimes reduced or absent	IgM	Usually reduced or absent
Mediators	———		
Induction	Sometimes negative	Mitogens	———
Elicitation	Sometimes all are negative	Ab titers	
		Isohemag-glutinins	Reduced or absent
Allograft	May be delayed	Schick test	May be positive
Lymphoid tissue biopsies		$1°$ Ab response	Reduced
		2^n Ab response	Reduced
Thymus	May be dystrophic	Lymphoid tissue biopsies	
		Lymph nodes	Lack plasma cells; follicular hyperplasia or hypertrophy may be present
		Intestine	Usually lack plasma cells; nodular lymphoid hyperplasia may be present

diseases.[135] Multiple primary malignancies in a single individual and an increased incidence of neoplasia in family members of CVI patients have also been recorded.[135] An association between the various gastrointestinal diseases in CVI and gastrointestinal malignancies has been suggested. The actual incidence of malignancy in CVI is about 4.3%, which is lower than many of the other immunodeficiency diseases, but is nevertheless important because of the relative frequency of the disease.[135]

Infantile X-linked Agammaglobulinemia (Bruton's)[203-210]

Bruton's disease is an X-linked immunodeficiency which becomes manifest at about 5 or 6 months of age with recurrent infections.[79,203] The most common infections include otitis media, otitis externa, sinusitis, bronchitis, meningitis, sepsis, and pneumonia. The prominent pathogens include pneumococci, streptococci, and *Hemophilus influenzae.*[203] Viral infections are usually handled uneventfully, but severe and even fatal viral infections do occur. *Giardia lamblia* infestation of the gut with resulting malabsorption is a frequent complication, and *Pneumocystis carinii* pneumonia has also been reported. Dermatitis is not infrequent. Gamma globulin therapy is beneficial, but severe infections still occur which require prompt and vigorous therapy. Overall, the prognosis remains poor.[203]

The immune defect is limited to the B-cell lineage.[203-206] Peripheral blood B-cell numbers are reduced or absent. Characteristically, all of the serum immunoglobulin classes are reduced or absent.[79] The onset of the disease at 5 or 6 months of age correlates with the decline in passively transferred maternal IgG. Transient hypogammaglobulinemia of infancy, a common self-limited immune deficiency, also occurs as the passively acquired IgG declines, and so can sometimes present a problem in differential diagnosis. The existing serum antibody titers and the primary and secondary antibody responses to most antigens are markedly deficient.[208,209] Immunization with bacteriophage ϕX174 has been found to be particularly useful in detecting abnormal antibody function since little response occurs to this potent allergen in Bruton's disease patients.[208] Biopsies of lymphoid tissues reveal a lack of plasma cells, and lymphoid follicles and germinal centers are absent from antigen stimulated nodes.[207] The pathogenesis can probably best be explained by a failure of the stem cells to differentiate into B-lymphocytes. Table 7-10 succinctly lists the immunologic observations.

Hodgkins disease and lymphosarcoma have been reported in X-linked agammaglobulinemia, but the incidence of malignancy is not strikingly high.[135,210] Fourteen malignancies arising in Bruton's patients have been recorded by the ICR.[135] They were predominantly of a lymphoreticular nature, which is characteristic for immunodeficiency disorders in general.

Table 7-10. Immunologic Findings in Bruton's X-Linked Agammaglobulinemia.

T CELL		B CELL	
Lymphocytes	Normal	B cells	Usually absent, normal in rare cases
T cells	Normal		
Mitogens	Normal	Ig's	
Antigens	Normal	IgG	Less than 100mg/100ml
MLC	Normal	IgM	Reduced or absent
Mediators	Normal	IgA	Reduced or absent
Induction	Normal	IgE	Reduced or absent
Elicitation	Normal	IgD	Reduced or absent
Allograft	Normal	Mitogens	———
Lymphoid tissue biopsies		Serum Ab titers	
		Isohemag-glutinins	Reduced or absent
Thymus	Normal	Schick test	Remains positive
		1° Ab response	Reduced or absent
		2° Ab response	Reduced or absent
		Lymphoid tissue biopsies	
		Bone marrow	Lacks plasma cells
		Lymph nodes	Lack plasma cells; follicles and germinal centers are absent from the cortex; hyperplasia of reticular may be seen
		Spleen	Lacks plasma cells
		Intestine	Lacks plasma cells

Selective IgA Deficiency[211-215]

Selective IgA deficiency is the most common of the primary immune deficiency states.[135] Cases may be sporadic, but both autosomal dominant and autosomal recessive inheritance have been established. Among apparently normal individuals, IgA deficiency has been found to occur in as many as one person in 500.[211] An incidence of one in 200 has been reported in selected populations, such as people with autoimmune or allergic disorders, people with recurrent infections, or the relatives of people with hypogammaglobulinemia. The clinical presentation is highly variable.[212-214] Many patients are discovered during a work-up for an autoimmune disease, and numerous autoimmune disorders have been reported to occur in association with IgA deficiency. They particularly include rheumatoid arthritis, systemic lupus erythematosus, thyroiditis, and pernicious anemia.[214] The autoimmune diseases themselves do not appear to be influenced by the lack of IgA, but run an unremarkable course. Allergic symptoms may be associated with selective IgA deficiency. Asthma may be of earlier onset and run a more chronic and severe course in the presence of IgA deficiency. Recurrent pulmonary diseases occur in IgA deficiency, including bronchitis, pneumonia, chronic obstructive pulmonary disease, and pulmonary hemosiderosis, but they are relatively mild when compared with the same pulmonary diseases in some of the other primary immunodeficiency states. Celiac disease is the most frequent gastrointestinal disease associated with selective IgA deficiency, but regional enteritis, ulcerative colitis, and pernicious anemia have all been reported.[212-214] Their course is generally the same as that in patients with normal serum IgA levels. Pulmonary and gastrointestinal diseases would be expected to be a problem because of the role of secretory IgA in the immunologic defense of those sites.

The sine qua non of the diagnosis of selective IgA deficiency is a low serum level of IgA. Usually less than 5 mg/100 ml is present. By definition, no other humoral or cell-mediated deficiencies are present. Other immune deficiency diseases such as ataxia telangiectasia, Nezelof's syndrome, and chronic mucocutaneous candidiasis have a dificiency of IgA, but they can be distinguished from selective IgA deficiency by the associated immunologic deficiencies in those conditions. There is a normal number of circulating B cells, including those with surface IgA.[212-214] Intestinal biopsies reveal a lack of IgA-contaning plasma cells, but may show a compensatory increase of IgM-secreting cells. Monomeric IgM may be present in increased amounts in both the serum and secretions. A few patients with selective IgA deficiency have had normal secretory IgA levels and the presence of IgA-secreting plasma cells in the intestinal wall. Autoantibodies are a common finding, being present in as many as 40% of selective IgA deficiency patients. Antibodies to human IgA have been reported, which may result in anaphylaxis when blood products containing IgA are given. In some cases, immunologic attrition of the T-cell system occurs late in the disease.[212-214] Table 7-11 records the immune findings.

In spite of the relative mildness of the clinical findings and immunologic deficiencies, an increased incidence of malignancy is present.[135] The ICR survey noted that 2.4% of 833 patients had cancer.[135] Two patients with multiple primary sites of malignancy were recorded. The median age at the time of diagnosis of malignancy in 15 cases was 30 years, much higher than many of the other primary immune deficiency diseases.[135] The cancers have been lymphoreticular, mesenchymal, and epithelial in origin, and it is notable that many of the epithelial tumors arose from sites usually protected by secretory IgA.[135]

Table 7-11. Immunologic Findings in Selective IgA Deficiency.

T CELL		B CELL	
Lymphocytes	Normal	B cells	Normal
T cells	Normal	Ig's	
Mitogens	Normal	IgA	Reduced or absent
Antigens	Normal	IgM	Normal
MLC	Normal	IgG	Normal
Mediators	Normal	IgE	Normal
Induction	Normal	IgD	Normal
Elicitation	Normal	Secretory IgA	May be normal, reduced, or absent
Allograft	Normal		
Lymphoid tissue		7S IgM	May be increased in serum or secretions
biopsies	Normal	Mitogen	Normal
		Ab titers	Normal
		1° Ab response	Normal
		2° Ab response	Normal
		Lymphoid tissue biopsies	
		Intestine	May lack IgA-producing cells
		Lymph nodes	Normal

Selective IgM Deficiency[216-220]

Selective IgM deficiency is a relatively rare primary immune deficiency disorder, whereas a secondary deficiency of IgM is about 20 times more common.[216] The mode of inheritance has not yet been definitively established. Recurrent infection is the usual presenting symptom, although in 19% of the cases there are no symptoms.[216] Meningeal, upper respiratory, and gastrointestinal infections are the most frequent, and sepsis is often a complication.[216-218] Pneumococci, meningococci, *H. influenzae*, and other gram-negative bacteria are the usual pathogens, but viruses may also be a problem. Extensive wart infections have been described, as also has a case of generalized, although not progressive, vaccinia.[219] Atopic dermatitis and autoimmune phenomena have an increased incidence of IgM deficiency.[216,220]

This disease is characterized by a marked reduction or absence of the immunoglobulin IgM level in the serum and by normal levels of the other immunoglobulin classes.[216] A reduced number of B cells bearing surface IgM is present both in the blood and in lymphoid tissues. There is little or no humoral immune response of the IgM class, and other classes of immunoglobulins may also show reduced responsiveness, but of a milder degree. Thus, the isohemagglutinins are usually absent. The Schick test may also remain positive despite immunization. Table 7-12 briefly enumerates these immune data.

The incidence of neoplasia in this syndrome is high, being in the range of 7 to 10%.[135,216] Lymphoreticular malignancies predominate, but others, including a neuroblastoma, have been described.[135] Three brothers in a single family with selective IgM deficiency developed lymphoreticular neoplasms, so familial cases do occur. The median age of onset of malignancy in the seven cases reported to the ICR was 11 years.[135]

Table 7-12. Immunologic Findings in Selective IgM Deficiency.

T CELL		B CELL	
Lymphocytes	Normal	B cells	B cells with surface IgM reduced or absent
T cells	Normal		
Mitogens	Normal	Ig's	
Antigens	Normal	IgM	Reduced or absent
MLC	Normal	IgG	Normal
Mediators	Normal	IgA	Normal
Induction	Normal	IgD	Normal
Elicitation	Normal	IgE	May be elevated
Allograft	Normal	Mitogen	————
Lymphoid tissue biopsies	Normal	Serum Ab titers	
		Isohemag-glutinins	Reduced or absent
		Schick test	Sometimes positive
		1° Ab response	Reduced or absent IgM response, other classes of Ig's may also be reduced
		2° Ab response	Same as above
		Lymphoid tissue biopsies	
		Lymph nodes	May have hypoplastic follicles; lack germinal centers
		Spleen	Same as above

Selective IgG Subclass Deficiencies[221-224]

Human IgG is divided into four subclasses, IgG1, IgG2, IgG3, and IgG4, with the relative abundance of approximately 61%, 30%, 5%, and 4%, respectively.[221] Genetically determined antigenic markers (Gm) present on the heavy chains of the immunoglobulins are associated with the specific subclasses. Most antigens elicit an antibody response in all four subclasses of IgG, but the response to some antigens is limited to a single subclass. Functional and metabolic differences among the subclasses are also present.[221]

IgG subclass deficiency was detected in patients who presented with an undue susceptibility to pyogenic infections and progressive pulmonary disease.[222] When many primary immunodeficiency diseases were screened for IgG subclass disturbances, abnormalities were found in many cases of CVI and some cases of Wiskott-Aldrich syndrome, Bruton's disease, and SCID.[223-224] It has not yet been possible to correlate a particular IgG subclass deficiency with specific clinical symptoms or laboratory findings. It is also not yet clear how to differentiate a primary deficiency of IgG subclasses from a defect which is secondary to another disease.

Because of the association of this defect with various other immune deficiency states, it has not been possible to establish a pattern in the immunological workup. An association with malignancy has likewise not been established.

X-linked Immunodeficiency with Hyper-IgM[225-227]

This is a rare syndrome characterized by diminished serum concentrations of the immunoglobulins IgG and IgA but normal to markedly elevated IgM and IgD.[79,225,226] Two forms are recognized, the X-linked cases seen only in males and "acquired" cases which are seen in both sexes. Affected patients usually present in the first years of life with recurrent pyogenic respiratory tract infections. The infections are usually less severe than in Bruton's disease, but sepsis may supervene and may be fatal.[225] Extensive wart infection[79] and *Pneumocystis carinii* pneumonia[203] have been recorded. Neutropenia, sometimes cyclic, if often observed and may be associated with hemolytic aremia or thrombocytopenia.[79] Hepatosplenomegaly and lymphadenopathy are also common.

The defects in the immune system are primarily localized in the B cells which apparently fail to complete their maturation sequence. They develop the capacity to synthesize and secrete IgM, but fail to make the switch to IgG and IgA.[227] Abnormal B cells are present in the circulation bearing surface IgM and IgD, but IgG- and IgA-bearing B cells are absent.[227] The abnormal cells secrete large amounts of IgM and can be further stimulated to secrete more IgM, but not IgG and IgA, by exposure to pokeweed mitogen. The serum IgM retains its usual heterogeneity, and normal IgM antibody responses occur to some antigens. Elevated levels of the isohemagglutinins may be seen. However, most antibody responses are deficient, particularly the secondary responses which are more highly dependent on IgG. The lymph nodes fail to form follicles and germinal centers, and the plasma cell reaction in lymph nodes is also impaired.[227] Table 7-13 lists the immunologic functions.

Malignancies have been recorded in X-linked immunodeficiency with hyper-IgM, and their incidence is of the same order of magnitude as in Bruton's X-linked hypogammaglobulinemia (1.5 and 0.7%, respectively, in the ICR survey).[135] The abnormal IgM-producing B cells sometimes develop into malignant lymphoproliferative diseases.[227]

Antibody Deficiency with Normal or Hyperimmunoglobulinemia[228-229]

This rare immune deficiency state is characterized by a failure of antibody responsiveness to many antigens in the face of normal or near normal levels of serum immunoglobulins.[203] IgM and IgA may be deficient. Repeated respiratory infections including otitis, tonsilitis, and pneumonia draw attention to these children whose siblings may also have increased susceptibility to infections.[203] An inheritance pattern has not yet been firmly established.

The fact that the serum immunoglobulin levels are often normal emphasizes the necessity of doing more than quantitative immunoglobulins when screening for immune deficiency states. Functional tests are necessary to reveal this abnormality. The isohemagglutinin titers may be low or absent. Antibody responses to many antigens are reduced or absent.[228,229] Isolated T-cell abnormalities may be present as well, including antigen stimulation, mediator release, and allograft rejection.[203] Lymphoid tissue biopsies are usually normal, although reduced numbers of plasma cells may be seen. Table 7-14 lists the immune functions.

An increased incidence of neoplasia, particularly lymphoreticular malignancies, has been recorded. In the ICR survey, 3 patients out of the 95 recorded had malignancies.[135] The median age at the diagnosis of malignancy was 9 years.

Hereditary Transcobalamin II Deficiency[230-231]

Hereditary transcobalamin II deficiency is a rare syndrome.[54,230,231] The inheritance is autosomal recessive. Clinically it is characterized by gastrointestinal and respiratory infections in the first months of life. A megaloblastic anemia with a low reticulocyte count, granulocytopenia, thrombocytopenia, and hemorrhages occur, but the serum B_{12} levels are normal. The diagnostic finding is the absence of the serum protein transcobalamin II whose function is the transport of vitamin B_{12}. The clinical symptoms can be reversed by frequent administration of large doses of intramuscular vitamin B_{12}.

The immunological abnormalities include low levels of the immunoglobulins and no antibody response to immunization.[54,230,231] B-cell differentiation ap-

Table 7-13. Immunologic Function in X-Linked Immunodeficiency with Hyper-IgM.

T CELL		B CELL	
Lymphocytes	Abnormal lymphocytoid cells present	B cells	Those bearing surface IgM and IgD normal or increased; IgG- and IgA-bearing cells absent; abnormal lymphocytoid cells secreting IgM present
T cells	Normal		
Mitogens	Normal		
Antigens	———		
MLC	Normal		
Mediators	Normal	Ig's	
Induction	Usually normal, but may fail to sensitize	IgA	Reduced or absent
		IgG	Reduced or absent
Elicitation	Normal	IgM	Usually markedly elevated, but may be normal
Allografts	———		
Lymphoid tissue biopsies	———	IgD	Usually elevated
		Mitogen	Blastogenesis and IgM secretion normal, but IgG and IgA synthesis induced by PWM reduced
		Serum Ab titer	
		Isohemagglutinins	May be elevated
		Schick test	Remains positive, but may become negative after repeated immunizations
		1° Ab response	Reduced; may have normal IgM response to some antigens
		2° Ab response	Reduced
		Lymphoid tissue biopsies	
		Nodes	Absence of lymphoid follicles and germinal centers (normal in the acquired form); reduced numbers of plasma cells
		Intestine	Reduced plasma cells
		Bone marrow	Reduced plasma cells
		Various tissues	May be infiltrated by abnormal lymphocytoid cells

Table 7-14. Immunologic Function in Antibody Deficiency
with Normal or Hyperimmunoglobulinemia.

T CELL		B CELL	
Lymphocytes	Normal	B cells	Normal
T cells	Normal	Ig's	
Mitogens	Normal	IgG	Usually normal, may
Antigens	Normal or may be reduced		be elevated
		IgM	Usually normal, may be reduced
MLC	Normal		
Mediators	Normal or may be reduced	IgA	Usually normal, may be reduced
Induction	——	Mitogen	Normal
Elicitation	Normal	Serum Ab titer	
Allograft	May be delayed	Isohemag-glutinins	Reduced or absent, sometimes normal
Lymphoid tissue biopsies	——	1° Ab response	Reduced or absent, some are normal
		2° Ab response	Reduced or absent, some are normal
		Lymphoid tissue biopsies	
		Lymph nodes	Normal, but may have decreased numbers of plasma cells

parently occurs normally and antigen-specific memory cells develop, but clonal expansion, maturation into plasma cells, and synthesis of antibodies are blocked by the unavailability of vitamin B_{12}. Lymphoid tissue biopsies therefore show an absence of plasma cells. T-cell-mediated immunity is normal. The immunologic abnormalities are reversed by treatment with vitamin B_{12}. The immune functions are summarized in Table 7-15.

No malginancies have been described.

Transient Hypogammaglobulinemia of Infancy[232-234]

This is a relatively common immunodeficiency disorder which is fortunately mild and transient.[232-234] It occurs in males and females equally and is occasionally familial.[234] Its onset is at a few months of age with multiple infections involving the skin, lungs, meninges, gastrointestinal tract, or respiratory tracts, often with one infection directly following another.[234] Gram-positive bacteria

Table 7-15. Immunologic Findings in Hereditary Transcobalamin II Deficiency.

T CELL		B CELL	
Lymphocytes	Normal	B cells	Normal
T cells	Normal	Ig's	
Mitogens	Normal	IgG	Reduced or absent
Antigens	———	IgM	Reduced or absent
MLC	Normal	IgA	Reduced or absent
Mediators	———	Mitogen	———
Induction	Normal	Serum Ab titer	———
Elicitation	Normal	1° Ab response	Absent
Allograft	———	2° Ab response	Absent
Lymphoid tissue biopsies		Lymphoid tissue biopsies	
		Bone marrow	Plasma cells absent

are the usual pathogens. The infections are of a lesser degree of severity than seen in other immune deficiency diseases, with upper respiratory infections and diarrhea being the most common. Spontaneous clinical recovery usually occurs at about 9–15 months of age, with no persisting abnormalities.[234]

Low levels of immunoglobulins are present in the serum.[232-234] The disease is apparently the result of a delay in the onset of gamma globulin synthesis by an infant. It therefore becomes evident when the transplacental IgG received from the mother declines and fails to be replaced by immunoglobulins synthesized by the child. Differentiation from infantile X-linked hypogammaglobulinemia is sometimes difficult. Lymphoid tissue biopsies can usually prove the diagnosis since lymph nodes have normal architecture and rectal biopsies show the presence of plasma cells in transient hypogammaglobulinemia. Normal levels of immunoglobulins in the serum and normal functional tests are present some time after spontaneous recovery, at approximately 2–4 years of age.[234] Table 7-16 summarizes the immunologic data.

No malignancies have been recorded.

Congenital Absence or Hypoplasia of the Thymus Parathyroids (DiGeorge's Syndrome)[235-240]

DiGeorge's syndrome is a congenital immune deficiency disease which results from a sporadic mutation. It becomes evident shortly after birth with abnormal

Table 7-16. Immunologic Function in Transient Hypogammaglobulinemia.

T CELL	B CELL	
Normal	B cells	Present
	Ig's	
	IgG	Reduced or absent
	IgM	Reduced or absent; may be normal
	IgA	Reduced or absent; may be normal
	Mitogens	———
	Serum Ab titers	Reduced or absent
	1° Ab response	Reduced or absent
	2° Ab response	Reduced or absent
	Lymphoid tissue biopsies	
	Lymph nodes	Normal architecture, but may have reduced plasma cells
	Intestine	Plasma cells are present
	Bone marrow	Reduced plasma cell numbers

facies, cardiac abnormalities such as truncus arteriosus or interrupted aortic arch, and hypocalcemic tetany resulting from hypoparathyroidism.[235-238] Those who survive the newborn period develop chronic and recurrent infections of a severe nature with most occurring in the respiratory or gastrointestinal tracts. Failure to thrive is common, and death occurs within about two years in most cases without treatment.[237]

The immunologic abnormalities are the result of hypoplasia or aplasia of the thymus and are frequently present at birth. They may improve or deteriorate with age.[235] Patients with some thymic tissue are termed *partial DiGeorge syndrome*, and the action of the remaining tissue accounts for the better cell-mediated immunity present in those cases.[239] The peripheral blood T cells are absent or reduced, and all of the functional tests of T cells are usually abnormal.[235] The thymic abnormality results in lymphocyte depletion from the thymus-dependent areas of the lymph nodes and spleen.[235,240] Some patients also have abnormalities in their humoral immunity, giving an immunological picture resembling SCID.[240] They have been termed *DiGeorge variant* and can be differentiated from SCID on the basis of the facies, cardiac, and parathyroid abnormalities. Those with complete aplasia of the thymus have a profound deficiency in T cells and T-cell functions. Thus there is a wide spectrum of findings.[238] Table 7-17 concisely lists these functions.

Malignancies are not frequently encountered in DiGeorge's syndrome. A nervous system tumor is recorded in the ICR.[135]

Episodic Lymphocytopenia with Lymphocytotoxin (Immunologic Amnesia Syndrome)[241-244]

This is a very rare autosomal recessive disorder with its onset early in life.[241,244] The patients develop severe recurrent bacterial and viral infections. Otitis media, tonsillitis, sinusitis, cellulitis, pneumonia, and bronchiectasis all occur. Eczema is a prominent feature and is frequently secondarily infected. Eczema herpetiformis has been reported. The usual pathogens include pneumococci, streptococci, and herpes simplex virus. Death, usually from overwhelming infection, occurs in childhood. The longest survival to date has been 11 years.[241,244]

There is a quantitative T-cell deficiency but, on functional testing, a combined immunodeficiency.[242,243]   A characteristic finding is an episodic profound

Table 7-17. Immunologic Findings in DiGeorge's Syndrome.

T CELL		B CELL	
Lymphocytes	Reduced or rarely normal	B cells	Proportionately increased
T cells	Reduced or absent	Ig's	Normal or rarely reduced
Mitogens	Reduced or absent	Mitogen	Normal or rarely reduced
Antigens	Reduced or absent	Serum Ab titers	Normal or rarely reduced
MLC	Reduced or absent	1° Ab response	Normal or rarely reduced
Mediators	Reduced or absent	2° Ab response	Normal or rarely reduced
Induction	Reduced or absent	Lymphoid tissue biopsies	
Elicitation	Reduced or absent		
Allograft	Delayed or absent	Lymph nodes B-cell areas normal	
Lymphoid tissue biopsies			
Lymph nodes	Lymphocyte depletion in thymus-dependent areas; reticulum cells prominent; normal plasma cells; germinal centers normal or increased		
Spleen	Lymphocyte depletion in thymus-dependent areas		
Thymus	Aplasia or hypoplasia		

lymphocytopenia which has been shown to be the result of a circulating lympho-cytotoxin. The immunosuppressive effect of this lymphocytotoxin is analogous to the antilymphocyte globulin which is used clinically for immunosuppression in transplant patients.[242,243]   Lymphocytotoxins with immunosuppressive effects have also been reported following a variety of viral illnesses and after vaccination.[242] The toxin is absent from the serum during the intervals of normal lymphocyte count.[241]   Generally there is a resemblance of the immunologic disorders to Wiskott-Aldrich syndrome, which has led to speculation that they may be related.[244]

Patients who survive long enough may develop malignancies. An aggressive reticulum cell sarcoma was reported. One patient out of eight (12.5%) reported to the ICR had a malignancy.[135]   Table 7-18 summarizes the immune findings.

Purine Nucleoside Phosphorylase Deficiency[245-252]

The enzyme purine nucleoside phosphorylase (NP) catalyzes the reaction convert-ing inosine to hypoxanthine. The metabolic pathway is demonstrated in Figure 7-2, which shows that NP is involved in the step just following that in which ADA

Table 7-18. Immunologic Findings in Immunologic Amnesia Syndrome.

T CELL (DEFECTS EPISODIC)		B CELL	
Lymphocytes	Episodic lymphocytopenia	B cells	———
		Ig's	
T cells	Reduced or absent	IgG	Normal or reduced
Mitogens	Reduced or absent; occasionally normal	IgA	Normal or reduced
		IgM	Normal or reduced
Antigens	Reduced or absent	Mitogens	———
MLC	Reduced or absent	Serum Ab titers	
Mediators	———	Isohemag-glutinins	Reduced
Induction	Usually absent		
Elicitation	Absent or reduced	1° Ab response	Reduced or absent
Allograft	———	2° Ab response	Reduced or absent
Lymphoid tissue biopsies		Lymphoid tissue biopsies	
Lymph nodes	Depletion of small lymphocytes from the thymus-dependent areas	Lymph nodes	Germinal centers and follicles normal
Spleen	Depletion of small lymphocytes from the thymus-dependent areas	Spleen	Germinal centers and follicles normal
		Bone marrow	Lymphoid hyperplasia

is active. It is interesting that ADA deficiency results in a combined T- and B-cell immunodeficiency, while NP deficiency results in an isolated T-cell deficiency. Red blood cells contain the enzyme and are commonly used in the measurement of its activity, but other tissues, including lymphocytes, also contain NP.[245,246]

The syndrome is very rare and is apparently transmitted as an autosomal recessive trait.[245] Bacterial infections begin in childhood and include otitis media, pneumonia, bronchiolitis, and diarrhea.[246] A severe yeast infection has been reported. Viral infections are especially severe, and include cytomegalovirus, vaccinia, and varicella. The latter two have proved fatal in patients.[247,248] Severe anemia may be a feature, making differentiation from the Diamond-Blackfan syndrome of congenital hypoplastic anemia difficult.[245] No skeletal abnormalities have been reported. The clinical course becomes progressively more severe with age, as does SCID.[246]

The immune deficiency is apparently limited to the T cells.[245-252] Circulating T cell numbers are moderately to greatly reduced, and mitogen stimulation, antigen stimulation, MLC, and skin tests are all reduced or negative. The B-cell system apparently functions normally, with normal serum immunoglobulins, normal PWM, and normal antibody responses to immunizing or infecting agents.[245-252] The immune functions are listed in Table 7-19.

REFERENCES

1. Harris, J.E., and Sinkovics, J.G.: *The Immunology of Malignant Disease* (2nd ed.). St. Louis, MO: C.V. Mosby, 1976, p. 411.
2. Penn, I.: Chemical immunosuppression and human cancer. *Cancer* 34:1474-1480, 1974.
3. Hoover, R., and Fraumeni, J.F., Jr.: Risk of cancer in renal transplant recipients. *Lancet* 2:55-57, 1973.
4. Gatti, R.A., and Good, R.A.: Occurrence of malignancy in immunodeficiency diseases, a literature review. *Cancer* 28:89-98, 1971.
5. Kersey, J.H., Spector, B.D., and Good, R.A.: Primary immunodeficiency diseases and cancer: the immunodeficiency-cancer registry. *Int. J. Cancer* 12:333-347, 1973.
6. Kersey, J.H., Spector, B.D., and Good, R.A.: Cancer in children with primary immunodeficiency diseases. *J. Ped.* 84:263-264, 1974.
7. Ehrlich, P.: Ueber den jetzigen stand der karzinomforschung. In: *The Collected Papers of Paul Ehrlich* (F. Himmelweit, Ed.). London: Pergamon Press, 1957, p. 550.
8. Drew, S. I.: Immunological surveillance against neoplasia; an immunological quandry. *Hum. Path.* 10:5-14, 1979.
9. O'Connor, G.T.: Persistent immunologic stimulation as a factor in oncogenesis with special reference to Burkitt's tumor. *Am. J. Med.* 48:279-285, 1970.
10. Cooper, M.D., Chase, H.P., Lowman, J.T., et al.: Wiskott-Aldrich syndrome. An immunologic deficiency disease involving the afferent limb of immunity. *Am. J. Med.* 44:499-513, 1968.
11. Halterman, R.H., Leventhal, B.G., and Mann, D.L.: An acute leukemia antigen: correlation with clinical status, *N. Eng. J. Med.* 287:1272-1274, 1972.

Table 7-19. Immunologic Function in Purine Nucleoside
Phosphorylase Deficiency.

T CELL		B CELL	
Lymphocytes	Severe lymphopenia	B cells	Normal
T cells	Greatly reduced	Ig's	Normal
Mitogens	Reduced or negative	Mitogen	Normal
Antigens	Reduced or negative	Serum Ab titers	
MLC	Reduced or negative	Isohemag-	Normal
Mediators	———	glutinins	
Induction	Reduced or negative	1° Ab response	Normal
Elicitation	Reduced or negative	2° Ab response	Normal
Allograft	———	Lymphoid tissue biopsies	
Lymphoid tissue biopsies		Bone marrow	Lymphopenia and sometimes erythroid hypocellularity
Lymph nodes	T-cell depletion; plasma cells abundant; germinal centers normal or absent		
Thymus	Hypoplastic; Hassall's corpuscles may be present		

12. Larson, D.L., and Tomlinson, L.J.: Quantitative antibody studies in man. III. Antibody response in leukemia and other malignant lymphomata. *J. Clin. Invest.* **32**:317–321, 1953.
13. Herberman, R.B., and Hollinshead, A.C.: Delayed cutaneous hypersensitivity reactions to extracts of human tumors. *NCI Monogr.* **37**:189, 1973.
14. Hersh, E.M., Whitecar, J.P., McCredie, K.B., et al.: Chemotherapy, immunocompetence, immunosuppression, and prognosis in acute leukemia. *N. Eng. J. Med.* **285**:1211–1216, 1971.
15. Jones, S.E., Griffith, K., Dombrowski, P., and Gaines, J.A.: Immunodeficiency in patients with non-Hodgkins lymphomas. *Blood* **49**:335–344, 1977.
16. Kirkpatrick, C.H.: Cancer and immunodeficiency diseases. *Birth Defects* **12**:61–78, 1976.
17. Spector, B.D., Perry, G.S., III, Gajl-Peczalska, K.J., et al.: Malignancy in children with and without genetically-determined immunodeficiencies. *Birth Defects* **14**:85–89, 1978.
18. Stiehm, E.R.: Immunodeficiency disorders: general considerations. In: *Immunologic Disorders in Infants and Children* (E.R. Stiehm and V.A. Fulginiti, Eds.). Philadelphia, PA: W.B. Saunders, 1973, p. 145.
19. Bloom, B.R., et al.: Evaluation of in vitro methods for characterization of lymphocytes and macrophages. In: *In Vitro Methods in Cell Mediated and Tumor Immunity* (B.R. Bloom and J.R. David, Eds.). New York: Academic Press, 1976, p. 3.

20. Hoffman, T., and Kunkel, H.G.: The E rosette test. In: *In Vitro Methods in Cell Mediated and Tumor Immunity* (B.R. Bloom and J.R. David, Eds.). New York: Academic Press, 1976, p. 71.

21. Balch, C.M., Lawton, A.R., and Cooper, M.D.: Preparation of heterologous antisera specific for human T cells. In: *In Vitro Methods in Cell Mediated and Tumor Immunity* (B.R. Bloom and J.R. David, Eds.). New York: Academic Press, 1976, p. 105.

22. Moretta, L., Webb, S.R., Grossi, C.E., et al.: Functional analysis of two human T-cell subpopulations: help and suppression of B-cell responses by T cells bearing receptors for IgM or IgG. *J. Exp. Med.* 146:184-200, 1977.

23. Evans, R.L., Breard, J.M., Lazarus, H., et al.: Detection, isolation, and functional characterization of two human T-cell subclasses bearing unique differentiation antigens. *J. Exp. Med.* 245:221-233, 1977.

24. Reinherz, E.L., and Schlossman, S.F.: Con A-inducible suppression of MLC: evidence for mediation by the TH_2 T cell subset in man. *J. Immunol.* 122:2335-1341, 1979.

25. Reinherz, E.L., Rubinstein, A., Geha, R.S., et al.: Abnormalities of immunoregulatory T cells in disorders of immune function. *N. Eng. J. Med.* 301:1018-1022, 1979.

26. Waldmann, T.A., Blease, R.M., Broder, S., and Krakauer, R.S.: Disorders of suppressor immunoregulatory cells in the pathogenesis of immunodeficiency and autoimmunity. *Ann. Int. Med.* 88:226-238, 1978.

27. Cunningham-Rundles, S., Hanse, J.A., and Dupont, B.: Lymphocyte transformation in vitro in response to mitogens and antigens. In: *Clinical Immunobiology* (F.H. Bach and R.A. Good, Eds.). Vol. 3. New York: Academic Press, 1976, p. 151.

28. Dupont, B., and Good, R.A.: Lymphocyte transformation in vitro in patients with immunodeficiency diseases: use in diagnosis, histocompatibility testing and monitoring treatment. *Birth Defects* 11:477-485, 1975.

29. Miller, S.D., and Jones, H.E.: Correlation of lymphocyte transformation with tuberculin skin-test sensitivity. *Am. Rev. Resp. Dis.* 107:530-538, 1973.

30. Kirkpatrick, C.H., Rich, R.R., and Bennett, J.E.: Chronic mucocutaneous candidiasis: model-building in cellular immunity. *Ann. Int. Med.* 74:955-978, 1971.

31. Bach, F.H.: Mixed leukocyte cultures: a cellular approach to histocompatibility testing. In: *Clinical Immunobiology* (F.H. Bach and R.A. Good, Eds.). Vol. 3. New York: Academic Press, 1976, p. 27.

32. Hayry, P., et al.: Allograft response in vitro. *Transplant Rev.* 12:91, 1972.

33. Dupont, B., Hansen, J.A., and Yunis, E.J.: Human mixed-lymphocyte culture reaction: genetics, specificity, and biological implications. *Adv. Immunol.* 23:107-202, 1976.

34. Wilson, D.B., and Nowell, P.C.: Quantitative studies on the mixed lymphocyte interaction in rats. *J. Exp. Med.* 133:442-453, 1971.

35. Rocklin, R.E.: Products of activated lymphocytes. In: *Clinical Immunobiology* (F. H. Bach and R.A. Good, Eds.). Vol. 3. New York: Academic Press, 1976, p. 195.

36. Rocklin, R.E., MacDermott, R.P., Chess, L., et al.: Studies on mediator production by highly purified human T and B lymphocytes. *J. Exp. Med.* 140:1303-1316, 1974.

37. Rocklin, R.E.: Products of activated lymphocytes: leukocyte inhibitory factor (LIF) distinct from migration inhibitory factor (MIF). *J. Immunol.* 112:1461-1466, 1974.

38. Rocklin, R.E., Meyers, O.L., and David, J.R.: An in vitro assay for cellular hypersensitivity in man. *J. Immunol.* 104:95-102, 1970.

39. Catalona, W.J., Taylor, P.T., and Chretien, P.B.: Quantitative dinitrochlorobenzene contact sensitization in a normal population. *Clin. Exp. Immunol.* 12:325-334, 1972.

40. Catalona, W.J., Taylor, P.T., Rabson, A.S., and Chretien, P.B.: A method of dinitrochlorobenzene contact sensitization: a clinicopathological study. *N. Eng. J. Med.* 286:399-402, 1972.

41. Blease, R.M., Strober, W., and Waldmann, T.A.: Immunodeficiency in the Wiskott-Aldrich syndrome. *Birth Defects* **11**:250–254, 1975.

42. Biggar, W.D., and Good, R.A.: Immunodeficiency in ataxia-telangiectasia. *Birth Defects* **11**:271–276, 1975.

43. Pinsky, C.M.: Cell-mediated testing: in vivo testing. In: *Clinical Immunobiology* (F.H. Bach and R.A. Good, Eds.). Vol. 3. New York: Academic Press, 1976, p. 97.

44. Palmer, D.L., and Reed, W.P.: Delayed hypersensitivity skin testing. I. Response rates in a hospitalized population. *J. Infect. Dis.* **130**:132–137, 1974.

45. Palmer, D.L., and Reed, W.P.: Delayed hypersensitivity skin testing. II. Clinical correlates and anergy. *J. Infec. Dis.* **130**:138–143, 1974.

46. Holden, M., Dubin, M.R., and Diamond, P.H.: Frequency of negative intermediate strength tuberculin sensitivity in patients with active tuberculosis. *N. Eng. J. Med.* **285**:1506–1509, 1971.

47. Heiss, L.I., and Palmer, D.L.: Anergy in patients with leukocytosis. *Am. J. Med.* **56**:323–332, 1974.

48. Kissmeyer-Nielsen, F., Olsen, S., Petersen, V.P., and Fjeldborg, O.: Hyperacute rejection of kidney allografts associated with preexisting humoral antibodies against donor cells. *Lancet* **2**:662–665, 1966.

49. Schubert, W.K., et al.: Homograft rejection in children with congenital immunological defects: agammaglobulinemia and Aldrich syndrome. *Trans. Bull.* **26**:125, 1960.

50. Fitch, F.W., and Hunter, R.L., Jr.: Histology of immune responses. In: *Immunological Diseases* (M. Samter Ed., 3rd ed.). Little Brown and Co., 1978, p. 81.

51. Gelfand, E.W., Biggar, W.D., and Orange, R. P.: Immune deficiency: evaluation, diagnosis, and therapy. *Ped. Clin. N. Am.* **21**:745–776, 1974.

52. Brozy, M.S., Schulte-Wissermann, H., Gilbert, E., et al.: Thymic morphology in immunodeficiency diseases: results of thymic biopsies. *Clin. Immunol. Immunopath.* **12**:31–51, 1979.

53. Hong, R., and Pellett, J. W.: Transcervical thymic biopsy in children with immunodeficiency. *J. Ped. Surg.* **13**:427–428, 1978.

54. Gupta, S., and Good, R.A.: Markers for human lymphocyte subpopulations in primary immunodeficiency and lymphoproliferative disorders. *Sem. Hemat.* **17**:1–29, 1980.

55. Ross, G.D.: Identification of human lymphocyte subpopulations by surface marker analysis. *Blood* **53**:799–811, 1979.

56. Robbins, D.L., and Gershwin, M.E.: Identification and characterization of lymphocyte subpopulations. *Sem. Arth. Rheum.* **7**:245–277, 1978.

57. Strober, S.: T and B cells in immunologic diseases. *Am. J. Clin. Path.* **68** (Suppl.): 671–678, 1977.

58. Dickler, H.B.: Lymphocyte receptors for immunoglobulin. *Adv. Immunol.* **24**: 167–214, 1976.

59. Chess, L., and Schlossman, S.F.: Human lymphocyte subpopulations. *Adv. Immunol.* **24**:213–241, 1977.

60. Gally, J.A.: The structure, genetics, and biological properties of immunoglobulins. In: *Immunological Diseases* (M. Samter, Ed., 3rd ed.). Little Brown and Co., 1978, p. 49.

61. Spiegelberg, H.L.: Biological activities of immunoglobulins of different classes and subclasses. *Adv. Immunol.* **19**:259, 1974.

62. Cassidy, J.T., and Nordby, G.L.: Human serum immunoglobulin concentrations: prevalence of Ig deficiencies. *J. Allergy Clin. Immunol.* **55**:35–48, 1975.

63. Solomon, A., and McLaughlin, C. L.: Immunoglobulin disturbances and their clinical significance. *Med. Clin. N. Am.* **57**:499-516, 1973.
64. Schur, P., Borel, H., Gelfand, E. W., et al.: Selective gamma-G globulin deficiencies in patients with recurrent pyogenic infections. *N. Eng. J. Med.* **283**:631-634, 1970.
65. Mancini, G., Carbonara, A.O., and Heremans, J.F.: Immunochemical quantitation of antigens by single radial immunodiffusion. *Immunochem.* **2**:235, 1965.
66. Spiegelberg, H.L.: The structure and biology of human IgD. *Immunological Rev.* **37**:3-24, 1977.
67. Pernis, B.: Lymphocyte membrane IgD. *Immunol. Rev.* **37**:210-218, 1977.
68. Preudhommen, J.-L., Brouet, J.-C., and Seligmann, M.: Membrane-bound IgD on human lymphoid cells, with special reference to immunodeficiency and immunoproliferative diseases. *Immunol. Rev.* **37**:127-151, 1977.
69. Buckley, R.H., and Fiscus, S.A.: Serum IgD and IgE concentrations in immunodeficiency diseases. *J. Clin. Invest.* **55**:157-165, 1975.
70. Waldmann, T.A., Polmar, S.H., Balestra, S.T., et al.: Immunoglobulin E in immunologic diseases. II. Serum IgE concentration of patients with acquired hypogammaglobulinemia, thymoma and hypogammaglobulinemia, myotonic dystrophy, intestinal lymphangiectasia and Wiskott-Aldrich syndrome. *J. Immunol.* **109**:304-310, 1972.
71. Buckley, R.H., and Becker, W.G.: Abnormalities in the regulation of human IgE synthesis. *Immunol. Rev.* **41**:288-314, 1978.
72. Hauptman, SP., and Tomasi, T.B.: The secretory immune system. In: *Basic and Clinical Immunology* (H.H. Fudenberg, D.P. Stites, J.L. Caldwell, and J.V. Wells, Eds.; 2nd ed.). Los Altos, CA: Lange Medical Publications, 1978, p. 205.
73. Greaves, M., Janossy, G., and Doenhoff, M.: Selective triggering of human T and B lymphocytes in vitro by polyclonal mitogens. *J. Exp. Med.* **140**:1-18, 1974.
74. Douglas, S.D., Hoffman, P.F., Borjeson, J., and Chessin, L.N.: Studies on human peripheral blood lymphocytes. III. Fine structural features of lymphocyte transformation by pokeweed. *J. Immunol.* **98**:17-30, 1967.
75. Huetteroth, T.H., and Litwin, S.D.: Differentiation of human lymphocytes by pokeweed mitogen in vitro: studies in normal and immunodeficient subjects. *Klin. Wschr.* **55**:743-749, 1977.
76. Stiehm, E.R.: Immunodeficiency disorders: general considerations. In: *Immunologic Disorders in Infants and Children* (E.R. Stiehm and V.A. Fulginiti, Eds.). Philadelphia, PA: W. B. Saunders, 1973, p. 145.
77. Gleich, G.J., Uhr, J.W., Vaughan, J.H., and Swedlund, H.A.: Antibody formation in dysgammaglobulinemia, *J. Clin. Invest.* **45**:1334-1340, 1966.
78. Ching, Y-C, Davis, S.D., and Wedgwood, R.J.: Antibody studies in hypogammaglobulinemia. *J Clin. Invest.* **45**:1593-1600, 1966.
79. Rosen, F.S., and Janeway, C.A.: The gamma globulins. III. The antibody deficiency syndromes. *N. Eng. J. Med.* **275**:709-715, 769-775, 1966.
80. Ochs, H.D., Davis, S.D., and Wedgwood, R.J.: Immunologic responses to bacteriophage ϕx 174 in immunodeficiency diseases. *J. Clin. Invest.* **50**:2559-2568, 1971.
81. Minor, D.R., Schiffman, G., and McIntosh, L.S.: Response of patients with Hodgkins disease to pneumococcal vaccine. *Ann. Int. Med.* **90**:887-892, 1979.
82. Thorbecke, G.J., Romano, T.J., and Lerman, S.P.: Regulatory mechanisms in proliferation and differentiation of lymphoid tissue with particular reference to germinal center development. *Prog. Immunol.* **3**:25-34, 1974.
83. DeVaal, O.M., and Seynhaeve, V.: Reticular dysgenesia. *Lancet.* **2**:1123-1125, 1959.
84. Gitlin, D., Vawter, G., and Craig, J.M.: Thymic alymphoplasia and congenital aleukocytosis. *Pediatrics* **33**:184-193, 1964.

85. Alonso, K., Dew, J.M., and Starke, W.R.: Thymic alymphoplasia and congenital aleukocytosis (reticular dysgenesis). *Arch. Path.* 94:179-183, 1972.

86. O'Reilly, R.M., Pahwa, R., Dupont, B., and Good, R.A.: Severe combined immuno-deficiency: transplantation approaches for patients lacking an HLA genotypically identical sibling. *Transplant. Proc.* 10:187-199, 1978.

87. Aiuti, F., Businco, L., Griscelli, C., Touraine, J., and Webster, A.D.B.: Improvements in methods of identifying patients with severe combined immunodeficiency and related syndromes. *Z. Immun. Forsch.* 153:95-106, 1977.

88. O'Reilly, R.J., Dupont, B., Pahwa, S., et al.: Reconstitution in severe combined immunodeficiency by transplantation of marrow from an unrelated donor. *N. Eng. J. Med.* 297:1311-1318, 1977.

89. Hitzig, W.H.: Congenital thymic and lymphocytic deficiency disorders. In: *Immunologic Disorders in Infants and Children* (E. R. Stiehm and V. A. Fulginiti, Eds.). Philadelphia, PA: W.B. Saunders, 1973, p. 215.

90. Meuwissen, H.J., Bach, F.H., Hong, R., and Good, R.A.: Lymphocyte studies in congenital thymic dysplasia. The one way stimulation test. *J. Paediat.* 72:177-185, 1968.

91. Dupont, B., and Good, R.A.: Lymphocyte transformation in vitro in patients with immunodeficiency diseases: use in diagnosis, histocompatibility testing, and monitoring treatment. *Birth Defects* 11:477-485, 1975.

92. Nezelof, C.: Thymid dysplasia with normal immunoglobulins and immunological deficiency. *Birth Defects* 4:104-115, 1968.

93. Lawlor, G.J., Jr., Ammann, A.J., Wright, W.C., et al.: The syndrome of cellular immunodeficiency with immunoglobulins. *J. Pediat.* 84:183-192, 1974.

94. Seeger, R.C., Robins, R.A., Stevens, R.H., et al.: Severe combined immunodeficieny with B lymphocytes: in vitro correction of defective immunoglobulin production by addition of normal T lymphocytes. *Clin. Exp. Immunol.* 26:1-10, 1976.

95. Giblett, E.R., Anderson, J.E., Cohen, F., et al.: Adenosine deaminase deficiency in two patients with severely impaired cellular immunity. *Lancet* 2:1067-1069, 1972.

96. Meuwissen, H.J., Pollara, B., Pickering, R.J., et al.: Combined immunodeficiency disease associated with adenosine deaminase deficiency. *J. Pediat.* 86:169-181, 1975.

97. Van der Weyden, M.B., and Kelley, W.N.: Adenosine deaminase and immune function. *Br. J. Haemat.* 34:159-165, 1976.

98. Hirschhorn, R., and Sela, E.: Adenosine deaminase and immunodeficiency: an in vitro model. *Cell. Immunol.* 32:350-360, 1977.

99. Carson, D.A., Goldblum, R., and Seegmiller, J.E.: Quantitative immunoassay of adenosine deaminase in combined immunodeficiency disease. *J. Immunol.* 118: 270-273, 1977.

100. Hirschhorn, R.: Adenosine deaminase deficiency and immunodeficiencies. *Fed. Proc.* 36:2166-2170, 1977.

101. O'Reilly, R.J., Pahwa, R., Dupont, B., and Good, R.A.: Severe combined immuno-deficiency: transplantation approaches for patients lacking an HLA genotypically identical sibling. *Transplant. Proc.* 10:187-199, 1978.

102. Goldblum, R.M., Schmalstieg, F.C., Nelson, J.A., and Mills, G.C.: Adenosine deaminase (ADA) and other enzyme abnormalities in immune deficiency states. *Birth Defects* 14:73-84, 1978.

103. Hirschhorn, R., Roegner, V., Jenkins, T., et al.: Erythrocyte adenosine deaminase deficiency without immunodeficiency. Evidence for an unstable mutant enzyme. *J. Clin. Invest.* 64:1130-1139, 1979.

104. Boder, E., and Sedgwick, R.P.: Ataxia telangiectasia: a familial syndrome of progressive cerebellar ataxia, oculocutaneous telangiectasia, and frequent pulmonary infection. *Pediatrics* 21:526-553, 1958.

105. Louis-Bar (Mme.): Sur an syndrome progessif comprenant des telangiectases capillaires cutanees et conjonctivales symetriques, a disposition naevoide et des troubles cerebellauex. *Confinia Neurol.* 4:32, 1941.

106. Syllaba, L., and Henner, K.: Contribution a l'independance de l'athetose double ideopathique et congenital atteinte famiale, syndrome dystrophique, signe du reseau vasculaire conjonctival integrite psychique. *Rev. Neurol.* 15:541-562, 1926.

107. Wells, C.E., and Shy, G.M.: Progressive familial choreoathetosis with oculocutaneous telangiectasia. *J. Neurol. Neurosurg. Psychiat.* 20:98-104, 1957.

108. Tadjoedin, M.K., and Fraser, F.C.: Heredity of ataxia telangiectasia (Louis-Bar syndrome). *Am. J. Dis. Child.* 110:64-68, 1965.

109. Reed, W.B., Epstein, W.L., Boder, E., and Sedgwick, R.: Cutaneous manifestations of ataxia-telangiectasia. *JAMA* 195:746-753, 1966.

110. Boder, E.: Ataxia-telangiectasia: some historic, clinical, and pathologic observations. *Birth Defects* 11:255-270, 1975.

111. McFarlin, D.E., Strober, W., and Waldmann, T.A.: Ataxia-telangiectasia. *Medicine* 51:281-314, 1972.

112. Williams, H.E., Demis, D.J., and Higdon, R.S.: Ataxia-telangiectasia. A syndrome with characteristic cutaneous manifestations. *Arch. Derm.* 82:937-942, 1960.

113. Boder, E., and Sedgwick, R.: Ataxia-telangiectasia: a familial syndrome of progressive cerebellar ataxia, oculocutaneous telangiectasia, and frequent pulmonary infection. *Arch. Derm.* 78:402-404, 1958.

114. Peterson, R.D.A., and Good, R.A.: Ataxia telangiectasia. *Birth Defects* 4:370-374, 1968.

115. Schalch, D.S., McFarlin, D.E., and Barlow, M.H.: An unusual form of diabetes mellitus in ataxia-telangiectasia. *N. Eng. J. Med.* 282:1396-1402, 1970.

116. Ammann, A.J., DuQuesnoy, R.J., and Good, R.W.: Endocrinological studies in ataxia-telangiectasia and other immunological deficiency diseases. *Clin. Exp. Immunol.* 6:587-595, 1969.

117. Aguilar, M.J., Kamoshita, S., Landing, B.H., Boder, E., and Sedgwick, R.P.: Pathological observations in ataxia-telangiectasia. *J. Neuropath. Exp. Neurol.* 27:659-676, 1968.

118. Scully, R.E., and McNeely, B.U.: Case record of the Massachusetts General Hospital, case #22-1975. *N. Eng. J. Med.* 292:1231-1237, 1975.

119. Bowden, D.H., Davis, P.G., and Sommers, S.C.: Ataxia-telangiectasia: a case with lesions of ovaries and adenohypophysis. *J. Neuropath. Exp. Neurol.* 22:549-554, 1963.

120. Solitare, G.B., and Lopez, V.F.: Louis-Bar's syndrome (ataxia-telangiectasia). *Neurology* 17:23-31, 1967.

121. Peterson, R.D.A., Cooper, M.D., and Good, R.A.: The pathogenesis of immunologic deficiency diseases. *Am. J. Med.* 38:579-604, 1965.

122. Peterson, R.D.A., Cooper, M.D., and Good, R.A.: Lymphoid tissue abnormalities associated with ataxia telangiectasia. *Am. J. Med.* 41:342-359, 1966.

123. Eisen, A.H., Karpati, G., Laszlo, T., et al.: Immunologic deficiency in ataxia telangiectasia. *N. Eng. J. Med.* 272:18-22, 1965.

124. Ammann, A.J., Cain, W.A., Ishizaka, K., et al.: Immunoglobulin E deficiency in ataxia telangiectasia. *N. Eng. J. Med.* 281:469-472, 1969.

125. Feigen, R.D., Vietti, T.J., Wyatt, R.G., et al.: Ataxia telangiectasia with granulocytopenia. *J. Ped.* 77:431-438, 1970.

126. McFarlin, D.E., and Oppenheim, J.J.: Impaired lymphocyte transformation in ataxia telangiectasia in part due to a plasma inhibitory factor. *J. Immunol.* 103:1212-1222, 1969.

127. Saxon, A., Stevens, R.H., and Golde, D.W.: Helper and suppressor T-lymphocyte leukemia in ataxia telangiectasia. *N. Eng. J. Med.* **300**:700–704, 1979.
128. Biggar, W.D., and Good, R.A.: Immunodeficiency in ataxia telangiectasia. *Birth Defects* **11**:271–274, 1975.
129. Epstein, W.L., Fudenberg, H.H., Reed, W.B., et al.: Immunologic studies in ataxia telangiectasia. *Int. Arch. Allergy* **30**:15–29, 1966.
130. South, M.A., Cooper, M.D., Wollheim, F.A., and Good, R.A.: The IgA system. II. The clinical significance of IgA deficiency: studies in patients with agammaglobulinemia and ataxia telangiectasia. *Am. J. Med.* **44**:168–178, 1968.
131. Ammann, A.J., and Hong, R.: Cellular immunodeficiency disorders. In: *Immunologic Disorders in Infants and Children* (E. R. Stiehm and V. A. Fulginiti, Eds.). Philadelphia, PA: W. B. Saunders, 1973, p. 236.
132. Polmar, S.H., Waldmann, T.A., Balestra, S.T., et al.: Immunoglobulin E in immunologic deficiency diseases. I. Relation of IgE and IgA to respiratory tract disease in isolated IgE deficiency, IgA deficiency, and ataxia telangiectasia. *J. Clin. Invest.* **51**:326–330, 1972.
133. Schulte-Wissermann, H., Gutjahr, P., Zebisch, P., et al.: Immunological investigations in two brothers with ataxia telangiectasia (Louis-Bar). *Eur. J. Ped.* **122**:93–102, 1976.
134. Kaufman, D.B., and Miller, H.C.: Ataxia telangiectasia: an autoimmune disease associated with cytotoxic antibody to brain and thymus. *Clin. Tox. Immunopath.* **7**:288–299, 1977.
135. Spector, B.D., Perry, G.S., and Kersey, J.H.: Genetically determined immunodeficiency diseases (GDID) and malignancy: report from the Immunodeficiency Cancer Registry. *Clin. Immunol. Immunopath.* **11**:12–29, 1978.
136. Hecht, F., Koler, R.D., Riggs, D.A., et al.: Leukemia and lymphocytes in ataxia telangiectasia. *Lancet* **2**:1193, 1966.
137. Pfeiffer, R.A.: Chromosomal abnormalities in ataxia telangiectasia (Louis-Bar syndrome). *Humangenetik* **8**:302–306, 1970.
138. Hecht, F., McCaw, B.K., and Koler, R.D.: Ataxia telangiectasia: clonal growth of translocation lymphocytes. *N. Eng. J. Med.* **289**:286–291, 1973.
139. Oxford, J.M., Harnden, D.G., Parrington, J.M., and Delhanty, J.D.A.: Specific chromosome observations in ataxia telangiectasia. *J. Med. Genet.* **12**:251–261, 1975.
140. McCaw, B.K., Hecht, F., Harnden, D.G., and Teplitz, R.L.: Somatic rearrangement of chromosome 14 in human lymphocytes. *Proc. Nat. Acad. Sci. USA* **72**:2071–2075, 1975.
141. Waldmann, T.A., and McIntire, K.R.: Serum alpha-fetoprotein levels in patients with ataxia telangiectasia. *Lancet* **2**:1112–1115, 1972.
142. Gotoff, S.P., Amirmokri, E., and Liebner, E.J.: Ataxia telangiectasia. Neoplasia, untoward response to x-irradiation, and tuberous sclerosis. *Am J. Dis. Child.* **114**:617–625, 1967.
143. Taylor, A.M.R., Metcalfe, J.A., Oxford, J.M., and Harnden, D.G.: Is chromatid-type damage in ataxia telangiectasia after irradiation at G_0 a consequence of defective repair? *Nature* **260**:441–443, 1976.
144. Weichselbaum, R.R., Nove, J., and Little, J.B.: Deficient recovery from potentially lethal radiation damage in ataxia telangiectasia and xeroderma pigmentosum. *Nature* **271**:261–262, 1978.
145. Hoar, D.I., and Sargent, P.: Chemical mutagen hypersensitivity in ataxia telangiectasia. *Nature* **261**:590–592, 1976.

146. Taylor, A.M.R., Rosney, C.M., and Campbell, J.B.: Unusual sensitivity of ataxia telangiectasia cells to Bleomycin. *Cancer Res.* 39:1046-1050, 1979.

147. Joncas, J.H.: Persistence, reactivation, and cell transformation by human herpes virus: herpes simplex 1, 2, (HSV-1, HSV-2), cytomegalovirus (CMV), varicella-zoster (VZV), Epstein-Barr virus (EBV). *Can. J. Microbiol.* 25:254-260, 1979.

148. Wiskott, A.: Familiaerer, angeborener Morbus Werlhofii? *Mschr. Kinderheilk.* 68: 212-216, 1937.

149. Aldrich, R.A., Steinberg, A.G., and Campbell, D.C.: Pedigree demonstrating a sex-linked recessive condition, characterized by draining ears, eczematoid dermatitis, and bloody diarrhea. *Pediatrics* 13:133-138, 1954.

150. Wolff, J.A.: Wiskott-Aldrich syndrome: clinical, immunologic, and pathologic observations. *J. Ped.* 70:221-232, 1967.

151. Bach, F.H., Albertini, R.J., Joo, P., et al.: Bone marrow transplantation in a patient with the Wiskott-Aldrich syndrome. *Lancet* 2:1364-1366, 1968.

152. Brand, M.M., and Marinkovich, V.A.: Primary malignant reticulosis of the brain in Wiskott-Aldrich syndrome. *Arch. Dis. Child.* 44:536-542, 1969.

153. Sellars, W.A., and South, M.A.: Wiskott-Aldrich syndrome with 18-year survival: treatment with transfer factor. *Am. J. Dis. Child.* 129:622-627, 1975.

154. Huntley, C.C., and Dees, S.C.: Eczema associated with thrombocytopenic purpura and purulent otitis media. Report of five fatal cases. *Pediatrics* 19:351-360, 1957.

155. Krivit, W., and Good, R.A.: Aldrich's syndrome (thrombocytopenia, eczema, and infection in infants). *J. Dis. Child.* 97:137-153, 1959.

156. Radl, J., Masopust, J., Houstek, J., and Hrodek, O.: Paraproteinaemia and unusual dysgammaglobulinemia in a case of Wiskott-Aldrich syndrome. An immunochemical study. *Arch. Dis. Child.* 42:608-614, 1967.

157. ten Bensel, R.W., Stadlan, E.M., and Krivit, W.: The development of malignancy in the course of the Aldrich syndrome. *J. Ped.* 68:761-767, 1966.

158. Model, L.M.: Primary reticulum cell sarcoma of the brain in Wiskott-Aldrich syndrome: report of a case. *Arch. Neurol.* 34:633-635, 1977.

159. Amiet, A.: Aldrich-syndrom. Beobachtung zweier Faelle. *Ann. Paediat.* 201:315-335, 1963.

160. Faraci, R.P., Hoffstrand, H.J., Witebsky, F.G., et al.: Malignant lymphoma of the jejunum in a patient with Wiskott-Aldrich syndrome. *Arch. Surg.* 110:218-220, 1975.

161. Berglund, G., Finnstroem, O., Johansson, S.G.O., and Moeller, K.L.: Wiskott-Aldrich syndrome: a study of six cases with determination of the immunoglobulins A, D, G, M, and ND. *Acta Paediat. Scand.* 57:89-97, 1968.

162. Groettum, K.A., Hovig, T., Holmsen, H., et al.: Wiskott-Aldrich syndrome: qualitative platelet defects and short platelet survival. *Br. J. Haemat.* 17:373-388, 1969.

163. Pearson, H.A., Shulman, N.R., Oski, F.A., and Eitzman, D.V.: Platelet survival in Wiskott-Aldrich syndrome. *J. Ped.* 68:754-760, 1966.

164. Krivit, W., Yunis, E., and White, J.G.: Platelet survival studies in Aldrich syndrome. *Pediatrics* 37:339-341, 1966.

165. Kuramoto, A., Steiner, M., and Baldini, M.G.: Lack of platelet response to stimulation in the Wiskott-Aldrich syndrome. *N. Eng. J. Med.* 282:475-479, 1970.

166. August, C.S., Hathaway, W.E., Githens, J.H., et al.: Improved platelet function following bone marrow transplantation in an infant with the Wiskott-Aldrich syndrome. *J. Ped.* 82:58-64, 1973.

167. Shapiro, R.S., Gerrard, J.M., Perry, G.S., III, et al.: Wiskott-Aldrich syndrome: detection of carrier state by metabolic stress of platelets. *Lancet* 1:121-123, 1978.

168. Cooper, M.D., Chase, H.P., Lowman, J.T., et al.: Wiskott-Aldrich syndrome: an immunologic deficiency disease involving the afferent limb of immunity. *Am. J. Med.* 44:499-513, 1968.

169. Spitler, L.E., Levin, A.S., Stites, D.P., et al.: The Wiskott-Aldrich syndrome: immunologic studies in nine patients and selected family members. *Cell. Immunol.* 19: 201-218, 1975.

170. Marinkovich, V.A.: The in vitro response of peripheral blood lymphocytes from patients with Wiskott-Aldrich syndrome. *Clin. Allergy* 2:69-78, 1972.

171. Heidelberger, K.P., and LeGolvan, D.: Wiskott-Aldrich syndrome and cerebral neoplasia: report of a case with localized reticulum cell sarcoma. *Cancer* 33:280-284, 1974.

172. Evans, D.K., and Holzel, A.: Immune deficiency state in a girl with eczema and low serum IgM: possible female variant of Wiskott-Aldrich syndrome. *Arch. Dis. Child.* 45:527-533, 1970.

173. Zinn, K.H., and Belohradsky, B.H.: Wiskott-Aldrich syndrome with verrucae vulgares. *Hautarzt* 28:664-667, 1977.

174. Gerety, R.J., Poplack, D.G., Hoofnagle, J.H., et al.: Hepatitis B virus infection in the Wiskott-Aldrich syndrome. *J. Ped.* 88:561-564, 1976.

175. Srivastava, R.N.: Wiskott-Aldrich syndrome. *Arch. Dis. Child.* 42:604-607, 1967.

176. Stiehm, E.R., and McIntosh, R.M.: Wiskott-Aldrich syndrome: review and report of a large family. *Clin. Exp. Immunol.* 2:179-189, 1967.

177. Kildeberg, P.: The Aldrich syndrome: report of a case and discussion of pathogenesis. *Pediatrics* 27:362-369, 1961.

178. Levin, A.S., Spitler, L.E., Stites, D.P., and Fudenberg, H.H.: Wiskott-Aldrich syndrome, a genetically determined cellular immunologic deficiency: clinical and laboratory responses to therapy with transfer factor. *Proc. Natl. Acad. Sci. USA* 67:821-828, 1970.

179. Mackie, R.M., Alcorn, M.J., Stevenson, R.D., et al.: Wiskott-Aldrich syndrome with partial response to transfer factor. *Br. J. Derm.* 98:567-571, 1978.

180. Millikan, L.E.: Wiskott-Aldrich syndrome: a treatable immune disorder. *Mo. Med.* 70:764-767, 1973.

181. Root, A.W., and Speicher, C.E.: The triad of thrombocytopenia, eczema, and recurrent infections (Wiskott-Aldrich syndrome) associated with milk antibodies, giant cell pneumonia, and cytomegalic inclusion disease. *Pediatrics* 31:444-454, 1963.

182. Canales, L., and Mauer, A.M.: Sex-linked hereditary thrombocytopenia as a variant of Wiskott-Aldrich syndrome. *N. Eng. J. Med.* 277:899-901, 1967.

183. Diaz-Buxo, J.A., Hermans, P.E., and Ritts, R.E., Jr.: Wiskott-Aldrich syndrome in an adult. *Mayo Clin. Proc.* 49:455-459, 1974.

184. Blease, R.M., Strober, W., Brown, R.S., and Waldmann, T.A.: The Wiskott-Aldrich syndrome: a disorder with a possible defect in antigen processing or recognition. *Lancet* 1:1056-1061, 1968.

185. Oppenheim, J.J., Blease, R.M., and Waldmann, T.A.: Defective lymphocyte transformation and delayed hypersensitivity in Wiskott-Aldrich syndrome. *J. Immunol.* 104:835-844, 1970.

186. Blease, R.M., Oppenheim, J.J., Seeger, R.C., and Waldmann, T.A.: Lymphocyte-macrophage interaction in antigen induced in vitro lymphocyte transformation in patients with the Wiskott-Aldrich syndrome and other diseases with anergy. *Cell. Immunol.* 4:228-242, 1972.

187. Blease, R. M., Strober, W., and Waldmann, T. A.: Immunodeficiency in the Wiskott-Aldrich syndrome. *Birth Defects* 11:250-254, 1975.

188. Radl, J., Dooren, L.J., Morell, A., et al.: Immunoglobulins and transient paraproteins in sera of patients with the Wiskott-Aldrich syndrome: a followup study. *Clin. Exp. Immunol.* 25:256-263, 1976.

189. Ammann, A.J., and Hong, R.: Cellular immunodeficiency disorders. In: *Immunologic Disorders in Infants and Children* (E.R. Stiehm and V.A. Fulginiti, Eds.). Philadelphia, PA: W.B. Saunders, 1973, p. 242.

190. Bruce, R.M., and Blease, R.M.: Monoclonal gammopathy in the Wiskott-Aldrich syndrome. *J. Ped.* 85:204-207, 1974.

191. Kreuger, G.R.F., Malangren, R.A., and Beard, C.W.: Malignant lymphomas and plasmacytosis in mice under prolonged immunosuppression and persistent antigenic stimulation. *Transplantation* 11:138-144, 1971.

192. Takemoto, K.K., Rabson, A.S., Mullarkey, M.F., et al.: Isolation of papovavirus from brain tumor and urine of a patient with Wiskott-Aldrich syndrome. *JNCI* 53: 1205-1207, 1974.

193. Geha, R.S., Schneeberger, E., Merler, E., and Rosen, F.S.: Heterogeneity of "acquired" or common variable agammaglobulinemia. *N. Eng. J. Med.* 291:1-6, 1974.

194. Kopp, W.L., Trier, J.S., Stiehm, E.R., and Foroozan, P.: "Acquired" agammaglobulinemia with defective delayed hypersensitivity. *Ann. Int. Med.* 69:309-317, 1968.

195. Douglas, S.D., Goldberg, L.S., and Fudenberg, H.H.: Clinical, serologic, and leukocyte function studies on patients with histopathic "acquired" agammaglobulinemia and their families. *Am. J. Med.* 48:48-53, 1970.

196. Hermans, P.E., Diza-Buxo, J.A., and Stobo, J.D.: Idiopathic late onset immunoglobulin deficiency: clinical observations in 50 patients. *Am. J. Med.* 61:221-237, 1976.

197. Hermans, P.E., Huizenga, K.A., Hoffman, H.N., et al.: Dysgammaglobulinemia associated with nodular lymphoid hyperplasia of the small intestine. *Am. J. Med.* 40: 78-80, 1966.

198. Twomey, J.J., Jordan, P.H., Jarrold, T., et al.: The syndrome of immunoglobulin deficiency and pernicious anemia: a study of 10 cases. *Am. J. Med.* 47:340-350, 1969.

199. Battle, W.M., and Brooks, F.P.: Adenocarcinoma of the stomach with common variable immunodeficiency syndrome. *Arch. Int. Med.* 138:1682-1684, 1978.

200. Hermans, P.E., and Huizenga, K.A.: Association of gastric carcinoma with idiopathic late onset immunoglobulin deficiency. *Ann. Int. Med.* 76:605-609, 1972.

201. Ciccimarra, F., Rosen, F.S., Schneeberger, E., and Merler, E.: Failure of heavy chain glycosylation of IgG in some patients with common, variable agammaglobulinemia. *J. Clin. Invest.* 57:1386-1390, 1976.

202. Gafni, J., Michaeli, D., and Heller, H.: Idiopathic acquired agammaglobulinemia associated with thymoma. *N. Eng. J. Med.* 263:536-541, 1960.

203. Davis, S.D.: Antibody deficiency diseases. In: *Immunologic Disorders in Infants and Children* (E.R. Stiehm and V.A. Fulginiti, Eds.). Philadelphia, PA: W.B. Saunders, 1973, p. 184.

204. Cooperband, S.R., Rosen, F.S., and Kibrick, S.: Studies on the in vitro behavior of agammaglobulinemic lymphocytes. *J. Clin. Invest.* 47:836-847, 1968.

205. Geha, R.S., Rosen, F.S., and Merler, E.: Identification and characterization of subpopulations of lymphocytes in human peripheral blood after fractionation on discontinuous gradients of albumin. *J. Clin. Invest.* 52:1726-1734, 1973.

206. Abdou, M.I., Casella, S.R., Abdou, N. L., and Abrahamsohn, I.A.: Comparative study of bone marrow and blood B cells in infantile and acquired agammaglobulinemia. *J. Clin. Invest.* 52:2218-2224, 1973.

207. Cooper, M.D., Lawton, A.R., and Bockman, D.E.: Agammaglobulinemia with B lymphocytes: specific defect of plasma-cell differentiation. *Lancet* 2:791-794, 1971.

208. Ochs, H.D., Davis, S.D., and Wedgwood, R.J.: Immunologic responses to bacteriophage ϕX174 in immunodeficiency diseases. *J. Clin. Invest.* 50:2559-2568, 1971.

209. Ching, Y-C, Davis, S.D., and Wedgwood, R.J.: Antibody studies in hypogammaglobulinemia. *J. Clin. Invest.* 45:1593-1600, 1966.

210. Gellman, E.F., and Vietti, T.J.: Congenital hypogammaglobulinemia preceding Hodgkin's disease: a case report and review of the literature. *J. Ped.* 76:131-133, 1970.
211. Hobbs, J.R.: Immune imbalance in dysgammaglobulinemia type IV. *Lancet* 1:110-114, 1968.
212. Ammann, A.J., and Hong, R.: Selective IgA deficiency. In: *Immunologic Disorders in Infants and Children* (E.R. Stiehm and V.A. Fulginiti, Eds.). Philadelphia, PA: W.B. Saunders, 1973, p. 199.
213. Ammann, A.J., and Hong, R.: Selective IgA deficiency: presentation of 30 cases and a review of the literature. *Medicine* 50:223-236, 1971.
214. Ammann, A.J., and Hong, R.: Selective IgA deficiency and autoimmunity. *Clin. Exp. Immunol.* 7:833-838, 1970.
215. Arnold, R.R., Cole, M.F., Prince, S., and McGhee, J.R.: Secreting IgM antibodies to Streptococcus mutans in subjects with selective IgA deficiency. *Clin. Exp. Immunol.* 8:475-486, 1977.
216. Hobbs, J.R.: IgM deficiency. *Birth Defects* 11:112-116, 1975.
217. Hobbs, J.R., Milner, R.D.G., and Watt, P.J.: Gamma-M deficiency predisposing to meningococcal septicemia. *Br. Med. J.* 4:583-586, 1967.
218. Faulk, W.P., Kiyasu, W.S., Cooper, M.D., and Fudenberg, H.H.: Deficiency of IgM. *Pediatrics* 47:399-404, 1971.
219. Chandra, R.K., Kameramma, B., and Soothill, J.F.: Generalized nonprogressive vaccinia associated with IgM deficiency. *Lancet* 1:687, 1969.
220. Stoelinga, G.B.A., van Munster, P.J.J., and Sloff, J.P.: Antibody deficiency, dysimmunoglobulinemia type 5. *Acta Paediat. Scand.* 58:352-362, 1969.
221. Morell, A., Skvaril, F., and Barandun, S.: Serum concentrations of IgG subclasses. In: *Clinical Immunology* (F.H. Bach and R.A. Good, Eds.). New York: Academic Press, 1976, p. 37.
222. Schur, P.H., Borel, H., Gelfand, E.W., et al.: Selective gamma-G globulin deficiencies in patients with recurrent pyogenic infections. *N. Eng. J. Med.* 283:631-633, 1970.
223. Yount, W.J.: Imbalances of IgG subclasses and gene defect in patients with primary hypogammaglobulinemia. *Birth Defects* 11:99-107, 1975.
224. Morell, A., Skvaril, F., Radl, J., et al.: IgG-subclass abnormalities in primary immune deficiency diseases. *Birth Defects* 11:108-116, 1975.
225. Stiehm, E.R., and Fudenberg, H.H.: Clinical and immunologic features of dysgammaglobulinemia type I: report of a case diagnosed in the first year of life. *Am. J. Med.* 40:805-815, 1966.
226. Hobbs, J.R., Russell, A., and Worlledge, S.M.: Dysgammaglobulinemia type IV C. *Clin. Exp. Immunol.* 2:589-599, 1967.
227. Geha, R.S., Hyslop, N., Alami, S., et al.: Hyperimmunoglobulin-M deficiency (dysgammaglobulinemia): presence of IgM-secreting plasmacytoid cells in peripheral blood and failure of IgM-IgG switch in B cell differentiation. *J. Clin. Invest.* 64:385-391, 1979.
228. Blecher, T.E., Soothill, J.F., Voyce, M.A., and Walker, W.H.G.: Antibody deficiency syndrome: a case with normal immunoglobulin levels. *Clin. Exp. Immunol.* 3:47, 1968.
229. Rothback, C., Nagel, J., Rabin, B., and Fireman, P.: Antibody deficiency with normal immunoglobulins. *J. Ped.* 94:250-253, 1979.
230. Hakami, N., Neiman, P.E., Canellos, G.P., and Lazerson, J.: Neonatal megaloblastic anemia due to inherited transcobalamin II deficiency in two siblings. *N. Eng. J. Med.* 285:1163-1170, 1971.
231. Hitzig, W.H., Dohmann, U., Pluss, H.J., and Vischer, D.: Hereditary transcobalamin II deficiency: clinical findings in a new family. *J. Ped.* 85:622-628, 1974.

232. Janeway, C.A., and Gitlin, D.: Gammaglobulins. *Adv. Ped.* 9:65, 1957.
233. Fudenberg, H.H., and Fudenberg, B.R.: Antibody to hereditary human gammaglobulin (GM) factor resulting from maternal-fetal incompatibility. *Science* 145:170-171, 1964.
234. Miller, M.E.: The immunodeficiencies of immaturity. In: *Immunologic Disorders in Infants and Children* (E.R. Stiehm and V.A. Fulginiti, Eds.). Philadelphia, PA: W.B. Saunders, 1973, p. 168.
235. Lischner, H.W., and Huff, D.S.: T cell deficiency in DiGeorge syndrome. *Birth Defects* 11:16-21, 1975.
236. Lischner, H.W.: DiGeorge syndrome(s). *J. Ped.* 81:1042-1044, 1972.
237. Hitzig, W.H.: Congenital thymic and lymphocytic deficiency disorders. In: *Immunologic Disorders in Infants and Children* (E.R. Stiehm and V.A. Fulginiti, Eds.). Philadelphia, PA: W.B. Saunders, 1973, p. 215.
238. Conley, M.E., Bechwith, J.B., Maucer, J.F.K., and Tenckhoff, L.: The spectrum of the DiGeorge syndrome. *J. Ped.* 94:883-890, 1979.
239. Pabst, H.F., Wright, W.C., LeRiche, J., and Stiehm, E.R.: Partial DiGeorge syndrome with substantial cell-mediated immunity. *Am. J. Dis. Child.* 130:316-319, 1976.
240. Gatti, R.A., Gershanik, J.J., Levkoff, A.H., et al.: DiGeorge syndrome associated with combined immunodeficiency. *J. Ped.* 81:920-926, 1972.
241. Kretschmer, R., August, C.S., Rosen, F.S., and Janeway, C.A.: Recurrent infections, episodic lymphopenia, and impaired cellular immunity: further observations on "immunologic amnesia" in two siblings. *N. Eng. J. Med.* 281:285-290, 1969.
242. Kreisler, M.J., Hirata, A.A., and Terasaki, P.I.: Cytotoxins in disease III: antibodies against lymphocytes produced by vaccination. *Transplantation* 10:411-415, 1970.
243. Gelfand, E.W., Parkman, R., and Rosen, F.S.: Lymphocytotoxins and immunologic unresponsiveness. *Birth Defects* 11:158-162, 1975.
244. Ammann, A.J., and Hong, R.: Cellular immunodeficiency disorders. In: *Immunologic Disorders in Infants and Children* (E.R. Stiehm and V.A. Fulginiti, Eds.). Philadelphia, PA: W.B. Saunders, 1973, p. 266.
245. Giblett, E.R., Ammann, A.J., Wara, D.W., et al.: Nucleoside phosphorylase deficiency in a child with severely defective T cell immunity and normal B cell immunity. *Lancet* 1:1010-1013, 1975.
246. Polmar, S.H.: Metabolic aspects of immunodeficiency disease. *Sem. Hemat.* 17:30-43, 1980.
247. Ammann, A.J., Wara, D.W., and Allen, T.: Immunotherapy and immunopathologic studies in a patient with nucleoside phosphorylase deficiency. *Clin. Immunol. Immunopath.* 10:262-269, 1978.
248. Vivelizier, J.L., Hamet, M., Ballet, J.J., et al.: Impaired defense against vaccinia in a child with T-lymphocyte deficiency associated with inosine phosphorylase defect. *J. Ped.* 92:362, 1978.
249. Biggar, W.D., Giblett, E.R., Ozere, R.L., et al.: A new form of nucleoside phosphorylase deficiency in two brothers with defective T cell function. *J. Ped.* 92:354-357, 1978.
250. Carpella-de Luca, E., Aiuti, F., Lucarella, P., et al.: A patient with nucleoside phosphorylase deficiency, selective T cell deficiency, and autoimmune hemolytic anemia. *J. Ped.* 93:1000-1003, 1978.
251. Gelfand, E.W., Dosch, H.M., Biggar, W.D., et al.: Purine nucleoside phosphorylase deficiency: studies of lymphocyte function. *J. Clin. Invest.* 61:1071-1080, 1978.
252. Stoop, J.W., Zegers, B.J.M., Hendricks, G.F.M., et al.: Purine nucleoside phosphorylase deficiency associated with selective cellular immunodeficiency. *N. Eng. J. Med.* 296:651, 655, 1977.

8
Sebaceous Neoplasia and Visceral Cancer (Torre's Syndrome) and Its Relationship to the Cancer Family Syndrome

Henry T. Lynch, M.D., Patrick M. Lynch, J.D., Judith A. Pester, M.D.
and Ramon M. Fusaro, M.D., Ph.D.

INTRODUCTION

The history of medicine has many examples of disorders whose physical signs were unknown or incompletely known for a period of time after the cancer association was recognized. For example, in the family originally reported by Gardner,[1] the abnormal dentition that was a component of the polyposis–epidermal cyst-osteoma complex was not recognized until after the feature had been documented in unrelated families[2] and further study of the original kindred.[3] In our own studies, kindreds with malignant melanoma clustering were initially thought to lack precancerous signs. Several family reports[4,5] of a multiple atypical mole precursor to melanoma (FAMMM syndrome) have now established the addition of a new cancer-associated ganodermatosis to the existing roster (see Chapter 9).

Of more immediate interest to this discussion has been the recent suggestion[6] of an association between the relatively obscure disorder, Torre's syndrome,[7-20] and the more frequently encountered cancer family syndrome (CFS).[21-38] We shall describe studies performed to date on these disorders and our basis for believing that Torre's "syndrome" is merely an expression of the pleiotropic gene responsible for the CFS.

Summary of Torre's Syndrome Characteristics

Although there have not been a great many case reports of Torre's syndrome, the clinical similarities of the respective cases have been striking: (1) There have been multiple cutaneous lesions involving sebaceous gland neoplasia, but including also, in a given patient, a wide range of squamous and basal cell lesions with greater or lesser degrees of sebaceous cell differentiation; (2) There is early onset of visceral cancers, predominantly of the gastrointestinal tract; (3) One finds multiple, synchronous or metachronous occurrence of such visceral lesions; (4) Even when their internal malignancies are invasive or show evidence of metastases, such patients have exceptional survival; the infrequency of metastases as a sequelae of invasive malignancy may itself be a central feature of the syndrome; (5) The occurrence of comparatively rare duodenal malignancy in several patients described suggests that it too may be an integral component of the syndrome; (6) The fact that several of the reported family histories are suggestively positive for visceral malignancy and for vairably described cutaneous lesions supports the notion that a heritable factor may be involved.

TORRE'S SYNDROME

In 1967, Torre reported the case of a 57-year-old man with asymptomatic papular, waxy lesions of the face, trunk, and scalp, variously documented as "sebaceous adenomas," "sebaceous carcinomas," and "basal cell epitheliomata with sebaceous differentiation."[7] Almost incidentally, the patient was reported to have had a primary carcinoma of the ampulla of Vater (age 48) and a primary carcinoma of the colon (age 51); no mention was made of presence or absence of a family history of either the unusual skin lesions or the internal cancer.

Earlier in 1967, Muir, Yates-Bell, and Barlow[8] reported the rather striking case of a patient with at least seven internal carcinomas associated with multiple molluscum sebaceum (keratoacanthoma). Specifically, the patient was diagnosed with a moderately differentiated squamous cell carcinoma of the larynx (Broder's Grade III) at age 37, followed by diagnosis of four, apparently primary, carcinomata located predominantly in the proximal colon, as well as three benign colonic polyps. At age 41, two primary malignancies of the duodenum, including a periampullary carcinoma that obscured the ampulla itself, were noted. It was stated that ". . .this patient's growths may have been of low malignancy, though this was not suggested by their histologic appearance." In other words, the authors found it remarkable that none of the rather invasive tumors had metastasized. During the six-year period prior to, and all during, this previously described sequence of events, the patient had been diagnosed with recurrent, multiple molluscum sebaceum of the face, none described as cancerous. The lesions ranged ". . .from hyperplasia of a group of follicles with hyperkeratosis of the lining epithelium. . .to that of the fully developed keratoacanthoma in which numerous hyperkeratotic follicles had merged into a crater-like mass . . . . The base of the lesion showed regular downgrowths of squamous epithelium forming keratin and associated with a heavy infiltrate of chronic inflammatory cells in the adjacent dermis." Yet another lesion was histologically described as a sebaceous adenoma, ". . . a highly differentiated sebaceous gland tumour composed of irregular lobules consisting of a peripheral layer of generative basal cells with a central mass of mature sebaceous cells."

In 1974, Bitran and Pellettiere[9] reported a woman who also had multiple sebaceous adenomas but who, rather than developing multiple gastrointestinal neoplasia, manifested at age 33 an epidermoid carcinoma of the vulva followed at age 43 by an adenocarcinoma of the endometrium, metastatic to the lung. Unlike the earlier reports, this woman did have evidence of frank metastases from the primary lesion, but as in the earlier cases, she recovered uneventfully, despite the originally poor prognosis.

In 1971, Bakker and Tjon A Joe[10] reported the first case of Torre's syndrome in which a family history was reported (father of the patient died of colon cancer). At age 43, the reported patient manifested a well-differentiated squamous cell carcinoma of the cheek which, on independent evaluation, appeared more like a benign keratoacanthoma. The following year, at age 44, a large, ulcerating carcinoma of the ascending colon was diagnosed, invading the fatty mesocolon but with no nodes involved. Nine years later, a sebaceous gland carcinoma of the back was excised followed by 18 similar lesions in the ensuing years, appearing on the back, breast, face, and extremities. At age 63, a carcinoma of the transverse colon was diagnosed and, at age 65, an anaplastic carcinoma of the stomach. In discussing etiology, the authors state that "the factor responsible for this predisposition to tumor formation in this special place (sebaceous cells) remains uncertain. Extrinsic physical and chemical agents cannot perhaps be totally excluded but seem improbable; a chronic disease of the sebaceous gland and hair sheath cells that could have given rise to a precancerous state can be reasonably excluded. Therefore, a hereditary predisposition seems to be the most important factor and becomes, in our view, quite acceptable because the only cases of multiple tumors of sebaceous glands described in the literature were seen in patients with multiple tumors in widely different organs." They conclude that their case, as well as those of Torre[7] and Muir et al.[8] "are examples of a rare syndrome, characterized by the occurrence of multiple lesions of the skin, partly sebaceous gland tumors and partly keratoacanthoma, in patients with multiple tumors of the internal organs, mostly of a low grade of malignancy."

In 1973, Rulon and Helwig[11] reviewed 105 cases of sebaceous neoplasia from the Armed Forces Institute of Pathology charts and found five patients who had also had internal cancer. The five cases were similar in that each involved cutaneous lesions of widely varying histologic appearance and each had multiple visceral carcinomas, typically of the proximal colon, with each case showing prolonged survival.

In 1974, Jakobiec[12] reported a patient who, in addition to the characteristic sebaceous adenomas and keratoacanthomas, exhibited a fungating carcinoma of the rectosigmoid at age 49. This patient's family history was the most striking reported up to that time, in that the father had a benign fibrous growth of the colon at age 36, and also had skin lesions described as squamous cell carcinomas, basal cell epithelioma, and pseudoepitheliomatous hyperplasia in his 60s. At age 65, a right hemicolectomy was performed on the father for carcinoma, followed at age 69 by a left hemicolectomy for a second colonic carcinoma.

In 1974, Sciallis and Winkelmann[13] reported two cases of Torre's syndrome. The first patient, a white male, presented with sebaceous adenoma of the temple at age 42, followed by sebaceous adenoma of the upper back at age 55, basal cell carcinoma and sebaceous adenoma of the chest at age 56, and two sebaceous adenomas of the forehead at age 57. Sebaceous hyperplasia of the nasolabial fold was also reported to have occurred at age 57. At age 53, a Grade III adenocarcinoma of the cecum was diagnosed. No polyposis was evident. No recurrence of the tumor was reported. The father of this patient was reported to have had an adenocarcinoma of the colon at age 40 and lived to age 77. The patient could not recall whether or not the father had cutaneous lesions.

The second case was a white female who, at age 57, manifested a Grade III adenocarcinoma of the hepatic flexure, without invasion. At age 60, a sebaceous adenoma was removed from the occipital region of the scalp. There was reported to have been no recurrence of either the colonic or cutaneous lesions. The family history was not reported.

Also in 1974, Leonard and Deaton[14] reported the case of a white female who, at age 47, was diagnosed with carcinoma of the descending colon, invading the muscularis but without evidence of lymph node metastases. At age 52, squamous cell carcinoma of the vocal cord was diagnosed, and at age 56, a noninvasive adenocarcinoma of the enodmetrium was treated; none of the lesions recurred. Between the ages of 55 and 63, six sebaceous adenomas and squamous cell carcinomas of the skin were removed from the left breast, anterior chest wall, neck, left arm, and back. The family history was quite significant in that the mother was reported to have had carcinoma, as were six of ten sibs; the lesions included two carcinomas of the cervix, one of the colon, three that were "other gastrointestinal," and one cancer whose primary site was unknown.

In 1976, Reiffers et al.[15] reported a case of a 45-year-old Swiss male diagnosed with multiple sebaceous hyperplasia, benign adenoacanthoma, keratoacanthoma, and squamous cell epitheliomas, primarily of the face. Previously, at age 34, an adenocarcinoma of the sigmoid colon with a second primary located more proximally in the colon were diagnosed. At age 43, an epidermoid cancer of the external auditory meatus was detected; a micropolyp of the rectosigmoid was removed at this time. A villous adenoma of the colon was removed at age 45 at approximately the same time that the multiple skin lesions appeared. This patient presented with a most remarkable and informative family history, describing for the first time in the literature of Torre's syndrome the degree of variable expressivity that can occur. The patient's brother died at age 33 of intestinal cancer and was reported to have had none of the cutaneous lesions observed in the proband. Conversely, their father mainfested cutaneous lesions, reported to have been quite similar to those observed in the proband, yet did not manifest intestinal cancer.

Also in 1976, Tschang et al.[16] reported the following case: a 40-year-old white female underwent a hysterectomy for endometrial carcinoma, followed at age 46 by a Duke's A adenocarcinoma of the rectum and a Duke's B adeno-carcinoma of the sigmoid colon. One of the resected colonic lesions involved the periureteral soft tissue and ileal wall. Between ages 48 and 50, two sebaceous adenomas and two keratoacanthomas were removed from her face. At age 54, lesions described as keratoacanthoma (left cheek) and basal cell carcinoma (infraorbital) were excised. Her family history was also significant in that her father and seven of his ten siblings were reported to have died of abdominal malignancy. Of the patient's four siblings, one had endometrial carcinoma and skin lesions, of undertermined type.

The one example of a patient with multiple sebaceous gland tumors who showed evidence of polyposis was that reported by Lynn-Davies et al.[18] in 1974. At age 48, a white male was diagnosed by sigmoidoscopy as having "many sessile and pedunculated polypoid tumors, varying in size between 1 and 2 cm, beginning at the anal verge." Radiography and subsequent laparotomy demonstrated "multiple polyposis of the large bowel." A 6 × 5 cm, well-differentiated papillary adenocarcinoma was detected in the cecum. Several regional lymph nodes were extensively replaced with secondary adenocarcinoma. During the 25 years prior to this time, multiple asymptomatic tumors of the forehead, face, and upper trunk had gradually increased in size and number. Skin biopsies performed at approximately the same time as the colon surgery showed the lesions to be sebaceous adenomata. Two years later, a 1 cm osteoma of the right tibia was shown on skeletal survey. The patient died at age 52 and at autopsy was found to have massive metastatic adenocarcinoma of the liver. Additional findings included exostosis of the right calcaneus and right tibia, neural hamartoma of the right adrenal medulla, and solitary chromophobe adenoma of the pituitary.

The patient's sister had had a carcinoma of the large bowel removed 20 years previously at age 26; although no further details were provided, there had apparently been no recurrence. Another sister manifested multiple cutaneous lesions of the forehead, face, and upper trunk and, although small and less numerous than those observed in her brother, they had the same microscopic appearance. Evaluation of the colon showed only a small (4 mm) sessile adenomatous polyp of the rectum. Although the patients in this report bear a superficial resemblance to the expression seen in Gardner's syndrome, the noncystic nature of the sebaceous lesions and the lack of polyposis in the sister with cutaneous lesions may serve to distinguish these cases from the typical expression of Gardner's syndrome.

In an excellent review of differential diagnosis of sebaceous tumors, Sciallis and Winkelman[13] differentiated the sebaceous adenoma/sebaceous gland carcinomas that occur in Torre's syndrome from several other disorders (see also Table 8-1). The sebaceous nevus of Jadassohn is distinguished on the basis of its congenital onset. Senile sebaceous hyperplasia lacks stromal reaction or atypical keratinization; moreover, the authors found no relationship to gastrointestinal malignancy in a review of 50 cases from the Mayo Clinic with 10-year follow-up. A review by Nickel and Reed,[39] cited by Sciallis and Winkelmann, would delete adenoma sebaceum from classification as a sebaceous gland disorder. Nevertheless, for completeness, the disorder has been listed in Table 8-1.

Recently, Anderson reported a family in which four of five patients with colonic or small bowel cancer supposedly had skin tumors consistent with Torre's syndrome.[19] One patient, a male, was diagnosed at age 49 with duodenal carcinoma, and three basal cell carcinomas which were treated between ages 48 and 49. A second member of this family was diagnosed with carcinoma of the sigmoid colon at age 70; between ages 73 and 91, he had multiple skin lesions classified as basal cell carcinoma, sebaceous hyperplasia, keratoacanthoma, and actinic and seborrheic keratoses. A third male relative was diagnosed with carcinoma of the rectosigmoid colon at age 43 and was found at age 51 to have "multiple hyperkeratotic lesions." The status of the fourth patient was not discussed in Anderson's text.

In no case did there appear to be histopathologic verification of the more unusual lesions associated with Torre's syndrome (i.e., sebaceous adenoma, epithelioma, and carcinoma) which characterized the earlier case reports. It is entirely possible that independent dermatopathologic review of existing slides and tissue sections, coupled with intensive screening of affected and high risk patients, might have disclosed such cases in the family reported by Anderson. This issue is stressed because it is apparent that a consensus is lacking as to precisely what cutaneous lesions are actually associated with visceral neoplasms in Torre's syndrome. Because lesions such as basal and squamous cell carcinomas, and actinic and seborrheic keratoses, are so common in older age groups, they cannot (and should not) serve as evidence that the syndrome exists in any given patient.

One of the most insightful case reports of Torre's syndrome was that of Householder and Zeligman,[20] who reported the following cases:

Case 1: The patient was diagnosed at age 59 with a keratoacanthoma, sebaceous adenoma, and later a sebaceous carcinoma and another sebaceous adenoma. At age 64, a second keratoacanthoma was removed and in the following three years, two sebaceous epitheliomas were removed. At age 39, the cecum was removed because of cancer, and at age 53, cancer of the transverse colon was resected. In later years, several isolated adenomatous polyps were removed.

Case 2: A 71-year-old woman had a 20-year history of a lesion ultimately diagnosed as a sebaceous adenoma. At age 45, carcinoma of the uterus was diagnosed and at age 59, the colon was resected for adenocarcinoma.

Table 8-1. Differential Diagnosis.*

DISORDER	
Torre's syndrome[6-20]	Single or multiple sebaceous neoplasia, associated with early onset and multiple primary visceral cancer (typically GI) in absence of polyposis. Prolonged survival common. Familiality suggested but not rigorously evaluated
Cancer family syndrome[21-38]	Early onset, multiple primary visceral cancer (predominantly proximal colon and endometrial) in absence of polyposis. Prolonged suvival common. Some patients show evidence of sebaceous neoplasia. Familial clustering repeatedly documented as consistent with autosomal dominant genetic transmission
Signs of Leser-Trelat[43-44]	"Sudden appearance and rapid increase in size and number of seborrheic keratoses" secondary to internal cancer (usually adenocarcinoma and frequently of the stomach). As in acanthosis nigricans,[45] skin changes postulated to be result of latent genetic abnormality which is only expressed in the presence of a highly malignant carcinoma
Gardner's syndrome[46]	Colonic polyposis as of familial polyposis coli (hereditary basis well established). Sebaceous cyst as leading skin sign; also osteomas (mandible, maxilla, skull, common sites), abnormal dentition, abdominal fibrosis; (less frequently) desmoid tumors, periampullary malignancy
Perifollicular dermal fibroma with colon polyps[47,48]	Multiple dermal perifollicular fibromas, appearing as skin tags (one family report). Associated isolated adenomatous colon polyps
Tuberous sclerosis[49] (epiloia, Bourneville's disease)	Autosomal dominant inheritance. Cerebral cortical nodules (neural deficiency, epilepsy, death before age 20 common). Angiofibromas (adenoma sebaceum) at nasolabial folds; shagreen patches; ash leaf depigmentation; retinal tumor; rhabdomyosarcoma; skeletal abnormality; kidney and heart tumors
Nevoid basal cell carcinoma syndrome[50]	Multiple nevoid basal cell cancers, frontal bossing, hypertelorism, bone cysts, bifid ribs, agenesis of corpus callosum, brachymetacarpalism, palmar pits, endocrine anomalies, medulloblastoma, jaw fibrosarcoma, ameloblastoma, ovarian fibroma. Autosomal dominance well established. No significant GI or other adenocarcinoma association
Generalized keratoacanthoma[51]	Diffuse eruptive keratoacanthomas with pruritus and mucous membrane involvement but without internal malignancy. Multiple or solitary keratoacanthoma with squamous carcinoma of larynx,[52] rectum, and anus.[53] May in fact be related to Torre's syndrome except that sebaceous lesions and adenocarcinomas are not expressed

*Several of the disorders listed are clearly not examples of sebaceous gland activity, hereditary disease, or gastrointestinal tract cancer associations, but have been listed in the interest of providing a broader background.

Both patients were reported to have had positive family histories of colon cancer, though no information was available regarding the status of relevant skin lesions in close relatives. Householder and Zeligman suggested that the key feature of Torre's syndrome was the occurrence of sebaceous neoplasia with visceral cancer and that keratoacanthoma was frequent, though not invariably present. Thus, these authors suggested that the patient could not be classified as having Torre's syndrome on the basis of visceral neoplasm and keratoacanthoma alone, but that sebaceous neoplasia is essential. The authors disagreed with several earlier commentaries which had suggested that the skin lesions were in some way a consequence of visceral malignancy; Householder and Zeligman's review indicated that roughly one-third of the reported patients had had sebaceous neoplasia prior to the onset of colonic and other visceral cancer and that, in this respect, there was some predictive value in the lesions themselves. Commenting upon the predictive potential of sebaceous adenomas and carcinomas, these authors suggested that any patient presenting with such a skin lesion should be evaluated for possible presence of visceral cancer. Finally, because of the frequent suggestion of positive family histories, loosely documented though they were, the presence of Torre's syndrome in a given patient was considered adequate indication for evaluation and screening of close relatives. However, the report did not specify the need for stool guaiac and barium enema as means of achieving early detection of colorectal cancer, the most frequently occurring visceral malignancy.

Summary and Classification of Skin Lesions

Previous case reports of Torre's syndrome (Table 8-2) described a range of cutaneous lesions, including sebaceous adenoma, sebaceous epithelioma, sebaceous carcinoma, keratoacanthoma, and a variety of lesions encountered frequently in older individuals, such as seborrheic and actinic keratoses, as well as typical basal and squamous cell carcinomas. Obviously, the sebaceous lesions and, to a lesser extent, the keratoacanthomas, when coupled with visceral malignancy, form the core criteria for Torre's syndrome. The remaining skin lesions appear to have been catalogued mainly for purposes of completeness. It seems unlikely that one would classify a patient as having Torre's syndrome if that patient had, in addition to visceral malignancy, only the more commonly encountered skin lesions described above.

The Cancer Family Syndrome

The following paragraphs will suggest that Torre's syndrome represents a variant of the much more frequently encountered cancer family syndrome. Although the Creighton group has contributed a number of case reports of the

Table 8-2. Case Reports.

| | CUTANEOUS MANIFESTATIONS AND VISCERAL CARCINOMA | | | |
SOURCE	SEBACEOUS ADENOMAS	OTHER SKIN LESIONS*	VISCERAL TUMORS AND CARCINOMAS	FAMILY HISTORY OF TUMORS
Muir et al.[8]	Multiple	Keratoacanthomas	Larynx, colon, duodenum	
Torre[7]	Multiple	Sebaceous carcinoma, sebaceous BCC, SCC	Ampulla of Vater, colon	
Rulon and Helwig[11]				
Case 1	10	Keratoacanthoma, sebaceous hyperplasia, SCC	Colon	
Case 2	2	Sebaceous BCC	Renal pelvis, urinary bladder	Father: carcinoma of colon and prostate
Case 3	11	Benign keratosis, dermatofibroma	Colon, ureter	
Case 4	8	Epidermal cysts	Colon, stomach	Sister: carcinoma of breast; brother: carcinoma of colon, colon polyps, carcinoma of bladder; brother: carcinoma of liver
Case 5	2	Sebaceous BCC	Colon	
Bitran and Pellettiere[9]	8	Sebaceous epithelioma, SCC of vulva	Endometrium	
Bakker and Tjon A Joe[10]	19	Keratoacanthomas	Colon, stomach	Father: carcinoma of colon

Table 8-2. (Cont.)

Sciallis and Winkelmann[13]				
Case 1	5	BCC, sebaceous hyperplasia	Ileocecal valve	Father: carcinoma of colon
Case 2	1	None	Colon	Negative
Jakobiec[12]	17	Keratoacanthoma, sebaceous hyperplasias, sebaceous BCC	Rectosigmoid	Father: carcinoma of colon
Leonard and Deaton[14]	6	SCC	Colon, larynx, endometrium	Carcinoma of colon, cervix, gastrointestinal tract
Tschang et al.[16]	5	Keratoacanthomas, BCC	Endometrium, rectum, sigmoid colon	Father: carcinoma; sister: carcinoma of endometrium
Reiffers et al.[15]	5	Keratoacanthoma, sebaceous epitheliomas, sebaceous hyperplasias, SCC	Rectosigmoid, colon	Brother: carcinoma of colon
Householder and Zeligman[20]				
Case 1	2	Keratoacanthomas, sebaceous epitheliomas, sebaceous carcinoma, carcinoma of adnexal origin	Colon, duodenum	Father: carcinoma of colon; mother: carcinoma of uterus; brother: carcinoma
Case 2	1	None	Colon, uterus	Mother: carcinoma of liver; son: carcinoma of rectum
Poleksic[17]	None	Keratoacanthoma, SCC	Colon, prostrate, esophagus	

Table 8-2. (Cont.)

Lynne-Davies and Brown[18]				
Case 1	Multiple	None	Colon	Sister: carcinoma of colon
Case 2	Multiple	None	Colon	
Anderson[19]				
Case 1	None	BCC	Duodenal	All three patients from same kindred
Case 2	None	BCC, sebaceous hyperplasia, keratoacanthoma	Colon	
Case 3	None	SCC	Colon	
Our patients				
(C-113) (III-3)	None	Sebaceous epithelioma	Distal colon, proximal colon, endometrium, rectum	Numerous blood relatives with cancers of CFS type[22]
(C-197) (III-2)	None	Sebaceous epithelioma	Endometrium, proximal colon	Numerous blood relatives with cancers of CFS type
(C-197) (III-1)	1	Keratoacanthoma	Rectum, distal colon	Numerous blood relatives with cancers of CFS type
(C-200) (III-11)	1	SCC	None	Numerous blood relatives with cancers of CFS type[25]
Family "G" of Warthin (same patient as Bitran and Pellettiere[9])	8	SCC of vulva, sebaceous epithelioma	Endometrium	Numerous blood relatives with cancers of CFS type

*Sebaceous BCC indicates basal cell carcinoma with sebaceous differentiation; BCC, basal cell carcinoma; SCC, squamous cell carcinoma.

CFS[21-25,28,36,38] and described the nuances of its clinical expression in some detail, the world literature in fact contains many additional documentations of the synrome.[26,27,29-33] Unlike case reports of Torre's syndrome, studies of the CFS typically describe malignant neoplastic lesions over multiple generations and involve, in some cases, dozens of similarly affected family members. Segregation patterns of tumor transmission are compatible with an autosomal dominantly inherited factor.

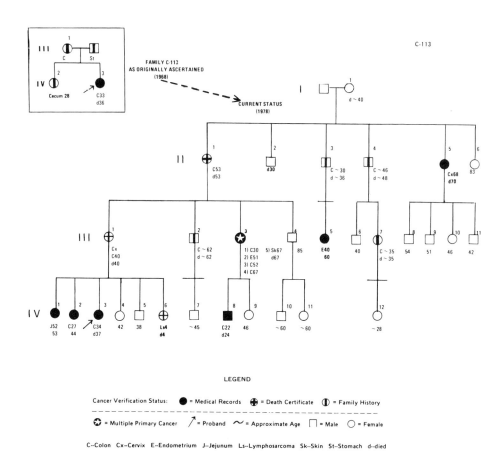

Figure 8-1. Pedigree of a family with cancer family syndrome in which patient III-3 had multiple carcinomas of the colon and endometrium, and manifested cutaneous lesions of Torre's syndrome.

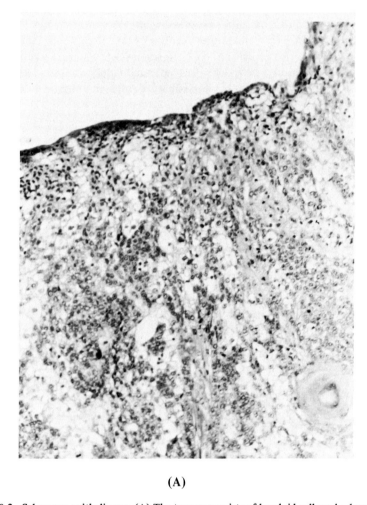

(A)

Figure 8-2. Sebaceous epithelioma: (A) The tumors consists of basaloid cells and sebaceous cells (H & E, 100×, original magnification). (B) Basaloid cells are present which show sebaceous cell differentiation (H & E, 100×, original magnification). (C) The tumor consists of basaloid (germinative) cells with evidence of sebaceous maturation (H & E, 160×, original magnification). (D) Some mature sebaceous cells are present (H & E, 250×, original magnification).

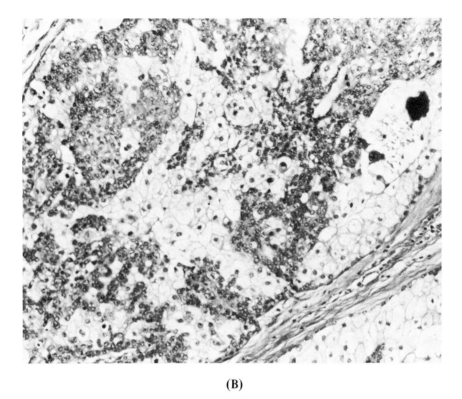

(B)

Figure 8-2 (Continued)

Since Warthin's original report of Family G,[27] characteristics of the CFS have been crystallized and include the following:

1. There is an early age of onset of colonic, endometrial and, to a lesser extent, ovarian,[34] stomach, and breast[35] adenocarcinoma — the mean age being approximately 45 years.[28,36]
2. The tumor complex is expressed vertically in representative pedigrees in a pattern consistent with autosomal dominant transmission.[36]
3. An extraordinary frequency of multiple primary visceral malignancy (approaching 50%) is seen in affected members of CFS kindreds.[37,38]
4. Colonic malignancy appears in great excess at the proximal colon (an average of 65% are so situated in affected families as compared to 20–40% in the general population.)[40,41]
5. There is significant improvement in survival of affected patients despite invasive or metastatic cancer.[38]

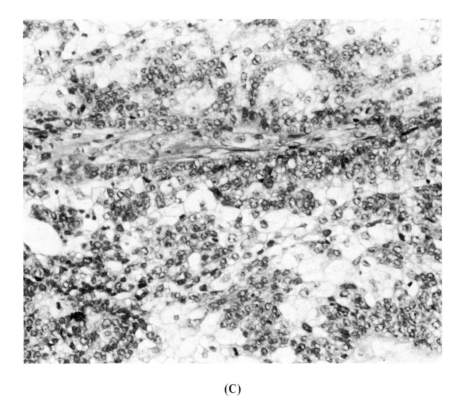

(C)

Figure 8-2 (Continued)

Unlike Torre's syndrome, patients afflicted with the CFS have not heretofore been believed to manifest evidence of a cutaneous phenotype.

Review of the literature on Torre's syndrome suggested striking parallels between its clinical expression and that of individual patients with the CFS, the only significant differences being the mentioned lack of a cutaneous phenotype in the CFS and the sparse documentation of family history in Torre's syndrome. These apparent differences may be rather misleading for two reasons: (1) the family history is one of the most poorly documented aspects of the typical patient history,[42] and (2) benign cutaneous lesions are not invariably documented in a routine physical examination. In the evaluation of a patient critically ill because of the presence of visceral malignancy, such features routinely escape detection. For these reasons, we undertook a review of our extensive files pertaining to the CFS (over 5,000 total relatives comprising 26 families)

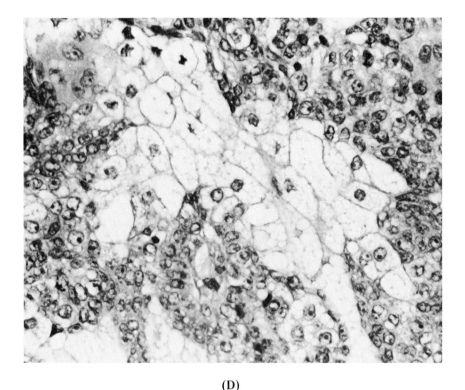

(D)

Figure 8-2 (Continued)

in order to determine whether or not there might, in fact, be hitherto unrecognized examples of Torre's syndrome in supposed CFS patients. Despite the poor evaluations of the skin in available charts, this search was immediately rewarded by the discovery of patients from several families showing the full clinical spectrum of Torre's syndrome.[6] These cases are described as follows (with pedigrees and pathology on following pages):

Family C-113 (Figure 8-1): Patient III-3 manifested an invasive adenocarcinoma of the cecum at age 30. Following right hemicolectomy, an ileotransverse anastomosis was accomplished. At age 50, total abdominal hysterectomy with bilateral salpingo-oophorectomy was performed for adenocarcinoma of the endometrium, the tumor penetrating two-thirds of the thickness of the myometrium but with no serosal involvement. The patient received postoperative irradiation. Six months later, at age 51, she underwent a segmental colonic resection for carcinoma of

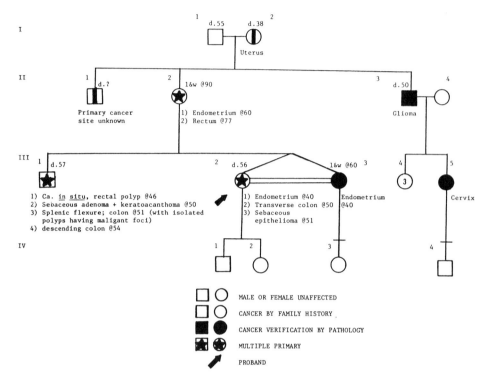

Figure 8-3. Pedigree of a family with cancer family syndrome. Note that the proband (III-2) was diagnosed as having colon and endometrial carcinoma as well as a sebaceous epithelioma.

the distal transverse colon in which the tumor penetrated the muscularis mucosae and submucosal tissue but did not invade the muscularis externa. At age 67, the patient received a diagnosis of carcinoma of the rectum, histologically verified. During the same hospitalization, a sebaceous epithelioma with basal cell differentiation was excised from the patient's right flank (Figure 8-2 A through D). Previously (age 51), she was treated for multiple seborrheic keratoses and at age 66 for keratoses of the forehead. Further details were unavailable. Six months after that resection for rectal cancer, the patient expired of metastases, presumably from the primary tumor.

Patient IV-1 was diagnosed with carcinoma of the jejunum at age 52. Sebaceous cysts of the face were diagnosed clinically at age 53. Her sister, IV-2, had a carcinoma of the cecum at age 27. At age 44, papillomatous lesions of the back and cheek were noted.

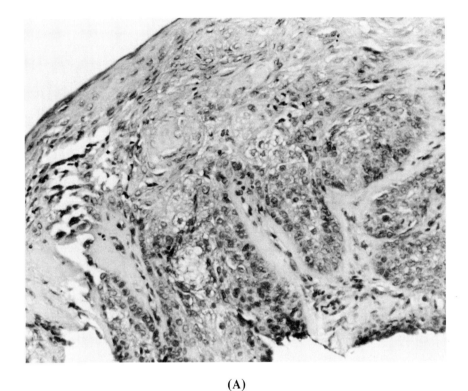

(A)

Figure 8-4. Sebaceous epithelioma: (A) The tumor consists mainly of basaloid cells with focal sebaceous differentiation (H & E, 160X, original magnification). (B) A few mature sebaceous cells are present (H & E, 250X, original magnification). (C) Basaloid cells and mature sebaceous cells are evident (H & E, 250X, original magnification).

Family C-197 (Figure 8 3): Patient III-2 (the proband) had, at age 40, a carcinoma of the endometrium, followed ten years later by an invasive carcinoma of the proximal transverse colon. One year later, at age 51, a sebaceous gland carcinoma of the neck was excised as an outpatient procedure (Figure 8-4 A through C). The patient's identical twin sister (III-3) developed a carcinoma of the endometrium, just three months before the same diagnosis was made in her sister. This patient has not manifested colon cancer nor does she admit to having cutaneous lesions. The brother (III-1) of these sisters was diagnosed as having a malignant rectal polyp at age 46 and an invasive colonic adenocarcinoma at the splenic flexure at age 51. At age 50, he was reported to have a sebaceous carcinoma and squamous cell carcinoma of the eyebrow and temple. Reevaluation

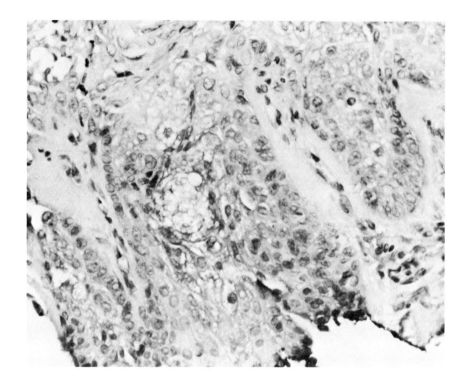

(B)

Figure 8-4 (Continued)

of these lesions showed them to be a sebaceous adenoma (Figure 8-5 A through C) and a keratoacanthoma. Finally, the mother of these siblings (II-2) was diagnosed at age 60 with carcinoma of the endometrium and at age 77 with carcinoma of the rectum. She is living and well at age 90.

Family C-200 (Figure 8-6): This family provides an example of a patient (III-11, currently age 48) who has manifested several of the cutaneous stigmata of Torre's syndrome, but who has not manifested visceral carcinoma to date. At age 43, a sebaceous adenoma of the face was removed (Figure 8-7 A and B). Five months later, a well-differentiated squamous cell carcinoma of the skin of the nose was removed. Soon thereafter, a fibroepithelial polyp of the left ear was excised. While it was stated that the patient has had no evidence of visceral malignancy to date, a mucinous cystadenoma of the left ovary was removed at age 42.

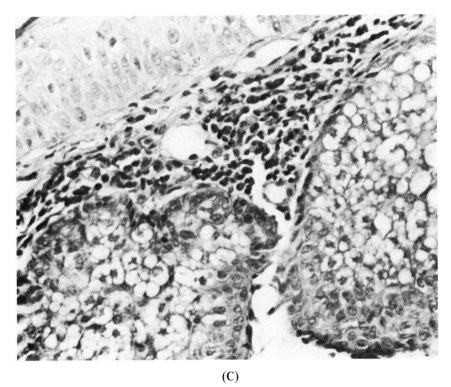

(C)

Figure 8-4 (Continued)

Family G of Warthin[27] (Figure 8-8): At age 33, a 57-year-old white female was treated for an epidermoid carcinoma of the vulva. At 43 years of age, she had an adenocarcinoma of the endometrium treated with intracavity radiotherapy. Concurrently, a pneumonectomy for a left hilar mass confirmed a metastatic adenocarcinoma consistent with an endometrial primary tumor. She subsequently underwent a hysterectomy and bilateral salpingo-oophorectomy. At age 42, prior to the diagnosis of endometrial carcinoma, she had a waxy, papular, sebaceous adenoma of the abdomen excised. During a 14-year period, she had eight sebaceous adenomas and sebaceous epitheliomas excised from her skin. Her case was presented as an example of Torre's syndrome by Bittran and Pellettiere.[9] No mention of family history was given in their report. Through the kindness of Dr. Pellettiere, who at our request made additional contact with this patient, we learned that she was a member in the direct genetic line of descent of Family

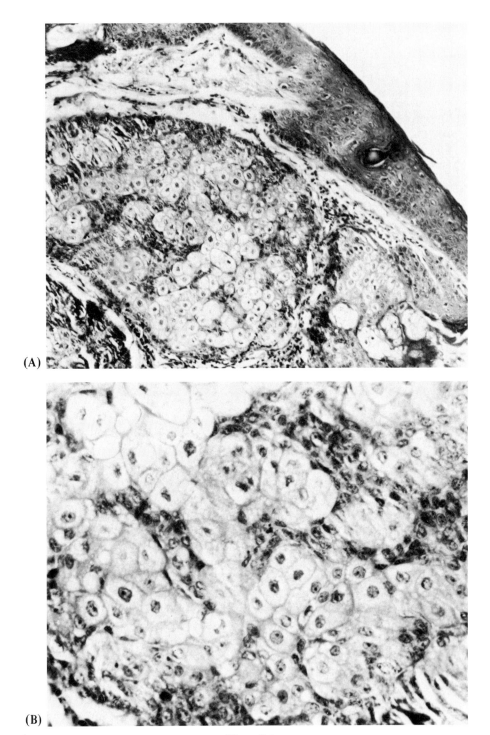

Figure 8-5.

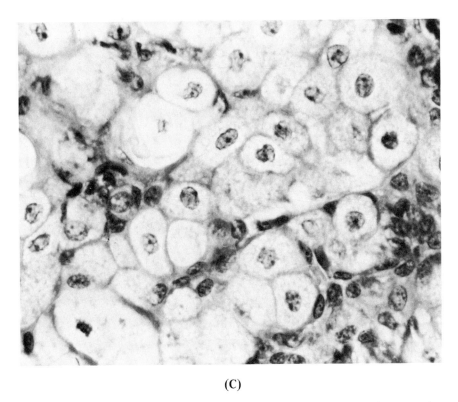

(C)

Figure 8-5. Sebaceous adenoma: (A) The tumor consists predominantly of mature seba-ceous cells (H & E, 100X, original magnification). (B) Mature sebaceous cells and a few ger-minative cells (H & E, 160X, original magnification). (C) Mature sebaceous cells (H & E, 400X, original magnification).

G of Warthin (the original CFS kindred), a family which has been under study for more than 75 years. It is of further interest that this patient, although ex-tremely knowledgeable about her family history, had not disclosed any of these facts to her husband or to her four children, each of the latter being at 50% risk for the CFS.

CONCLUSION

The coexistence of sebaceous skin lesions, early onset visceral carcinoma, and prolonged survival in patients from families with the CFS clearly integrates Torre's syndrome as a phenotypic component of the CFS. For this reason, the

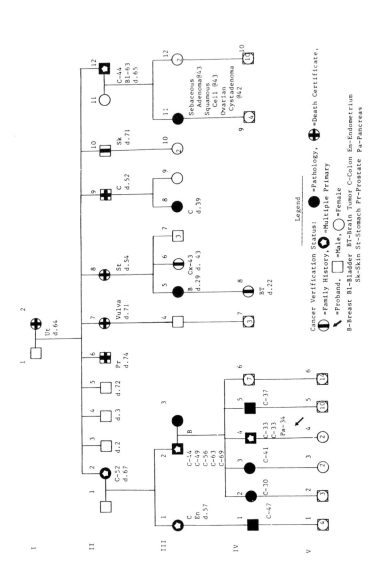

Figure 8-6. Pedigree of a family with cancer family syndrome. One of the members (III-11) has manifested several cutaneous stigmata of Torre's syndrome, but has not had visceral carcinoma.

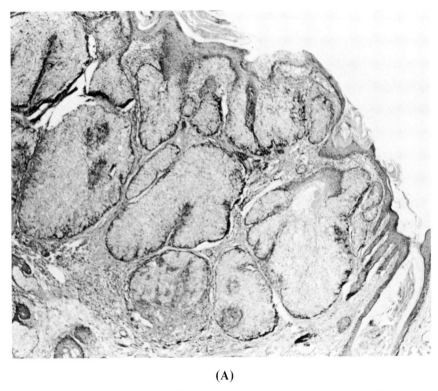

(A)

Figure 8-7. Sebaceous adenoma: (A) The tumor consists of several lobules of mature sebaceous cells (H & E, 25X, original magnification). (B) Mature sebaceous cells (H & E,
100X, original magnification).

CFS may now be considered a cancer-associated genodermatosis, albeit one in
which the cutaneous signs are not always fully penetrant.

In light of this linkage with Torre's syndrome, all CFS kindreds should be
reevaluated with particular attention to the integument, in order to learn what
fraction of patients with the syndrome actually manifest the cutaneous stigmata.
Conversely, meticulous attention to family history should be devoted to any patient with Torre's syndrome. Any patient with the cutaneous lesions, with or
without a known family history of cancer, should be screened for visceral cancer.

The natural history of the cutaneous signs must be critically scrutinized in an
effort to isolate the factors that elicit these cutaneous signs, i.e., primary vs sec-

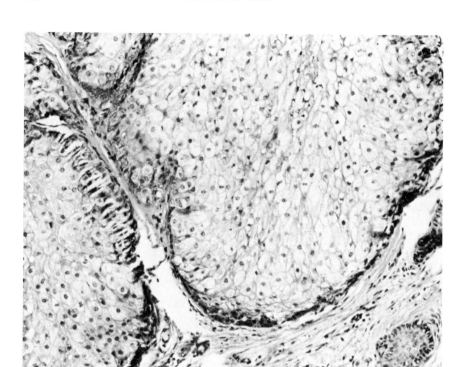

(B)

Figure 8-7 (Continued)

ondary manifestations of underlying cancer. Perhaps patients at risk for the CFS are unusually susceptible to certain environmental factors which might promote the development of the cutaneous signs. Eventual recognition of subclinical markers may one day aid in the identification of patients destined to express internal cancers.

As is so often true in medicine, new observations lead to an ever-increasing array of perplexing questions as well as opportunities for study of more basic issues in the biology of disease, in this case, cancer. We believe that the identification of a cutaneous marker in the CFS presents such questions and opportunities.

REFERENCES

1. Gardner, E.J., and Stephens, F.E.: Cancer of the lower digestive tract in one family group. *Am. J. Hum. Genet.* 2:41, 1950.
2. Fader, M., Kline, S.N., Sputz, S.S., and Zubrow, H.J.: Gardner's syndrome (intestinal polyposis, osteomas, sebaceous cysts) and a new dental discovery. *Oral Surg.* 15 (2):153–172, 1962.

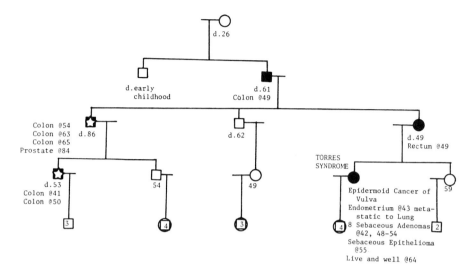

Figure 8-8. Pedigree of a sibship from a large family with cancer family syndrome. One of the females with endometrial carcinoma also had multiple sebaceous adenomas and epitheliomas excised from her skin.

3. Gardner, E.J.: Followup study of a family group exhibiting dominant inheritance for a syndrome including intestinal polyps, osteomas, fibromas, and epidermal cysts. *Am. J. Hum. Genet.* **14**:376–390, 1962.

4. Lynch, H.T., Frichot, B.C., and Lynch, J.F.: Familial atypical multiple mole-melanoma syndrome. *J. Med. Genet.* **15**:352–356, 1978.

5. Clark, W.H., Reimer, R.R., Greene, M., Ainsworth, A.M., and Mastrangelo, M.J.: Origin of familial malignant melanomas from heritable melanocytic lesions. *Arch. Derm.* **114**:732–728, 1978.

6. Lynch, H.T., Lynch, P.M., Fusaro, R., and Pester, J.: The cancer family syndrome: rare cutaneous pheontypic linkage of Torre's syndrome. *Arch. Int. Med.* **141**:607–611, 1981

7. Torre, D.: Multiple sebaceous tumors. *Arch. Derm.* **98**:549–551, 1968.

8. Muir, E.G., Yates-Bell, A.J., and Barlow, K.A.: Multiple primary carcinomata of the colon, duodenum, and larynx associated with keratoacanthoma of the face. *Br. J. Surg.* **54**(3):191–195, 1967.

9. Bitran, J., and Pellettiere, E.V.: Multiple sebaceous gland tumors and internal carcinoma: Torre's syndrome. *Cancer* **33**:835–836, 1974.

10. Bakker, P.M., Tjon A Joe, S.S.: Multiple sebaceous gland tumors with multiple tumors of internal organs, a new syndrome? *Dermatologica* **142**:50–57, 1971.

11. Rulon, D.B., and Helwig, E.B.: Multiple sebaceous neoplasms of the skin: an association with multiple visceral carcinomas, especially of the colon. *Am. J. Clin. Path.* **60**:745–752, 1973.

12. Jakobiec, F.A.: Sebaceous adenoma of the eyelid and visceral malignancy. *Am. J. Ophthalmol.* **78**(6):952–960, 1974.

13. Sciallis, G.F., and Winkelmann, R.K.: Multiple sebaceous adenomas and gastrointestinal carcinoma. *Arch. Derm.* 110:913-916, 1974.

14. Leonard D.D., and Deaton, W.R.: Multiple sebaceous gland tumors and visceral carcinomas. *Arch. Derm.* 110:917-920, 1974.

15. Reiffers, J., Laugier, P., and Hunziker, N.: Hyperplasies sebacees, keratoacanthomes, epitheliomas du visage et cancer du colon (une nouvelle entite?). *Dermatologica* 153: 23-33, 1976.

16. Tschang, T.P., Poulos, E., Ho, C.K., Kuo, T.T.: Multiple sebaceous adenomas and internal malignant disease: a case report with chromosomal analysis. *Hum. Path.* 7(V):589-594, 1976.

17. Poleksic, S.: Keratoacanthoma and multiple carcinomas. *Br. J. Derm.* 91:461-463, 1974.

18. Lynne-Davies, G., and Brown, J.: Multiple sebaceous gland tumors associated with polyposis of the colon and bony abnormalities. *Can. Med. Assoc. J.* 110:1377-1379, 1974.

19. Anderson, D.E.: An inherited form of large bowel cancer (Muir's syndrome). *Cancer* 45:1103-1107, 1980.

20. Householder, M.S., and Zeligman, I.: Sebaceous neoplasms associated with visceral carcinomas. *Arch, Derm.* 116:61-64, 1980.

21. Lynch, H.T., Lynch, P.M., and Harris, R.E.: Minimal genetic findings and their cancer control implications: a family with the cancer family syndrome. *JAMA* 236(6): 582-584, 1978.

22. Lynch, H.T., and Lynch, P.M.: The cancer family syndrome: a pragmatic basis for syndrome identification. *Dis. Colon Rect.* 22(2):106-110, 1979.

23. Lynch, H.T., and Krush, A.J.: The cancer family syndrome and cancer control. *Surg. Gyn. Obstet.* 132:247-250, 1971.

24. Lynch, H.T.: Familial cancer prevalence spanning eight years (Family N). *Arch. Int. Med.* 134:9321-938, 1974.

25. Lynch H.T., Swartz, M., Lynch, J., and Krush, A.J.: A family study of adenocarcinoma of the colon and multiple primary cancer. *Surg. Gyn. Obstet.* 134:781-786, 1972.

26. Williams, C.: Management of malignancy in "cancer families." *Lancet* 1:198-199, 1978.

27. Warthin, A.S.: Hereditary with reference to carcinoma. *Arch. Int. Med.* 12:546-555, 1913.

28. Lynch, H.T., Harris, R.E., Organ, C.H., Guirgis, H.A., Lynch, P.M., Lynch, J.F., and Nelsen, E.J.: The surgeon, genetics, and cancer control: the Cancer Family Syndrome. *Ann. Surg.* 16:434-440, 1977.

29. Boland, R.C.: Cancer family syndrome: a case report and literature review. *Dig. Dis.* 23(5):25s-27s, 1978.

30. Dubosson, J.D., Klein, D., Pettavel, J., Rey, Ch.-D.: Syndrome dy cancer familial a travers 4 generations. *Schweiz. Med. Wschr.* 107:587-881, 1977.

31. Cannon, M.M., and Leavell, B.S.: Multiple cancer types in one family. *Cancer* 19(4): 538-540, 1966.

32. Butt, H., and Schumacher, M.: Mehrfachkarzinome bei familiarer Haufung von Genital und Intestinalkarzinomen. *Deutsche. Med. Wschr.* 11(12):468-471, 1971.

33. Savage, D.: A family history of uterine and gastrointestinal cancer. *Br. Med. J.* 2: 341-343, 1956.

34. Lynch, H.T., and Lynch, P.M.: Tumor variation in the cancer family syndrome: ovarian carcinoma. *Am. J. Surg.* 138:439-442, 1979.

35. Lynch, H.T., Krush, A.J., and Guirgis, H.A.: Genetic factors in families with combined gastrointestinal and breast cancer. *Am. J. Gastroent.* **59**(1):31-49, 1973.
36. Lynch, H.T., Guirgis, H.A., Harris, R.E., Lynch, P.M., Lynch, J.F., Elston, R.C., Go, R.C.P., and Kaplan, E.: Clinical, genetic, and biostatistical progress in the cancer family syndrome. In: Frontiers of Gastrointestinal Research (P. Rozen, Ed.). Basel: S. Karger, 1979, pp. 142-150.
37. Lynch, H.T., Harris, R.E., Lynch, P.M., Guirgis, H.A., and Lynch, J.F.: The role of heredity in multiple primary cancer. *Cancer* **40**:1849-1854, 1977.
38. Lynch, H.T., Bardawil, W.A., Harris, R.E., Lynch, P.M., Guirgis, H.A., and Lynch, J.F.: Multiple primary cancers and prolonged survival. *Dis. Colon Rect.* **21**(3): 175-168, 1978.
39. Nickel, W.R., and Reed, W.B.: Tuberous sclerosis: special reference to the microscopic alterations in the cutaneous hamartomas. *Arch. Derm.* **85**:209-224, 1962.
40. Lynch, P.M., Lynch, H.T., and Harris, R.E.: Hereditary proximal colonic cancer. *Dis. Colon Rect.* **20**(8):661-668, 1977.
41. Anderson, D.E., and Romsdahl, M.M.: Family history: a criterion for selective screening. In: *Genetics of Human Cancer* (J.J. Mulvihill, R.W. Miller, and J.F. Fraumeni, Jr., Eds.). New York: Raven Press, 1977, pp. 257-268.
42. Lynch, H.T., Follett, K.L., Lynch, P.M., Albano, W.A., Mailliard, J.A., and Pierson, R.: Family history in an oncology clinic: implications concerning cancer genetics. *JAMA* **242**:1268-1272, 1979.
43. Curth, H.O., Hilberg, A.W., and Machachek, G.F.: The site and histology of the cancer associated with malignant acanthosis nigricans. *Cancer* **15**(2):364-382, 1962.
44. Safai, B., Grant, J.M., and Good, R.: Cutaneous manifestations of internal malignancies (II): the sign of Leser-Trelat. *Int. J. Derm.* **17**(6):494-495, 1978.
45. Liddell, K., White, J.E., and Caldwell, I.W.: Seborrheic keratoses and carcinoma of the large bowel (three cases exhibiting the sign of Leser-Trelat). *Br. J. Derm.* **92**: 449-452, 1975.
46. Gardner, E.J., and Richard, R.C.: Multiple cutaneous and subcutaneous lesions occurring simultaneously with hereditary polyposis and osteomatosis. *Am. J. Hum. Genet.* **5**:139-147, 1953.
47. Hornstein, O.P., Knickenberg, M., and Morl, M.: Multiple dermal perifollicular fibromas with polyps of the colon: report of a peculiar clinical syndrome. *Acta Hepato-Gastroent.* **23**:55-58, 1976.
48. Hornstein, O.P.: Generalized dermal perifollicular fibromas with polyps of the colon. *Hum. Genet.* **33**:193-197, 1976.
49. Reed, W.D., Nickel, W.R., and Campion, G.: Internal manifestations of tuberous sclerosis. *Arch. Derm.* **87**:715-728, 1963.
50. Anderson, D.E., Taylor, W.B., Falls, H.F., and Davidson, R.T.: The nevoid basal cell carcinoma syndrome. *Am. J. Hum. Genet.* **19**:12-22, 1967.
51. Winkelmann, R.E., and Brown, J.: Generalized eruptive keratoacanthoma. *Arch. Derm.* **97**:615-617, 1968.
52. Chapman, R.S., and Finn, O.A.: Carcinoma of the larynx in two patients with keratoacanthoma. *Br. J. Derm.* **90**:685-688, 1974.
53. Stewart, W.M., Lauret, P., Hemet, J., Thomine, E., and Gueville, R.M.: Keratoacanthomes multiples et carcinomes visceraux: syndrome de Torre. *Ann. Derm. Venereal Paris* **104**:622-626, 1977.

9
Genetic Heterogeneity and Malignant Melanoma

*Henry T. Lynch, M.D., Ramon M. Fusaro, M.D., Ph.D.
and Judith A. Pester, M.D.*

INTRODUCTION

In their review of the genetics of malignant melanoma, Green and Fraumeni[1] cite an 1820 report by Norris[2] which is possibly the first description of a melanoma-prone family. This involves a 59-year-old male with cutaneous malignant melanoma (CMM) whose father died 30 years before him, also of CMM. It is of interest that the patient reportedly had multiple moles, as did his father and his brothers. There were no further reports dealing with familial melanoma until that of Cawley in 1952,[3] when he described this disease in a father and two of his three children. It has since become apparent that a hereditary form of malignant melanoma exists.[3-9] The majority of studies of familial melanoma have involved variable sized series of consecutively ascertained melanoma probands. The frequency of melanoma was then evaluated in their families and compared with controls. Lacking almost uniformly in these earlier studies were detailed clinical descriptions of the families, including cancer of all anatomic sites, associated diseases, and/or cutaneous anomalies. Therefore, it is not surprising that heterogeneity in familial melanoma has only recently been appreciated, as noted by Lynch and his associates.[5,6]

The purpose of this chapter is severalfold: (1) to provide a detailed updating of our ongoing clinical-pathological-genetic investigations of four families who manifest the familial atypical multiple mole-melanoma syndrome (acronym FAMMM) as reported by Lynch and colleagues[10,11] (also referred to as the B-K mole syndrome by Clark and associates[12,13]), and (2) to discuss other issues in familial malignant melanoma, including hereditary intraocular melanoma and its occassional association with cutaneous malignant melanoma and, finally, the spontaneous regression of metastatic malignant melanoma.

MATERIALS AND METHODS

Our standard protocol for cancer genetic investigations has been employed in studies of familial melanoma.[7,8] Briefly, this protocol incorporates the use of detailed questionnaires which are mailed to all of the proband's maternal and paternal informative relatives once clinical-genetic and pathologic evaluation of melanoma has been completed in the proband. Extension of the pedigree includes a search for cancer of all anatomic sites, in addition to documentation of all major causes of morbidity and mortality. A detailed description of the cutaneous phenotype is emphasized. Whenever possible, personal examinations of these relatives are then performed by a clinical oncologist-geneticist and a dermatologist. Suspicious cutaneous lesions are then biopsied. A registered nurse interviews each patient in order to update and to corroborate information obtained from the questionnaires. All primary medical and pathology documents are then secured, including pathology slides, for review by our collaborating dermatopathologist.

FAMILY STUDY RESULTS

Family 1: The proband (Figure 9-1, IV-4) was first described by Lynch and Krush in 1968.[4] At that time, the proband was age 26 and he had had four histologically verified CMMs on the skin of his legs, arms, and torso. A fifth malignant melanoma (nodular, Clark's level IV) was diagnosed on his mid-back during this examination. The patient had reddish hair, light complexion, blue eyes, and he had had very heavy sun exposure, having worked as a lifeguard in high school and college as well as being a collegiate swimmer. He was noted to have multiple moles and reported a similar cutaneous phenotype in his siblings (Figure 9-1, IV-5, 6). However, the significance of the FAMMM phenotype was not recognized at that time; the family was subsequently evaluated in 1977 and reported as an example of the FAMMM syndrome.[10,11]

A most recent evaluation of the proband and several of his relatives was accomplished in 1979 when the proband was age 38. Figure 9-2 shows a front view and Figure 9-3 shows a close-up view of the proband's back. His clinical lesions were extremely varied, and were mostly on the trunk and proximal areas of the extremities.

There were very few lesions on the exposed areas of the face and neck. The vast majority were regular, tan- to brown-colored macular lesions which were under 1 cm in diameter. In addition, there were many regular and irregular macular and papular lesions, some of which were almost black in color. These appeared to be ordinary nevi. One lesion which was atypical was seen on several areas of the trunk and was less than 1 cm, macular erythematous, and oval. At the periphery of the lesions, there were tan to brown macular areas within the regular oval perimeters. The atypical mole in Figure 9-3 (see arrow) was

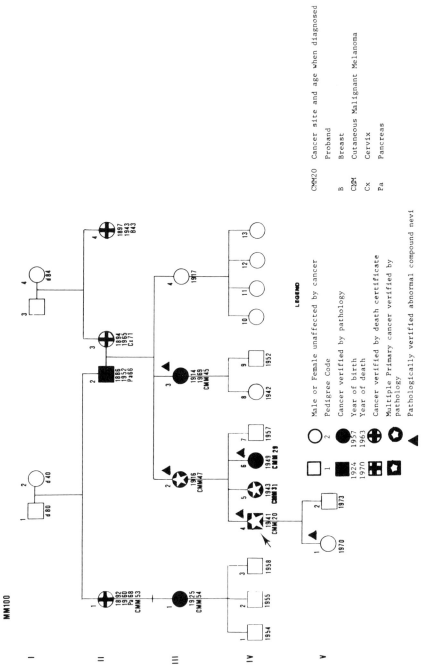

Figure 9-1. Family 1 showing a pedigree of the familial atypical multiple mole-melanoma (FAMMM) syndrome consistent with an autosomal dominant mode of inheritence.

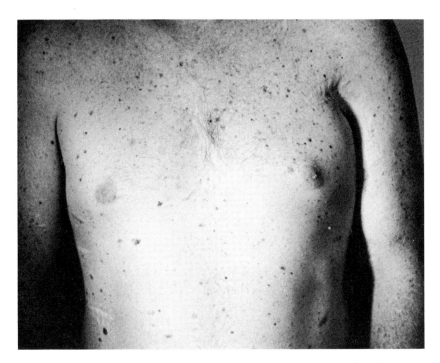

Figure 9-2. Front view of the proband in Family 1. Note the presence of multiple moles, several of which are strikingly atypical.

biopsied and histologically showed features compatible with a FAMMM mole. The skin lesion was a compound nevus (Figure 9-4). The melanocytes at the epidermal-dermal junction showed evidence of mild dysplasia. The papillary dermis (Figure 9-5) showed fibroplasia and new blood vessel formation. The amount of chronic inflammatory cells in the papillary dermis was minimal. Figures 9-6 and 9-7 show histologic sections of another lesion manifesting similar changes. Figure 9-8 is a superficial spreading malignant melanoma (Clark's level II). Note the lymphocytic infiltrate present in the papillary dermis. During the interim, the proband has had four additional CMMs all histologically verified, for a total of nine CMMs during a period of 18 years.

The proband's daughter (Figure 9-1, V-1) was examined in 1977, when she was age 7 years. She showed several brown moles on the skin of her back, all of which were round and regular (Figure 9-9A). It is noteworthy that her parents stated that these lesions began to appear around age 2. Particular attention was given to this possible age of onset of mole appearance in that the proband's mother stated that this seemed to be the age of onset of moles in her three chil-

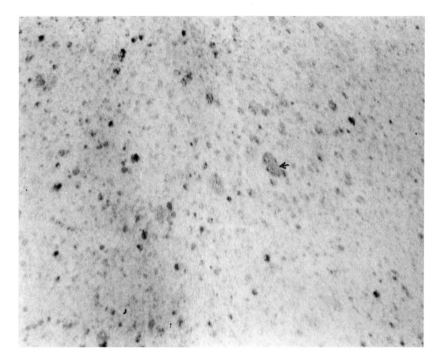

Figure 9-3. Close-up view of the skin of the back of the proband from Figure 9-1. The arrow indicates an atypical mole which histologically showed findings consistent with a familial atypical multiple mole-melanoma mole as shown in Figures 9-4 and 9-5.

dren (Figure 9-1, IV-4,5,6). This girl had shown normal growth and development, and was of average intelligence. Examination in 1979 at age 9 years (Figure 9-9B) showed a striking evolution of the lesions on her back as evidenced by the appearance of new moles. The lesions were few in number. They appeared to be ordinary macular and papular nevi with varying shades of tan and brown coloration. One of these lesions was 1 cm in diameter, and appeared papular and larger than the other lesions but was not atypical in clinical appearance. This lesion was excised (arrow) and histologic findings were consonant with a FAMMM mole. This was a compound nevus (Figure 9-10). There was moderate dysplasia of melanocytes, located at the epidermal-dermal junction. The papillary dermis (Figure 9-11) showed evidence of fibroplasia and a moderate infiltrate of mature appearing lymphocytes.

One of the proband's sisters (Figure 9-1, IV-5) was examined by one of us (HTL) in 1977 when she was age 33. This woman showed a cutaneous pheno-type which was virtually identical to that described in her brother. She has had four histologically verified CMMs, the first of these diagnosed in 1974. We

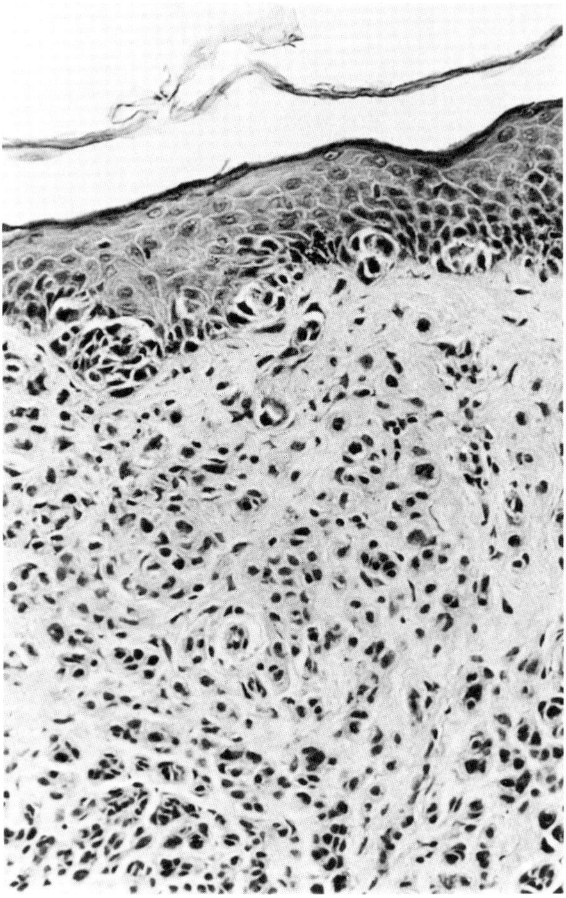

Figure 9-4. Compound nevus with melanocytic dysplasia at dermal-epidermal junction, fibroplasia of papillary dermis, and minimal chronic inflammation (H & E, 115×).

diagnosed her fourth CMM (histologically verified) on her back in 1977. A second sister (Figure 9-1, IV-6) was not personally examined by us. However, the history indicates that she also showed a cutaneous phenotype which was strikingly similar to her brother (the proband) and her sister. Because of this history, we strongly encouraged this 29-year-old woman to be evaluated by a dermatologist who excised multiple moles which, upon examination by us, showed the characteristic findings of the FAMMM histology. In addition, an unsuspected CMM was removed from her left flank.

The mother (Figure 9-1, III-2) of these patients was examined by one of us (HTL) in 1977 when she was age 60. She had her first CMM at age 47 and a

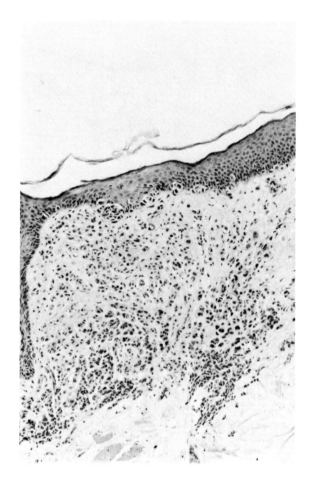

Figure 9-5. Fibroplasia of papillary dermis and minimal lymphocytic infiltrate (H & E, 233×).

second one at age 56. Her history indicated that multiple atypical moles had previously been excised. Our examination did not reveal the presence of atypical moles. However, histologic review of the previously excised moles showed some of them to be consistent with the FAMMM mole.

The proband's maternal aunt (Figure 9-1, III-3) had a history of a cutaneous phenotype consistent with the FAMMM syndrome. Histopathologic review of these moles showed findings consistent with the FAMMM mole. She had a histologically verified CMM at age 45 and died from metastases at age 55.

The proband's 54-year-old second cousin (Figure 9-1, III-1) did not show any evidence of the FAMMM phenotype. However, she had a histologically verified CMM at age 54. Her mother (Figure 9-1, II-1) had a CMM by history at age 53

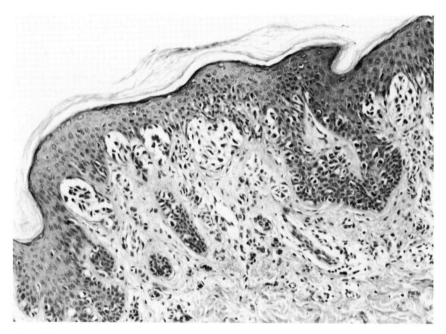

Figure 9-6. Severe dysplasia of melanocytes at dermal-epidermal interface (H & E, 500×).

and died of pancreatic carcinoma by medical history at age 68. We do not have knowledge of her cutaneous phenotype. The proband's grandfather (Figure 9-1, II-2) died of histologically verified pancreatic carcinoma at age 66. We do not have a reliable history of his cutaneous phenotype.

Findings in this family showed vertical transmission of the FAMMM phenotype (FAMMM moles and/or CMM) through four generations (Figure 9-1, II-1, III-2, IV-4,5,6, and V-1) with verification of FAMMM moles in several of these patients, including the proband's daughter (Figure 9-1, V-1), thereby showing three generations of FAMMM moles (histologically verified). The proband showed unusual tolerance to CMM as evidenced by his survival in the face of nine verified CMMs, one of which was a nodular malignant melanoma, Clark's level IV, during an 18-year period.

Family 2: The proband (Figure 9-12, III-1) was examined by a dermatology colleague who reported that she showed multiple atypical moles consistent with our original description of the FAMMM syndrome.[11] She had two verified CMMs at age 22. Our pathology review of her moles showed characteristic features of a FAMMM mole (Figure 9-13).

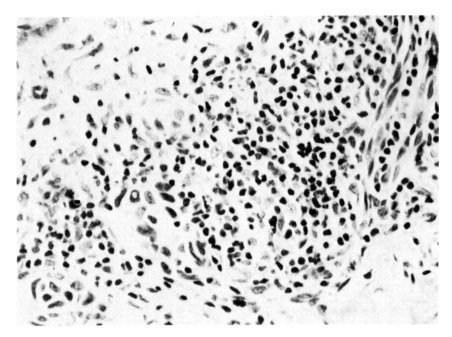

Figure 9-7. Lymphocytic infiltrate in papillary dermis and some neovascularization (H & E, 800×).

This patient's 20-year-old brother (Figure 9-12, III-3) had three histologically verified CMMs. He had a cutaneous phenotype by history which was characteristic of the FAMMM syndrome. Review of the pathology report of his atypical moles showed them to be consistent with FAMMM histology as reviewed by Dr. Wallace Clark. A sister of these patients (Figure 9-12, III-4) had a CMM by history at age 26.

The proband's father (Figure 9-12, II-2) had a CMM by history at age 30. This patient had a history of multiple atypical moles. It is of interest that the proband's mother (Figure 9-12, II-3) had a history of CMM at age 48. She allegedly does not have multiple moles, though we have not examined her. Consanguinity is absent. This is therefore an example of connubial melanoma. Melanoma by history was present in the proband's paternal grandmother (Figure 9-12, I-3) and histologically verified in the proband's maternal grandfather (Figure 9-12, I-4). A continuation study of this family is in progress by the National Cancer Institute.

Family 3: The proband (Figure 9-14, III-1) had histologically verified CMM at age 54. Our examination did not reveal any evidence of the FAMMM cutaneous

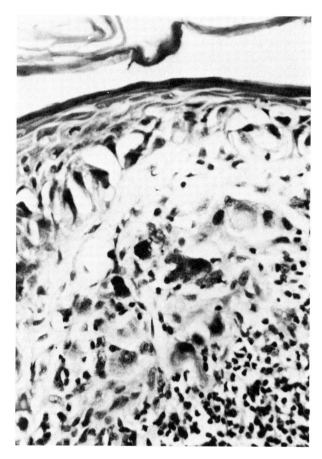

Figure 9-8. Superficial spreading malignant melanoma, Clark's level II. Lymphocytic infiltrate present in papillary dermis (H & E, 1250×).

phenotype. This patient died of metastatic malignant melanoma at age 61. One of her brothers (Figure 9-14, III-3) did not show any evidence of atypical moles; however, we diagnosed a basal cell carcinoma from the skin of his neck. A second brother (Figure 9-14, III-4) had histologically verified carcinoma of the lung and died from this disease at age 52. We did not have an opportunity to examine this patient. A third brother (Figure 9-14, III-5) had CMM by history at age 53, and a second (histologically verified) primary malignant neoplasm of the lung. He died from the latter at age 62. We did not have information about his cutaneous phenotype.

A 70-year-old sister of the proband (Figure 9-14, III-6) was examined by us and was found to be completely negative for the FAMMM phenotype and for

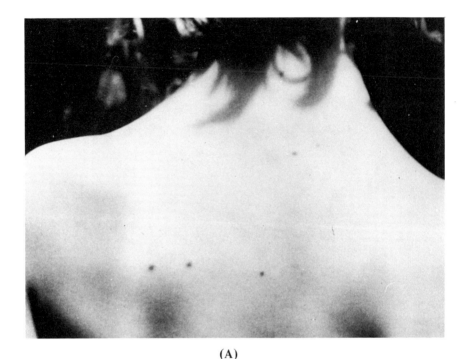

(A)

Figure 9-9. This figure shows the proband's daughter (A) at age 7 and (B) subsequently, at age 9. Note the increasing evidence of moles during this two-year interval with a prominent lesion (see arrow) which was also papular and slightly larger than the other lesions and which histologically was found to be a familial atypical multiple mole-melanoma mole as shown in Figures 9-10 and 9-11.

any cancer. However, it is noteworthy that she had a daughter (Figure 9-14, IV-4) who had a CMM histologically verified at age 23, and multiple atypical moles consistent clinically and histologically with the FAMMM phenotype. This woman also had a daughter (Figure 9-14, V-1) who showed a cutaneous phenotype consistent with the FAMMM syndrome (Figure 9-15A). She was examined by us at age 17, at which time multiple biopsies were obtained of the atypical moles, with findings histologically consistent with FAMMM moles (Figure 9-16). Another lesion from the same individual showed the FAMMM histologic characteristics (Figures 9-17 and 9-18). It is of interest that two years following our examination, the patient developed a Clark's level IV malignant melanoma at the site of a prior biopsy of a FAMMM mole (Figure 9-15B, see arrow).

Her two brothers (Figure 9-14, V-2,3) were examined by us and each had clinical and histologic evidence of the FAMMM phenotype. The proband's nephew (Figure 9-14, IV-6) had histologically verified Hodgkin's disease at age 28.

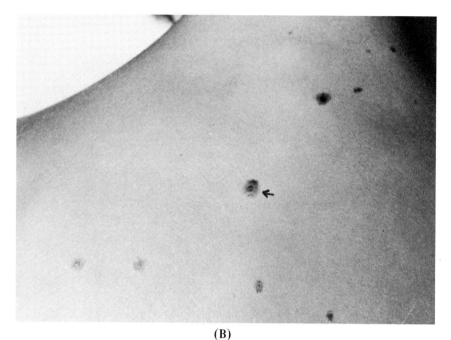

(B)

Figure 9-9 (Continued)

A niece of the proband (Figure 9-14, IV-5) had a history of more than 30 atypical moles which had been surgically removed but not yet examined by us. This patient has two children (Figure 9-14, V-4,5) with clinical and histologic findings consistent with the FAMMM phenotype.

In summary, this family showed clinical and histologic evidence of the FAMMM syndrome in members of two generations and CMM verified in three generations. A noteworthy aspect of the pedigree is the fact that one of these patients (Figure 9-14, III-6) showed no evidence of the FAMMM syndrome, yet she was the progenitor of this syndrome and had two siblings (Figure 9-14, III-1,5) with CMM. In addition, one of her children who was normal (Figure 9-14, IV-5) had two children with the FAMMM phenotype; thus, through two generations of normal individuals (Figure 9-14, III-6 and IV-5), the abnormal trait was passed and manifested in the third generation (Figure 9-14, IV-4 and V-5).

Family 4: This Dutch kindred (Figure 9-19) had been previously described.[14] The present study of the kindred was initiated when a Dutch ophthalmologist (Jendo A. Oosterhuis, M.D.) evaluated one of the relatives (Figure 9-19, IV-24) who manifested bilateral intraocular melanoma and multiple CMMs. On the

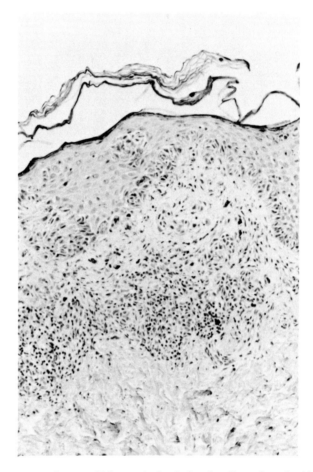

Figure 9-10. Compound nevus. Melanocytic dysplasia primarily at dermal-epidermal inter-face. Prominent lymphocytic infiltrate in papillary dermis (H & E, 148X).

suspicion of their manifesting the FAMMM syndrome, three members of our team, Drs. Fusaro and Lynch, and Jane Lynch, R.N., visited the family in Leiden, Holland and, in collaboration with their family physicians and the sub-ject ophthalmologist, personally evaluated eight relatives who were either pre-viously affected with melanoma or who, by virtue of their position in the pedi-gree, appeared to be at high risk for this disease. Cutaneous biopsies were performed on five of these individuals in an attempt to remove at least one mole from each patient. Clinical findings on three of these patients were very suggestive of the FAMMM syndrome. Two additional members were highly suspect of having the FAMMM cutaneous expression. Pathologic study was per-

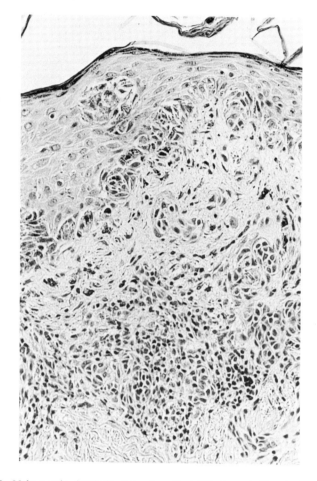

Figure 9-11. Melanocytic dysplasia. Lymphocytic infiltrate and fibroplasia of papillary dermis (II & E, 22/X).

formed independently by a dermatopathologist (JP) who, at the time, was not aware that the patients were suspected of having the FAMMM syndrome. In two members (Figure 9-19, V-24 and V-26) who were clinically diagnosed as FAMMM, the histology was confirmatory.

The skin lesion from the abdomen of patient V-24 was a compound nevus (Figure 9-19, V-24). The melanocytes at the dermal-epidermal junction showed mild dysplastic change. The papillary dermis showed some fibroplasia and new blood vessel formation. There was a focal perivascular chronic inflammatory cell infiltrate.

MM-110

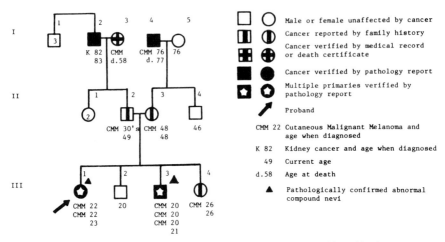

Figure 9-12. Pedigree of Family 2 showing malignant melanoma manifested in three generations with connubial malignant melanoma in the parents of the sibship of generation II.
Multiple primary melanomas, early age of onset, and familial atypical multiple mole-melanoma
moles were noted in the proband and her brother.

Histologic sections from four previously removed moles of another member
of the pedigree (Figure 9-19, V-26) showed nevocellular compound nevi with
mild to moderate dysplastic change of the melanocytes at the dermal-epidermal
junction. There was some mild fibroplasia, new blood vessel formation, and
chronic inflammation within the papillary dermis (Figures 9-20 through 9-22).
The histology of these lesions was suggestive of FAMMM moles. In summary:
(a) there was a moderate concordance between pathology and clinical evaluation
of the FAMMM syndrome in one of the patients; (b) in a second patient examined
by us, we did not see clinical evidence of atypical moles. However, this patient
had previously removed moles which showed suggestive FAMMM histologic
characteristics. Finally, this family is noteworthy for a most extraordinary occurrence of bilateral intraocular melanoma and multiple primary cutaneous malignant melanomas in one of the patients (Figure 9-19, IV-24). There was also a
spectacular array of cancers of other anatomic sites, some in association with
double primaries, including both malignant melanoma and noncutaneous malignancy in relatives throughout the kindred. This family will be the subject of a
separate publication in the *British Journal of Cancer*.

Table 9-1 is a summary of the histologic observations of FAMMM moles in
these four kindreds. We have compared them with descriptions of histopathology
of the B-K mole described by Clark and associates.[10]

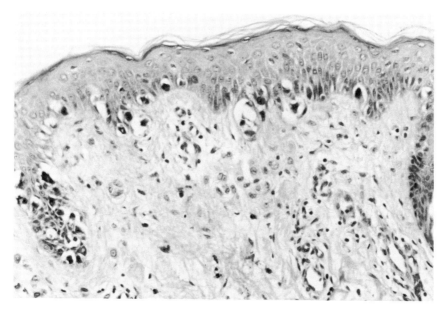

Figure 9-13. Compound nevus with marked dysplasia of melanocytes at D-E interface. Fibroplasia and capillary proliferation of papillary dermis, few chronic inflammatory cells are noted (H & E, 240×).

Intraocular Malignant Melanoma

Primary intraocular malignant melanoma (IOM) comprises a relatively small proportion of all occurrences of malignant melanoma. Nevertheless, IOM is the most common malignant neoplasm of the eye. This lesion occurs most frequently after the fifth and sixth decades of life, and it is extremely rare in children. There is a racial predilection for IOM in that, like CMM, it occurs most frequently in Caucasians and is rare in Negroes.[15] In addition, the frequency of IOM in men and women is the same. The clinical behavior of metastases in IOM is highly unpredictable. Some patients may have a fulminant course, while in others, as many as 20 or more years may elapse after enucleation of the affected eye before widespread dissemination occurs.[16] The principal site of metastasis is to the liver and, in some circumstances, this may be the only site of metastases, giving rise to a false impression that it is a separate primary tumor; in other patients, virtually every organ and tissue of the body, again as in CMM, may ultimately be involved with metastatic disease. The etiology of IOM is unknown. Several studies[17-25] have shown the disease to cluster in families consistent with a hereditary etiology.

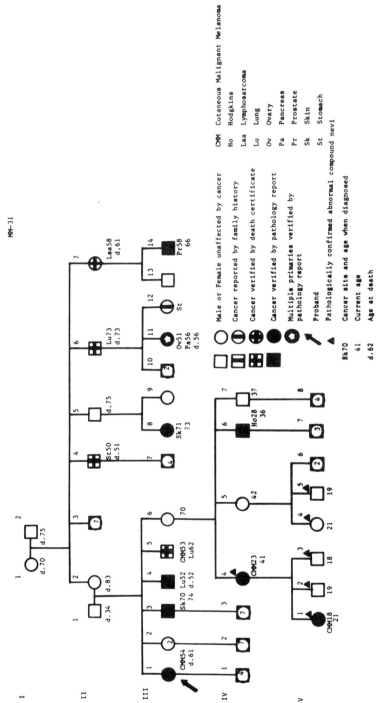

Figure 9-14. Pedigree of Family 3 showing malignant melanoma verified in three generations with histologic verification of familial atypical multiple mole-melanoma moles in individuals affected with malignant melanoma as well as individuals at risk for this disease. Noteworthy is patient III-6, who at age 70 had no evidence of malignant melanoma and whose phenotype did not show presence of atypical moles, yet she had siblings affected with malignant melanoma and she was the progenitor of two generations of affected individuals.

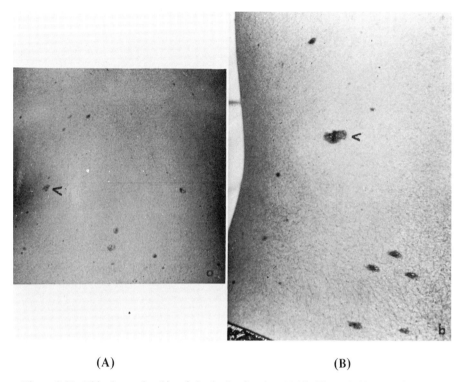

(A)   (B)

Figure 9-15. This shows the skin of the back of patient V-1 in Figure 9-14. (A) The arrow shows an atypical mole which pathologically was a familial atypical multiple mole-melanoma mole, from biopsy at age 17. (B) Two years later, at age 19, this lesion has progressed (arrow) and biopsy showed histologic evidence of a Clark's level IV malignant melanoma.

Lynch[22] surveyed the medical records of 45 patients with histologically diagnosed IOM at the University of Texas M.D. Anderson Hospital and Tumor Institute in Houston, Texas between March 1944 and September 1966. Only one patient in this group had an affected relative (Figure 9-23). Specifically, this was a 61-year-old proband (Figure 9-23, II-1) with verified IOM whose 58-year-old sister (Figure 9-23, II-4) also had histologically verified IOM. A second family (Figure 9-24), independently referred, and not part of this medical records review, involved a 34-year-old white female (the proband, Figure 9-24, III-2) with verified IOM, whose paternal grandfather (Figure 9-24, I-1) was affected with IOM by history and whose paternal uncle (Figure 9-24, II-6) had histologic verification of IOM. The patient's father (Figure 9-24, II-4) did not show evidence of IOM, though his three remaining siblings (sisters) had histologically confirmed cancer. One of these individuals had cholangiocarcinoma of the liver at age 65 (Figure 9-24, II-1), another paternal aunt (Figure 9-24, II-2) had histo-

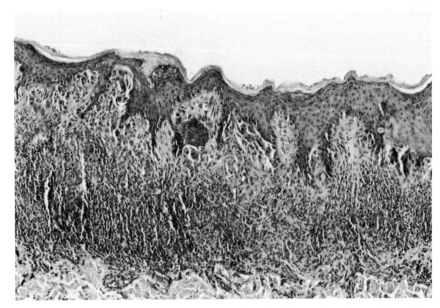

Figure 9-16. Marked dysplasia of melanocytes at dermal-epidermal interface and in papillary dermis. Note the marked lymphocytic infiltrate in the papillary dermis (H & E, 83×).

logically verified adenocarcinoma of the stomach at age 67, and the third paternal aunt (Figure 9-24, II-3) had histologically verified adenocarcinoma of the rectum at age 64.

None of the relatives of the patients with IOM in either of these two families showed evidence of CMM. Findings from these two subject families, as well as those reported from the world literature (Figure 9-25), were consistent with an autosomal dominant mode of inheritance for the hereditary variety of IOM.

In a subsequent study, Lynch and Krush[26] described two families (Figure 9-26) wherein IOM did occur in association with CMM. In one family, a 61-year-old female (Figure 9-26A, II-1) had verified IOM and her 51-year-old sister (Figure 9-26A, II-2) had verified CMM. In the second family, a 74-year-old male (Figure 9-26B, I-1) had verified IOM and his 44-year-old son (Figure 9-26B, II-1) had verified CMM. In an unpublished study (Figure 9-27) which is still in progress, Lynch[27] studied a family from North Carolina. The proband (Figure 9-27, II-1) is a 65-year-old female who had a CMM diagnosed at age 52 and subsequently at age 60 developed colon cancer. Her 68-year-old sister (Figure 9-27, II-4) has had many benign skin lesions excised and developed a CMM at age 45, carcinoma of the breast at age 61, and a basosquamous cell carcinoma of the skin at age 66. A brother (Figure 9-27, II-3) had prostate carcinoma diagnosed at age 66 and died at age 69 of metastatic disease. A sister (Figure 9-27, II-2) at age 60 de-

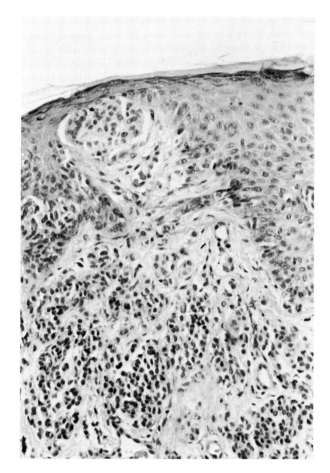

Figure 9-17. Dysplasia of melanocytes at dermal-epidermal interface. Lymphocytic infiltrate noted in papillary dermis (H & E, 500×).

veloped a spindle cell type melanoma of the left eye and expired two years later. There was no evidence of the FAMMM syndrome in this family.

Finally, IOM (bilateral) has also been described in a patient with von Recklinghausen's neurofibromatosis.[28]

Spontaneous Regression of Metastatic Malignant Melanoma

An exceedingly perplexing problem in cancer biology pertains to the relatively rare phenomenon of its spontaneous regression. In a previous review of spontaneous regression of cancer from 1900 to 1960, Everson and Cole[29] documented

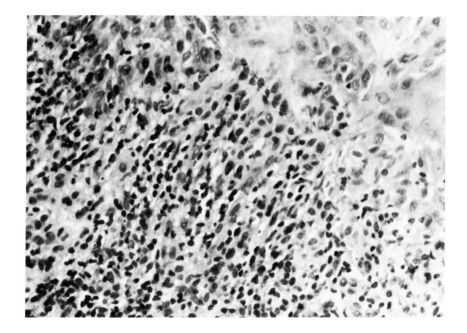

Figure 9-18. Marked lymphocytic infiltrate present in papillary dermis (H & E, 800×).

176 cases of which 19 were examples of spontaneous regression of malignant melanoma. More than half of all of the occurrences of spontaneous regression were of four tumor types: hypernephroma, neuroblastoma, choriocarcinoma, and malignant melanoma.

Nathanson[30] reviewed the subject of spontaneous regression of malignant melanoma since 1900. He observed 33 patients with a total regression of malignant melanoma. Of these cases, 27 were well-documented examples of spontaneous regression of metastatic malignant melanoma.

We[31] studied a family with xeroderma pigmentosum (XP) wherein five of nine siblings were affected with this disease (Figure 9-28). The family was of further interest in that the proband (Figure 9-28, II-4), when initially seen by us at age 17, had pathologic evidence of metastatic malignant melanoma. No therapy was administered. In addition, his then 22-year-old sister (Figure 9-28, II-2) had had a past history of cutaneous malignant melanoma of the skin of her temple, excised at age 21. Subsequently, she presented with metastatic malignant melanoma, which was untreated. We reevaluated this family about ten years later and shall describe those salient aspects dealing with the genesis of spontaneous regression of metastatic melanoma in these two individuals.[32]

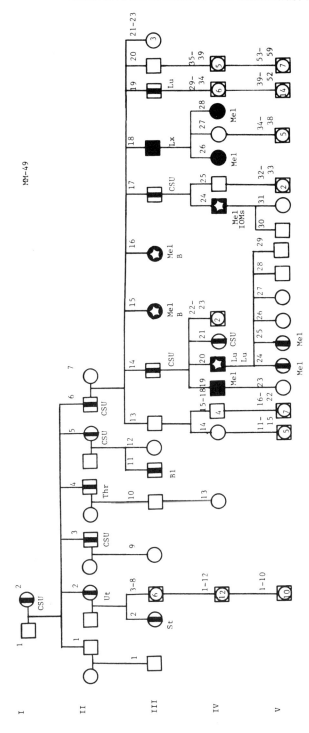

Figure 9-19. Family 4 showing a pedigree which has the cutaneous and histologic findings of the familial atypical multiple mole-melanoma syndrome. In addition to multiple cutaneous melanomas and bilateral intraocular melanomas, this family has a varied assortment of systemic cancers, some in association with double primaries.

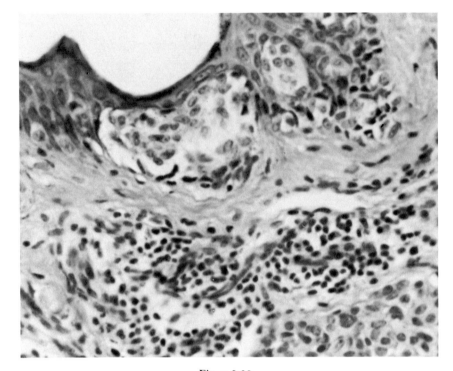

Figure 9-20.

Figures 9-20 through 9-22. Compound Nevus. Melanocytic dysplasia at the dermal- epidermal junction, chronic inflammation in the papillary dermis, new blood vessel formation, and fibroplasia (H & E, 40×).

Case 1: The proband (Figure 9-28, II-4) was a 28-year-old white male, in whom the diagnosis of XP was established at seven years of age. A program of sunlight avoidance was then instituted. He was examined by one of us (HTL) in 1966 and his past history has been reviewed previously.[31] On reexamination in 1975, we observed the patient to show the typical features of XP (hyper- and hypopigmentation, as well as multiple lentigines and ephelides) over the integument, but not over the bathing trunk area. There was evidence of ichthyosis vulgaris on the extensor surfaces of the limbs. In June 1966, at age 17, a primary malignant melanoma was excised from the right forearm. Three months later, a second surgical procedure at this same anatomic site revealed deep metastatic malignant melanoma (Figures 9-29 and 9-30). A histopathologic examination at the patient's hospital at that time revealed "postsurgical persistence of malignant melanoma in the skeletal muscle of the right forearm . . . . Foci of malignant melanoma were also present within tissue coming from under the fascia." No

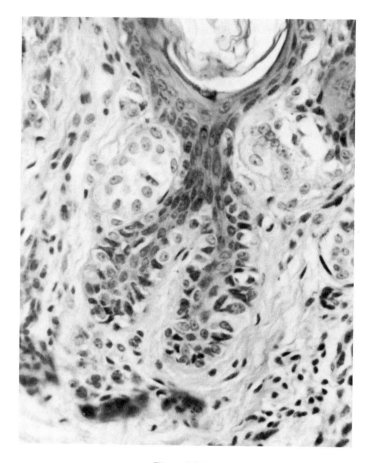

Figure 9-21.

further surgery or therapy was administered. The remainder of the physical examination was unremarkable; specifically, there was no visceral or cutaneous evidence of metastatic malignant melanoma. The patient is still surviving, is healthy, shows no sequelae of malignant melanoma, had graduated from college, is married, and is raising a family.

Case 2: This patient (Figure 9-28, II-2) was the 33-year-old sister of the proband. She received a diagnosis of XP at age 13, at which time a program for avoidance of sunlight was started. She was later examined by one of us (HTL) in 1966, at age 22, as part of a family study.[31] She had had at least 25 basal and squamous cell carcinomas of her skin. A superficial spreading malignant melanoma was excised from the skin of her right temple in 1965. There was no evidence of

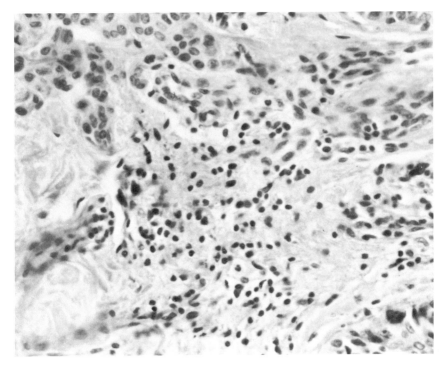

Figure 9-22.

malignant melanoma at the time of our examination. In December 1967, at age 23, a lesion involving the skin of the left lower knee, 1.6 × 0.8 × 0.4 cm deep, was excised. A report of a histologic examination at the patient's hospital stated it was a "malignant melanoma, primary configuration; the base and margins of the resected skin were free of tumor." No further excision of the area was done. Approximately ten months later, the patient was reexamined, at which time there was edema of the leg and increased pigmentation in the region of the old scar on the left knee. It is of interest that the patient gave a history of dehiscence of the wound after the previous surgery. There were two nodes in the left inguinal area measuring approximately 1.5 cm in diameter, and in the medial aspect of the middle third of the left thigh, subcutaneous nodes were found which measured approximately 0.5 cm in diameter.

A groin dissection was performed. Superficial and deep femoral lymph nodes were excised, with the largest measuring 3.3 cm × 2.2 cm × 1.4 cm in depth. These lymph nodes appeared to be involved with malignant melanoma.

Microscopic examination showed that two of the six external iliac nodes contained metastatic malignant melanoma. Of 14 superficial and deep femoral

Table 9-1. Comparison of Histologic Features of Nevi in the FAMMM Syndrome and the B-K Mole Syndrome.

FAMMM SYNDROME	B-K MOLE SYNDROME
Compound nevus	Compound nevus
Melanocytic dysplasia (mild to severe)	Atypical melanocytic hyperplasia
Fibroplasia – papillary dermis (variable)	Fibroplasia – papillary dermis
Lymphocytic infiltrate – papillary dermis (variable: may or may not be present)	Lymphocytic infiltrate – papillary dermis
Histology not always similar to a regressing malignant melanoma or halo nevus	Histology like a regressing malignant melanoma or halo nevus

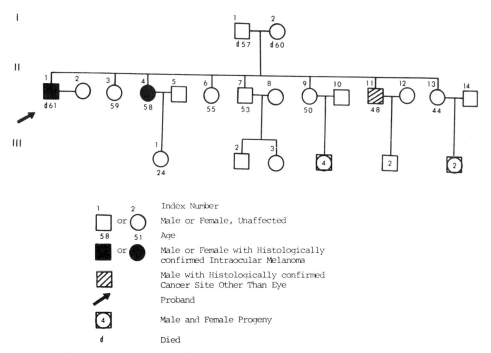

Figure 9-23. Pedigree of two siblings with histologically confirmed intraocular malignant melanoma. (From H.T. Lynch et al., Heredity and malignant melanoma. *Cancer* 21:119–125, 1968)

nodes, 4 contained metastatic malignant melanoma. The accompanying skin from the left knee showed two small foci of junctional nevi. Each of these areas showed some cellular atypia of the melonocytes and an associated inflammatory reaction. However, these lesions did not show histologic evidence of malignant

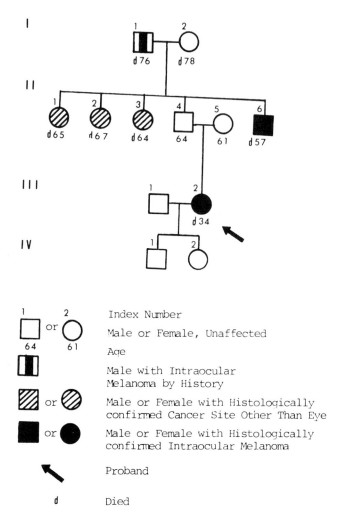

Figure 9-24. Pedigree of a family with intraocular melanoma present in three generations. Note that carcinoma is present in several other siblings in generation II. (From H.T. Lynch et al., Heredity and malignant melanoma. *Cancer* 21:119–125, 1968)

melanoma. It was believed that the previous malignant melanoma removed from the skin of the left knee ten months before the groin dissection was apparently the primary site for the multiple nodal metastases. No further treatment was given to this patient.

Two months later, during January 1968, a lesion involving the skin, measuring 2.0 × 1.7 × 1.0 cm in depth, was excised from the soft tissue of the knee. This comprised a firm, dark-colored piece of tissue which, on microscopic exami-

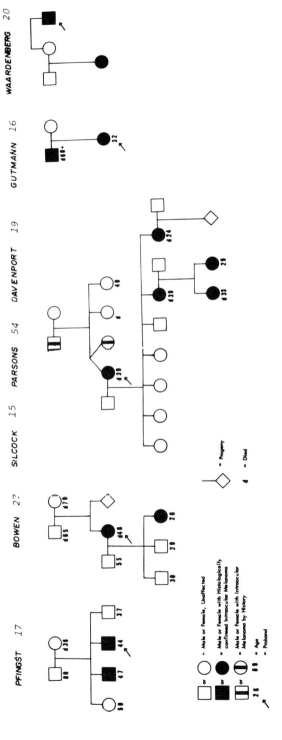

Figure 9-25. Abbreviated pedigrees of four families from the literature with intraocular melanoma. (From H.T. Lynch et al., Heredity and malignant melanoma. *Cancer* 21: 119–125, 1968)

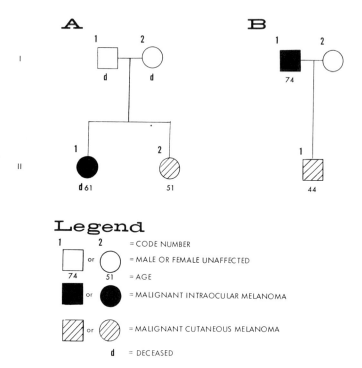

Figure 9-26. Pedigrees of two families wherein intraocular melanoma occurred in association with cutaneous melanoma.

nation, was found to be a subcutaneous nodule composed of several circumscribed lobules of metastatic malignant melanoma. Lymphoid tissue present within this area suggested that the nodule may originally have been a lymph node which was now largely replaced by malignant melanoma. The pathology diagnosis was metastatic malignant melanoma.

Concurrent with these observations, there was histological evidence of foamy-laden histiocytes within a lymph node containing metastatic malignant melanoma (Figure 9-31). In an adjacent area outside the lymph node (Figure 9-32), there were capillary proliferation and chronic inflammatory cells, chiefly lymphocytes. These observations could be interpreted as histological evidence of the spontaneous regression of the metastatic malignant melanoma which was apparent clinically.

After the groin dissection, the edema of her leg began to resolve. She showed progressive improvement in her health. She has since had three normal pregnancies, with the most recent occurring in 1977. The patient has not been personally examined by us since our initial evaluation in 1966. However, we have been able to retrieve medical documents from physicians and from members of

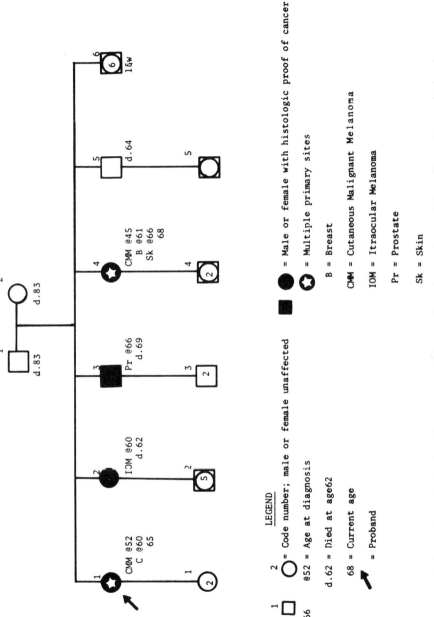

Figure 9-27. Pedigree of a family with cutaneous and intraocular melanoma in association with carcinoma of other sites.

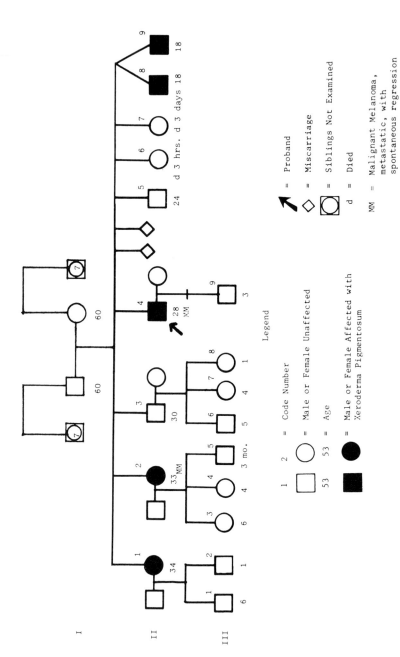

Figure 9-28. Pedigree of a family with xeroderma pigmentosum in which two affected siblings manifested metastatic malignant melanoma and spontaneous regression. (From H.T. Lynch et al., Spontaneous regression of metastatic malignant melanoma in two sibs with xeroderma pigmentosum. *J. Med. Genet.* 15(5):357–362, 1978).

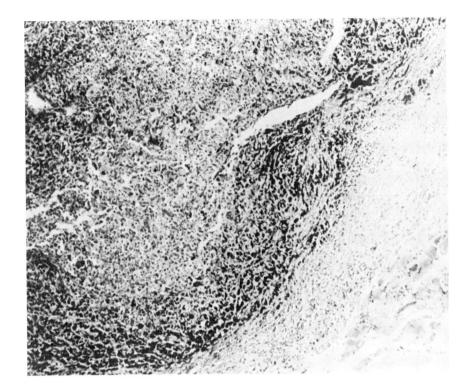

Figure 9-29. Low power view of metastatic melanoma nodules (*upper left*) in fibrous connective tissue adjacent to skeletal muscle (*lower right*). (From H.T. Lynch, et al., Spontaneous regression of metastatic malignant melanoma in two sibs with xeroderma pigmentosum. *J. Med. Genet.* 15(5):357–362. 1978).

the family, including her parents. All of these reports indicate that the patient is apparently in an excellent state of health. The affected area of the right leg has apparently returned to normal. Unfortunately, the patient has steadfastly refused any further participation in our investigation.

Comments. Spontaneous regression of metastatic malignant melanoma in a sister and brother affected with XP, who have survived 13 and 15 years, respectively, in the absence of therapy, poses a challenge for interpretation of pathogenetic mechanisms contributing to this unusual phenomenon. In the study in question, one area of a lymph node containing metastatic malignant melanoma showed several features of possible spontaneous regression, namely foamy-laden histiocytes, capillary proliferation, and a chronic inflammatory infiltrate. The lymphocytic infiltrate in this area, devoid of malignant cells, suggests that perhaps an

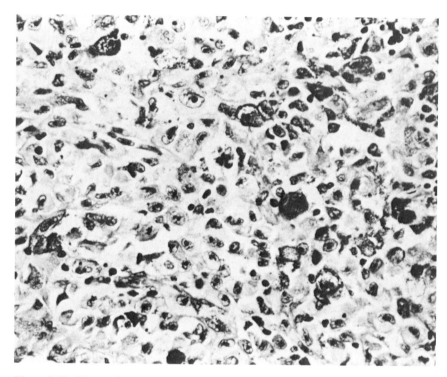

Figure 9-30. Metastatic melanoma nodule composed of cytologically malignant, pleimorphic, melanocytic cells, many heavily pigmented. (From H.T. Lynch, et al., Spontaneous regression of metastatic malignant melanoma in two sibs with xeroderma pigmentosum. *J. Med. Genet.* 15(5):357–362, 1978).

immunological mechanism was at work. These histologic features and their potential immunologic significance for tumor regression have been well documented.[33]

Nathanson's[30] review uncovered two patients with XP who underwent spontaneous regression of malignant melanoma (one with regression of a primary and one with regression of *metastatic* malignant melanoma). Combining Nathanson's 27 cases of spontaneous regression of metastatic malignant melanoma (one with XP), with our 2 cases gives approximately a 10% frequency of spontaneous regression of metastatic malignant melanoma in patients with XP. The question that comes immediately to mind is, Does the genotype for XP, a known multifaceted hereditary disease with impaired DNA repair mechanisms, and with skin as the principal cancer target organ, somehow incredibly also foster a message to be learned from this experiment of nature? This question, of course, raises certain etiological considerations relevant to the survival of the species in

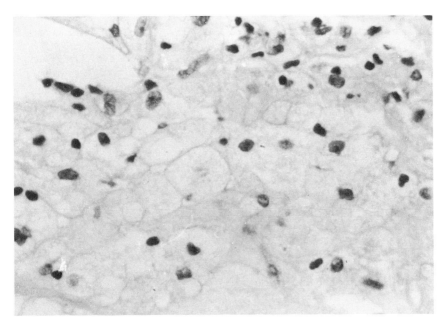

Figure 9-31. Area of foamy histiocytes within a lymph node containing metastatic malignant melanoma (H & E, 237X). (From H.T. Lynch, et al., Spontaneous regression of metastatic malignant melanoma in two sibs with xeroderma pigmentosum. *J. Med. Genet.* 15(5):357–362, 1978).

an evolutionary sense. This reasoning is not unlike explanations given for the favorable response to *Plasmodium falciparum* in heterozygote carriers of the gene for sickle cell anemia,[34] the so-called thrifty genotype for diabetes mellitus,[35] and the heterozygous advantage for other genetic traits.

Should this reasoning be plausible, the study of XP could have profound implications for the comprehension of control mechanisms in certain forms of cancer. Conceivably, such information could be applied to problems in carcinogenesis in the general population.

Anderson[36] has postulated that patients with the familial variety of malignant melanoma may show a better prognosis than nonfamilial (sporadic) occurrences of this disease. As already discussed, we have documented cases of hereditary melanoma in the familial atypical multiple mole-melanoma syndrome which show excellent survival in the face of multiple primary malignant melanomas.[11] Finally, unusual survival from multiple primary malignant neoplasms, particularly adenocarcinomas of the colon and endometrium in advanced stages, has been observed in patients with autosomal dominantly inherited cancer family syndrome.[37]

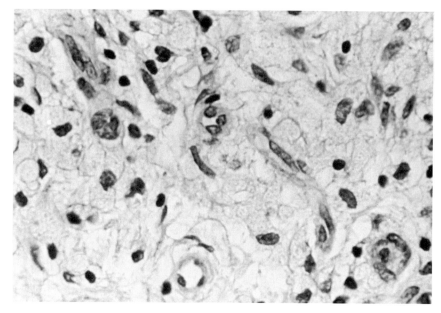

Figure 9-32. View from area adjacent to that seen in Figure 9-31 showing capillary proliferation and chronic inflammatory cells, chiefly lymphocytes (H & E, 237X). (From H.T. Lynch, et al., Spontaneous regression of metastatic malignant melanoma in two sibs with xeroderma pigmentosum. *J. Med. Genet.* 15(5):357–362).

It is noteworthy that infections have frequently been observed in patients who have undergone spontaneous regression of cancer.[30] This may have been important in our 33-year-old patient who experienced dehiscence of her surgical wound.

We urge investigators to study areas such as hormonal factors, immunological competency, viral host interactions, bacterial infections, and possibly other pertinent phenomena, in order to explain mechanisms of cancer toleration in patients with XP. This knowledge might ultimately yield clues to the comprehension of the pathogenesis and natural history of certain forms of cancer in the general population.

DISCUSSION

The frequency of malignant melanoma has been increasing remarkably in recent years in many reporting centers throughout the world,[38] thereby posing an important public health problem. This increased occurrence has been particularly noteworthy in those latitudes with heavy sun exposure which are inhabited by a population at increased risk by virtue of light pigmentation and Celtic ancestry. Queensland, Australia has been such as area where the combination of prolonged sunlight exposure and a high risk population has resulted in a marked excess of this disease. Fortunately, Australia also has had a group of highly motivated clinicians; this fact, in combination with disease excess, has led to pertinent epidemiologic studies.[39]

Studies dealing with the genetics of malignant melanoma in man,[5] as in the case of practically all varieties of cancer,[8] have been aided significantly by animal studies. For example, Gordon,[40] in studies on hybrid fish, showed melanoma risk to be enhanced in the F_1 cross between one parent carrying a macromelanophore-spotting gene (*Xiphophorous masculatus*) and the other parent from a strain lacking this gene (*Xiphophorous helleri*). When a back-cross was made between the F_1 hybrid and the parent strain from which the spotting gene originated, melanoma developed which was less severe than that occurring in the hybrid, presumably resulting from a protective effect of the residual genotype of *Xiphophorous masculatus*. Finally, a back-cross to the parental strain which lacked the macromelanophore gene resulted in severe melanosis and melanoma in progeny inheriting the macromelanophore-spotting gene but lacking "protection" from the residual genotype of the *Xiphophorous helleri* parent. This work and others on the genetic and biochemical basis of malignant melanoma at the infrahuman level have involved the pine snake, *Drosophila*, swine, dogs, horses, and cattle.[41]

At the human level, earlier studies of familial melanoma failed to give attention to clinical-pathologic differences relevant to cutaneous phenotype or associated cancer. For example, Anderson[9] studied an aggregate of 74 documented pedigrees of familial malignant melanoma and concluded that the genetics of this disease were complex and that they probably involved several autosomal loci, in addition to a possible cytoplasmic component transmitted through carrier women. Southerland[42] identified 18 families prone to melanoma and suggested that the genetics were consistent with an autosomal dominant gene showing incomplete penetrance. Wallace et al.[43] studied 42 melanoma pedigrees and concluded that polygenic inheritance provided a more acceptable explanation for the genetics of this disease. Gleicher and associates[44] reviewed the world literature on the subject and found 92 reported examples of familial melanoma. They concluded that an autosomal dominant mode of inheritance would provide the best explanation for the majority of these reports. The fact that genetic conclusions differed in these several malignant melanoma family studies is consonant with our own observation of extant genetic heterogeneity in this disease.[6]

We have described the clinical-pathologic-genetic features in four families with the FAMMM syndrome. Vertical transmission, including father to son, of CMM and/or FAMMM moles was verified. There was no significant sex predilection. There was a broad spectrum of clinical signs which characterized the phenotype. These ranged from an apparent lack of disease expression in one of our genetically informative patients (Figure 9-14, III-6) to florid manifestations in the proband in Family 1 (Figure 9-1, IV-4). The sum total of these observations is compatible with an autosomal dominant gene showing marked variable expressivity.

The absence of disease in an alleged gene carrier in the hereditary retinoblastoma model has recently been discussed by Matsunaga.[45] He has inferred, given the relatively high frequency of resistant carriers of the retinoblastoma gene, that genes determining host resistance to retinoblastoma are nonspecific and may affect the growth of tumors in general. If this were the case, one might expect penetrance and expressivity of cancer of all sites among relatives. In other words, these observations are in agreement with the hypothesis that patients at high cancer risk may harbor in their genotypes an array of cancer-resistant genes (so-called suppressor genes) which could have a major effect on penetrance of the cancer component of the phenotype. This hypothesis therefore suggests the presence of polygenic systems independent of the major cancer-predisposing gene which has a more general effect on cancer susceptibility or resistance. We believe that this reasoning could explain the so-called skipped generation as evidenced in our informative, unaffected gene carrier patient discussed above. We have observed this phenomenon in other dominantly inherited cancer syndromes.[8]

There may be a broad tumor spectrum in the FAMMM syndrome. For example, study of Family 4 has disclosed findings which strongly suggest that the deleterious FAMMM gene may predispose to a variety of *other* histologic forms of cancer, in addition to cutaneous malignant melanoma. A report by Bellet et al[46] establishes a precedent for this line of reasoning in the FAMMM syndrome. Specifically, these investigators showed concurrent intraocular melanoma and cutaneous melanoma in a patient who probably had the FAMMM syndrome. Note that in Family 4, we observed an apparent excess of carcinoma of the breast, stomach, urinary bladder, lung, and larynx. In addition, a single patient showed bilateral intraocular melanoma and multiple cutaneous malignant melanomas, each of which was believed to represent separate primary malignant melanomas.

We realize the limitations which are necessarily imposed when observations are restricted to a single pedigree. However, the increased frequency of cancer of multiple anatomic sites in this kindred should compel the documentation of cancer of *all* anatomic sites in every family showing pathologic and/or clinical manifestations consistent with the FAMMM syndrome. It is only through such efforts as these that the full tumor spectrum of this probably pleiotropic gene might be understood.

Finally, we have underway the investigation of a family in which the proband, a 28-year-old female, has histologically verified cutaneous malignant melanoma and a separate primary squamous cell cancer of the oral cavity. Her father had histologically verified malignant melanoma at age 28 years, cancer of the prostate at age 54 years, and a squamous cell carcinoma of the lung at age 57 years. He has multiple moles. His brother has histologically verified cutaneous malignant melanoma. We have a history of other individuals in the family showing cutaneous features which are suggestive of the FAMMM phenotype. This study will be subsequently published.

Sites of predilection of CMM in our kindreds favored unexposed areas of the body. This was in contrast to their more frequent occurrence in sun-exposed areas in the sporadic variety of malignant melanomas.[47] The CMMs in our FAMMM patients were exclusively of the superficial spreading or nodular variety, with a depth of invasion ranging from Clark's level I to IV.

The natural history of this disease was also variable. There was evidence of the onset of FAMMM moles in childhood in Family 1. Malignant melanomas were of strikingly early age of onset and often multiple with a lifelong susceptibility to these lesions in the face of apparent unusually long survival. Prolonged survival may be a characteristic of hereditary forms of malignant melanoma.

PATHOLOGY

Four unrelated families have been investigated, and within each family, the skin lesions from several members have been studied.

All of the patients studied have varying numbers of melanocytic nevi. These may be compound, junctional, or intradermal nevi. However, most of the moles are recognized as compound nevocellular nevi. Of those that are compound nevi, a significant number show varying degrees of dysplasia of the melanoctyes. The junctional nevi also show varying degrees of dysplasia, although most of these are mild changes. In reviewing these compound nevi, there is variation in the degree of dysplasia between families and within families. Some of the family members exhibit many compound nevi which show dysplasia, while others do not exhibit the same degree of dysplasia of the melanocytes.

The proband of Family 1 (Figure 9-1, IV-4) shows the most significant abnormal changes in the nevi. Most of his lesions show varying degrees of dysplasia of melanocytes at the dermal-epidermal (D-E) junction. There also is fibroplasia, and chronic inflammation of the papillary dermis. This patient also has had the greatest number of cutaneous malignant melanomas (nine over a 17-year period). The proband's mother also shows dysplasia of the compound nevi and she also has manifested two CMMs. The daughter (Figure 9-1, V-1) of the proband has had one clinically larger than usual mole in comparison to others present and this shows dysplasia of the melanocytes at the D-E junction, fibroplasia, and chronic inflammation of the dermis. A sister (Figure 9-1, IV-6) and a maternal aunt (Figure 9-1, III-3) shows a lesser degree of melanocytic dysplasia.

The proband in Family 2 (Figure 9-12, III-1) shows similar dysplasia of the melanocytes with a small amount of accompanying chronic inflammation and fibroplasia of the dermis.

The proband in Family 3 (Figure 9-14, V-1) appears to show the greatest degree of dysplastic melanocytes within her compound nevi. The changes are noted at the D-E junction. Again, many of these compound nevi show fibroplasia and chronic inflammation within the papillary dermis. The two brothers of the proband (Figure 9-14, V-2,3) also show melanocytic dysplasia of their lesions, but this appears to be not quite as severe as occurred to the proband. The mother (Figure 9-14, IV-4) of the proband also shows dysplasia of the melanoctyes within her lesions. However, most of these are only graded as mild dysplastic changes. Many of her lesions are intradermal nevi and thus should not be considered to be premalignant. Two cousins (Figure 9-14, V-4,5) of the proband also (within their skin lesions) show only mild atypical changes of the melanocytes.

The patients in these families demonstrate a large number of abnormal compound nevi. However, it appears as if some members in these families are affected more significantly than others. These lesions showed melanocytic dysplasia or atypical melanocytic hyperplasia which range from mild to severe changes. The papillary dermis in most of these lesions shows some fibroplasia, new blood vessel formation, and a chronic lymphocytic infiltrate. In some instances, the fibroplasia and chronic inflammation are moderate to marked. The histopathology of the FAMMM moles shows them to be compound nevocellular nevi with varying degrees of dysplasia of the melanocytes. There appears to be considerable variation in the degree of dysplasia in nevi between and within families. Specifically, certain members exhibited compound nevi which showed marked dysplasia, while other relatives demonstrated a lesser degree of dysplasia of the melanocytes.

The histologic appearance of such lesions favors the interpretation that this pattern is consistent with an immune response in the host and the subsequent changes that are seen in the evolution of such lesions. This pathologic process may be an expression of a similar event that occurs in halo nevi or a regressing malignant melanoma.

The histopathologic features seen in these nevi are similar to the changes in moles from patients manifesting the B-K mole syndrome as described by Clark and associates.[12,13] These authors use the term *atypical melanocytic hyperplasia*. This term is considered to be synonymous with melanocytic dysplasia. Histologically, one sees individual melanocytes or clusters of melanocytes that show cytologic abnormalities. These atypical melanocytes are seen primarily at the D-E interface. These then are melanocytes which show some premalignant change, although the exact potential for malignant change is not known.

Several members of these families also show the development of junctional nevi and intradermal nevi. Again, the melanocytes within the junctional nevi show varying degrees of dysplasia.

A serious dilemma exists relevant to the pathogenesis of the FAMMM mole with specific reference to its benign versus its malignant propensity. This therefore poses a crucial question for management, namely, Which moles do you biopsy on the basis of clinical inspection and then, after histologic study, which will require wider excision? Unfortunately, this issue has not yet been fully resolved from the pathology standpoint.

The families have also demonstrated the development of several malignant melanocytic tumors. Of the four members in Family 1 (Figure 9-1), we have evaluated pathology on 11 malignant lesions (CMMs). Three are classified as premalignant melanosis (SSMM, Clark's level I); six are classified as superficial spreading malignant melanoma (Clark's levels II and III). The proband demonstrates four superficial spreading malignant melanomas and these are Clark's level II. One sister has a superficial spreading malignant melanoma, Clark's level II, and the mother of the proband has a superficial spreading malignant melanoma, Clark's level III. Two of the malignant tumors are diagnosed as nodular malignant melanomas. The proband shows a nodular malignant melanoma, Clark's level IV, and a sister of the proband shows a Clark's level III.

CLINICAL DESCRIPTION: SUMMARY OF CUTANEOUS PHENOTYPE

The clinical expression of the multiple nevi and atypical moles in this syndrome is extremely variable. Those patients with the full cutaneous expression have, on inspection, 100–1,000 nevi of varying shades of brown and black. The sizes fluctuate from a few millimeters to several centimeters. The face is conspicuously spared. Scattered through this maze of clinically regular-appearing nevi are atypical-appearing nevi ranging in size from less than 5 mm to more than 10 mm. Their color is not uniform and includes shades of brown, tan, black, and pink. The latter color helps distinguish them. In addition, these macular-papular atypical lesions usually have irregular borders which are not clinically distinct in outline. Thus, there appear to be two discrete populations of nevi present. The atypical lesions may be the only lesions present in some patients and may number less than five or ten.

While the descriptive terminology of the FAMMM syndrome emphasizes its association with atypical moles and malignant melanoma, we believe that it is prudent to give additional attention to other cancer associations. For example, in Family 1 (Figure 9-1), there were occurrences of pancreatic carcinoma in siblings in the direct genetic line, while lung cancer and Hodgkin's disease occurred in informative relatives in Family 3 (Figure 9-14). Family 4 showed cancer of the breast, lung, larynx, stomach, urinary bladder, and uterus in addition to IOMs and CMMs in a single patient. It will be important that all reports of the FAMMM syndrome include a painstaking appraisal of cancer of *all* anatomic sites so that patterns of tumor associations, should they exist, might be recognized. It is also imperative that we explore possible relationships between the FAMMM syndrome and other familial/hereditary varieties of malignant melanoma, in addition to sporadic malignant melanoma. In short, a question that requires more meticulous study is, What is the clinical, pathologic, and etiologic significance of the FAMMM syndrome relevant to oncology in general and to all etiologic varieties of malignant melanoma in particular?

MANAGEMENT

An important question pertains to the philosophy of treatment of FAMMM-affected patients. One particularly wonders about the role of conservative vs radical treatment of the malignant melanomas. This question must be tempered by the unusually benign clinical course which has been documented in certain of our patients. Another issue pertains to the need for restriction of solar radiation exposure in patients manifesting the FAMMM syndrome. Relevant to this concern, we must consider data which suggest that malignant melanoma (lentio maligna melanoma excepted) may differ from other varieties of skin cancer in that it may be elicited by intense and shorter periods of solar radiation exposure as opposed to the more frequent finding of cumulative lifetime sun exposures in nonmelanoma skin cancer. It has been speculated that a putative "solar circulating factor" may be etiologic in certain malignant melanomas occurring in non-sun-exposed areas.[48] In the case of the FAMMM syndrome, this could seemingly be heralded by the presumptive genetic proclivity to carcinogenesis in the atypical moles.

The de novo occurrences of melanoma in certain patients at high risk but lacking FAMMM moles is of interest. This could represent a chance occurrence. However, we believe it most likely represents heterogeneity as evidenced by cancer manifestation of this putative dominant pleiotropic gene which has not expressed the atypical mole component of the syndrome in a fraction of the patients. This problem is in some respects similar to that of dominantly inherited Gardner's syndrome in which colon cancer may occur in a patient who may lack the cutaneous and/or osseous component of this cancer-associated genodermatosis. These considerations are discussed since it has been suggested[12,13] that the pathology findings in the atypical moles are essential for diagnosis of this hereditary malignant melanoma-associated syndrome. We prefer to consider the pathology of the moles as only one, albeit important, component of the syndrome; nevertheless, its presence or absence is not mandatory for diagnosis of the FAMMM syndrome. We believe it is prudent to base the diagnosis on the sum total of the clinical and pathological findings in concert with the pedigree. We emphasize this point since, soberingly, family history has been sorely neglected in most clinical cancer studies.[49]

Recognition of the cutaneous phenotype is an exceedingly important component of the management program. One must particularly consider variability in its expression. Detailed family history will aid greatly in casting clinical findings in their proper perspective since members who are at high risk for the genotype can often be identified even when only minimal aberrations are present in the skin. Biopsy-proven FAMMM histology in an atypical mole will add confidence to the diagnostic suspicion.

We believe that patients showing the FAMMM phenotype should be provided with detailed information about the natural history of the FAMMM syndrome. Such an educational program should include acquainting the patient with clinical examples of moles which demonstrate the variable stages in the transition to malignant melanoma. We provide our patients with laminated cards which they can carry in their wallets and which describe the salient characteristics of lesions which may be consonant with the differing varieties of clinical presentations of CMM. We review the material on these cards with the patients initially and then periodically thereafter so that they are well acquainted with the significance of changes in moles. Ideally, these patients should be under the care of an informed dermatologist who is well acquainted with the syndrome. They should see this specialist about four times a year, and any moles which are suspicious or have changed in character during the interim from one visit to the next should be biopsied.

Clark and his associates have progressively altered the terminology of the FAMMM syndrome. In their original description, they referred to the FAMMM group as the B-K Mole Syndrome.[12] Subsequently, they renamed the disorder the Dysplastic Nevus Syndrome (DNS),[50] by expanding the concept on a histologic basis to include not only the familial patients with the histologically aberrant nevi, but also those sporadic malignant melanoma patients who show nevi with the same histology. They now have designated the DNS as the "Large Atypical Nevus Syndrome (LANS)" with familial and sporadic subtypes.[51] Even though the LANS terminology appears to emphasize the clinical description, it uses the histology of the nevi to bridge the two clinical areas, familial and sporadic subtypes. This is problematic in that the entire spectrum of histologic findings are not always uniformly present in FAMMM patients who have atypical nevi. The clinical expression of the nevi in the FAMMM pedigrees ranges phenotypically from no nevi through small nevi to large atypical nevi. We are therefore concerned that Clark's terminology may have confused, if not obscured, the distinctiveness of the FAMMM syndrome, which must be considered with respect to several parameters, i.e., clinical, histologic, and genetic. It is the latter which clearly separates the FAMMM phenotype and must be emphasized in the management of the high cancer risk in the pedigree. This is shown in our pedigrees reported here, in that some patients do not have the FAMMM cutaneous phenotype, but still develop malignant melanomas, not only of the skin, but the eye. In addition, the occurrence of malignancies in other organs in these patients clearly separates the FAMMM group as needing high cancer risk management.

In conclusion, families of the type we have described should serve as excellent models for studies of genetic-environmental interaction in carcinogenesis, as well as for investigation of the role of immunologic factors in its control. Finally, we do not know with certainty at this time what fraction of all malignant melanomas might be hereditary and herein, quantitatively, what subset of the hereditary variety might represent the FAMMM syndrome.

SUMMARY

Detailed clinical-pathologic-genetic studies have been performed on four kindreds showing the FAMMM syndrome. Findings showed vertical transmission, including father to son, of cutaneous malignant melanoma and/or FAMMM moles. There was no significant sex predilection. Of interest was a broad spectrum of clinical signs characterizing the phenotype which ranged from an apparent lack of disease expression to minimal, more moderate, and florid manifestations. The most extreme examples were in a patient who developed nine separate primary CMMs and in a second who had bilateral intraocular melanomas and multiple CMMs. The histopathology of the FAMMM moles show them to be compound nevocellular nevi with varying degress of dysplasia of the melanocytes, fibroplasia, and chronic inflammation within the papillary dermis. Of further interest was marked variation in the degree of melanocytic dysplasia in moles between and within families. Other facets of hereditary melanoma, including intraocular melanoma, have been discussed. Emphasis has been given throughout to the need for detailed description of cutaneous phenotype and cancer of all anatomic sites in the study of hereditary melanomas.

ADDENDUM

Through the courtesy of R.R. Hook, Ph.D., University of Missouri at Columbia, we have had an opportunity to evaluate malignant melanoma in the Sinclair miniature swine colony (Oxenhandler, R.W., Adelstein, E.H., Haigh, J.P., Hook, R.R., Jr., Clark, W.H.: Malignant melanoma in the Sinclair miniature swine: an autopsy study of 60 cases. *Amer J Pathol* 96:707–714, 1979). Interestingly, these animals have an excess of congenital malignant melanoma, multiple primary melanoma, multiple nevi, and a high rate of spontaneous regression of malignant melanoma. Preliminary evaulation of their premelanotic nevi by us showed histologic similarities to FAMMM moles. These animals should provide an excellent model for the study of the FAMMM syndrome.

REFERENCES

1. Greene, M.H., and Fraumeni, J.F.: The hereditary variant of malignant melanoma. In: *Human Malignant Melanoma* (W.A. Clark, Jr., et al., Eds.). New York: Grune and Stratton, 1979, pp. 139–66.
2. Norris, W.: A case of fungoid disease. *Edinb. Med. Surg. J.* 16:562–565, 1820.

3. Cawley, E.P.: Genetic aspects of malignant melanoma. *Arch. Derm. Syph.* **65**: 440–450, 1952.

4. Lynch, H.T., and Krush, A.J.: Heredity and malignant melanoma: implications for early cancer detection. *Can. Med. Assoc. J.* **99**:17–21, 1968.

5. Lynch, H.T., and Frichot, B.C.: Skin, heredity, and cancer. *Sem. Oncol.* **5**:67–84, 1978.

6. Lynch, H.T., Frichot, B.C., Lynch, P., Lynch, J., and Guirgis, H.A.: Family studies of malignant melanoma and associated cancer. *Surg. Gyn. Obstet.* **141**:517–522, 1975.

7. Lynch, H.T.: *Skin, Heredity and Malignant Neoplasms*, Flushing, NY: Medical Examination Publ. Co., 1972, pp. 239.

8. Lynch, H.T.: *Cancer Genetics*, Springfield, IL: Charles C. Thomas Co., 1976, pp. 639.

9. Anderson, D.E.: Clinical characteristics of the genetic variety of cutaneous melanoma in man. *Cancer* **28**:721–725, 1971.

10. Frichot, B.C., and Lynch, H.T.: A new cutaneous phenotype in familial malignant melanoma. *Lancet* **1**:864–865, 1977.

11. Lynch, H.T., Frichot, B.C., and Lynch, J.F.: Familial atypical multiple mole-melanoma syndrome. *J. Med. Genet.* **15**:352–356, 1978.

12. Clark, W.H., Reimer, R.R., Greene, M., Ainsworth, A.M., and Mastrangelo, M.J.: Origin of familial malignant melanoma from heritable melanocytic lesions: the B-K mole syndrome. *Arch. Derm.* **114**:732–728, 1978.

13. Reimer, R.R., Clark, W.H., Greene, M.H., Ainsworth, A.M., and Fraumeni, J.F.: Precursor lesions in familial melanoma. *JAMA* **239**:744–746, 1978.

14. Lynch, H.T., et al.: Family studies of malignant melanoma and associated cancer. *Surg. Gyn. Obstet.* **141**:517–522, 1975.

15. Hogan, M.J., and Zimmerman, L.E.: *Ophthalmic Pathology, an Atlas and Textbook* (2nd ed.). Philadelphia, PA: W.B. Saunders, 1962, pp. 413.

16. Allen, J.C., and Jaeschke, U.H.: Recurrence of malignant melanoma in an orbit after 28 years. *Arch. Opthal.* **76**:79–81, 1966.

17. Silcock, A.O.: Hereditary sarcoma of eyeball in three generations. *Br. Med. J.* **1**: 1079, 1892.

18. Gutman, G.: Casuistischer Beitrag zur Lehre von den Geschwulsten des Augapfels. *Arch. Augenheilkunde.* **31**:158, 1895.

19. Pfingst, A.O.: Melanosarcoma of the choroid occurring in brothers. *Arch. Ophthal.* **50**:431, 1921.

20. Davenport, R.C.: A family history of choroidal sarcoma. *Br. J. Ophthal.* **2**:443, 1927.

21. Bowen, S.F., Jr., Brady, H., and Jones, V.L.: Malignant melanoma of eye occurring in two successive generations. *Arch. Ophthal.* **71**:805, 1964.

22. Lynch, H.T., Anderson, D.E., and Krush, A.J.: Heredity and intraocular malignant melanoma: study of two families and review of forty-five cases. *Cancer* **21**(I): 119, 1968.

23. Parsons, J.H.: *The Pathology of the Eye.* Vol. 2, Histology; Part II. New York: Putnam, 1905, pp. 496, 497.

24. Tucker, D.P., Steinberg, A.G., and Cogan, D.G.: Frequency of genetic transmission of sporadic retinoblastoma. *Arch. Ophthal.* **57**:532–535, 1957.

25. Green, G.H., Hong, W.K., Everett, J.R., Bhutani, R., and Amick, R.M.: Familial intraocular malignant melanoma: a case report. *Cancer* **41**:2481–2483, 1978.

26. Lynch, H.T., and Krush, A.J.: Heredity and malignant melanoma: implications for early cancer-detection. *Can. Med. Assoc. J.* **99**:17, 1968.

27. Lynch, H.T.: in preparation, 1981.
28. Gartner, S.: Malignant melanoma of the choroid and von Recklinghausen's disease. *Am. J. Ophthal.* **23**:73-78, 1940.
29. Everson, T.C., and Cole, W.H.: *Spontaneous Regression of Cancer.* Philadelphia, PA: Saunders, 1966.
30. Nathanson, L.: Spontaneous regression of malignant melanoma: a review of the literature on incidence, clinical features, and possible mechanisms. Conference of Spontaneous Regression of Cancer. *NCI Monograph* **44**:67-77, 1976.
31. Lynch, H.T., Anderson, D.E., Smith, J.L., Jr., et al.: Xeroderma pigmentosum, malignant melanoma, and congenital ichthyosis: a family study. *Arch. Derm.* **96**: 625-635, 1967.
32. Lynch, H.T., Frichot, B.C., III., Fisher, J., Smith, J.L., Jr., and Lynch, J.: Spontaneous regression of metastatic malignant melanoma in two siblings with xeroderma pigmentosum. *J. Med. Genet.* **15**:357-362, 1978.
33. Bodurtha, A.J., Berkelhammer, J., Kim, Y.H., Laucius, J.F., and Mastrangelo, M.J.: A clinical, histologic, and immunologic study of a case of metastatic malignant melanoma undergoing spontaneous regression. *Cancer* **37**:735-742, 1976.
34. Livingstone, F.B.: *Abnormal Hemoglobins in Human Populations: A Summary and Interpretation.* Chicago, IL: Aldine, 1967.
35. Neel, J.F.: Diabetes mellitus: a thrifty genotype rendered detrimental by "progress?" *Am. J. Hum. Genet.* **14**:353-362, 1962.
36. Anderson, D.E.: Clinical characteristics of the genetic variety of cutaneous melanoma in man. *Cancer* **28**:721-725, 1971.
37. Lynch, H.T., Bardawil, W.A., Harris, R.E., Lynch, P.M., Guirgis, H.A., and Lynch, J.F.: Multiple primary cancer and prolonged survival: familial colon and endometrial cancer. *Dis. Colon Rect.* **21**:165-168, 1978.
38. Doll, R.: An epidemiologic perspective of the biology of cancer. *Cancer Res.* **38**: 3573-3583, 1978.
39. Davis, N.C.: Cutaneous melanoma: the Queensland experience. *Curr. Prob. Surg.* **13**:1-63, 1976.
40. Gordon, M.: Hereditary basis of melanosis in hybrid fishes. *Am. J. Cancer.* **15**: 1495-1532, 1931.
41. Siciliano, M.J., and Perlmutter, A.: Maternal effect on development of melanoma in hybrid fish of the genus Xiphophorous. *JNCI* **49**(2):415-421, 1972.
42. Southerland, E.M.: Familial melanoma. *Proc. IX Int. Pigment. Cell Conf.* Houston 60, 1975.
43. Wallace, D.C., Exton, L.A., and McLeon, S.R.C.: Genetic factor in malignant melanoma. *Cancer* **27**:1262, 1971.
44. Gleicher, N., Cohen, C.J., Deppe, G., and Gusberg, S.B.: Familial malignant melanoma of the female genitalia: a case report and review. *Obstet. Gyn. Surv.* **84**: 1-15, 1979.
45. Matsunga, E.: Hereditary retinoblastoma: delayed mutation or host resistance? *Am. J. Hum. Genet.* **40**(IV):406-424, 1978.
46. Bellet, R.E., et al.: Primary choroidal and cutaneous melanomas occurring in a patient with the B-K mole syndrome phenotype. *Am. J. Ophthalmol.* **89**:567-570, 1980.

47. Kripke, M.L.: Speculations on the role of ultraviolet radiation in the development of malignant melanoma. *JNCI* **63**:541-545, 1979.

48. Lee, J.A., and Merrill, J.M.: Sunlight and the aetiology of malignant melanoma: a synthesis. *Med. J. Aust.* **2**:846-857, 1970.

49. Lynch, H.T., Follett, K.L., Lynch, P.M., Albano, W.A., Mailliard, J.A., and Pierson, R.L.: Family history in an oncology clinic: implications for cancer genetics. *JAMA* **242**:1268-1272, 1979.

50. Elder, D.E., Goldman, L.I., Goldman, S.C., Greene, M.H., Clark, W.H.: Dysplastic nevus syndrome: a phenotypic association of sporadic cutaneous melanoma. *Cancer* **46**:1787-1794, 1980.

51. Bondi, E.E., Clark, W.H., Elder, D., DuPont, G., and Greene, M.H.: Topical chemotherapy of dysplastic melanocytic nevi with 5% fluorouracil. *Arch. Derm.* **117**: 89-92, 1981.

10
Biochemical Aspects of Cancer-associated Genodermatoses

John A. Johnson, Ph.D.

INTRODUCTION

Rationale of this Report

Much specific detail has been included for the benefit of readers who wish a refresher on specific topics. Another advantage of this approach is that it provides a background for some speculative lines of reasoning. General reviews and summary tables have been cited in introductions to specific subjects. Specific data, and authors' conclusions, have been cited, and attempts have been made to develop unifying concepts and suggestions. Some of these constructions may be wrong, because of either lack of awareness of crucial data in the literature or failure to consider all aspects of the subject. However, the objective is always to stimulate: to provoke discussion, to encourage others to take a broader look at specialized areas of interest, to invoke the performance of experiments designed to elucidate basic concepts.

I have the unique opportunity to discuss the molecular biology of hereditary skin disease from the viewpoint of one versed in skin metabolism, and will exploit it to the fullest. This report is wide ranging and, hopefully, contains items of interest to a variety of readers. Comments and suggestions, pro and con, from interested readers are solicited.

General Comments

The biochemistry of genodermatoses and cancer covers many broad areas, such as skin metabolism, genetics, etiology of cancer, methodology for studying cancer, and rationale for therapy. These general areas will be discussed briefly in this introduction, but the report will concentrate on: (1) biological effects of ultraviolet radiation (UVR), (2) methods for assessing DNA damage and repair, and (3) genodermatoses involving sensitivity to sunlight and/or defects in the repair of DNA. The rationale for this approach is based on the accumulating evidence that cancer arises from one or more mutations, which in turn are the consequence of misrepair (or nonrepair) of damaged DNA. Multiple pathways of DNA repair have been studied with bacterial systems, and the availability of UVR mutants has enabled investigators to examine these mechanisms in detail. Much of the information gained has been extrapolated to the behavior of mammalian cells, in great part a result of the existence of the human UVR mutant, the genodermatosis called *xeroderma pigmentosum* (XP). Patients with XP are extremely sensitive to sunlight and develop multiple UV-induced cutaneous carcinomas at an early age. The discoveries by Cleaver in 1968[1] that fibroblasts from XP patients have a reduced ability to repair damaged DNA, and by de Weerd-Kastelein et al.[2] in 1972 that patients with XP may be classified into different complementation groups, have triggered a profusion of investigations into the mechanisms of DNA repair in mammalian cells. These efforts are proceeding at an increasing rate, and have expanded to include studies of other genodermatoses which exhibit sensitivity to sunlight and/or defects in DNA repair.

In order to keep the number of references within a reasonable limit, current reports will be cited. From these, the interested reader can obtain citations to much of the earlier literature. Several current general references are also recommended.[3-11]

Skin Metabolism. Skin undergoes most of the metabolic processes of other tissues and, therefore, can mirror systemic disorders. In addition, since skin may be easily collected without harming the donor, it is the ideal tissue for investigation of human metabolism. Likewise, skin tumors are readily accessible for study.

It should be recognized that skin is a heterogeneous tissue: it consists of a large, relatively inert dermis, a metabolically active epidermis, and various appendages (hair follicles, sweat glands, etc.). The dermis is important to biochemists because its cells (fibroblasts) are easy to collect and culture, and because they often reflect systemic metabolic derangements. The etiology of many hereditary disorders has been elucidated by investigating the metabolic behavior of cultured fibroblasts. The epidermis is continuously renewing itself and is therefore metabolically active (particularly the dividing cells of the basal layer). Since epidermal slices may be collected without harm from humans, this tissue should also be of interest to biochemists. The recent development of techniques for establishing pure epidermal cell cultures and for culturing explants will greatly expand the experimental use of this tissue.

In summary, those of us interested in the metabolism of skin consider it the ideal tissue for conducting definitive biochemical and physiological experiments with humans. Skin metabolism will not be discussed in detail here, but comments concerning unique biochemical aspects will be made where appropriate. The interested reader is referred to several reviews for further information.[12-15]

Genetics. Biochemists are usually not concerned with the technical aspects of this subject. However, to understand the association of hereditary disorders and cancer, one must have some knowledge of chromosomal terminology and aberrations. Regarding autosomal recessive dermatoses, the biochemist may be able to suggest or develop tests for detecting heterozygotes who may be at increased risk for cancer.

Etiology of Cancer. Dermatologic investigators are attuned to the current consensus that many cancers are caused by environmental factors, since skin is exposed to a multitude of noxious agents. The multiple-hit theory of tumor induction is attractive in the consideration of genodermatoses and cancer. Thus, the phenotype of skin disorder may reflect a genetic aberration which constitutes the initial "hit." Individuals carrying this genotype will obviously be at increased risk upon exposure to environmental agents.

From a perusal of the literature, it appears that dermatologists have not been greatly concerned with the association of genodermatoses and cancer unless the latter involves the skin. There is considerable interest in "cutaneous signs of internal malignancy," but the burden of investigation of genetic associations has been borne largely by internists, oncologists, and epidemiologists. Alerting the dermatologic community to relationships between genodermatoses and cancer in general will serve the twofold purpose of encouraging dermatologists to look for, and report, such associations, and to counsel patients about the need for periodic examination for cancer.

Unique Aspects of Skin Cancer. Most skin cancers arise in the epidermis and are readily treated by surgery or local therapy. They rarely metastasize or kill the host (the notable exception being malignant melanoma) and therefore do not generate the public concern that other forms of cancer do.

Since skin is chronically exposed to UVR and visible light for the lifetime of the individual, the most important environmental factor in the etiology of skin cancer is UVR. And because skin and cutaneous tumors are conveniently located, in vitro and in vivo experiments involving exposure to light are easy to perform. Consequently, much of the information concerning skin carcinogenesis relates to ultraviolet induction of tumors. Also, the genodermatoses most likely to be recognized as being associated with cancer are those in which patients exhibit sensitivity to sunlight and consequent early development of multiple skin tumors. Thus, the "sun-sensitivity" disorders have been exhaustively documented and studied.

Methodology. Investigation of genodermatoses and cancer involves many techniques of interest to the biochemist, such as detection of chromosomal aberrations, evaluation of defects in DNA synthesis and repair, and detection of "tumor markers." The development of new techniques and the critical evaluation of established ones are subjects for ongoing investigations.

Rationale for Therapy. By understanding the biochemistry of rapidly dividing cells, investigators have discovered agents which are selectively toxic to tumors. Knowledge of the metabolism of drugs permits the design of chemotherapeutic agents which may be activated in situ in tumor cells. A tumor marker, if truly unique for a specific cancer type, might be used to trigger the host's immunologic response to the tumor. Alternatively, antibodies to a unique antigen may be coupled to a cytotoxic agent and employed to "home in" on inaccessible cancers. Ability to quantitate plasma tumor marker levels may be of value in early detection of tumors, prognosis, selection of therapy, and monitoring of therapeutic response.

BIOLOGICAL EFFECTS OF ULTRAVIOLET RADIATION

Fundamental Concepts

In dealing with the biological action of UVR and visible light, one should consider the regions included in the sunlight spectrum, i.e., 290-400 nm (UV) and 400-700 nm (visible). Photobiologists refer to three UV regions: UV-A (320-400 nm, long UV), UV-B (290-320 nm, short UV) and UV-C (below 290 nm). The boundary between UV-A and UV-B, at 320 nm, is a convenient reference for dermatologists, because this is the cutoff point for ordinary window glass. Thus, a photosensitive patient who develops symptoms when exposed to sunlight through glass is judged sensitive to long UVR and/or visible light. Wavelengths below 290 nm are absorbed by ozone in the stratosphere and therefore do not occur in terrestrial sunlight. This region is of interest to biologists, however, because experiments are often conducted with germicidal lamps which emit an energy peak at 254 nm. Several important aspects about sunlight impinging on skin must be considered:

1. The energy content of electromagnetic radiation varies inversely as the wavelength. Thus the shorter the wavelength, the greater the damage to biological systems. In fact, UV-B is referred to as the sunburn region, because it is responsible for the physical trauma resulting from overexposure to the sun. The UV-A region is relatively innocuous, except when a photosensitizer is present. Many compounds (e.g., psoralens) absorb energy in this region and transfer it to a cellular component in such a manner that an exaggerated photoresponse occurs. The PUVA treatment for psoriasis and other skin disorders is based on this rationale: PUVA = psoralen + UV-A. This point is worth noting, because analogous experiments have

been conducted with lymphocytes and fibroblasts. In general, when considering exposure of skin to sunlight, we are dealing with an energy range of 40 to 100 kcal/mole photons, corresponding to wavelengths of 700 to 290 nm. Since the higher end of this energy range is sufficient to break some covalent bonds, UV-B can cause chemical alterations in sensitive organic molecules. A more pronounced effect will be observed with UVR at 254 nm, a point which must be considered when experiments are conducted at that wavelength. (The fact that UVR at 254 nm is germicidal speaks for its destructive potential.) Much more drastic alterations result from irradiation with γ-rays such as x-rays and ^{60}Co emissions. These radiations are of much shorter wavelength and higher energy content than UVR, and are referred to as ionizing radiation because of their potential for breaking chemical bonds.

2. The energy content of sunlight decreases rapidly below 400 nm, to zero at 290 nm. Therefore, the total content of the UV-B region is much less than that of the UV-A region. Despite this, the shorter wavelengths are so biologically effective that most of the destructive action of sunlight results from UV-B.

3. The penetration of UVR into skin varies inversely with the wavelength. Proteins have a broad absorption band at 280 nm, and thus filter out the most energetic wavelengths of UV-B. Epidermal melanin screens both UV-A and UV-B, and affords moderate protection to fair-skinned persons and much greater protection to pigmented individuals. Thus, the latter are less susceptible to actinic damage and have a much lower incidence of UV-induced skin cancer. This subject was discussed in detail by Kaidbey et al.[16] Because energy must be absorbed before a photobiological response can occur, and because of the selective absorption of UV-B in the epidermis, most of the destructive action of sunlight occurs in that tissue. The situation is different for persons sensitive to UV-A, however, since longer wavelengths penetrate to the dermis. Thus, in erythropoietic protoporphyria, the classic hereditary disorder of long-UV photosensitivity, the first observable histologic change after irradiation occurs near the dermal capillaries.

4. In addition to the selective absorption of UV-B in the epidermis, one must consider the fact that epidermal cells are closely packed, whereas dermal fibroblasts are widely scattered. Consequently, the carcinogenic potential of sunlight or UV-B is expressed in the induction of mainly squamous and basal cell carcinomas rather than dermal sarcomas. Although fibroblast cultures are easy to establish and conduct experiments with, and have provided much valuable information about genodermatoses involving sunlight sensitivity, one must keep in mind that such experiments are not at all comparable to the natural state of sunlight impinging on human skin.

5. Another consideration which is difficult to compensate for in the laboratory is that ambient conditions such as heat, wind, and humidity affect the actinic and carcinogenic potential of UVR.[17]

Structure of DNA

Before discussing the effects of UVR on DNA, it may be helpful to review some basic features. A DNA strand consists of a backbone of deoxyribose units attached by 3', 5'-phosphodiester bonds. Because of the 3', 5'-linkage, each strand is directional; i.e., one can read from the 5' to the 3' end. Each sugar moiety has one of four nitrogenous bases (the purines — guanine and adenine, and the pyrimidines — cytosine and thymine) attached to it by an N-glycosidic bond. Two complementary strands (in which one has guanine and the other, cytosine; one has adenine and the other, thymine) associate in a double helix to form the DNA molecule with the attached bases oriented into the center of the helix. The strands are antiparallel and are held together by hydrogen bonding between opposing bases. The double helix is further stabilized by base stacking; i.e., the essentially planar rings of adjacent bases in each strand are oriented parallel to each other. These features may explain several phenomena of base damage and repair:

1. Enzymic or spontaneous cleavage of N-glycosidic bonds produces apurinic or apyrimidinic DNA. The phosphodiester bonds of sugar units devoid of bases are labile, so that the strand can be nicked by alkaline media.
2. Sobell et al.[18] described a phenomenon of DNA breathing and drug intercalation which may explain the photo-sensitizing action of certain psoralens. In this process, a small segment of DNA partially unwinds, leaving an open space in the double helix which still allows base pairing between opposite strands. The heterocylic rings of each base pair are coplanar, and the rings of adjacent base pairs are in parallel planes. This arrangement provides a "slot" that the planar quinoxaline ring of echinomycin fits snugly into (see Figures 1 and 5 of reference 18). It is easy to visualize the furocoumarin ring of a psoralen inserting into such a slot, where it could act as an efficient photosensitizer: the paired bases, which are normally shielded within the DNA helix, will be exposed and will be in close proximity to the psoralen ring.
3. Adjacent pyrimidine bases may be in the appropriate orientation for photodimerization, and the DNA breathing process may periodically expose them to photons.

Because both DNA strands are copied simultaneously during replication, and because all known DNA polymerases copy only in the 3' to 5' direction of the template (i.e., 5' to 3' in the daughter strand), the antiparallel orientation of the strands lends great complexity to semiconservative replication. This subject has been reviewed in detail by Gefter.[19] Briefly, one can visualize a nick in one strand, with the free end rapidly unwinding from the intact partner, and a "replication fork" moving along the DNA molecule. Continuous synthesis of a daughter strand occurs in one template, but continuous synthesis of the other strand requires assembly of *Okazaki fragments* from the replication fork in a direction opposite to its movement and rapid joining of these fragments.

In addition to the complexities outlined above, one must consider that DNA in its natural state is associated with histones and nonhistone proteins, and is folded in itself in a complex fashion. Information about this complicated arrangement of DNA and proteins may shed light on the observation that repair of UVR-induced pyrimidine dimers does not occur uniformly along the DNA molecule[20] and on the fact that fibroblasts of various XP patients exhibit the same defect in ability to nick DNA at a damaged site, yet are able to "cure" each other in cell fusion experiments.

To further complicate the picture of DNA synthesis and repair, one must now consider the occurrence of *introns* in eukaryotic cells.[21] Introns are intervening DNA segments within a gene, which are copied along with the gene segments during transcription. The overlarge RNA copy is then cut and patched so that the product is a complementary copy of the gene. Introns are a recent discovery; Crick[21] attributes the origin of the concept to publications arising from the Cold Spring Harbor Symposium of 1977. They apparently do not exist in prokaryotic DNA, since one would have expected their discovery long ago. This point underscores the frequent admonition of molecular biologists that much of our understanding of DNA replication and repair in mammalian cells is extrapolated from studies of prokaryotic systems, and therefore must be accepted with reservations. The subject of introns is too new to know whether they serve physiological functions, or whether some may be nonfunctional vestiges of evolutionary processes. The latter alternative might provide some understanding of why even normal human fibroblasts can tolerate long-lived pyrimidine dimers and remain viable.[22]

Effects of Ultraviolet Radiation on DNA

The action of UVR on chromatin involves damage to protein as well as to DNA. However, the cell is continuously replacing damaged proteins, and it appears to have adequate capability to repair UV-induced damage. On the other hand, injury to DNA results in loss of genetic information, and accurate repair is required if the integrity of the cell is to be maintained. Thus, consideration of induction of cancer by UVR is focused on its effects on DNA. Much of the voluminous literature regarding clinical implications of the action of UVR on living systems is concentrated on the induction and repair of pyrimidine dimers.

Such efforts have yielded much valuable information and undoubtedly will continue to do so. However, it may be timely to consider whether more subtle types of UVR-induced DNA damage should be investigated. With this thought in mind, it is appropriate to review some basic reactions catalyzed by UVR. The extreme complexity of these interactions has been reviewed by Smith.[23]

Base Damage. Base damage can involve chemical alterations, dimerization, and photocatalyzed addition of endogenous compounds (e.g., amino acids). In accord with Smith's comment that pyrimidines are about ten times more sensitive to damage by UVR than purines, this discussion will also be limited to photochemical reactions of pyrimidines. Reactions will be discussed as though they occurred with free nitrogenous bases, but one should keep in mind that many of them have been verified to occur in DNA strands.

Photohydration. Photohydration involves addition of water across the 5,6 double bond of pyrimidines, and can be reversed by elimination of water. Photohydration of cytosine labilizes the amino group attached to the ring. Oxidative deamination and regeneration of the double bond will leave a uracil moiety (the characteristic base of RNA).

Photooxidation. Photooxidation of the methyl group of thymine yields 5-formyluracil. The reactive aldehyde group can form a Schiff base with a free amino group of a protein, thus cross-linking DNA to protein.

Photodimerization. The major pyrimidine dimer produced by UVR is the cyclobutane type, i.e., the bases are joined at their 5 and 6 positions to form a cyclobutane ring. Other types of pyrimidine adducts are produced in much lower yields, but in general their biological significance is not known. In theory, cyclobutane-type dimers may include all possible combinations of cytosine (C) and thymine (T): C-C, C T, and T-T. As will be discussed later (see "Xeroderma Pigmentosum: Experimental Detection of Pyrimidine Dimers"), it may be important to investigate the relative proportions of these dimers in UV-irradiated DNA.

Addition of Hydroxyl Radicals. Irradiation of DNA with UVR produces a minor product, 5,6-dihydroxydihydrothymine (thymine glycol); greater amounts are produced by γ-radiation. Saturation of the 5,6 double bond labilizes the N-glycosidic link, so that mild treatment of DNA containing these lesions releases free base. Alkaline treatment also cleaves the heterocyclic ring, forming acetol,[24] which provides an assay for thymine glycol (see "Ataxia Telangiectasia: Biochemical Studies of Defective Repair").

Chain Breaks. Chain breaks require cleavage of phosphodiester bonds or carbon-carbon bonds in the sugar moiety. The energy content of UV-B is sufficient to produce only low yields of breaks. As implied earlier, ionizing radiation is of sufficient energy to efficiently break DNA strands. Smith[23] pointed out that one should not think of chain breaks as being of a single type. Cleavage of the phosphodiester link may occur at the 3' bond with one deoxyribose moiety or at the 5' link with the adjacent sugar unit. Likewise, cleavage of the 4',5' bond or the 3',4' bond of deoxyribose will produce strand breaks. Obviously, cleavage at these different sites will yield several types of chain breaks with different groups on the DNA ends. Thus, several enzymes with different specificities will be required to repair such damage.

Carcinogenic Action of Ultraviolet Radiation

Induction of Skin Cancer. Photocarcinogenesis in humans and animals has been reviewed by Epstein.[25] The primary carcinogenic region of sunlight is UV-B, and the skin-damaging effects of UV-B are potentiated by UV-A. The evidence linking chronic exposure to sunlight with induction of skin cancers in man is circumstantial, since controlled experiments have not been performed with humans. However, there is strong epidemiological evidence implicating sunlight in induction of basal and squamous cell carcinomas, and suggestive data for certain types of cutaneous melanoma.

Photosensitizers such as 8-methoxypsoralen (8-MOP) and porphyrins cause acute phototoxic responses to UV-A, and chronically exposed photosensitized animals develop skin cancers. One might wonder about the incidence of skin cancer in humans photosensitive to UV-A; their lifelong avoidance of the sun to minimize skin damage probably reduces their risk of cutaneous cancer. Another consideration is that the acute response of a photosensitized epidermal cell to UVR may kill the cell rather than transform it into a malignant species. The PUVA therapy for psoriasis may be the human analogue of animal experiments with UV-A. Investigators employing this regime have stressed the need to assess the risk-benefit ratio for each patient, and to employ PUVA only for severe cases not amenable to other forms of therapy. However, in a two-year prospective study of 1,373 patients receiving PUVA therapy,[26] the incidence of basal and squamous cell carcinomas was 2.6 times that expected for a matched control population. The elevated risk of cancer was restricted to patients who had a history of exposure to ionizing radiation or had a previous cutaneous carcinoma. One must recognize, however, that two years constitute a short interval in the usual induction period for human skin cancers; if patients without cancer risk factors are maintained on PUVA therapy, they may also exhibit an increased incidence of skin cancer.

Effect of Ultraviolet Radiation on Host Resistance to Cancer. Many skin cancers produced by chronic exposure of mice to UVR are highly antigenic and are rejected when transplanted into syngeneic hosts.[27] However, if the prospective host is subjected to a short course of exposure to UVR, it is unable to reject the tumor. The immunologic aspects of this phenomenon were discussed by Kripke and Fisher[28] and by Fisher.[29] They suggested that chronic exposure to UVR may facilitate the growth of tumors of diverse etiology, and demonstrated the enhanced survival of B16 melanoma in UV-irradiated mice. This observation may help explain the indirect association of sunlight with human melanoma, as reflected in the occurrence of tumors at body sites not exposed to the sun. Another important observation bearing on this question was reported by Rosdahl.[30] She observed that chronic exposure of mice to UV-B caused a long-lasting increase in number of melanocytes in both irradiated and unirradiated ears. The results were interpreted to suggest UVR induction of a systemic melanocyte-stimulating factor, rather than destruction of a growth-controlling chalone. Roberts et al.[31] produced tumor susceptibility in mice by treating them with subcarcinogenic doses of 8-MOP and UV-A. The implications of this report for PUVA therapy of humans should be examined. The above-cited reports remind one of the "solar circulating factor," postulated by Lee and Merrill[32] as an etiologic factor in nodular melanoma.

Doses of Ultraviolet Irradiation: Experimental vs Therapeutic

Much of the literature concerning UV-induced DNA damage deals with irradiation of cultured fibroblasts. Doses of UV-B from a few to several hundred joules per square meter have been employed. In order to place this in perspective, one might consider the approximate dose ranges employed in phototests on humans (Table 10-1). Although the International Dose Unit is J/m^2, it is more convenient to cite phototest doses of UV-B in mJ/cm^2, and of UV-A in J/cm^2. The thousandfold difference in units reflects the much greater biological effectiveness of UV-B compared to UV-A. The minimal erythemal dose of UV-B (20–50 mJ/cm^2, or 200–500 J/m^2) is at the high end of the experimental dose

Table 10-1. Experimental Doses of Ultraviolet Radiation for Humans.*

Minimal erythema dose, UV-B	20-50	mJ/cm^2
Minimal erythema dose, UV-A	20-50	J/cm^2
Minimal phototoxic dose, UV-A, after:		
Oral psoralen	2-5	J/cm^2
Topical psoralen	.2-.5	J/cm^2

*Phototest values provided by Dermer.[33]

range. It must be noted, however, that in vivo, only a fraction of the incident UV-B reaches the basal cells and fibroblasts. Experimental radiation doses are sometimes given in ergs per square millimeter; a convenient conversion reminder is: 100 ergs/mm^2 = 10 J/m^2. Since UVR at 254 nm is often employed to study DNA damage, it may be helpful to relate this radiation to sunlight. In terms of lethal effects on a UV-sensitive strain of *E. coli*, one minute of noontime sunlight in Dallas in late fall is equivalent to 0.1 J/m^2 UVR at 254 nm.[34] Cleaver[35] employed this figure to estimate that one hour of midday sunlight in April in San Francisco is equivalent to 10 J/m^2 of UVR at 254 nm, in terms of survival of normal human fibroblasts. Trosko et al.[36] calculated that on the basis of amount of pyrimidine dimers formed in human amnion cells, five hours of sunlight in August in East Lansing is equivalent to 60 J/m^2 UVR at 265 nm. Andrews[37] recently reported the relative lethality of UV-B, UV-A, and UV-254, in terms of survival of lymphoblast lines from patients with xeroderma pigmentosum. To cause growth inhibition equivalent to that of a given dose at 254 nm, required 5–10 times as much UV-B and 5–10 $\times$ 10^4 times as much UV-A.

PATHWAYS OF DNA REPAIR

Smith[38] has reviewed this subject with regard to bacterial DNA repair; Hewitt and Meyn[39] discussed the applicability of bacterial models to mammalian cells. Since bacterial mutants deficient in various repair steps are available, bacterial mechanisms are known in greater detail than are those for mammalian cells. The classical human mutant, the XP fibroblast, has been extremely useful in clarification of excision repair of pyrimidine dimers in mammalian cells. The information presented in this section has been obtained by study of bacterial systems, but much of it has been validated for eukaryotic cells.

Three basic repair processes have been documented. (1) Repair in situ may occur spontaneously, as in dehydration of pyrimidine photohydrates, or it may be performed enzymically, as in *photoreactivation.* Photoreactivation involves splitting of cyclobutane-type pyrimidine dimers under the influence of visible light. (2) *Excision repair* (dark repair) requires removal of the damaged DNA segment and replacement with undamaged nucleotides. This pathway has been observed as a means of replacing pyrimidine dimers, and also of repairing other DNA lesions induced by radiation and chemicals. (3) In *postreplication repair* (S-phase repair), the DNA lesions are bypassed during replication, leaving gaps in the daughter strands which are subsequently filled.

Photoreactivation

Photoreactivation (PR) has been investigated in detail by Sutherland.[40] It was thought for some time that photoreactivating enzyme (PRE) did not occur in mammalian cells, until Sutherland isolated PRE from human leukocytes. She noted that its action spectrum extended to at least 600 nm, which includes the output of yellow bulbs commonly used as safelights. Sutherland et al.[41] observed that the action spectrum for human fibroblasts was the same as that for the purified enzyme. This property and the fact that cell culture conditions influence PRE activity[42] explain why others had not detected the enzyme. Compared to other mechanisms for pyrimidine dimer repair, PR capacity is low. However, when considered in the context of total repair capacity of the cell, PR may be a contributory factor in defective repair. In the assessment of other pyrimidine dimer repair pathways or in the evaluation of the effect of unrepaired pyrimidine dimers on a biological response, prior exposure of cells to white light (i.e., photoreactivation) affords a useful control experiment.

Excision Repair

Defects in DNA which are amenable to excision repair include pyrimidine dimers, single-strand breaks, and base damage. Grossman et al.[43] have reviewed dimer excision repair.

Short-patch Repair. This is the classical mechanism for prereplication replacement of pyrimidine dimers. It requires: (1) incision of the DNA strand near the damaged site by an endonuclease; (2) excision of 30 or fewer nucleotides, including the pyrimidine dimer, by a 5′-exonuclease (alternatively, an oligonucleotide containing the damaged site may be cleaved off by an endonuclease); (3) replacement of the missing nucleotides, using the intact strand as a template, by a DNA polymerase; (4) joining of the newly synthesized segment to the original strand by a polynucleotide ligase. Step 3 may precede step 2, or they may occur simultaneously. The phenomenon of *liquid holding recovery* occurs in UV-irradiated *E. coli* cells, which exhibit much higher survival if they are held in the dark in buffer for several hours before plating on nutrient medium. Experiments with mutants suggest that the mechanism for recovery is short-patch repair.

Long-patch Repair. This involves the removal and replacement of about 1,500 nucleotides and is dependent on the growth medium.

Repair of Single-strand Breaks. Since UVR is not sufficiently energetic to initiate many strand breaks in DNA, this type of repair is usually not considered in examining the effects of UVR or sunlight on living systems. On the other hand, x-rays produce numerous strand breaks and extensive base damage. The extreme sensitivity of patients with ataxia telangiectasia to x-rays has stimulated considerable interest in repair of these types of DNA damage. Experiments with bacterial mutants indicate that single-strand breaks are repaired by the same short-patch and long-patch mechanisms described above. Obviously, the incision step is not required. However, Waldstein[44] and Cleaver[45] pointed out that x-rays induce breaks which usually do not have the 3'-OH ends required for action of DNA polymerase or ligase. Consequently, enzymic modification of the 3' terminus is required.

Repair of X-ray-induced Base Damage. Two modes of repair are possible: *nucleotide* excision and *nucleoside* excision. The former is analogous to repair of pyrimidine dimers but is difficult to study because no convenient assay for this type of damage has been developed. Nucleoside excision involves removal of the damaged base by a DNA glycosylase, leaving an apyrimidinic or apurinic site. An enzyme specific for uracil and others specific for alkylated bases in DNA have been reported. A specific endonuclease cleaves the site of base removal, and subsequent repair is assumed to occur as in the usual mode of excision repair. It is likely that cells must have repair capability in order to counteract the low level of spontaneous depurination (about 10/min per cell)[46] and the slow spontaneous production of uracil moieties. Recently, Deutsch and Linn[47] reported a repair capacity in human fibroblasts which does not require excision repair — purine insertase. A purified preparation eliminated alkaline-labile sites in an apurinic DNA substrate, in the presence of guanine or adenine. Specificity of base insertion appears to depend on the orientating effects of base stacking and hydrogen bonding, since the insertase preparation introduces the purine appropriate for the specific lesion in the apurinic DNA substrate. Thus, depurinated poly(dA-dT) accepted adenine but not guanine, and depurinated poly(dG-dC) accepted only guanine. The reaction does not appear to require a high-energy cofactor, which raises the possibility that the stabilizing factors of base stacking and hydrogen bonding of the entering purine provide enough energy to form the N-glycosidic bond. And if fidelity is dictated by the amount of energy expended, this type of repair is error prone. It is of interest that caffeine, which inhibits error-prone repair in other systems, also inhibits insertase activity.

Repair of Chemical Adducts. Various chemicals react with bases in DNA to form mono- or diadducts (cross-links), particularly under the influence of UVR. These lesions are probably removed by excision repair processes. Cleaver et al.[48] suggested that opposite ends of a cross-link are repaired by different mechanisms, possibly by base removal and nucleoside excision on one strand followed by nucleotide excision on the other.

Postreplication Repair

As pointed out by Lehmann,[49] postreplication repair (PRR) does not truly represent repair, since it provides accurate synthesis of complete DNA daughter strands in the presence of damaged sites in the template. Two general modes of replication past a damaged site may be visualized:[50] (1) Replication skips the site and the gap in the daughter strand is filled in later, either by de novo synthesis or by recombination with the opposite parental strand. The several steps involved in the latter process have been outlined by Lavin.[51] (2) Replication stops at the damaged site but continues on the intact parental strand. When the daughter strand is sufficiently elongated, branch migration (backward movement) occurs, allowing the daughter chains to fold and pair up. The terminal segment of the elongated daughter strand serves as a template for the other, thus permitting insertion of nucleotides complementary to the damaged segment of the parental strand. Replication on both parental strands then proceeds in normal fashion.

Higgins et al.[52] considered the consequences of branch migration (also known as strand displacement) and made two predictions: (1) It is well known that bromodeoxyuridine (BrUdR) will substitute for thymine during DNA replication, and the resulting daughter strands will be heavier than normal DNA. Parent/daughter duplexes arising from semiconservative replication will have intermediate density. If branch migration occurs during PRR in the presence of BrUdR, the isolation and shearing of DNA undergoing repair will produce many fragments of intermediate density and some heavy ones. The latter will represent paired daughter strands which had been in the process of repair replication when the DNA was sheared. (2) If the fraction containing DNA of intermediate density is examined by electron microscopy, one should observe four-pronged replicating structures which have one arm considerably shorter than the other. The authors verified both predictions for human cells treated with a DNA-damaging agent (see Figure 4 of their report for impressive electron micrographs).

In UV-irradiated excision deficient cells, the lengths of newly synthesized daughter strands are approximately the same as the distance between pyrimidine dimers in the parental DNA. As time after irradiation increases, daughter strand length increases until it attains that of unirradiated cells. It has been estimated that the daughter strand gaps constitute the absence of about 1,000 nucleotides. It has not been firmly established that these gaps are actually opposite DNA damage sites, although there is some experimental support for such orientation.

In the interest of completeness, one should mention *SOS repair*, the error-prone DNA-polymerizing activity induced in *E. coli* by a variety of agents and which is responsible for UV mutagenesis.[53] Little or nothing is known about the relevance of this system to DNA repair in eukaryotic cells.[54]

Repair Error as a Factor in Mutagenesis and Carcinogenesis

Studies with bacterial mutants suggest that excision repair (short-patch) is error free, whereas PRR is error prone. Mutants defective in long-patch excision repair are not mutable by UV irradiation, while mutants with defective short-patch excision repair undergo mutations. Since the latter must rely on error-prone PRR to maintain viability, it is concluded that repair errors lead to mutations. Boiteux et al.[55] discussed mutagenesis by mispairing and nonpairing DNA lesions. To expand this concept, most ultimate carcinogens are mutagenic; therefore, errors in DNA repair may lead to carcinogenesis. Zajdela and Latarjet[56] provided partial confirmation of this concept in vivo, with mice subjected to chronic UV irradiation. When caffeine or theophylline (known inhibitors of PRR) were applied to the skin before irradiation, the incidence of skin cancer was reduced 48%. On the other hand, topical reductone or chloroquine (considered inhibitors of excision repair) did not affect tumor incidence. Topical uridine (a strong UV absorber) had no effect, thus establishing that the effect of caffeine or theophylline did not result from physical screening of UVR. Since both agents cause elevation of intracellular cyclic AMP by inhibition of phosphodiesterase, one might wonder if this were the mechanism of inhibition of cancer induction. However, topical application of dibutyryl cyclic AMP or a more potent diesterase inhibitor did not influence the action of UVR.[57]

Xeroderma pigmentosum may be a human example of the association of repair errors and carcinogenesis. Fibroblasts from persons with the classical form of the disorder exhibit defective excision repair, and patients develop multiple skin carcinomas at an early age. Conscientious lifelong avoidance of sunlight may reduce the incidence of skin cancer.[58] Another human example might be derived from the ongoing multicenter study of PUVA patients referred to earlier (see "Carcinogenic Action of Ultraviolet Irradiation"). It would be of interest to know if any of the 30 subjects who developed skin carcinomas were heavy coffee drinkers. In fact, it might be worthwhile to investigate the incidence of skin cancer in heavy users of caffeine-containing beverages in the general population.

METHODOLOGY FOR MEASURING DNA DAMAGE AND REPAIR

In reviewing the literature, one encounters a profusion of methods for assessing DNA damage and repair. Various techniques will be reviewed, but this section is not intended to be exhaustive. Cleaver[59] discussed and evaluated various methods in detail, and Hanawalt[60] provided convenient tables for comparison of assay procedures for excision repair and for postreplication repair. Cleaver outlined the suitability of several methods for studying excision repair. Paterson[61] evaluated various assay methods based on the use of lesion-specific enzymes. Techniques will be discussed with appropriate applications, but the reader should recognize that a given technique may be employed to examine more than one repair mechanism. In general, the techniques have been applied to fibroblasts and, occasionally, to lymphocytes and other cells. It is appropriate to discuss terminology.[62] A repair process is named according to the technique employed to monitor insertion of a new DNA segment. Thus, *unscheduled DNA synthesis* refers to detection of ^{3}H-TdR incorporation radioautographically; *radiation-stimulated synthesis*, to isolation of DNA and determination of its radioactivity. *Repair replication* refers to analysis via isopycnic gradients or bromouracil photolysis, and *dimer excision* involves hydrolysis of isolated DNA and chromatographic isolation of photoproducts.

Unscheduled DNA Synthesis

Cultured cells are exposed to a DNA-damaging agent (e.g., chemical carcinogen) and pulse labeled with tritiated thymidine (^{3}H-TdR). The amount of ^{3}H-TdR incorporated into DNA is assessed either by radioautography or by isolation of the DNA and counting its radioactivity. Radioautography permits one to localize the sites of DNA synthesis. Cleaver (in Figure 13 of reference 59) illustrated the localization of DNA synthesis in nuclei irradiated with a UV microbeam. He also pointed out that comparison of unscheduled DNA synthesis (UDS) between different cell types is difficult because different pool sizes and rates of turnover will influence the amount of ^{3}H-thymidine incorporated. These differences can be minimized by blocking thymidine monophosphate synthesis with fluorodeoxyuridine (FUdR).

Quantitation of DNA synthesis by radioautography requires tedious counting of silver grains, whereas measurement of incorporated radioactivity in DNA is easy to perform. However, unless a synchronous cell culture is employed, even a pulse label of ^{3}H-TdR will catch some cells in S-phase (i.e., semiconservative replication). This is corrected for in radioautographs by ignoring the heavily labeled cells. In quantitating DNA radioactivity, one may allow for semiconservative replication by comparing results with a control culture subjected to identical experimental conditions except exposure to the DNA-damaging agent. However, replication entails much more efficient incorporation of thymine than does UDS and is usually blocked with an agent such as hydroxyurea. This technique has merit, but one must be aware that the blocking agent itself may introduce uncontrollable error.

Use of synchronous cell cultures appears ideal in theory, but complicates the experimental protocol and raises the concern that the steps employed to obtain synchrony may alter the metabolism of the cell. On the other hand, synchronous cultures would allow examination of the DNA-damaging effects of agents during different phases of the cell cycle. Lymphocytes are amenable to this technique, because they are predominantly in the G_0 phase in whole blood. Synchronous fibroblast cultures might be conveniently obtained by employing fibroblast growth factor (FGF), as suggested by Gospodarowicz.[63] This factor permits cells to grow in the presence of plasma rather than serum (thus more closely approximating the in vivo state) and, when added to a culture of resting cells, causes them to resume growth simultaneously. The commercial availability of FGF (Collaborative Research, Inc.) renders this approach feasible.

Both purines and pyrimidines will serve as radiotracers for DNA synthesis,[59] but purines undergo multiple metabolic fates. It is natural to employ ^{3}H-TdR, since it will distinguish DNA synthesis from RNA synthesis. As will be noted later (see "Experimental Detection of Pyrimidine Dimers: Nature of UV-induced Dimers"), the use of cytidine as a radiotracer may provide information about information and repair of pyrimidine dimers.

Lastly, it must be emphasized that measurement of UDS reflects incorporation of thymidine into DNA by processes other than semiconservative replication, but reveals little about the repair mechanisms involved. After UV irradiation of human fibroblasts, most of the incorporation of radioactivity measured as UDS is observed before much loss of pyrimidine dimer is detected.[64] This temporal difference may in part represent the greater sensitivity of radioautography. One may also wonder if at least some fraction of UDS represents incision at the damage site and insertion of nucleotides, while the dimer-containing terminus is still attached to the damaged DNA strand.

Repair Replication

This process is defined as the insertion of small patches in DNA molecules during repair of UV-induced damage. Patch sizes can be estimated from studies of radioautographs, but more direct techniques are available.[59]

Isopycnic Gradient Centrifugation. This method is also known as buoyant density centrifugation or equilibrium density centrifugation. It is based on the fact that BrUdR will substitute for thymidine in DNA synthesis and repair, and it enables one to distinguish semiconservative replication from low levels of repair replication. Semiconservative replication will produce DNA molecules with the daughter strand containing BrUdR instead of TdR, and the molecules will have a higher density than normal DNA. Molecules which have only undergone repair replication will not contain enough BrUdR units to be much denser than normal. Equilibrium centrifugation on a cesium chloride density gradient will resolve a heavy and light band of DNA. For quantitation of repair replication, cells are incubated in ^{3}H-BrUdR for a short interval, and radioactivity of the light band is measured. The use of hydroxyurea to block semiconservative repair improves resolution, but studies have been conducted without it. In the latter instance, isopycnic analysis is performed on single-stranded DNA on alkaline gradients.

Bromouracil Photolysis. This technique provides a precise estimate of patch size in repair replication and has validated results obtained by other methods.[59] Irradiation of BrUdR-containing DNA with UVR at 313 nm produces strand breaks and alkali-labile regions. In a typical experiment, cells are prelabeled with ^{3}H-TdR, irradiated with UVR, and allowed to grow in BrUdR for a given interval.

The need for hydroxyurea during BrUdR incorporation has been argued pro and con. After BrUdR treatment, the cells are irradiated at 313 nm and analyzed on alkaline sucrose gradients.

Column Chromatography. Scudiero et al.[65] reported a rapid method for quantitating excision repair. Cells are incubated in the presence of ^{3}H-TdR, hydroxyurea, and a DNA-damaging agent. The cells are then lysed, and the lysate is incubated with ribonuclease and pronase. After shearing to reduce DNA size, the lysate is chromatographed on BND-cellulose. The fraction eluting in $1M$ NaC1 is monitored for increased radioactivity resulting from repair synthesis.

Removal of Pyrimidine Dimers

Excision repair of UV-induced pyrimidine dimers may be monitored by direct quantitation of dimers or by determining the number of sites sensitive to enzymes specific for dimer sites in damaged DNA.

Radiochromatographic Dimer Assay. Cells are prelabeled with ^{3}H-TdR and, at various intervals after irradiation, are lysed and extracted with 5% trichloroacetic acid. The insoluble chromosomal DNA is hydrolyzed with formic acid to yield free bases and photoproducts, and subjected to chromatography (paper, thin layer, or column). The percent of total DNA radioactivity in the dimer fraction is interpreted as a measure of the number of dimers present at the time of cell lysis; the rate of decrease of dimer radioactivity after irradiation reflects the kinetics of the specific repair process responsible for dimer removal. Paterson[61] pointed out that the amount of dimer formation at UVR doses below 5 J/m[2] (the upper limit for good survival of mammalian cells) is too low for accurate quantitation. Presumably, analysis of DNA hydrolysate from a sufficient number of cells by column chromatography will resolve this problem. The method has been employed to monitor excision on DNA lesions other than dimers, but one must be aware that some photoproducts (e.g., cytosine hydrate) are not stable to acid hydrolysis.

An alternate approach is to monitor the release of pyrimidine dimer from cellular DNA by analyzing the fraction soluble in 5% trichloroacetic acid. This requires resolution of some technical problems, such as isolation of a radiopure fraction in the presence of a relatively large amount of radioactive thymine and establishing whether acid-soluble, dimer-containing oligonucleotides represent excision repair segments or isolation artifacts.

Detection of Endonuclease-sensitive Dimer Sites. Enzymes which cleave DNA at pyrimidine dimer sites are called UV endonucleases. Dimers are detected by enzymic cleavage of dimer sites in damaged DNA and resolution of the products by alkaline sucrose gradient centrifugation. Analysis of the loss of endonuclease susceptibility of DNA from cells incubated for increasing intervals after UV irradiation provides an indirect measure of the kinetics of excision repair. Paterson[61] has outlined two basic protocols:

1. In vitro assay involves prelabeling a control culture of cells with ^{14}C-TdR and a second with ^{3}H-TdR. The latter is exposed to UVR, and both cultures are incubated for a selected interval to allow repair to occur. The cultures are combined, lysed, and coextracted to yield a mixture of [14]C- and ^{3}H-labeled DNA. Duplicate aliquots are incubated, one in the presence, and the other in the absence, of purified *M. luteus* UV endonuclease. Each digest is centrifuged in alkaline sucrose gradients, and fractions are subjected to double-label counting. The ^{14}C radioactivity of unirradiated DNA and the radioactivity profiles of the sample not treated with endonuclease permit appropriate corrections and calculations to be made to attain an estimate of the number of dimers in irradiated DNA at the time of cell lysis.
2. In vivo assay, as noted by Paterson, is a phrase employed to distinguish this intracellular assay from the above extracellular (in vitro) one.* The procedure is similar to that above, except that after UV irradiation and incubation, cells are treated to render their membranes permeable to endonuclease and are incubated directly with the enzyme. After this incubation, the cells are lysed on alkaline sucrose gradients and analyzed as described above. For mammalian cells, two freeze-thaw cycles will permeabilize membranes sufficiently to permit entry of endonuclease.[66]

A drawback of endonuclease analysis is that not all pyrimidine dimer sites are detected, as compared to radiochromatographic estimation of dimer content. This is particularly true of the in vivo assay, where endogenous ligases may rejoin endonuclease-induced nicks or where chromosomal proteins may shield regions of DNA from endonuclease attack. Nevertheless, after summarizing values from the literature, Paterson estimated that the yield of endonuclease-sensitive sites after irradiation at 254 nm is about $2.5/10^8$ daltons/J/m^2. This value agrees well with total dimer content obtained by radiochromatographic isolation.

An advantage of endonuclease analysis is that it is sensitive enough to monitor DNA damage caused by sublethal doses of UVR in normal human fibroblasts. Repair deficient Chinese hamster V79 cells were investigated by van Zeeland,[66] employing the in vivo assay with T4 endonuclease V. Damage to DNA at UVR

---

*The reader should be alert to the use of "in vivo" in reports of DNA damage and repair. Statements containing the phrase often refer to results obtained with live, cultured cells and do not necessarily relate to metabolic events in the intact donor of the cells.

doses below 1 J/m² was detected, but only about 50% of the induced dimer sites were sensitive to enzymic nicking. It is of interest that, despite incomplete enzymic cleavage, the number of endonuclease-sensitive sites increased linearly up to a UVR dose of 5 J/m². Other advantages of his technique are: (1) by use of endonucleases of appropriate specificity, other types of DNA damage may be studied; (2) each of the three basic repair processes (excision repair, postreplication repair and photoreactivation) may be examined; (3) the cells under study are not exposed to cytotoxic agents such as hydroxyurea, BrUdR, or FUdR.

In general, repair endonucleases appear to recognize topological deformations at damaged sites, and the nature of the lesion is of secondary importance. However, purified *M. luteus* enzyme and bacteriophage T4 endonuclease V are specific for pyrimidine dimer sites. Although all dimer types are recognized, there is some evidence that T-T dimer is preferred to C-C. Dimer specificity may be an area for additional study. For example, the incomplete detection of dimer sites by *M. luteus* endonuclease, compared to radiochromatographic isolation of dimers, may result from the resistance to enzymic attack of sites containing T-C or C-T dimers. (Because of the directionality of the DNA strand, 5' T-C will look different from 5' C-T.) On the other hand, if the number of pyrimidine dimers is calculated from the radioactivity of a chromatographic fraction with the assumption that all of the label arose from T-T dimers, one may underestimate the original dimer content of damaged DNA. Note that since both endonuclease analysis and radiochromatographic assay employ radiolabeled thymidine as a tracer, they provide no information about C-C dimers. Although this dimer type may be quantitatively unimportant in UV-damaged DNA, its possible biologic effects on eukaryotic cells have not been studied in detail.

Postreplication Repair

Exposure of cultured mammalian cells to UVR doses above 5 J/m² inhibits semiconservative replication. By definition, PRR occurs during DNA replication and has therefore been studied in great detail. The phenomenon of PRR (also known as S-phase recovery) has been discussed briefly (see "Pathways of DNA Repair"). Since knowledge of methodology is important in understanding some aspects of this subject, techniques will be discussed further in this section. Two basic mechanisms will be examined.

Gapped Synthesis. This process leaves gaps in daughter strand segments at sites of template damage, and requires filling of gaps either by de novo synthesis or by recombinational exchange with the opposite parental DNA strand. The latter process also requires de novo synthesis to fill the gaps produced in the parental strand, employing its newly synthesized daughter sequence as a template. The techniques employed to study gap filling have been described above and are based on analysis of the molecular weight distribution of replicated DNA at various intervals after UV irradiation. Hanawalt[60] provided a convenient tabulation of procedures. Cells are incubated with ^{14}C-TdR to label parental DNA. After irradiation, incubation with ^{3}H-TdR labels daughter DNA and provides a measure of de novo synthesis. Sedimentation analysis in alkaline sucrose gradient, performed on cells at various times after irradiation, yields information concerning how rapidly daughter strand segments are rejoined into intact strands. Meyn and Fletcher[67] monitored daughter strand length by alkaline elution on polyvinyl chloride filters. Although the method does not provide estimates of molecular weights, it is simple to perform and elution profiles are easy to interpret.

The extent of recombinational repair may be examined by use of a UV endonuclease as a probe for dimer sites in daughter DNA. Detection of such lesions in daughter strands is difficult to interpret, because they may represent UV damage to growing strands in cells that were in the S-phase during irradiation.[68] This problem can be resolved by examining synchronous cell cultures, as was done by D'Ambrosio and Setlow.[69] They observed that when Chinese hamster V79 cells were subjected to 10 J/m^2 of UVR in G_1, about 0.1 dimer per 10^8 daltons was produced in daughter strands, whereas irradiation of S-phase cells yielded about 1.2 dimers per 10^8 daltons. On the other hand, Meneghini and Menck[70] blocked replication with hydroxyurea during irradiation of normal and XP fibroblasts, and still observed dimers in daughter DNA. Other experimental data were also consistent with transfer of 10–20% of parental DNA (containing dimers) to daughter strands.

Bypass Replication. Since the process involves production of daughter strands without gaps, it requires that synthesis stop at a template lesion until some other mechanism provides the daughter segment complementary to the damaged site so that replication can resume. The temporary halting at damage sites may be responsible for the reduced rate of semiconservative replication after UV irradiation. The technique of DNA fiber radioautography provides information about rate of movement of replicating forks and initiation of new replicons. Edenberg[71] studied semiconservative replication in UV-irradiated HeLa cells via density labeling with BrUdR, and replicon movement via fiber radioautography. He observed that after UVR doses below 5 J/m^2 (germicidal lamp), replication was inhibited at 1.5 hours but recovered completely by 6 hours. Analysis of DNA fibers was performed by subjecting cells to 10 J/m^2 UV irradiation, labeling them with ^{3}H-TdR, and preparing radioautographs. Lengths of radiolabeled DNA segments were estimated with a microscope equipped with an ocular micrometer. Three general mechanisms for inhibition of replication by UVR were proposed. (1) The rate of movement of replication forks is decreased.

(2) Replication stops at a DNA lesion (a), or pauses and reinitiates beyond the lesion (b). (3) Initiation of new replicons is inhibited. The data on segment length vs time after irradiation allowed Edenberg to distinguish between these mechanisms and was consistent with mechanism 2a: replication stopped at lesions for at least 90 minutes. Although fiber analysis provides no information concerning the nature of the lesions, the results of the density labeling experiments suggested they were pyrimidine dimers. Doniger[72] investigated the rate of fork movement in Chinese hamster cells after irradiation at 254 nm. A dose of 5 J/m^2 had no effect, whereas 10 J/m^2 caused a 40% decrease. Caffeine reduced the rate of rejoining of daughter strands (measured via alkaline sucrose gradient centrifugation), whereas it did not influence rate of fork movement. It should be noted that the present techniques for fiber analysis have not revealed whether the effect of a pyrimidine dimer is to slow synthesis of one daughter strand or both.[73] The concept of PRR involving branch migration (see "Pathways of DNA Repair") predicts that synthesis of both strands will be interrupted for some undetermined time at each damaged site in a parental strand.

Redefinition of PRR. Cleaver et al.[48] proposed that PRR should be viewed in the context of the effect of excision repair on semiconservative replication. They noted several aspects of DNA replication in damaged cells: (1) reduced rate of DNA synthesis, (2) transient reduction in size of daughter DNA, and (3) linkage of daughter segments into parental-sized DNA. The primary response of normal cells to UV irradiation is reduced DNA synthesis. This may be a consequence of blocking of replicon initiation by the nicks produced during excision repair. Irradiation of excision defective and XP variant fibroblasts produces daughter segments which are smaller than normal, but the rate of rejoining is unchanged. The authors concluded that PRR may not in fact exist, but the inhibitory effect of caffeine requires further study. In a subsequent report, Park and Cleaver[74] expanded this concept to elucidate the action of caffeine and presented a model for events during DNA replication in UV-damaged mammalian cells. They concluded that conventional pulse-chase experiments do not uniquely define PRR, but that it can be defined in terms of blocking of DNA replication forks.

Photoreactivation

Sutherland[40] deserves credit for persistence in devising techniques for detecting photoreactivating enzyme in cells of placental mammals. Sutherland and Oliver[42] discussed three assays for PRE:

1. Bacterial transformation is very sensitive but may be subject to interference by cellular components.
2. The nuclease digestion method is rapid, specific, and sensitive. Although it requires highly purified ^{32}P-labeled DNA of high specific activity which

must be prepared frequently, the authors employ it routinely. The ^{32}P-DNA is irradiated with UVR to produce pyrimidine dimers, and two mixtures containing the extract of interest are prepared. One mixture is exposed to white light; the other is kept in the dark. Each sample is subjected to enzymic digestion to yield mixtures of inorganic phosphate, nucleotides, and dimer-containing oligonucleotides. The oligonucleotides are absorbed onto Norit A charcoal, washed, and counted for radioactivity.

3. The method employing ^{3}H-thymidine is more time consuming and less sensitive than nuclease digestion, but it may be the method of choice when only occasional assays are performed. Cells are prelabeled with ^{3}H-TdR, exposed to UVR, and either exposed (assay) or not exposed (control) to white light. Cells are hydrolyzed with hot formic acid, and evaporated to dryness, and each reconstituted residue is subjected to paper chromatography. Radioactivity of the area corresponding to pyrimidine dimers is measured. Sutherland and coworkers have demonstrated that this method yields results equivalent to those obtained with nuclease digestion and that the isolated dimer fraction has the properties of thymine dimer. It was stressed that when setting up an assay, the experimental conditions must be validated by analyzing a preparation with known PRE activity. As mentioned earlier, once PR is established for a cell type, the process can be employed to evaluate the effect of pyrimidine dimers on an observed response: if the response is diminished or eliminated by exposure to white light, it is probably mediated by dimers.

The PRE appears specific for cyclobutyl pyrimidine dimers, since it did not release psoralen from a cyclobutyl adduct with thymine.[75]

Repair of Damaged Bases

As noted earlier ("Pathways of DNA Repair: Repair of X-ray-induced Base Damage"), replacement of damaged bases is probably achieved by an excision repair process which is difficult to assay directly. The ability of cells to perform *nucleoside* excision can be examined indirectly by assaying for specific endonuclease activity. Linn and coworkers[76] reported that there are several activities in human fibroblasts which act on lesions produced by alkylating agents, uracil-DNA glycosylase, x-rays, or osmium tetroxide. It should be noted that, as discussed by Linn,[77] the term *AP endonuclease* (more formally, AP endodeoxyribonuclease) should refer to an enzyme which acts at both apurinic and apyrimidinic sites. At present, the specificity of these endonucleases is not known to the extent of being able to specify apurinic or apyrimidinic, and AP endonuclease must be interpreted in terms of the DNA substrate employed to detect the activity. Since DNA can be selectively depurinated under mild chemical conditions,[78] such a preparation may be employed as a substrate. Activity detected with this substrate will obviously represent apurinic activity. On the other hand, action of uracil-DNA glycosylase will produce an apyrimidinic substrate. Kuhnlein et al.[46] employed ^{3}H-TdR-labeled phage PM2 DNA which was subjected to conditions which released adenine and guanine. The number of apurinic sites was determined by the number of alkali-labile bonds. The AP endonuclease activity of a preparation was assayed by incubation with the depurinated DNA. The nicked DNA was selectively denatured, absorbed onto a nitrocellulose filter, and counted for radioactivity. After performing appropriate control experiments and making certain assumptions, the authors calculated endonuclease activity.

Tests of Cell Viability

Ultimately, one expects to relate a cellular biochemical flaw to some parameter of cell viability, which may reflect a clinical symptom in the patient. Several approaches for evaluating a cell's metabolic integrity will be briefly reviewed.

Colony forming ability (CFA) measures the ability of cells to grow after subjecting them to an experimental insult. For example, cultured cells are irradiated with UVR and a known number are transferred to a solid growth medium. The number of cells transferred is small enough that one can assume each colony which grows out arose from a single cell.

Host-cell reactivation (HCR) is a measure of the ability of a cell to repair damage in a virus which normally grows well in the cell. Thus, adenovirus 2 is subjected to UV irradiation, grown in human fibroblasts, and measured by a plaque assay.[79] A complementary technique is to monitor virus production in cells after the cells have been injured.[80]

Cell transformation may be assessed by the susceptibility of cells to morphologic transformation by viruses. For example, human fibroblast cultures are infected with murine or feline sarcoma virus and incubated for several days, and the transformed cell foci are counted.[81] Sutherland[75] monitored ability to grow in soft agar to assess the effect of irradiation on fibroblasts.

Cell fusion has been employed to segregate fibroblasts from patients with XP into several complementation groups. Cell strains from two individuals, which exhibit reduced UDS, are treated with an agent such as inactivated Sendai virus, allowed to fuse, and incubated with ^{3}H-TdR. A radioautograph reveals a variety of multinucleated cells. The nuclei exhibit heavy, medium, and light labeling corresponding to S-phase DNA synthesis, normal UDS, and reduced UDS. Since the object of the experiment is to determine whether the nuclei will "cure" or complement each other with regard to UDS, S-phase nuclei are ignored. For simplicity, binucleate cells will be discussed. Homokaryons contain nuclei from the same cell strain, and both nuclei will exhibit light labeling (reduced UDS). Heterokaryons contain one nucleus from each strain, and if both nuclei exhibit medium labeling, the patients from which the strains were derived are judged to belong to different complementation groups. Presumably, one nucleus is deficient in an enzyme or factor required for UDS, which is produced in excess in the other nucleus, and vice versa, so that they can restore normal UDS in each other. It is fortunate that the missing components are apparently freely diffusible through the cytoplasm. In their pioneering study, de Weerd-Kastelein[2] employed cell strains from patients of opposite sex and detected binucleate heterokaryons by observing a Barr body in one nucleus and the Y chromosome in the other.

GENODERMATOSES ASSOCIATED WITH CANCER

Surveys of Hereditary Cancer and of Genodermatoses

It is neither appropriate nor feasible to present a comprehensive overview of these broad areas. However, in searching the literature concerning specific areas of interest for this report, I encountered numerous extensive reviews. For the benefit of the reader who may desire a listing of such reports, they are cited here. They are grouped under general aspects of carcinogenesis,[82-85] familial cancer,[86-91] genetics and cancer,[92-102] and genodermatoses and cancer.[103-107] Reference 95 is the third report of an ambitious project to correlate data from worldwide reports on chromosomal aberrations and human neoplasms. Convenient tables of genodermatoses, mode of inheritance, and associated cancers are presented in references 101 to 106. In this book, the table in reference 103 has been updated by H.T. Lynch (see Chapter 1), and R.M. Fusaro and H.T. Lynch have discussed the cutaneous aspects of genodermatoses and cancer (Chapter 3).

Autosomal Recessive Genodermatoses

Many of the genodermatoses associated with cancer have a recessive mode of inheritance. The key question in terms of patient counseling and index of suspicion of cancer was first proposed by Swift in 1971[108]: Are heterozygous individuals at increased risk for cancer? Because of the long-term follow-ups required for prospective studies of human cancer, extensive surveys are probably not feasible. Retrospective studies present additional difficulties in the searching out of old records, validation of cancer reports, and evaluation of cancer risk factors. Such investigations become exceedingly difficult if there is no test for heterozygosity in members of a pedigree. Instead of assigning a yes or no rating to each member, one must employ a probability figure based on the relationship to the homozygous proband. Needless to say, the sample size required to define a statistical correlation with increased cancer risk will be much larger than if one could examine only the heterozygous members of a pedigree. Swift[109] estimated that a study based on probability of heterozygosity requires about five man-years of dedicated effort. Since the gene frequency for the heterozygous state is considerably higher than the homozygous expression of disease, even rare hereditary cancer disorders are numerically significant if heterozygotes are at increased risk. Therefore, development of convenient tests for heterozygosity should receive high priority in the study of genodermatoses associated with cancer.

Genodermatoses and Genetic Damage and Repair

Since genodermatoses associated with cancer are often characterized by increased sensitivity to UVR or ionizing radiation, and carcinogenesis implies genetic alterations, much effort has been directed to investigation of the effects of irradiation on cellular DNA and the ability of cells to repair damaged DNA. Several general reviews are recommended.[110-113] Robbins[114] updated the literature to mid-1979. Arlett and Harcourt[115] presented a table summarizing the sensitivity of various fibroblast strains to several DNA damaging agents; Lehmann et al.[116] tabulated repair parameters and caffeine sensitivities for cell lines from a variety of genodermatoses and other disorders. Cleaver et al.[117] tabulated a variety of responses to carcinogens for cells from patients with several genodermatoses.

XERODERMA PIGMENTOSUM

Because of the extreme sunlight sensitivity and early onset of multiple tumors in xeroderma pigmentosum, biochemical studies have been concentrated on the influence of UVR on XP cells. Numerous reports of investigations with other DNA-damaging agents are scattered throughout the literature, and Pawsey et al.[50] performed a valuable service by collecting and summarizing this information. Other current reviews of XP are also recommended.[22,118-126] Although studies of XP have provided a wealth of information concerning DNA damage and repair in humans, one must keep in mind that the disorder may not be a general model for carcinogenesis.[127] Tumors appear mainly on the skin of patients in response to a specific mutagen, UVR, which most tissues are not exposed to. On the other hand, UVR may have systemic effects, and in that context, response of XP cells to chemical carcinogens may represent a general phenomenon. It may also be noted that immunological impairment in XP has been reported.[22]

Cleaver et al.[62] suggested that in order to facilitate tracing cell lines from different laboratories to the original patients, a standard nomenclature should be employed. Each line is XP, followed by two numbers or letters relating to the first report of the culture, followed by two letters designating the laboratory of origin. Thus XP25RO represents strain 25, established in Rotterdam. It has also been suggested that cells from obligate heterozygotes (parents) be designated XPH-.[128] For convenience, a number of laboratory designations are listed in Table 10-2.

The use of standard nomenclature in publications was helpful in the preparation of this report, because it permitted correlation of current information with biochemical data obtained before complementation analysis was initiated. In several instances, authors provided sufficient cross-references to permit identification of the complementation groups of XP cells employed in early studies. (It would be a worthy project for someone with an extensive data base to assemble these cross-references into a concise compendium.)

Complementation Studies

Although they are clinically indistinguishable, one can distinguish two groups of XP patients biochemically: fibroblasts from patients with classical XP exhibit deficient excision repair, whereas those from XP variants do not. Since unscheduled DNA synthesis reflects (at least in part) excision repair, classical XP

Table 10-2. Designations for Sites of Origin of Xeroderma Pigmentosum Cell Lines.*

AA	Ann Arbor	KC	Kansas City	PW	Pollards Wood
BA	Baltimore	KO	Kobe	RO	Rotterdam
BE	Bethesda	LO	London	SD	San Diego
BI	Birmingham	MI	Miami	SE	Sendai
BR	Brighton	NA	Nagasaki	SF	San Francisco
CA	Cairo	NBi	Nairobi	SL	St. Louis
CH	Charentz[†]	NE	Newcastle	ST	Stockholm
CTO	Canada, Toronto	NY	New York	TA	Tel Aviv
EG	Egypt[‡]	OR	Oak Ridge	TE	Tehran
HE	Heidelberg	OS	Osaka	TO	Tokyo
HO	Houston	PA	Paris	WA	Washington state
JO	Johannesburg	PR	Pavia-Roma	WI	Wichita

*Some designations were assumed from the addresses of investigators who originated the cell lines. Letters may be used for cell lines other than XP; e.g., AT3BI represents the third ataxia telangiectasia strain, Birmingham.
[†]Russian Armenian.
[‡]Cell lines originally designated EG are now assigned the more specific code, CA (J.E. Cleaver, personal communication).

cells have reduced UDS and are therefore amenable to complementation studies. One can quantitate UDS from radioautographs by counting the number of silver grains over the nuclei of a large number of heterodikaryons, and comparing the mean with that of unfused XP cells in the same microscopic field and with that in normal cell cultures.[50,129] Pawsey et al.[50] obtained comparable results with a microphotometer and used it routinely as a more objective measure than visual counting.

In a collaborative study reported in 1975,[130] investigators from Rotterdam and from Bethesda (National Institutes of Health) exchanged XP fibroblast strains belonging to three and four complementation groups, respectively. The Rotterdam nomenclature was: DeSanctis-Cacchione, classical XP (severe), and classical XP (light to moderate); the NIH groups were labeled A, B, C, and D. Both laboratories verified that the DeSanctis-Cacchione strain belonged to group A, and the classical XP (severe), to group C. The third Rotterdam strain complemented all four NIH groups and was therefore assigned to group E. The authors suggested that the term *DeSanctis-Cacchione* no longer be used to denote a complementation group and that the groups be assigned letters A–E. They confirmed earlier studies which indicated that the rate of UDS was relatively constant in strains within the same complementation group, but could vary widely between groups. In a survey of 96 XP patients in Japan, Takebe and coworkers[120,131] reported that fibroblasts from a patient with very mild skin symptoms (XP23OS) complemented all five of the known complementation groups and, therefore, represented a new group, F. The Rotterdam investigators, in collaboration with investigators in Birmingham, England also detected a patient (XP2BI) whose cells were different from groups A–E.[121] In collaboration with the Japanese investigators, it was determined that the XP2BI strain complements XP23OS and, therefore, belongs in a new group, G.[131] Thus, there are at present seven known groups of repair deficient classical XP and a group of XP variants. Cleaver et al.[117] provided a convenient table of post-UV responses of cells from groups A–G and variant, based on dose modifying factor, UDS, loss of endonuclease-sensitive sites, and accumulation of strand breaks.

It appears that complementation of UDS by nuclei from different groups represents true recovery of repair capability. Kraemer et al.[130] cited reports to document that: (1) normal UDS in complemented nuclei is resistant to hydroxyurea; (2) complemented nuclei exhibit normal rates of pyrimidine dimer excision and repair replication; (3) heterokaryons with complementing nuclei exhibit normal host-cell reactivation of UV-irradiated adenovirus 2. On the other hand, the *kinetics* of complementation of XP nuclei reveal important differences between groups. Giannelli and Pawsey[132] distinguished two groups of classical XP strains, rapid (r) and slow (s), based on the rate of complementation with normal cells in the presence of cycloheximide to inhibit protein synthesis. They examined dikaryons to hexakaryons containing 1 normal and 1–5 XP nuclei,

1 male s-XP and 1–5 female r-XP nuclei, and 1 female r-XP and 1–5 male s-XP nuclei. They were thus able to evaluate gene dosage effects. The fascinating implications of these extensive studies will not be reviewed here, except to note that the investigators expressed the hope that ongoing studies will clarify the relationship between the r and s mutations and the various complementation groups. They also expect to help resolve the question of whether each complementation group represents a mutation at a different locus, or whether inter- and intragenic interactions of a smaller number of loci are involved. Pawsey et al.[50] have discussed the current status of these investigations.

In general, the levels of UDS are similar between affected numbers of the same kindred, and occur within fairly narrow ranges within complementation groups. An exception to this rule, XP8LO, was described by de Weerd-Kastelein et al.[133] This strain was assigned to complementation group A (UDS less than 5%), but exhibited 36% UDS after a UV dose of 5 J/m^2. Because of the relatively high UDS, it was difficult to distinguish heterokaryons. A novel labeling technique was employed: cells of one strain were incubated with carbon particles (India ink); the other, with latex spheres. Since considerable overlap in UDS may occur, Bootsma[121] cautioned that it is not reliable to assign a new XP strain to a complementation group based on clinical symptoms and UDS level. The quantitative radioautographic technique is sensitive enough to permit prenatal diagnosis of XP with amniotic cells.[134] The UDS levels of such cells and of fibroblasts from the voluntarily terminated fetus were in good agreement in two cases.[50] There are some associations of clinical symptoms with complementation group. For example, Pawsey et al.[50] summarized the results of their cell fusion studies and those of de Weerd-Kastelein et al.[2] and Kraemer et al.[130] They tabulated the total number of patients and the number of those with severe neurological symptoms by complementation group (neurological number in parenthesis): A, 11 (9); B, 1 (1); C, 13 (0); D, 6 (2); E, 1 (0). The sole member of group B also has features of Cockayne's syndrome. The clustering of neurologic patients in group A coincides with the very low levels of UV-induced UDS displayed by these cells.[112,119,130] It has been postulated that similar low levels of repair in neurons may explain the early onset of neurological symptoms. Since neurons do not divide, they require efficient DNA repair capability to maintain metabolic integrity in the face of numerous DNA-damaging insults during the life of the individual. Therefore, it has been proposed[135,136] that impaired DNA repair may lead to premature neuronal death and development of neurological symptoms. Likewise, severity of skin symptoms correlates roughly with level of UDS.[119,120]

Much has been written about the possible association between defective post-UV excision repair and early onset of multiple cutaneous carcinomas in patients with classical XP. Takebe et al.[120] pointed out that of the 96 patients examined by them, none with a UDS level of 5% or less was 30 years old or older. This suggests that patients with this UDS level, born earlier than 30 years before the investigation, had died. With the present high index of suspicion for XP, and the initiation of lifelong regimes of solar avoidance and photoprotection,[58] it is to be expected that the life span of younger individuals will be increased. It can be rationalized that cells deficient in excision repair, an error-free process, may have to rely more on error-prone postreplication repair and thus be at a higher risk for mutations and carcinogenesis. However, XP variants have normal excision repair and reduced PRR; yet they are as prone to development of skin cancer as classical XP patients. Perhaps the former have excision repair defects which have not yet been detected. As pointed out by Setlow,[110] our present biochemical methods may not be detecting defective repair of photoproducts which are quantitatively unimportant but biologically significant.

Complementation studies between classical XP cells and other human fibroblast strains have been conducted. As might be expected, normal and heterozygous cells restore UDS.[137] One might also expect XP variant cells to complement classical strains, but surprisingly, it appears this has never been done. If this oversight is indeed true, it should be corrected quickly. I see no a priori reason to assume that all variant strains will completely complement all classical types; some combinations might exhibit incomplete or no complementation. If this occurred with some fusion pairs, variants could be assigned to "noncomplementation" groups. The knowledge gained from fusion of all possible combinations could provide new insight into the nature of defective DNA repair in XP cells.

The PUVA protocol may be employed to study excision repair via UDS. Baden et al.[138] observed that XP cells exhibited no UDS after PUVA exposure which caused maximal response in control cells. At exposure doses which caused equivalent suppression of semiconservative DNA synthesis, UDS of control cells after PUVA was about half that after exposure at 254 nm. In the former instance, UDS does not represent excision of pyrimidine dimers. In fact, under the influence of UV-A, psoralens form a variety of photoadducts with pyrimidines in DNA (reviewed by Baden et al.). Consequently, although the probability seems low, it would be interesting to determine whether XP variant cells exhibit low UDS after PUVA treatment. If this were true, one could conduct complementation tests analogous to those which have delineated the groups in classical XP. It would be of at least academic interest to perform fusion studies with PUVA on classical XP cells as well.

Fused-cell preparations of XP variants can be examined by biochemical techniques to monitor a process that they are deficient in — postreplication repair. The results are not as clear-cut as those obtained for UDS of classical XP cells, because one must analyze a mixture of several types of multikaryons. Nevertheless, Jasper in Bootsma's group[121] observed restoration of PRR when normal cells were fused with XP variant, but not when different variant strains were fused. Thus, although it has been speculated that XP variants may constitute a heterogeneous repair group analogous to classical XP, they do not complement for PRR. Clinical heterogeneity is indicated by a rare form known as pigmented xerodermoid,[119] in which clinical symptoms do not appear until the second or third decade. Lymphocytes and epidermal cells from one patient were reported to have normal excision repair, but were deficient in PRR.[139] J.E. Cleaver (personal communication) has information that indicates pigmented xerodermoid is essentially identical to XP variant.

Biochemical Studies of Defective Repair

Many studies have been performed concerning all aspects of DNA repair in XP cells. (For a convenient overview of parameters of repair of classical groups A–E and variant, after irradiation or exposure to chemicals, see Table 1 in reference 140.)

Excision Repair. As noted by Setlow[110] similar estimates of post-UV repair defects in XP cells have been obtained by a variety of techniques. Reduced ability to remove purimidine dimers in classical XP fibroblasts has been demonstrated by reduction in loss of dimers from DNA, loss of dimer sites via BrUdR photolysis, and loss of UV endonuclease sensitive sites. Numerous studies have revealed a flaw in the initial step in excision repair, i.e., incision. Thus, Tanaka et al.[141,142] demonstrated that if XP cells of groups A–E were permeabilized with inactivated Sendai virus so they would accept T4 endonuclease V, the exogenous enzyme restored post-UV UDS to normal. Extracts of cells of groups A, C, and D excise dimers from UV-irradiated purified *E. coli* DNA.[143] However, extracts of group A cells were unable to remove dimers from their own UV-irradiated chromatin. On the other hand, UV-irradiated purified DNA from XP cells was susceptible to dimer excision by XP cell extracts. These results suggest that factors in addition to endonuclease are involved in the incision of chromatin DNA in mammalian cells. Variations in the levels or degree of interaction of these factors could account for the different complementation groups of classical XP. Giannelli[22] pointed out that pyrimidine dimers are long-lived lesions, even in normal cells, but they persist longer in repair deficient XP strains. The repair defect in the latter may therefore be quantitative rather than qualitative.

Postreplication Repair. In 1975, investigators from England and the Netherlands described a collaborative study which was the first to detect a biochemical repair defect in XP variant fibroblasts.[144] They reported that these cells converted newly synthesized DNA to high molecular weight DNA at a rate much slower than that of normal cells; i.e., they were deficient in PRR. A classical XP line (group C) exhibited an intermediate rate of repair. Caffeine drastically inhibited

PRR in variant cells but had little effect on normal ones, thereby facilitating identification of the former. As was the case for excision repair in classical XP cells, the defect in PRR was kinetic rather than absolute: after a UV dose of 12.5 J/m^2, normal fibroblasts completed daughter strand rejoining in 1.5 to 2.5 hours, whereas XP variants required 5 to 8 hours. In a later study, Lehmann et al.[116] extended their observations to five variant strains. They also reported that classical XP groups A–D exhibited a less severe defect in PRR, whereas group E cells had normal PRR. Of particular value, their Table 1 provides levels of PRR, excision repair, and cell survivial (with and without caffeine) for classical and XP variant cells, and for strains from patients with a variety of disorders involving sensitivity to UVR or γ-radiation, or development of multiple cancers. Fibroblast strains comprised three distinct categories, based on degree of deficiency in PRR: (1) XP variant, severe; (2) classical XP A–D, intermediate; (3) classical XP-E and all other strains tested, normal. Lehmann et al.[144] presented a model for the PRR defect in XP variants, based on the known ability of caffeine to bind to single-stranded DNA. Caffeine competes with as yet uncharacterized repair enzymes at the dimer or gap site. Enzymes in normal cells compete effectively, whereas one of these enzymes in XP cells is defective and has a reduced binding affinity. Therefore, gap filling is slower in the absence of caffeine and strongly retarded in its presence. An alternative model assumes two PRR mechanisms, one caffeine sensitive, the other caffeine resistant. The latter would be absent in defective cells.

Day[145] examined the effect of caffeine on host-cell reactivation of adenovirus-2. He observed that 4 mM caffeine inhibits reactivation in normal and XP variant fibroblasts, but not in excision deficient classical XP cells. Therefore, normal and XP variant cells have a caffeine-sensitive repair process which is either excision repair or a pathway involving a step in excision repair. The latter alternative, involving a repair step which might be shared by two or more repair processes, does not conflict with the models of Lehmann et al.[144] Fujiwara and Tatsumi[146] observed that caffeine concentrations up to 2 mM did not reduce post-UV survival of normal and excision deficient XP fibroblasts, but potentiated the UV killing of XP variant cells. Alkaline sucrose sedimentation revealed that UV-irradiated normal and classical XP cells produced small DNA segments in 1.5 hours and converted them to parental-size DNA in 4 hours, in the presence or absence of caffeine. In contrast, variant cells produced much smaller segments and rejoined them at a lower rate, which was strongly inhibited by caffeine. The authors also conducted density labeling studies (isopycnic centrifugation) with BrUdR, similar to those described by Higgins et al. (see "Pathways of DNA Repair: Postreplication Repair"). They also detected a heavy fraction in sheared DNA, one hour after UV irradiation of normal, classical XP, and variant cells. (Recall that heavy fragments represent paired daughter segments which were undergoing bypass repair via strand displacement when the DNA was sheared.)

A four-hour chase eliminated the heavy fraction in all cell types. Caffeine (2mM) inhibited this process slightly in normal and classical XP cells, and strongly in variant cells. Of interest, the heavy fraction was barely detectable in unirradiated normal and classical XP extracts, but constituted a significant peak in the centrifugation profile of the XP variant strain. This recalls the comment by Sutherland and Oliver[42] that, because fibroblasts may be injured by white light, their laboratory is illuminated with gold fluorescent lamps. The possibility that PRR deficient XP variants may be unable to perform efficient repair of light-induced DNA damage merits investigation.

Because daughter strand rejoining in normal and classical cells was not severely inhibited by caffeine, as measured by alkaline sucrose sedimentation and density labeling, Fujiwara and Tatsumi concluded that these strains have a caffeine-resistant bypass repair process. On the other hand, both experimental techniques demonstrated that variant cells perform bypass repair by a caffeine-sensitive mechanism. The authors suggested that bypass repair requires an additional polymerase which is caffeine resistant in normal and classical XP cells, and defective (caffeine sensitive) in XP variants. Fujiwara[147] assigned 12 XP variants to three subgroups based on caffeine sensitivity of replicative repair (number of patients in parenthesis): I, severe (3); II, moderate (3); and III, resistant (6). Association of caffeine-sensitive replication repair with skin carcinogenesis is suggested by the fact that carcinomas occurred in every patient in groups I and II but not in those of group III. One would like to know the ages and histories of UV exposure of patients in group III, before drawing a firm conclusion. A puzzling aspect of this study is that one patient's cells were caffeine sensitive (group I), whereas her affected sister's cells were resistant; the author commented that the latter state might transform to caffeine sensitivity.

Higgins et al.[52] observed four-pronged replicating structures in sheared DNA from XP cells (type unspecified) treated with N-acetoxy-2-acetylaminofluorene. It would be interesting to examine the effect of caffeine on these structures in DNA from UV-irradiated variant cells. One should keep in mind that the experimental conclusions discussed in this section may require modification in view of Cleaver's reinterpretation of PRR[48,74] discussed earlier (see "Methodology for Measuring DNA Damage and Repair: Redefinition of Postreplication Repair"). The reduced post-UV response of XP variant cells is interpreted in terms of an increased probability that a damaged DNA site will block a replication fork.

Photoreactivation. Enzymic monomerization of pyrimidine dimers in situ appears to be the ideal mode of repair of UV-B damage for human skin cells, which are chronically bathed in photoreactivating light (UV-A and visible). One may tend to discount the importance of this process in terms of the rate of dimer repair observed in vitro, compared to excision repair or PRR. However, with regard to genodermatoses involving sun sensitivity and early onset of multiple carcinomas, impaired PR may be of utmost importance. Sutherland's work verifying the presence of photoreactivating enzyme in mammalian cells may therefore have important clinical implications for such disorders as XP.

Sutherland et al.[148] measured PRE in fibroblast extracts, with ^{32}P-labeled phage DNA as substrate, and observed PRE activities in classical XP cells (groups A–E) that ranged from 0 (group B) to 50% (group E) of normal. (The group B patient also had Cockayne's syndrome.) They also demonstrated that an XP-A culture, which exhibited less than 2% UDS and 36% PRE, monomerized at least two-thirds of the pyrimidine dimers produced in cellular DNA by UVR (10 J/m^2 at 254 nm), after 30 minutes exposure to photoreactivating light. Mixing experiments established that the reduced PRE activity in XP extracts was not the result of an endogenous inhibitor. Sutherland and Oliver[149] reported that the PRE activity in four XP variant strains was 4 to 56% of normal. As rough approximations of total repair capacities, they summed activities (percent of normal) for UDS, PRR, and PRE activity (normal = 300). Cells from the XP variant with light to moderate symptoms tallied 173; the others, with more severe symptoms, scored 137, 141, and 143. It is fascinating that cells of a heterozygous mother of one unaffected and five XP offspring scored 234 because of low PRE activity (34%). Since XP heterozygotes exhibit no clinical symptoms of sun sensitivity, it appears that deficient PRE activity alone may not be biologically harmful.

Sutherland and Oliver[150] described a study of the inheritance pattern of PRE in XP families. By assaying PRE activity in XP patients and their parents (heterozygotes for XP), they determined relationships between persons with normal (PP), intermediate (Pp), and low (pp) PRE levels. Fibroblast strains were available from the American Type Culture Collection for the mother mentioned above, the unaffected father, one unaffected child, and three XP offspring. The PRE levels were consistent with simple inheritance, with the father (PP) and mother (Pp) having one unaffected child (PP) and three XP children (Pp). Thus, although the defective PRE allele need not be associated with the heterozygous XP state (father is PP), it appears to segregate with the homozygous XP offspring. The authors pointed out that the limited availability of cells from XP patients and their parents precludes thorough testing of the inheritance model. If a patient has low PRE activity (pp), one can predict that each parent will be pp or Pp but never PP. This was verified for three patient-mother combinations: the PRE levels of the patients (pp) were 11, 18, and 15, respectively; of the mothers (Pp), 41, 73, and 36, respectively. The PRE gene status of the patients was not correlated with UDS capability; the complementation groups (percent UDS) were D (25–55), B (3–7), and variant (100), respectively. As an aside, it might be mentioned that this information was not available in the report. However, the authors used the standard terminology recommended by Cleaver et al.,[62] and the data were readily obtained from a table (Complemented XP Cell Lines Available for Study) presented by Friedberg et al.[112] The affected individuals of the XP family discussed above were group C with 5–20% repair replication[58] and 15–25% UDS.[112] Sutherland and Oliver reemphasized their concept that total repair capacity may be the deciding factor in sun sensitivity and predisposition to skin cancer. They also stressed, "Conversely, individuals with a defect in one repair system may be clinically normal as long as the total repair capacity remains high relative to the burden of damage to the DNA." This comment is particularly germane to the concept of heterozygosity, cumulative DNA damage, and increased risk of cancer.

Repair of Apurinic DNA. As discussed earlier ("Methodology for Measuring DNA Damage and Repair: Repair of Damaged Bases"), nucleoside excision may be examined by assaying specific endonuclease activity. Kuhnlein et al.[46] assayed fibroblast extracts with ^{3}H-labeled apurinic phage DNA as the substrate. Classical XP (A, B, C, and E) and XP variant strains had 40–60% of normal enzyme levels, whereas group D extracts had 17%. Kinetic studies revealed that the endonuclease in group C extract exhibited normal apparent K_m, whereas extracts from group A and D cells had greatly reduced affinity for the DNA substrate, as evidenced by values of K_m six- to ninefold higher than normal. The authors noted that UV-damaged DNA contains few, if any, apurinic sites and that the endonuclease activity of normal cells is several orders of magnitude greater than the rate of spontaneous production of sites. However, the altered K_m values in strains A and D suggest that the steady-state concentration of apurinic sites may be 10- to 30-fold greater than normal. This consideration, and the fact that fibroblasts from groups A and C exhibit low host-cell reactivation[79] may relate to the neurological disturbances occurring in patients in groups A and C. Linn et al.[76] reported chromatographic separation of apurinic endonuclease from human fibroblasts into a low-K_m and a high-K_m fraction. Both fractions were present in extracts from normal, XP-A, and ataxia telangiectasia strains, but the low-K_m activity was missing in group D cells.

Bacchetti et al.[151] detected an endonuclease in extracts of human fibroblasts which recognized lesions in UV-irradiated DNA that were not pyrimidine dimers (photoreactivation did not reduce enzyme activity). Extracts from XP cells that exhibited no UDS had normal endonuclease activity. Hariharan and Cerutti[152] examined the excision of thymine glycol from UV- or γ-irradiated DNA. Nuclear preparations from cells of XP groups A–D removed the damaged base efficiently. The yield of UV-induced glycol was 3% that of pyrimidine dimer, a value similar to that reported by Bacchetti and Benne[153] for nondimer sites recognized by an endonuclease from calf thymus. The nondimer-specific enzyme in human fibroblasts may also recognize thymine glycol; if so, this type of lesion is not involved in the sensitivity of XP cells to UVR.

Studies Performed with Cell Nuclei. The exhaustive investigations conducted with intact fibroblasts from patients with XP have perhaps reached the point of diminishing return. Therefore, recently developed techniques for investigating nuclei from osmotically ruptured cells offer an exciting new look at DNA damage and repair. To be sure, the study of nuclei presents the danger that essential components may be leached out during isolation. This may be offset by the advantage of being able to investigate intranuclear events in the absence of cytoplasmic processes which may obscure the results.

Ciarrocchi and Linn[154] isolated nuclei from human fibroblasts which had been exposed to radiation or chemical carcinogens, and measured DNA repair via incorporation of tritiated deoxythymidine triphosphate (^{3}H-dTTP). The presence of the other deoxynucleoside triphosphates was required, as was magnesium ion, and incorporation of the label was enhanced by ATP. Appropriate control experiments established that dTTP was not degraded to a nucleoside before incorporation, as would be expected if intact cells were present. Results obtained with nuclei from fibroblasts exposed to UVR or chemical carcinogens were similar to those obtained by autoradiographic measurement of UDS in intact cells. Additional validation of the cell-free system was established by examining nuclei of XP cells: those from group A had no UV-induced repair, those from groups C and D had reduced levels, and those from XP variant had nearly normal repair. In an experiment analogous to that of Tanaka et al.[141] with permeabilized cells, T4 endonuclease V was added to nuclei of irradiated normal and repair deficient XP cells (groups A and C). After 4.5 J/m^2 UVR at 254 nm, repair was stimulated twofold in normal, and tenfold in XP, nuclei (the values for the latter were still less than normal). Irradiation at 40 J/m^2 produced so much DNA damage that all endonuclease-stimulated preparations yielded similar high repair values. It was not stated whether exogenous endonuclease activity was rate limiting in this instance. If it were not, one might conclude that some subsequent step in excision repair became rate limiting, and the XP nuclei were proficient in that activity. Stimulation of repair activity of normal nuclei by endonuclease was not observed by Tanaka with permeabilized cells. This difference might represent replacement of endogenous endonuclease lost during isolation of the nuclei. The authors pointed out that the cell-free system may be useful in the identification of agents which damage DNA, and in complementation studies with XP cells or other defective strains.

Smith and Hanawalt[155] performed studies similar to those of Ciarrocchi and Linn, with density labeled nuclei from UV-irradiated normal and XP-A fibroblasts. They observed that irradiation of isolated nuclei of normal cells induced the same level of repair as occurred in nuclei isolated immediately after irradiation of whole cells and that nuclei from irradiated XP-A cells did not exhibit repair. As noted above, T4 endonuclease V stimulated incorporation of ^{3}H-dTTP in both normal and XP nuclei. Density labeling allowed the authors to estimate that the size of the repair patches was about 35 nucleotides, in nuclei as well as in intact cells.

Comment. Nuclei from irradiated excision deficient XP cells may provide a specific assay for human fibroblast endonucleases. One might wonder, Why not employ a simpler system with purified, irradiated DNA? This point will be expanded in the following section, but it should be mentioned that in order to delineate the subtle differences which distinguish seven groups of excision deficient XP cells — at a single step, incision — it may be necessary to use a detection system mimicking the intracellular state.

Experimental Detection of Pyrimidine Dimers — Are Present Techniques Adequate?

To set the stage for this topic, it is appropriate to cite the introductory statement of the extensive review by Johnson[118] of UV induction of thymine-containing dimers in skin: "Neither the chemical nature, nor the anatomical site of a primary, specific molecular target for the effects of sunlight upon normal, lightly pigmented human skin has been unequivocally defined." He pointed out that irradiation of DNA with UVR also produces cytosine-containing dimers, but fortunately the majority of dimers formed are of the cyclobutane type containing thymine-thymine (T-T) or thymine-cytosine (T-C). Thus, experiments based on incorporation of ^{3}H-TdR will detect most UV-induced pyrimidine dimers, and every investigator employing these techniques tacitly accepts the validity of this conclusion. However, in dealing with the quandary of how classical XP fibroblasts can exhibit at least seven complementary repair flaws at a single step (incision), it may be productive to examine more closely the validity of this concept for DNA damage in *intact human cells.* A survey of the literature concerning the nature of UV-induced dimers reveals many reports of studies with irradiated purified DNA or with DNA from irradiated bacterial systems. Likewise, with few exceptions, the properties of dimer-specific endonucleases have been investigated with nonmammalian DNA or cells. In contrast, one should consider the conditions that exist when intact mammalian cells are irradiated. Proteins and nucleic acids in chromatin may undergo stacking interactions between aromatic amino acid side chains and nitrogenous bases. Intercalated amino acid rings can block dimerization[156] or alternatively, catalyze photomonomerization of existing dimers.[157] Since the aromatic rings probably exhibit selectivity for the adjacent bases they intercalate with, the proportions and types of pyrimidine dimers produced by irradiation of chromatin in eukaryotic cells may be entirely different from the pattern induced in isolated DNA or in DNA of prokaryotic cells.

Nature of UV-induced Dimers. Johnson[118] discussed several reports which provide unequivocal evidence that thymine-containing dimers are produced in skin exposed to UVR in vivo. However, the dose required for minimal dimer production is an order of magnitude greater than the minimal erythema dose. Therefore, in experiments designed to produce maximum response in cell cultures, one must consider that pyrimidine dimers and other photoproducts are produced in proportions and yields which may bear no relation to the structure of DNA damaged in vivo. For example, all possible cyclobutane dimers may be formed: T-T, T-C, C-T, and C-C. (Note that because of the directionality of the DNA chain, T-C and C-T may look different to a specific endonuclease.) Saturation of the 5,6 double bond of cytosine labilizes its amino group, as occurs with cytosine photohydrate (see "Biological Effects of Ultraviolet Irradiation: Effects of Ultraviolet Irradiation on DNA"), leading to formation of uracil. Therefore, in addition to the dimers listed, UV-damaged DNA may also contain T-U, U-T, and U-U. The need for a specific endonuclease to initiate excision repair at each dimer site would explain the existence of seven complementation groups in classical XP. Perhaps this view is too simplistic; other explanations (e.g., missing cofactors that are required for dimer excision) may be more plausible. However, the universal use of ^{3}H-TdR as a convenient indicator of pyrimidine dimer formation and repair precludes the possibility of gaining information about cytosine dimers in irradiated mammalian cells. Therefore, it seems imperative that experiments be conducted with human fibroblasts, similar to those performed by Setlow and Carrier[158] with E. coli DNA. By prelabeling the DNA with radioactive cytosine or thymine, they gained information about the distribution of UV-induced thymine- and cytosine-containing dimers, and about the dependence of the pattern on dose and wavelength of UVR. It is significant that at low doses at 265 nm, they consistently observed a higher production of C-T in intact cells than in DNA irradiated in vitro.

A different type of pyrimidine dimer, 6-4'-{pyrimidin-2'-one} –thymine has received little attention in irradiated mammalian cells. This compound arises as the hydrolysis product of a cytosine-thymine adduct present in irradiated DNA. Since, according to Wang and Varghese,[159] this adduct is stereochemically more favored than cyclobutane T-T, its presence and mode of repair should be investigated in irradiated human fibroblasts.

Are Pyrimidine Dimers the Ultimate Answer? Many investigators recognized that UVR causes nondimer damage in DNA; Feldberg[160] cited several reports to that effect. Also, chemical carcinogens can be broadly classified as UV-like or not, according to the type of mechanism required to repair the damage they induce in DNA. Thus, bacterial strains lacking UV-repair capacity are sensitive to 4-nitroquinoline-1-oxide (4-NQO). This carcinogen affects survival of normal human fibroblasts to the same extent as UVR and, like UVR, has an exaggerated effect on repair deficient XP cells.[161] Similarly, XP cells which exhibit reduced UDS via radioautography after UV irradiation, also have a reduced response to

4-NQO. The DNA lesions caused by 4-NQO are not pyrimidine dimers, as evidenced by the fact that T4 endonuclease V does not restore the reduced UDS in permeabilized XP cells treated with the carcinogen.[142] Therefore, DNA lesions other than pyrimidine dimers can reveal repair defects in XP cells. Another example was cited earlier in this section (see "Complementation Studies"): PUVA treatment of repair deficient XP fibroblasts results in reduced UDS.

The effects of agents such as 4-NQO and PUVA may be rationalized on the basis that they produce lesions which require excision repair, and deficiencies in endonuclease activity in XP cells show up in a manner similar to that displayed for pyrimidine dimers. By the same token, quantitatively minor UV-induced lesions may also be repaired inefficiently by XP cells. These lesions remain undetected either because of the use of ^{3}H-TdR for detection or because their effect is obscured by the use of large doses of UVR to maximize dimer formation. Early in his investigations, Cleaver[35] recognized that UVR doses employed experimentally were lethal to cells. Normal human fibroblasts exhibited 3% survival after 10 J/m^2 at 254 nm, and 0.14% after 20 J/m^2. At that early stage, it was appropriate to employ large doses of UVR because inefficient repair of pyrimidine dimers was the first observed defect in XP cells. Perhaps it is now appropriate to employ irradiation conditions more representative of sunlight impinging on human skin and to look for lesions other than pyrimidine dimers.

Studies of Cell Viability

Colony Forming Ability. Andrews et al.[135] determined CFA vs UVR dose of two XP variants and several strains each of groups A, C, and D. Survival of variant cells was only slightly less than normal, whereas survival of classical XP lines was segregated by group, in inverse relation to the degree of neurological abnormalities (NA) in the patients. Thus, group C cells (no NA) had intermediate survival; group D (severe NA), lower; and group A (more severe NA), lowest.

In a more extensive study,[136] the authors tabulated UDS, UV susceptibility, and donor NA for five normal, two variant, one XP-E, and six to eight strains each of groups A, C, and D. The XP-E cells had higher survival than the variants, whereas the CFAs of the other groups were segregated as in the earlier report. On the basis of these studies, the authors developed the hypothesis that greatly reduced post-UV CFA of fibroblasts reflects repair deficiencies in neurons, leading to premature neuronal death and early development of severe NA. Markedly reduced CFA also correlated with acute sun sensitivity. The UV sensitivity was identical for each member of a sibling pair in groups A, C, and D (two pairs), but CFAs varied within each group. It therefore appears that the same defective gene sequence is inherited in a given kindred, but not necessarily within a specific complementation group.

Robbins et al.[162] discussed unique features of fibroblasts from the only member of group B, a patient who also has Cockayne's syndrome (CS). This rare autosomal recessive disorder is characterized by acute sun sensitivity and neurological abnormalities. However, the CFA of group B cells was in a transition zone below the levels of non-neurological group C cells and above those of neurological group D cells. Andrews et al.[163] observed that fibroblasts from nine patients with CS exhibited normal post-UV UDS (group B cells have 3–7% of normal). The CS strains had reduced CFAs, but they occurred in the upper part of the region for group C cells. Thus, in CS, sun sensitivity and neurological abnormalities are not associated with greatly decreased post-UV CFA. It may be significant that patients with CS do not have a high incidence of skin tumors. The anomalously high CFA of the group B patient's cells suggests that her neurological abnormalities result from CS, not XP. Arlett et al.[164] demonstrated that caffeine enhanced the UV sensitivity of XP variant cells but did not affect post-UV CFA of repair deficient group A cells. Since, in the absence of caffeine, the latter are sensitive to UVR whereas variant cells are resistant, it appears that defective excision repair has a more serious effect on post-UV survival than does defective PRR.

Host-cell Reactivation. Day[79] employed the sensitive adenovirus 2 HCR system to evaluate repair capabilities of several cell strains. Normal and XP heterozygous cells exhibited the highest restoration of UV-damaged virus, group B and C cells had lesser capability, and group A and D cells exhibited the lowest HCR. The author noted that a UVR dose of 1,200 J/m^2 produces only 250 dimers in viral DNA, and the low amount of repair required for HCR is not sufficient to saturate the presumably lower repair activity of XP heterozygous cells. In a later report,[165] he noted that fibroblasts of patients from the five known XP variant kindreds had reduced HCR (60% of normal). The effect of PUVA treatment on adenovirus 2 was much more severe when host cells were from group A or D than when they were normal or XP variant fibroblasts.[166] Presumably, repair deficient XP cells are unable to remove psoralen monoadducts from viral DNA. This repair defect may be responsible for the high sensitivity of XP fibroblasts themselves to PUVA.[138] Aaronson and Lytle[167] studied HCR of the transforming DNA tumor virus, SV40. Transformed fibroblasts are not subject to growth restraints and are counted as multilayered colonies in a field of contact-inhibited untransformed cells. The growth of irradiated SV40 in two classical XP strains was much less than normal.

Cell Transformation. The susceptibility of XP cells to transformation by feline sarcoma virus was investigated by Chang.[81] This system is a sensitive indicator of cellular repair defects and yielded a rough correlation between transformability and extent of deficiency in excision repair. However, it may be too sensitive to unavoidable variation in experimental conditions, as evidenced in the widespread in numbers of transformed cells for three XP siblings. Hall and Tokuno[168] observed that irradiation of SV40 virus increased the transformation frequencies of two XP variant cell lines. Normal and heterozygous variant fibroblasts exhibited the same degrees of transformation by irradiated or unirradiated virus.

Use of Various Cell Types to Study Xeroderma Pigmentosum

Fibroblasts. Skin fibroblasts can be easily cultured and manipulated, and interesting strains are stored in cell repositories for the use of all investigators. Two organizations store fibroblast strains from probands and family members representing numerous hereditary disorders: (1) American Type Culture Collection (ATCC), 12301 Parklawn Drive, Rockville, MD 20852; (2) Human Genetic Mutant Cell Repository, Institute for Medical Research, Copewood and Davis Streets, Camden, NJ 08103. These repositories serve an extremely important function for researchers interested in autosomal recessive disorders, because in some instances cells from the obligate heterozygous parents are available. For example, Sutherland and Oliver[150] studied the inheritance pattern of PRE with strains from the ATCC, that arose from skin biopsies of the classic XP family which has been monitored by Lynch and colleagues for many years.[169] Cell cultures were available from the father (CRL1167), mother (CRL1165), a son (XP2BE), twin sons (XP8BE and XP9BE), and an unaffected son (CRL1168) The Camden repository also has cultures from the XP patients and from another son (XP4SL). Cells from the proband and both parents of two other families are stored in the Camden repository. Hashem et al.[170] recently tabulated, by complementation group or variant, 16 XP cell stocks available from the above-mentioned repositories and 41 strains in the Department of Human Genetics, Rotterdam and the MRC Cell Mutation Unit, Brighton.

Without question, the availability of diverse strains of skin fibroblasts from patients with XP and other genodermatoses has contributed greatly to our basic knowledge about DNA damage and repair in man. On the other hand, it must be kept in mind that neoplasms associated with genodermatoses rarely involve dermal fibroblasts. It is therefore reassuring to know that the biochemical flaws detected in fibroblasts have also been observed in other cell types.

Epidermal Cells. Two years after Cleaver[1] first reported defective post-UV repair replication in fibroblasts from patients with XP, Epstein et al.[171] confirmed his results in vivo, in the same patients. After a subject was exposed to UV-B, ^{3}H-TdR was injected intradermally into the irradiated and adjacent unirradiated skin. Biopsies were collected one hour later, and autoradiographs were prepared. Autoradiographs from irradiated skin of normal subjects revealed that about 50% of the epidermal and upper dermal cells had the sparse nuclear labeling characteristic of UDS. In contrast, skin sections from two patients with DeSanctis-Cacchione syndrome exhibited no post-UV UDS, and fibroblasts of a patient with no neurological symptoms exhibited only 4% UDS. These results agreed with those of Cleaver, who observed no post-UV increase in labeling indices of fibroblast cultures from the three patients, and no increase in repair replication via density labeling. However, an important additional piece of information is available from the in vivo study: the *basal cells* of the patient with no neurological defects exhibited UDS which was 24% of normal. This observation underscores the point that in studying the etiology of cutaneous carcinomas in patients with XP, we should be examining the effects of UVR on epidermal cells, not fibroblasts. In vivo repair replication was estimated for basal cells of patients with several other disorders of sun sensitivity and/or cancer-prone skin.[172] (Cleaver, in reference 35, published a similar table for post-UV repair replication of fibroblasts.) Radioautographs revealed that the UV dose required to demonstrate UDS in vivo was large, 13.6×10^6 ergs/cm^2 of UV-B (1.36 J/cm^2), corresponding to about three minimal erythema doses.[172] The relevance of reduced UDS to in vivo recovery of human epidermis from acute UV injury is unclear. Epstein et al.[172] reported that injured skin of XP patients appear to heal normally, but tumor formation may occur within a few weeks after irradiation.

Jung[173] performed the in vitro analogue of the experiments of Epstein et al. Skin slices from patients with pigmented xerodermoid (XP variant) were irradiated and incubated with ^{3}H-TdR. Radioautographs revealed normal repair activity in epidermal cells. Robbins and colleagues[174,175] recognized that since the epidermis is the primary site of clinical disease and neoplasia in XP, one should verify that epidermal cells exhibit the same DNA repair features as fibroblasts. They isolated epidermal cells from skin slices of control persons and patients with XP, subjected the cells to UVR, and estimated UDS by radioautography. Epidermal cells from a patient, whose lymphocytes and fibroblasts were earlier shown to have reduced post-UV UDS, also exhibited a low level. For a patient later shown to be XP variant, his epidermal cells, lymphocytes, and fibroblasts all had normal UDS.

Baden et al.[138] demonstrated that guinea pig epidermis is capable of in vivo excision of psoralen photoadducts. Within 12 hours after PUVA treatment of the animal, 54% of the photoadduct in epidermal DNA was removed, and only 8% remained after 72 hours. Taichman and Setlow[176] measured loss of dimer-specific endonuclease-sensitive sites after UV irradiation of normal human keratinocyte and fibroblast cultures, and observed similar repair rates in the two cultures.

Other Cells. Friedberg et al.[112] cited studies demonstrating defective DNA repair in blood lymphocytes, lymphoblast lines, and conjunctival cultures from XP patients. Robbins et al.[140] pointed out that since it is often difficult to grow enough fibroblasts to perform biochemical studies, long-term lymphoblast lines may be more appropriate. At that time, they had developed XP-C strains which demonstrated reduced post-UV UDS. Their aim was to develop lymphoblast lines for each XP form; the Human Genetic Mutant Cell Repository now has at least one line for each of groups A–E and variant.

Ideas for Investigating Xeroderma Pigmentosum and Carcinogenesis

It becomes quickly apparent to anyone surveying the literature that most investigations of XP fibroblasts have been concerned with using these convenient mutants to study basic mechanisms of DNA damage and repair — the amount of effort devoted to the study of carcinogenesis is minuscule in comparison. In hopes of stimulating interest in the latter type of investigation, some basic considerations will be presented.

Most genodermatoses associated with cancer involve neoplasms of noncutaneous tissues. For these disorders, the use of convenient fibroblast cultures to study carcinogenesis is entirely appropriate. However, for XP, the major association with cancer appears to involve the transformation of epidermal cells under the influence of UVR.

Suitability of Epidermal Cells for Investigation of Carcinogenesis. The nearly exclusive use of fibroblasts to study carcinogenesis in XP has obscured a very important concept: the pluripotential basal cell is far different from every other human cell type in its ability to change its pattern of differentiation. One need only consider the healing of a shallow wound to understand the versatility of this cell. Epithelialization of the wound floor occurs not only by migration of epidermal cells from the wound edges, but by recruitment of basal cells from every transected hair follicle and sweat duct. Once confluency is attained, the cells attach to newly synthesized basement membrane and, thereafter, divide and differentiate into normal epidermal keratinocytes. Thus, cells which originally produced hair keratin or formed the lining of sweat ducts become reprogrammed into epidermal basal cells.

These considerations strongly suggest that investigators interested in XP and carcinogenesis should employ keratinocyte cultures. Although these cells are more difficult to establish and maintain than fibroblasts, culture techniques have been refined to the extent that durable, functional cell populations can be prepared. Kitano[177] recently reviewed this subject in detail and presented a cogent description of cells proliferating until confluency is obtained, stratifying and differentiating into keratinocytes, and eventually desquamating into the medium. It may even be possible to conduct experiments with basal cell preparations: Stanley et al.[178] observed that basal cells in epidermal cell suspensions selectively adhere to collagen coatings on glass slides.

Exposure Conditions. Investigators often subject cell cultures to UVR at the highly destructive wavelength of 254 nm. It is understandable that one wishes to maximize biological response when investigating DNA damage and repair, but this may not be appropriate in studies of cell transformation and carcinogenesis. It is not surprising that fibroblasts survive destructive doses of UV-C when only a fraction of the induced pyrimidine dimers are repaired. Cell culture conditions are designed to maximize cell survival and, in that context, may not reflect the in vivo state. In addition, one must consider that the human epidermis in vivo is subjected to chronic exposure to sunlight (UV-B, UV-A, visible, and infrared) and artificial light (UV-A and visible). Under those conditions, epidermal DNA may be in a delicate balance between damage caused by sporadic exposure to UVR, visible light, and heat; continuous repair by at least two mechanisms (excision and PRR); and discontinuous repair by PR. Therefore, relatively small perturbations in amount of DNA damage may reveal significant differences in behavior between cells of XP complementation groups and/or XP variants. In this same vein, perhaps heterozygous XP cells will respond in a manner intermediate between those of normal and homozygous cells.

In view of these comments, it may be worthwhile to conduct experiments by exposing cells to sunlamps or a solar simulator.[179] As a starting point, investigators with established culture procedures might consider exposing fibroblasts to alternate light sources (with the reservation that one may ultimately wish to employ keratinocyte cultures). Some studies have been conducted with sunlight. Cleaver[35] demonstrated repair synthesis after exposure of normal human fibroblasts to 6 hours of midday sunlight in April in San Francisco. The sunlight dose was enormous; Cleaver calculated that exposure for one hour would kill 97% of the fibroblasts (i.e., one hour of sunlight is equivalent to 10 J/m^2 UVR at 254 nm). Trosko et al.[36] exposed human amnion cells to sunlight and measured amounts of pyrimidine dimers formed. Again the dose was high; the amount of dimers produced after 5 hours exposure was equivalent to 60 J/m^2 UVR at 265 nm.

Is Defective DNA Repair Responsible for Carcinogenesis in XP? Obviously, defective DNA repair is not an obligatory factor in carcinogenesis, since many tumor cells do not exhibit detectable repair flaws.[180] Neither can impaired excision of pyrimidine dimers be the ultimate answer in XP, because XP variants are as cancer prone as classical XP patients. It has been proposed that reduced repair capability allows chronically induced UV damage to accumulate, eventually leading to the mutation resulting in carcinogenesis. This concept is testable. Epidermal slices are readily collectable from humans without harm, and there are established techniques for isolating epidermal DNA. Is the pyrimidine dimer content of epidermis from XP patients higher than normal? It appears that all that is required to answer this crucial question is development of a sensitive, nonradiochemical assay for dimers. (It may not be feasible to attempt to label sufficient human epidermal DNA in vivo.)

Along the same line, one might assay the levels of uracil in DNA from XP epidermis. It is intriguing that although it is well known that uracil is continuously formed in DNA by spontaneous deamination of cytosine, and assay methods for uracil-DNA glycosylase are available, apparently no enzyme studies have been conducted with cells from XP patients (however, see Epilogue). Of particular interest would be an investigation similar to that described by Sirover.[181] He reported a tenfold induction of uracil-DNA glycosylase in human lymphocytes stimulated with phytohemagglutinin. In contrast to the effects of pyrimidine dimers, which may retard DNA replication or result in error-prone repair, uracil in DNA may exert a direct mutagenic effect. Since uracil pairs with adenine instead of guanine, semiconservative replication of a DNA segment which originally contained cytosine may result in a purine substitution. This point mutation, if it occurred in a critical segment of a strand, might trigger carcinogenesis. Alternatively, efficient repair enzymes such as uracil-DNA glycosylase plus apyrimidinic endonuclease (or cytosine insertase?) may keep DNA uracil levels low enough in normal cells to minimize the chance of tumor formation. For those interested in the study of uracil formation and repair, epidermis from relatively hairless mammals (man, white pig, etc.) should be the tissue of choice. If DNA uracil is inimical to metabolic integrity, epidermal cells should have efficient repair mechanisms. An obvious avenue of study is to measure DNA uracil levels in sun-exposed and unexposed epidermis of normal individuals and patients with XP.

It might be noted that whatever the mechanism(s) for cell transformation in epidermis in man, the tumor-control processes break down frequently. Despite the fact that abnormal cells may be removed by migration to the skin surface and desquamation, skin cancers appeared to account for more than half of all malignant neoplasms in the United States.[182] In addition, nonmalignant proliferating units (actinic keratoses, moles, freckles, etc.) are common.

Study of Epidermal Tumor Cells. Since the major clinical concern for patients with XP is constant surveillance for development of cutaneous carcinomas, it is disappointing to note that the voluminous literature on XP contains few references to biochemical studies of tumor cells from these patients. This dearth of information is surprising in view of the fact that cutaneous tumors are often treated by surgery, thus ensuring a convenient supply of tissue, and tumor cells are easy to culture and maintain. To be sure, the basal and squamous cell carcinomas and the cutaneous melanomas developing in individuals with XP are histologically identical to tumors removed from humans without XP. *However, the parental cell(s) of the malignant entity carried a heritable flaw in DNA repair which most likely is expressed in the tumor cells.* This was verified by Robbins et al.[183] who demonstrated that basal cell carcinoma cells from an XP variant exhibited UV-induced UDS at least as great as the patient's fibroblasts.

On the other hand, tumor cells from an XP-C patient, whose lymphocytes and fibroblasts had 15–25% UDS, exhibited very low UDS. Likewise, Setlow and Regan[184] observed that amelanotic melanoma cells from an XP patient had the same low response to the chemical agent N-acetoxy-2-acetylaminofluorene (AAAF) as did classical XP fibroblasts. It is also noteworthy that SV40-transformed XP cells exhibited the same lack of repair replication as did the original strain.[185]

Since malignant XP cells have the same repair defects as their parental cells, the former may be exquisitely sensitive to chemotherapeutic agents that one would not usually consider for treatment of skin cancer. The implications of this concept for treatment of metastatic malignant melanoma in XP patients (the major cause of their early death) are obvious. It would be relatively easy to screen a host of DNA-damaging agents for specific toxicity to XP melanoma cells. To be sure, the therapeutic index of a specific agent may be low, but life-threatening circumstances justify extreme measures. Also, mild chemotherapy after removal of a cutaneous melanoma might prevent recurrence and/or metastasis. Thus, by capitalizing on an inherited flaw in tumor cells, one might prolong the life span of patients with XP.

An even more exciting area for biochemical and immunological investigation was revealed by Lynch and colleagues. They described spontaneous regression of metastatic melanoma in two sibs with XP,[186] and unusual survival of a patient with familial atypical multiple mole-melanoma (FAMMM) syndrome, who developed seven documented primary melanomas.[187] Do these individuals mount an exaggerated immune response to their melanoma cells? Does their serum contain an agent toxic to their melanoma cells? If so, is it toxic to melanoma cells in general?

The Heterozygous State in Xeroderma Pigmentosum

As discussed earlier ("Genodermatoses Associated with Cancer: Autosomal Recessive Genodermatoses"), an important question regarding recessive genodermatoses associated with cancer is whether heterozygous individuals are at increased risk. Many investigators have cited the need for a convenient test for heterozygosity in order to conduct definitive epidemiologic studies; lack of such a test greatly complicates the statistical approach. Additional confounding factors arise in the study of XP, because the biological endpoint (skin cancer) arises from the cumulative effects of chronic, lifelong exposure to sunlight. Thus, one must correct for geographic areas of residence, skin pigmentation, and history of sunlight exposure.

Tests for the heterozygous state in many hereditary disorders are performed by assaying for intermediate levels of a metabolite or enzyme (i.e., a gene product). Since there is no known metabolite abnormality in XP cells, and knowledge about DNA repair in human fibroblasts is not sufficiently advanced to permit direct assay of repair enzymes, investigators have attempted to assess heterozygosity on the basis of intermediate levels of a *process*, i.e., repair capacity.

Biochemical Studies. Numerous reports have listed values for UDS or repair replication in fibroblasts from obligate heterozygous parents of classical XP patients.[128,188] Pawsey et al.[50] reported values for 13 heterozygotes and reviewed the literature. Although reduced repair capacity has often been observed in heterozygous cells, many strains exhibit normal repair. Cleaver[189] reported that fibroblasts from the parents of an XP patient exhibited normal excision repair up to a UV dose of 7 J/m². Beyond that level, amount of repair leveled off, whereas repair in normal cells continued to rise. Apparently, the amount of DNA damage induced by doses above 7 J/m² saturated the repair systems in heterozygous cells. Unfortunately, this relationship is not general; one of four heterozygous strains tested at 22 J/m² had normal repair.

Day[79] observed that cells from parents of XP patients (groups A–D) conducted normal host cell reactivation of irradiated adenovirus 2. Coppey et al.[80] investigated the kinetics and dose dependence of recovery of fibroblasts from UV irradiation, in terms of production of herpes simplex virus 1. They detected some differences between actions of normal and heterozygous cells, suggesting the possibility of developing a test for heterozygosity.

Tests for the Heterozygous State. Cleaver[124] mentioned a method of detecting heterozygous XP cells based on the frequency of mutation induced by ethyl methanesulfonate, but considers it too difficult for routine use.

Giannelli and Pawsey[137] conducted an extensive study of radioautographic UDS in multinucleate heterokaryons in fused-cell preparations. They concluded that nuclei from normal fibroblasts could complement more nuclei from cells of a classical XP patient than could those from a parent of an XP patient. In other words, their results clearly distinguished heterozygous from normal cells on the basis of "complementing capacity." From the results of kinetic studies, the authors suggested that an enzyme-acceptor complex may be involved in DNA repair and that the enzyme in classical XP cells may have reduced affinity for the receptor. The suggestion that the enzyme is not a monomer (consists of different units?) may accommodate complementation between different classical XP groups. This elegant study appears to represent a definitive test for heterozygosity in classical XP, but it may require too much expertise and effort for general use.

Maher et al.[190] described the synergistic effect of caffeine on the cytoxicity of UVR or aryl hydrocarbon epoxides in XP strains. Hydrocarbon-epoxide adducts to DNA appear to be repaired by the same mechanism involved in repair of UV damage. Caffeine potentiated, in a dose-dependent manner, the toxicity of

UVR or chemical agents to XP variant cells, and had little or no influence on effects of the agents on classical XP strains. The differential effect of caffeine should be investigated with cells of parents of XP variants.

Ahmed and Setlow[191] examined excision repair in cells from patients with classical XP (groups, C, D, and E) and from XP variants. Similar results were obtained with three techniques: radioautographic UDS, BrUdR photolysis, and loss of pyrimidine dimer sites sensitive to UV endonuclease. Saturation doses of UVR and AAAF were determined for each cell type, and these doses were then employed in combination. Two repair patterns were observed: (1) total repair in excision proficient cells (normal and XP variant) was additive; (2) total repair in classical XP cells was much less than additive, or even less than treatment with UVR or chemical agent alone. The additive effects of saturation doses of UVR and AAAF in repair proficient cells suggest that DNA damage induced by the two agents is repaired by different pathways. On the other hand, the authors pointed out the AAAF damage resembles UV damage in type of excision repair (long patch) and effects on classical XP cells. In view of these observations, it seems worthwhile (if it has not already been done) to determine the saturation dose of AAAF for cells from parents of classical XP patients, as a test for heterozygosity. If this survey does not yield definitive results, combinations of UVR and AAAF should be evaluated.

What Type of Study Will Provide a Convenient Test for Heterozygosity? As implied earlier, tests for heterozygosity usually depend on the effects of gene dosage on levels of a gene product. Thus, normal (wild type) cells with genotype +/+ will have normal levels; heterozygous cells +/-, intermediate levels; and homozygous -/-, little or no product. If the extreme sun sensitivity and high incidence of cutaneous carcinoma in patients with XP results from reduced activity of an enzyme or cofactor involved in repair of UV-damaged DNA, it is imperative that these components be identified and characterized. This statement is not to belittle the extensive past and present efforts of many investigators to accomplish that goal. Instead, I repeat the suggestion presented earlier in this section ("Biochemical Studies of Defective DNA Repair: Studies Performed with Cell Nuclei"): nuclei from irradiated repair deficient XP cells (alternatively, permeabilized cells) should provide convenient detection systems for repair factors in normal human fibroblasts, thus rendering it feasible to isolate and purify these components. The seven classical XP groups and XP variants afford a versatile array of detection systems, each one possibly specific for a different repair factor. If XP nuclei lived up to this promise, the information gained would constitute a breakthrough in basic understanding of repair of UV-damaged DNA in man and would provide convenient tests for heterozygosity in all types of XP. A current abstract by Lambert et al.[192] describes a method of screening human lymphoblasts for multiple endonucleases. Nucleoplasmic and chromatin-protein fractions are subjected to isoelectric focusing, and bands equilibrating at various pH regions are assayed for endonuclease activity. This technique is very sensitive, yet adaptable to large-scale fractionations. Coupling of this procedure with the detection systems afforded by XP nuclei might provide rapid identification and isolation of defective DNA repair factors in a variety of aberrant cells.

In the meantime, while definitive techniques for quantitating gene products are being developed, one might investigate the effect of retinoids on DNA repair of fibroblasts from XP patients and heterozygotes. Some of these chemotherapeutic agents are being employed for the treatment of disorders of keratinization.[193] An agent potent enough to reprogram aberrant keratinocytes might have an intermediate effect on DNA repair in heterozygous fibroblasts.

Are Heterozygotes at Risk for Cancer? We are indebted to Swift and colleagues for their persistence in pursuing this question in the absence of a convenient test for heterozygosity. Swift and Chase[194] identified 31 XP families and constructed extensive pedigrees, including nonblood relatives (spouses) for controls. Questionnaires, hospital records, and death certificates were collected for 2,597 blood relatives and spouses. Relatives with a probability of heterozygosity of 0.67 or one had a statistically significant higher prevalence of nonmelanoma skin cancer than did spouse controls. The prevalence in all blood relatives living in southern states was significantly higher than spouse controls, whereas no difference was observed between relatives and spouses living in other areas. The 30 blood relatives with verified nonmelanoma skin cancer belonged to 13 families. However, the number of carcinomas was concentrated in four families which had a large number of members aged 30 years or older, who resided in the southern part of the United States.

The authors detected no malignant melanomas in blood relatives. They pointed out that, since the incidence of basal and squamous cell carcinoma is several times higher than that of cutaneous melanoma in XP homozygotes, a predisposition of heterozygotes for melanoma might not be detected in their study group.

The number of observed deaths of relatives from lung, stomach, and prostate cancers was higher than expected, and the authors recommended caution because of the small number in each category and the possible influence of factors other than segregation of the XP gene. On the other hand, they noted there have been no reports of these cancers in XP homozygotes or of usual incidences in XP families.

Lastly, the authors reemphasized the need for a test for heterozygosity and suggested a systematic comparison of various methods, with a large number of obligate heterozygotes. A suggestion is in order: each investigator, when establishing a fibroblast strain from a patient with XP, should make every effort to obtain skin biopsies from *both* parents and from siblings. The Camden repository and ATCC have 19 cell stocks from parents of XP patients and several from unaffected siblings. Only three proband/father/mother combinations are available.

Cumulative Actinic Damage — Implications for Black
Patients with Xeroderma Pigmentosum

It seems likely that accumulation of unrepaired lesions in epidermal DNA of XP patients eventually leads to induction of carcinoma. In addition to abundant biochemical data suggesting such an etiology, there is evidence that replacement of sun-damaged epidermis of XP patients retards the appearance of new tumors. Since the skin of black XP patients contains sufficient melanin to screen out much of the damaging UVR of sunlight,[16] one would expect cutaneous carcinomas to occur at a later age in blacks than in lightly pigmented patients. The serious clinical implications of this point will be discussed later. Psoralens have been administered to promote a natural tan in Caucasian XP patients, in hopes of providing protection against UVR. Varying degrees of success have been reported, but Reed's experience seems definitive.[195] He reported that six XP patients treated by him all developed a greater number of malignancies.

Therapeutic Replacement of Damaged Epidermis. Topical 5-fluorouracil (5-FU) has been employed to prevent or retard the induction of carcinomas in XP patients.[196,197] This chemotherapeutic agent destroys precancerous and cancerous epidermal lesions, while at the same time permitting new epidermis to grow and replace the neoplastic tissue. Gleason[198] reported the five-year arrest of facial tumors in a patient with XP by total reconstruction of her face with split-thickness skin grafts from her thighs. Epstein et al.[199] observed that no tumors had developed in areas of a patient's face that had been dermabraded seven years earlier. They also noted that an area of the thigh, which had provided epidermis for a skin graft ten months previously, did not exhibit the generalized freckling of adjacent epidermis. On the basis of this observation, they removed dermatome slices of skin from other areas of the thighs that were prone to development of neoplasms.

Comment. The relevance of defective repair of UV-induced DNA damage in the etiology of skin cancer has been argued pro and con, even with regard to XP. The reports discussed above establish that replacement of actinically damaged epidermis by new epidermis, or by less severely damaged tissue, retards the development of UV-induced neoplasms. The fact that donor sites on the thighs respond favorably suggests that nonactinic factors, such as frequent washing and use of cosmetics, are not the major inducers of the multiple tumors which occur on the face. Therefore, the clinical and biochemical evidence provide mutual support for the premise that UVR acts as a carcinogen rather than a co-carcinogen for most patients with XP. This concept may require modification for black patients.

Xeroderma Pigmentosum in Blacks. Although dermatology textbooks often refer to the occurrence of XP in all races, there are few reports of XP in blacks. Another textbook comment stresses the prevalence of oculocutaneous symptoms in XP. An important racial distinction is that XP is usually diagnosed from skin symptoms in lightly pigmented patients, whereas the presenting features in blacks are often eye lesions in very young children. Before discussing clinical reports, it is revealing to review the history of XP, as presented by Bellows et al.[200]

Xeroderma pigmentosum was first described by Hebra and Kaposi in 1874, and by 1943 about 460 cases had been reported.[201] In contrast, the first report of XP in blacks was presented by Loewenthal and Trowell in 1938.[202] One of the authors' opening comments is appropriate: "The reason for this report is the occurrence of the condition in three members of a family of African negroes – a race which has hitherto been presumed to be immune from the disease because of the lavish amount of cutaneous pigment present in its individuals." By 1974 only 15 affected blacks had been reported.[201] Ocular complications in XP include lid tumors, ectropion, keratitis, and corneal opacities. Frequency of eye involvement has been reported as low as 30% and as high as 80%. The higher figure is appropriate for black patients,[200] who often develop bilateral corneal opacities at an early age.

Loewenthal and Trowell[202] described XP in three of five full-blooded black brothers in Uganda. Skin lesions appeared at about age 1½, followed soon after by ocular trouble. The patients' skin had the normal dark pigmentation of their race, with numerous hyper- and hypopigmented macules on the limbs and trunk. It was customary for children of their tribe to wear no clothing. Significantly, the two older patients each had a hard, pedunculated tumor on the tip of the tongue. One tumor was diagnosed histologically as " . . . a fibroma with a somewhat large proportion of active cells, as though malignancy were to be looked for later." The two older children (ages 3½ and 8) had diffuse leukoma of both corneas; the youngest (age 2½) had a severe keratitis with early leukoma.

Bellows et al.[200] reported ocular manifestations in three siblings of a family in Haiti. The first case, 6 years old, was seen in 1971. He had had widespread cutaneous nodules since age 3, but presented with an enlarging mass arising from the left orbit. His right cornea was opaque. The mass on the left eye was removed, but subsequent recurrence necessitated enucleation. Histologic features of the mass were suggestive of angiosarcoma, with prominent indications of squamous cell carcinoma (SqCC) at the margins. The second case, age 4, was seen at the same time as her brother. She had a mass arising from the inferior temporal limbal region of the right globe, extending into the cornea. Fifteen months later, both her corneas were opaque. The third case, age 6 months, had normal cutaneous and ocular findings in 1971. Fifteen months later, he had marked photophobia, reddened conjunctiva and hazy corneas; hyperpigmented macules were present on his face and extremities.

Freedman[203] performed corneal transplants on two brothers and a cousin (ages 13, 16, and 30, respectively) from South Africa. Each patient exhibited mild skin symptoms but had been blind since 2 years of age because of corneal opacities. Histologic examination of the corneal buttons removed from graft sites revealed bullous changes in the epithelium, partial destruction of Bowman's membrane, presence of blood vessels, and irregular stroma. The author considers full-thickness transplants to be preferable to split-thickness grafts, to avoid possible future complications from the host's corneal endothelial cells. At the time of the report, each graft had remained clear for six months. In a classic study relating ocular changes to cumulative actinic damage, Freedman observed another XP patient from age 8 months to 2 years. The earliest change (one year old) was invasion of blood vessels from the limbus into the lower half of the cornea. These vessels regressed, leaving a corneal opacity. A similar process occurred in the upper half of the cornea, until the whole cornea was opaque at age 2. The chronological sequence of events suggests that the unprotected lower half of the cornea acquired sufficient actinic damage to become clinically apparent in one year, whereas the upper half of the cornea received enough protection from the eyelid to delay the process.

In the first report of XP in a black person in the United States, Hananian and Cleaver[204] described a patient in Miami. It is remarkable that the patient's fibroblasts have been stored in the Camden repository, but a clinical report was not presented until now. The authors suggested that the cell line be designated XP1MI. The patient exhibited the following sequence of symptoms: skin and eye abnormalities at age 6½, basal cell carcinoma (BCC) of cheek and nose at age 13, severely reduced vision resulting from bilateral corneal haziness at age 17. She also had BCCs at the latter age. The coexistence of systemic lupus erythematosus (SLE) could have been coincidental or could be related to the XP condition (excessive sunlight exposure can trigger SLE attacks). The patient's fibroblasts exhibited reduced DNA repair (20–30%), consistent with their assignment to group C by other investigators.

Plotnick,[205] in Michigan, described mucocutaneous and ocular lesions in two brothers (ages 21 and 29) and a sister (age 12). The oldest patient was first seen at age 9 (1961) by an ophthalmologist, and a SqCC of the right sclerolimbal margin was removed. In 1963, a warty lesion was excised from the tongue, and SqCC was again diagnosed. The patient was seen in 1969 for a lesion on the bulbar conjunctiva, which was removed and determined to be SqCC. A large number of "black freckles" on the patient's face alerted the ophthalmologist to consult a dermatologist, who diagnosed XP. In 1971, at the age of 19, the patient exhibited the first skin lesions severe enough to require treatment: a BCC of the nose and a SqCC in situ (Bowen) of the lower eyelid were removed. A SqCC of the eyebrow was excised in 1976. The younger brother was seen at age 12 in 1969; and a SqCC in situ was removed from the left cornea. Pigmentation anomalies on the face led to a diagnosis of XP. In 1974, a SqCC in situ was removed from the right cornea. Like his brother, at about age 20 (1977), the patient had skin lesions: SqCCs were excised from the lower lip, right cheek, and dorsum of the nose. The youngest patient was seen by a dermatologist in 1975 at age 10. At that time, a lesion excised from the cheek was diagnosed as lentigo maligna. One year later, an invasive SqCC was removed from the tip of her tongue. In 1977, a second lesion identified as lentigo maligna was removed from the nose. Lastly, 20 months after removal of the first, a second invasive SqCC was excised from the tip of the tongue. The author pointed out that development of SqCCs of the tongue suggests that UVR may not be the only inducer of neoplasia in XP. Alternatively, UVR may be acting systemically (see "Biological Effects of Ultraviolet Irradiation: Effect of Ultraviolet Radiation on Host Resistance to Cancer") as a co-carcinogen with an environmental agent (spicy food?).

Clinical Implications of XP in Blacks. The most important factor in successful treatment of XP is early diagnosis and immediate institution of rigorous, lifelong avoidance of UVR. Clinical aspects of the articles cited above were discussed in detail to impress upon the reader the insidious, disabling features of XP in blacks. It is ironic that the high level of photoprotection afforded by cutaneous melanin in black children delays bringing them to the attention of a physician until irreversible eye damage has occurred. The prevailing theme throughout the above-cited reports is that skin symptoms of black children with XP are not severe enough to alarm the parents and, only when ocular lesions appear, is there sufficient motivation to seek medical help. The situation in underdeveloped tropical areas must be particularly severe. Full-blooded black children there are accustomed to spending much time in the sun, with little or no protective clothing. Lack of skin manifestations severe enough to raise suspicion of disease, and inadequate medical facilities, probably doom XP patients to early blindness and reduced survival. The situation may be somewhat less serious in developed countries in temperate latitudes, if the index of suspicion for XP can be raised in ophthalmologists. The patients described by Plotnick[205] in Michigan illustrate this point. The oldest was first seen by an ophthalmologist at 9 years of age, and twice more over a period of eight years. At the last visit (age 17), pigmentary changes raised the suspicion of XP. A diagnosis of XP was also made in a younger brother (age 12) at that time and, subsequently, in a younger sister at age 10. It is significant that cutaneous carcinoma did not appear in the brothers until ages 19 or 20 (the sister has not yet attained this age). It is imperative that when XP is diagnosed in a black, all siblings be examined for cutaneous and ocular manifestations. Biochemical studies of lymphocytes or fibroblasts are justified if the siblings are too young to exhibit skin symptoms. There has been a question of whether XP can be diagnosed in blacks by clinical and histologic examination; this point was addressed by Targowsky and Loewenthal[206] in 1956. Biochemical verification of the diagnosis is advisable for all black patients.

A possible area of clinical concern is that, although XP in general is a rare disorder, the incidence in blacks is unknown. The paucity of published reports and the likelihood that many individuals with XP are never seen by a physician familiar with the disease suggest that epidemiologic studies will underestimate its incidence in blacks.

Biochemical Implications of XP in Blacks. The unusual occurrence of SqCC on the tip of the tongue in black patients was noted above.[202,205] This point is worth stressing, because in spite of the fact that mucocutaneous findings are often cited in clinical descriptions of XP, molecular biologists tend to fixate on cutaneous (i.e., UV-induced) carcinoma. Perhaps we have reached a point of nonprofitability in the study of repair of UV-damaged DNA by XP cells and need a fresh approach. Knowledgeable investigators may derive inspiration from the clinical manifestations of Plotnick's patients: SqCCs of the tongue appeared at an earlier age (10–13 years) than did cutaneous tumors (19–20 years).[205] Another tantalizing phenomenon was reported long ago by Bell and Rothnem.[207] Two brothers with XP each developed a SqCC of the lower lip at ages (13 and 16 years) when no skin keratoses or tumors had appeared.

The racial predilection for classical XP groups (i.e., North Americans and Europeans for group C; Orientals for group A) suggests that complementation studies with fibroblasts from black patients should be performed. Although not readily apparent from the literature, several lines have been studied and assigned to groups A and C (J.E. Cleaver, personal communication). Cleaver (personal communication) recently detected a black XP variant.

There are scattered references in the literature to a partial X-linkage in XP. Although the available data for blacks are limited, the five reports discussed above listed nine males, three females, and two patients of unspecified sex. If a partial X-linkage occurs in blacks, patients should be examined for glucose-6-phosphate dehydrogenase (G6PD) status. Fialkow[208] presented an extensive review on the analysis of G6PD variants to evaluate the clonal origin of tumors. The X-linked G6PD occurs predominantly in the B form in Caucasians, whereas 30–40% of black males have a variant, type A. About 40% of black females are heterozygous for G6PD A/B. In accord with the Lyons hypothesis of random but permanent inactivation of the X chromosome, about half of a heterozygous female's cells will produce G6PD-B only; the others, G6PD-A. It would be of at least academic interest to examine the G6PD pattern of tumors from heterozygous black females with XP. If only one enzyme type is present, the presumption is that the tumor arose from a single transformed cell (as predicted by Fialkow); if both forms are present, a multi-cellular origin is indicated. As an aside, G6PD is detected as a dimer, A_2 or B_2. If the hybrid AB were detected, it would mean that the inactive X chromosome had been turned on in a cell. This phenomenon has not been detected in the numerous neoplasms studied to date, but XP is an unusual disorder. To date, two sisters, XP1NBi and XP2NBi, have been classified as G6PD type B.

Does Xeroderma Pigmentosum Occur in the American Indian?

Xeroderma pigmentosum has been reported in many human populations: e.g., American, Western European, Arab, East Asian, Japanese, African black, Russian Armenian; a notable exception is the American Indian. The single MEDLINE entry regarding XP in this race cited an excellent review by Reed[209] on genetics and photo-dermatoses. He discussed hereditary polymorphous light eruption (HPLE) in the American Indian; XP was reviewed in a separate section, with no reference to it occurring in the American Indian. If XP does not occur in this race, the genetic implications may be important. For example, one might conclude that the mutation leading to the XP gene occurred after the ancestral migration which separated the American Indian from other human races. Furthermore, the XP mutation must be an extremely improbable event, or it would have appeared in the American Indian. These considerations imply that the mutation is in a section of DNA which is critically important for life; possibly most mutations in this area are lethal and therefore do not contribute to the XP gene pool. It is therefore important that information about XP in an American Indian (at least one parent must be full blooded) be promptly reported. Because of its genetic isolation, the American Indian race is of considerable interest to investigators of hereditary disease. For example, HPLE, a hereditary photosensitivity, is distributed among Indians of North, Central, and South America. The HPLE gene may have developed some time after the ancestral migration to North America, since tribes of the Atlantic Coast and Pacific Northwest appear to be free of the disorder.

Comment. The absence of reports of XP in American Indians may simply reflect low clinical suspicion and/or lack of medical attention. It is premature to speculate further, but if it were established that XP does not occur in this race, one could estimate a maximum mutation rate for the XP gene. Since this value would be considerably lower than Takebe's[210] estimate of 10^{-6} to 10^{-5}, it would require reassessment of the assumptions made in calculating mutation rates in humans. Alternatively, one might wonder if something in the American Indian's genetic makeup renders an XP mutation lethal, even in a heterozygote. It may be significant that HPLE appears to be unique for this race and involves photosensitivity.

OTHER GENODERMATOSES ASSOCIATED WITH CANCER

The genodermatoses, ataxial telangiectasia (AT), Fanconi anemia, and Bloom's syndrome, exhibit common features such as chromosomal instability, predisposition to cancer, and defective DNA repair.[211]   They have been studied as models of spontaneous carcinogenesis, but as pointed out by Weichselbaum and Little,[127] associated neoplasia is usually hematopoietic and/or lymphoreticular. Furthermore, these disorders (especially AT) are characterized by immunologic disturbances. Accordingly, information concerning possible repair flaws and their relation to carcinogenesis should be interpreted in the context of impaired immunologic surveillance or defense. The authors consider familial retinoblastoma to be a good model for the study of DNA repair and carcinogenesis, since it has no recognized immune defects. They presented an up-to-date discussion of defects in repair of x-ray damage in fibroblasts from such patients.

Cockayne's syndrome is not specifically associated with cancer, but it is of interest within the scope of this report for several reasons: (1) it occurs concurrently with XP in the single known patient of complementation group B; (2) fibroblasts are sensitive to UVR and chemical agents, and exhibit DNA repair defects; (3) the clinical hallmark of this disease is extreme sun sensitivity. Familial cutaneous malignant melanoma, strictly speaking, is not a genodermatosis *associated* with cancer; it *is* cancer. However, internal cancers are also associated with this disorder.[103] It will be discussed here in order to attempt to relate biochemical theory to spontaneous regression of melanoma, especially in patients with XP. The hereditary disorder psoriasis will receive some attention. Not only is this disease a fascinating example of nonmalignant, uncontrolled proliferation, but it may have a *negative* association with cancer. Hereditary total albinism is associated with skin cancer because patients do not produce sufficient melanin to affort normal protection against UVR. As in XP, the increased incidence of carcinomas and melanomas in albinos is not familial cancer per se, but rather a secondary consequence of a hereditary inability to cope with UVR in normal fashion. Lastly, the possible relationship of nerve growth factor to neurofibromatosis will be analyzed.

Ataxia Telangiectasia

The radiosensitivity associated with AT was discovered when patients given x-ray therapy suffered severe tissue damage in the radiation field. This clinical clue has led investigators to study the nature of γ-induced DNA damage and mechanisms of repair of these lesions in human cells. The clinical symptoms and biochemical aspects of AT were thoroughly discussed in a current review.[212] Friedberg et al.[112] summarized the available data about responses of numerous AT cell lines to various DNA damaging agents. The current terminology is analogous to XP (e.g., AT3BI is third strain, Birmingham), and the authors provided cross-references to earlier designations. In general, AT cells are the ionizing radiation analogue of XP cells. With some exceptions, they exhibit mutually exclusive responses to DNA-damaging agents: if one strain is sensitive, the other is not; if one exhibits deficient repair, the other is proficient; etc.

Complementation Studies. Genetic heterogeneity was suspected in AT on the basis of clinical and biochemical evidence. Paterson et al.[213] confirmed this by measuring the ability of heterokaryons from fused strains to repair γ-induced DNA damage. Of the three repair deficient strains tested, two were assigned to group A and one to group B. Repair proficient AT strains constitute a third group, analogous to XP variant. It appears there are no other reports of complementation studies of AT cells, in spite of the indications of genetic heterogeneity. I agree with Paterson and Smith[212] that these studies should receive high priority.

It would be of interest to fuse AT and XP cells, as suggested by Lynch and Frichot;[103] fusion with XP variant fibroblasts might be especially informative. The fact that AT strains are γ-sensitive and XP cells are UVR-sensitive suggests that such studies would be unrewarding. However, XP and AT cells exhibit similar responses to some chemicals[212] and, therefore, might complement each other if the appropriate DNA-damaging agent were employed. Furthermore, in analogy with the earlier suggestion for XP nuclei (see "Xeroderma Pigmentosum: What Type of Study Will Provide a Convenient Test for Heterozygosity?"), intact XP cells provide eight different detection systems for complementation analysis of other repair defective strains. Such analyses should be implemented for every hereditary disorder involving defective DNA repair.

Effects of Gamma Radiation on DNA. Before discussing biochemical studies of repair of γ-induced DNA damage, it may be appropriate to review the effects of ionizing radiation. Because of its high energy content, γ-radiation causes formation of single- and double-strand breaks (SSB, DSB) and extensive base damage. A DSB may represent separate events in close proximity on opposite strands, but there is evidence it may result from a single event.[214] At any rate, it is apparent that DSB are formed much less frequently than SSB.[214,215] Not surprisingly, DSB are lethal,[216] since it is difficult to visualize a repair mechanism that does not require an intact template segment on the complementary strand. Single-strand breaks and damaged bases are repaired by the same mechanisms outlined for repair of UV-induced damage. Obviously, SSB do not require the incision step before initiation of excision repair, but the 3' terminus may require tailoring. In most x-ray-induced breaks, a base is lost.[215] Presumably, bond cleavage occurs in a deoxyribose unit rather than at the phosphodiester link. The nature of γ-induced DNA damage may be summarized by listing the major differences between it and the effects of UVR: (1) single-strand breaks are much more common; (2) extensive base damage occurs, especially photohydration of the 5,6 bond of pyrimidines;[217] (3) pyrimidine dimers are not a prominent feature of γ-induced damage.

Hutchinson[215] reported that interaction of x-rays with DNA involves release of energy packets averaging 100 eV, producing clusters of radiochemical events in a small volume. From the literature, he estimated the efficiency of DSB formation in oxygenated cells as $0.1-0.2$ break/10^9 daltons-krad, which is reduced by a factor of two or three in the absence of oxygen. The frequency of SSB production is about ten times greater. Cole et al.[216] observed that γ-irradiation of Chinese hamster ovary cells released 70 eV per SSB, and 2,700 eV per DSB produced, verifying that frequency of DSB formation is much less than that of SSB. At doses below 20 krad, SSB were completely rejoined, whereas DSB were repaired efficiently after doses up to 60 krad. It might be instructive to relate doses to UVR. One rad is equivalent to 100 ergs of energy absorbed per gram of tissue; 1 krad = 0.01 J/g. For a confluent layer of fibroblasts 10 μm thick, with assumed density of 1 g/cm^3, 1 g is equivalent to 0.1 m^2. Accordingly, 1 krad = 0.1 J/m^2. If the limiting dose for cell survival is that for effective repair of DSB, 60 krad = 6 J/m^2. The latter figure is comparable to one cited earlier: 10 J/m^2 UVR at 254 nm killed 97% of normal human fibroblasts (see 'Xeroderma Pigmentosum: Exposure Conditions"). Experiments with ionizing radiation are conducted at doses of a few hundred rads to 300 krad. (Contrast this with yearly exposure of humans to environmental radiation of less than a rad.)

A final point to be clarified involves γ-radiation sources (x-rays and ^{60}Co are frequently used). The description of x-rays is in terms of kilovolts applied to the apparatus. As a rule of thumb, the energy of the x-ray beam is about one-third the applied voltage. Radioactive emitters are characterized by the maximum energy of the emitted photons, e.g., 1.25 keV (average) for ^{60}Co. These two types of radiation cannot be compared directly except in terms of total doses (kilorads). Because cells may be subject to a dose rate effect, authors usually report the dose rate of their source.

Biochemical Studies of Defective Repair. Little[218] proposed two types of DNA lesions in x-ray-irradiated cells: (1) those which lead to cell death, probably because of unrejoined breaks, and (2) those which cause mutation and transformation, probably resulting from base damage and misrepair. Hutchinson[219] noted that far less is known about repair of SSB than about repair of pyrimidine dimers. The main reason for this paucity of information is that γ-radiation produces relatively few breaks (1-5/10^9 daltons-krad x-rays), and cells may only tolerate a few breaks (CFA of mammalian cells is halved after only 100 rads). Hutchinson reviewed methods for measuring SSB repair. In general, they are based on alkaline sedimentation or elution, and analysis of DNA molecular weight at various intervals after irradiation. It should be noted that these techniques monitor rejoining of breaks but do not detect misrepair.

Paterson et al.[213] subjected normal human cells, and strains from ten AT patients of unrelated kindred to ^{60}Co radiation (25-100 krad). Irradiation was conducted in the absence of oxygen to increase the proportion of base defects to SSB. In accord with the findings of others, AT cells were proficient in rejoining SSB. On the other hand, six of the ten strains studied had defective excision repair. These strains appear to be the γ-radiation counterpart of classical XP cells, with the repair defect at some step other than incision. The authors also pointed out that repair proficient AT cells responded to radiation in a manner similar to responses of XP variant cells to UVR, thus suggesting the former may also have defective PRR. They proposed a novel application: since chemical DNA-damaging agents may be classified as UV-like, γ-like (radiomimetic), or both, AT and XP cells could be used to screen any number of environmental agents as possible mutagens or carcinogens. Sheridan and Huang[220] developed a method sensitive enough to detect one SSB per 10^9 daltons, permitting quantitation of repair at doses below 400 rads. Even at this low dose, six AT strains exhibited a normal rate and extent of repair of SSB. Therefore, the radiosensitivity of AT cells does not appear to be the result of an inability to repair SSB.

As noted earlier, the major type of base damage from ionizing radiation involves addition of hydroxy radicals to the 5,6 bond of pyrimidines, causing labelization of the N-glycosidic bond.[217,221] Accordingly, radiation produces apyrimidinic sites, which in turn are alkali labile. Radiomimetic alkylating agents also cause loss of pyrimidines, and loss of bases can occur spontaneously at $37°$.[221] Similar base-labilizing reactions affect purines as well. The most studied form of base-damage repair in AT cells is removal of thymine glycol (5,6-dihydroxydihydrothymine), abbreviated t'. The efficiency of t' formation in oxygenated human lung fibroblasts is $0.5/10^9$ daltons-krad, compared to 1.9 SSB/10^9 daltons-krad.[221] In contrast, the yield in adenovirus 5 DNA after 500 J/m^2 UVR at 250 nm was 78 t'/10^9 daltons.[153] On the basis that 1 krad = 0.1 J/m^2 (see "Effects of γ-radiation on DNA," earlier in this section), the corresponding value for UVR is 0.02 t' 10^9 daltons. Harriharan and Cerutti[24] developed an assay based on the fact that mild alkaline treatment of t'-containing DNA removes the damaged bases and cleaves them to yield acetol. Prelabeling the DNA with ^{3}H-(methyl)-TdR provides a means of quantitating the acetol produced. Whole cell sonicates of five AT fibroblast strains displayed normal capabilities to remove t' from chromatin which was isolated from normal and AT cells and subjected to γ-radiation.[222] Two of the AT strains had earlier been shown to have defective post-γ excision repair. The authors concluded that t' lesions are not involved in the lethal action of ionizing radiation on human fibroblasts.

The repair of apyrimidinic and/or apurinic γ-induced lesions by AT cells is a likely area of investigation. These lesions can arise by direct cleavage of the N-glycosidic bond or, indirectly, by modification of the nitrogenous bases. Sheridan and Haung[223] measured the AP endonuclease activity of six AT strains representing repair deficient groups A and B, and repair proficient variants. All cell types had somewhat reduced activity (77%). However, they estimated that this activity was much greater than that required to repair apurinic sites arising spontaneously.

Some brief remarks about radiomimetic agents are in order. Bleomycin induces chromosomal abnormalities and extensive DNA damage in lymphocytes.

Taylor et al.[224] cited reports that it causes release of bases, destruction of deoxyribose, and production of SSB and DSB. They demonstrated that treatment of four strains of AT lymphocytes with bleomycin caused chromosomal aberrations much higher than those of normal cells and greatly reduced cell survival. They suggested that the elevated sensitivity of AT cells to bleomycin may represent defective rejoining of a fraction of DNA strand breaks. Ahmed and Setlow[225] performed experiments analogous to those reported for XP cells (see "Xeroderma Pigmentosum: Tests for the Heterozygous State"), with AT cells and other strains. Saturating doses for excision repair were determined for UVR and AAAF. Cells were then treated with both agents at those doses. Both repair deficient and proficient AT lines exhibited additive repair, suggesting proficiency in excision repair of damage from either agent.

Gamma-induced Chromosomal Aberrations. Lymphocytes from AT patients provide a means of studying the relationship of γ-induced DNA lesions and their effects on chromosomal and chromatid breaks and translocations. Lymphocytes are particularly useful, because they can be harvested in G_0 phase and followed through the cell cycle for one or more divisions. Also, detection of cytogenetic abnormalities is a much more sensitive indicator of DNA damage than biochemical assay.[220] This fascinating topic will not be reviewed here, except to point out that AT lymphocytes develop 10-20 times the normal number of chromatid-type aberrations after low doses of radiation, and to refer the interested reader to an extensive current review.[226]

The Heterozygous State in AT. As with other autosomal recessive disorders associated with cancer, one would like to have a convenient test for heterozygosity in AT. Chen et al.[227] developed a method which afforded a clear distinction from normal for the heterozygous strains tested. They subjected lymphoblastoid lines to oxic radiation and monitored CFA and trypan blue exclusion. The average CFA for heterozygotes (parents of AT patients) was statistically lower than normal, with possibly some overlap of individual values. Trypan blue exclusion, however, clearly separated six heterozygous from eight normal and five homozygous strains. A clinically normal sibling of an AT patient had an intermediate response and was tentatively judged to be heterozygous. The authors cautioned that because of the existence of complementation groups, some heterozygous lines may not exhibit intermediate responses. This concern may prove baseless as additional AT strains are tested. Also, if cells from the parents of an AT patient respond in a heterozygous manner, one may reasonably expect that other heterozygous members of the kindred will be identifiable. This hypothesis is testable by continuing to examine lymphocytes from unaffected siblings as well as from AT patients — accumulation of sufficient data should reveal a simple Mendelian inheritance of the mutated gene. Paterson et al.[228] monitored CFA and repair replication of AT fibroblasts after hypoxic γ-irradiation. Of the seven heterozygous strains tested, five exhibited intermediate CFA values. Three of these were tested for postirradiation repair replication and again had intermediate responses. In contrast to the observations of Chen et al., these three strains exhibited normal sensitivity to oxic irradiation. Paterson et al. suggested that lymphoblasts may be inherently better than skin fibroblasts for quantitating radiosensitivity of AT heterozygotes. In view of the immunologic abnormalities and preponderance of lymphoreticular cancer in AT patients, I agree.

Swift and colleagues conducted painstaking epidemiologic studies of AT families, without benefit of a definitive test for heterozygosity. From a study of 1,639 members of 27 families, Swift et al.[229] estimated that AT heterozygotes under age 45 had a fivefold greater chance than normal of dying from a malignant neoplasm. On this basis, Swift[109] estimated that over 5% of all persons dying from cancer before age 45 may carry the AT gene. Daly and Swift[230] have expanded the earlier work and presented an informative discussion of epidemiologic factors related to cancer in AT families.

Immunologic Aspects of AT. This topic has been discussed by J.C. Vance in Chapter 7 of this book; a few comments from a biochemist's veiwpoint will be presented here. Clinical and histologic aspects of AT were reviewed by Boder;[231] Biggar and Good[232] discussed immunodeficiencies. Weichselbaum and Little[127] presented the interesting concept that a nonimmunologic defect, faulty base repair, may be responsible for the slightly increased incidence of solid tumors in AT patients and the occurrence of solid tumors in heterozygotes. Swift's observation that heterozygotes under age 45 are at increased risk for cancer may indicate that slightly defective base repair may shorten the induction time for action of environmental carcinogens.

The therapeutic effectiveness of human lymphocyte dialysate (transfer factor) has been evaluated for a number of immunologic disorders. Treatment of four AT patients with transfer factor (weekly for two months) produced some enhancement of immunologic parameters, but no definite clinical improvement.[233] One wonders if transfer factor would provide anything other than palliative relief for patients with hereditary disorders.

An interesting aspect of AT is that patients often exhibit hyperglycemia and insulin resistance. Bar et al.[234] observed an 80–85% decrease in receptor affinity for insulin of monocytes from two AT patients. In contrast, normal affinities were observed for the patients' cultured fibroblasts, and for monocytes and fibroblasts from the parents and an unaffected sibling. Preincubation of human lymphocytes with an immunoglobulin-enriched fraction of patient plasma caused reduced insulin affinity. Thus, AT patients appear to have a circulating factor which alters the properties of insulin receptors on cell membranes.

Serum α-fetoprotein (AFP) levels are greatly elevated in patients with AT;[235,236] unfortunately, presumed heterozygotes have normal values rather than intermediate ones. It would be worth screening all available blood specimens of AT patients and their siblings by immunofluorescence, as reported by Keller et al.[237] for members of cancer-prone families. All subjects had normal AFP levels, but 43% of the blood specimens exhibited surface-bound antigen on the monocytes. Blood from cancer patients without a family history of cancer did not have positive-staining monocytes. It is likely that surface-bound AFP occurs on monocytes of AT patients and perhaps on those of heterozygotes. If the latter were true, immunofluorescence would provide a rapid, convenient test for heterozygosity.

Fanconi Anemia

Fanconi anemia (FA) is characterized by congenital abnormalities, aplastic anemia, chromatid-type aberrations, chromosome rearrangements, and high incidence of leukemia and other neoplasms. Neoplasia is not a major cause of death in FA patients because of their shortened life span, but it may be a significant factor in heterozygotes. Current evidence, however, indicates that if heterozygotes are at increased risk for a specific cancer type, it may be such a rare tumor that a very large number of relatives would have to be studied to detect the increase.[238] Although the mode of inheritance is thought to be autosomal recessive, reports of a high ratio of affected to unaffected siblings suggest caution. Clinical, cytogenetic, and biochemical heterogeneity indicate that complementation groups may exist. A new type of FA variant occurring in black sisters has been reported.[239]

Biochemical Studies. Fibroblasts from FA patients have been reported to have normal activity of apurinic endonuclease,[240] normal excision repair of UV-induced dimers,[241] and additive repair of damage from saturating doses of UVR and AAAF.[225] Although impaired removal of γ-induced thymine glycol has been reported,[221] the major area of biochemical interest appears to be repair of DNA cross-links. Fujiwara and Tatsumi[242] pointed out that FA lymphocytes are highly susceptible to chromosomal breakage by cross-linking agents such as mitomycin C, PUVA, and nitrogen mustard. They observed that three FA fibroblasts lines were very sensitive to killing by mitomycin C and concluded that the most sensitive strain may be incapable of excising the first half of the cross-link. The differing degrees of repair deficiency in FA strains indicated that complementation groups may exist. Fornace et al.[243] observed that fibroblasts from a patient with FA had normal DNA repair and cell survival after treatment with mitomycin C, suggesting this patient may belong to another complementation group. Hirsch-Kauffmann et al.[244] studied various steps in repair of UV-induced DNA damage in lymphocytes and fibroblasts from an FA patient and the heterozygous mother. Fibroblasts exhibited normal activities for endonuclease incision, repair synthesis, and exonuclease removal of photoproducts. However, the patient's lymphocytes exhibited low ligase activity, whereas heterozygous cells had intermediate activity.

The Heterozygous State. Auerbach and Wolman[245] have developed a test which clearly distinguishes lymphocytes of heterozygous FA persons from normal cells. The difunctional alkylating agent, diepoxybutane, does not affect chromosomes in normal cells but causes a fivefold increase in breakage in heterozygous cells.

Bloom's Syndrome

Bloom's syndrome (BS), an autosomal recessive disorder, involves stunted growth, sun sensitivity, and high frequency of chromosomal aberrations. The latter include a tenfold elevation of sister chromatid exchanges (SCEs) and characteristic elevated numbers of quadriradials. The Bloom's Syndrome Registry, established by German, has accumulated records of 71 patients from the first description of the disease in 1954 through the end of 1976.[246] The objective of this continuing project is surveillance of patients and heterozygotes for cancer.

Biochemical Studies. As noted by German,[211] defective DNA repair has not been demonstrated in BS, and consequently many negative studies have not been published. Normal extent and rate of repair of SSBs induced by x-rays have been reported,[247] as have normal responses to UVR and/or AAAF.[225] Selsky et al.[248] reported that one of three fibroblast strains exhibited decreased HCR of UV-irradiated herpes simplex virus; the cells themselves did not have increased sensitivity to UVR. Caffeine did not affect HCR post-UV survival of the three cell lines. Because of the lack of evidence for defective DNA repair in BS cells, German[211] proposed a new class of disorders in which DNA repair mechanisms are intact, but cellular factors cause increased DNA damage. He outlined several scenarios: (1) in normal cells, low levels of environmental agents and cellular factors cause some DNA damage which may be efficiently repaired, or misrepaired to create some mutations; (2) excessive exposure of normal cells to environmental agents overwhelms the repair systems, leading to mutations; (3) excessive cellular factors in a diseased cell (such as BS) overwhelm the repair systems. In the same publication, Tice et al.[249,250] presented experimental evidence that BS cells may indeed produce an agent or agents that damage DNA. When fibroblasts from a BS patient and a control were cocultivated, the SCEs were significantly elevated in control cells but not in the BS fibroblasts. This suggests that the latter cells secreted a DNA-damaging agent whose action on DNA of control cells was detected via the sensitive SCE detection system. However, Schonberg and German[251] were unable to reproduce these results, and Rudiger and colleagues[252] observed that BS cells cocultivated with normal cells had reduced SCEs, suggesting the latter provided a diffusible factor missing in the former.

Cockayne's Syndrome

Cockayne's syndrome (CS) is transmitted in an autosomal recessive manner, and exhibits arrested growth and extreme sun sensitivity. Although CS is not associated with increased risk of cancer, it is of interest because of its occurrence in the single member of XP complementation group B.

Biochemical Studies. Wade and Chu[253] examined CFA of ten CS strains and strains from four parents, after treatment with physical and chemical agents. The CS strains exhibited increased sensitivity to UVR, 4-NQO, and AAAF (inducers of long-patch repair), but not to x-rays, ethyl methanesulfonate, or acridine mustard (short-patch repair). Heterozygous cells had intermediate sensitivity to UVR, and caffeine did not decrease the post-UV CFA of CS cells. Andrews et al.[163] reported that nine CS strains had normal post-UV UDS but decreased CFA. Extrapolation of the survival curves (Figure 1 to Figure 4) of their report describing CFA of XP cells[136] showed that the range of UV sensitivity of CS cells was below that of control and XP variant cells, and overlapped the high portion of the XP-C region. Thus, although patients with CS are very sun sensitive, their fibroblasts exhibit only moderate sensitivity to UVR. The survival curve for XP-B cells was not presented, but Robbins et al.[140] reported that preliminary experiments indicated this curve may be intermediate between those of groups C and D strains. The implications for post-UV CFA and neurological abnormalities in the XP-B patient have been discussed (see "Xeroderma Pigmentosum: Colony Forming Ability").

There have been conflicting reports about post-UV DNA repair in CS cells. Schmickel et al.[254] reported they were unable to demonstrate a consistent defect in repair synthesis in CS cells in which replication synthesis was blocked. Irradiated cells from two patients with CS exhibited normal pyrimidine dimer removal.

Does the XP-B Patient Represent a Distinct Complementation Group? It is curious that although this patient's fibroblasts are one of the first strains to be assigned a complementation group by the discoverers,[255] no additional XP-B strains have been identified. The coexistence of CS suggests that one should carefully consider whether this patient truly represents a distinct complementation group. This point was anticipated by Takebe et al.[256] and by Friedberg.[257] The question to be asked is, Can the combined effects of the XP and CS genes account for very low post-UV UDS and ability to complement classical groups A and C-G? On the basis of available information, the answer is perhaps. If any reader has information, pro or con, concerning the validity of the following comments, I would appreciate receiving it.

One might consider that XP-B cells are actually XP variant whose DNA repair characteristics are altered by interaction of the unidentified repair defect resulting from the CS gene. Two specific repair properties[116] which are not characteristic of variant cells require explanation: (1) very low UDS (3-7%); and (2) intermediate, rather than low, PRR. I have no explanation for the low UDS of XP-B cells except to remind the reader that reduced ^{3}H-TdR incorporation does not identify the step involved in defective excision repair. Consequently, in an XP cell carrying the repair defect resulting from the CS gene, reduced UDS may have a different connotation than it does for XP groups A and C–G. Cleaver's definition of PRR (see "Methodology for Measuring DNA Damage and Repair: Redefinition of Postreplication Repair," earlier in this chapter) might explain why XP-B cells exhibit intermediate (rather than low) PRR. The reduced rate of DNA replication in UV-irradiated cells (normal or XP) probably results from the prevention of replicon initiation by strand breaks produced during excision repair. Consequently, changes in DNA synthesis in classical and variant cells may be considered secondary results of interactions between replication and repair, rather than primary defects in PRR. Whatever the interaction that results in low PRR in XP variant cells (which have normal excision repair), one might expect that if excision repair were greatly reduced (e.g., via influence of the CS gene in XP-B cells), the observed PRR would be higher than normally exhibited by variant cells. In other words, fewer strand breaks than normal would be produced, allowing initiation of a larger number of replicons. Even though perhaps operating at a reduced rate, the greater number of replicons could reflect higher PRR than is observed for XP variant cells with normal excision repair.

In view of the above comments, fusion of XP-B and CS cells would be enlightening. Unfortunately, apparently only one study with XP cells has been reported.[258] In that investigation, CS cells complemented XP strain A (M.H. Wade, personal communication). Fusion of XP-B and XP variant cells might be of interest in a reverse sense — would an XP-B nucleus in a heterodikaryon inhibit UDS in the variant nucleus?

Why Aren't Patients with CS at Increased Risk for Skin Cancer? This question is posed in order to clarify an important semantic distinction which may be overlooked by molecular biologists. In a genodermatosis such as XP, *sun sensitivity* often denotes increased incidence of cutaneous carcinoma; in that context, all XP patients are sun sensitive. To a clinical dermatologist, the phrase means photosensitivity, i.e., increased photoresponse leading to damage and death of epidermal cells. In fact, photosensitive individuals may have *decreased* incidence of skin cancer. (To my knowledge this has not been investigated.) These persons practice lifelong avoidance of the sun, and the effect of sunlight on their epidermal cells is to kill, rather than transform, them. Patients with CS have photo-dermatitis at an early age, which becomes less severe with time.[259] Thus, they are photosensitive and may not have a cellular defect in DNA repair at all. The coexistence of CS in the XP-B patient is naturally of interest, but the somewhat reduced post-UV CFA of CS cells is not impressive for several reasons: (1) the experiments were conducted with fibroblasts; (2) the survival curves fall in the upper region of XP-C cells, whose donors may or may not be photosensitive; (3) the cells were irradiated with UVR at 254 nm.

Familial Cutaneous Malignant Melanoma

Present knowledge about the hereditary disorder, familial cutaneous malignant melanoma (CMM), has been reviewed and updated by Lynch et al. in a current report.[260] They reported that family members exhibited the usual characteristics of hereditary cancer, i.e., very early onset of tumors which were often multiple. Unexposed areas of skin were often the sites of CMM, to a greater extent than occurs in nonhereditary melanoma. The authors suggested that prolonged survival may be a feature of familial CMM; their original patient with FAMMM syndrome has now had nine separate CMMs over an interval of 18 years. Familial CMM will not be discussed in detail in this section. Rather, mechanisms of control of melanocyte proliferation and the interrelationships of melanoma, halo nevi, and vitiligo will be examined. The occurrence of CMM in patients with XP is, strictly speaking, a secondary consequence of the sensitivity of XP epidermis to UVR and, therefore, is not truly familial melanoma. However, the spontaneous regression of metastatic malignant melanoma in XP patients is of interest in the context of Burnet's elegant hypothesis linking intrinsic mutagenesis to the pathogenesis of XP. For information about the processes involved in cancer metastasis, the reader is referred to a current thorough review by Poste and Fidler.[261] The authors made the point that whether a tumor arises from a single cell or multiple cells, by the time it reaches a size that is clinically detectable, it contains subpopulations with a wide range of metastatic capability. This concept bears directly on development of amelanotic melanomas.

Control of Melanocyte Proliferation. Fortunately, it appears that immunologic and nonimmunologic processes act in concert to exert rigorous control of growth of melanocytic tumors. Otherwise, CMMs might be as common as cutaneous carcinomas. Lerner pointed out some time ago that quinoidal melanin precursors are cytotoxic to melanocytes and thus constitute an intracellular self-destruct system, should uncontrolled proliferation begin. Alternatively, melanomas are highly antigenic and often trigger a cytotoxic immune response in the host. Immunologic destruction of melanoma cells, in turn, releases metabolites which are toxic to neighboring cells. Halo nevi are considered benign melanocyte proliferative units which are undergoing regression. The cytotoxic processes causing regression of a nevus also affect neighboring melanocytes, thus producing a non-pigmented halo around the resolving lesion. Halos are also noted around some regressing CMMs, and the rejection processes involved may be severe enough to cause general destruction of melanocytes, resulting in vitiligo in other skin areas. Vitiligo itself may be the result of an autoimmune process.[262-264] These and other considerations led Lerner and Nordlund[265] to suggest that perhaps vitiligo should be induced in patients after removal of a primary CMM, to prevent recurrence and/or metastasis. Presumably, one would stimulate the patient's immune response to melanocytes to the extent that vitiligo developed, and in this condition of increased surveillance, aberrant melanocytes would be quickly destroyed. Experimental verification of this concept was recently presented by Chavin et al.[266] They reported that subcutaneous administration of hydroquinone (a selective toxin for melanocytes) to mice decreased the number of "takes" of transplanted melanoma and increased the survival time of the animals.

Cooke et al.[267] described a melanoma-specific protein (MSP) which provides a unifying basis for abnormal melanocyte metabolism. This protein is excreted in the urine of individuals with malignant melanoma, actively developing halo nevi, and very active vitiligo; it is not found in the urine of patients with malignancies other than melanoma. The authors suggest MSP is a marker of active immunologic destruction of nevus cells (presumably also of melanocytes and melanoma cells). In a related study, Bennett and Copeman[268] demonstrated by indirect immunofluorescence that sera of patients with halo nevus or malignant melanoma contain antibodies that bind to cytoplasmic components of both halo nevus and melanoma cells. Identical cytoplasmic staining patterns were obtained with the melanoma-specific antiserum employed to detect MSP. How can one relate a single gene product, the "non-self" MSP, to these three diverse melanocytic processes? The following comments are speculative, but perhaps will provide clues for future studies. The MSP is probably synthesized in undetectable amounts in normal melanocytes. Melanocytes are widely dispersed in an immunologically privileged site, the epidermis, which is separated from the circulation and lymphatics by a basement membrane. Consequently, synthesis and release of minute quantities of MSP do not trigger a host response. In familial vitiligo, a defective gene may cause melanocytes to synthesize and/or excrete sufficient MSP to initiate production of cytotoxic antibodies. Once initiated, the process is autocatalytic: antibodies destroy cells, releasing more MSP, triggering more antibody production, etc. A similar rationale would explain vitiligo caused by topical melanocyte-damaging agents. Mutations leading to halo nevus and melanoma do not affect MSP directly. However, cellular components are produced in excess in proliferating tissue, and dying cells release products which eventually reach the circulation. (Since MSP is excreted in the urine, it obviously enters the circulation.) The MSP, then, may be the key element in host surveillance for melanoma.

Sober et al.[269] addressed the interesting question of amelanotic melanoma. It is their impression that an amelanotic tumor arises in a small area of a pigmented primary lesion and that subsequent metastases are amelanotic. This concept may be expanded. Cutaneous melanomas often present as a multihued mass, with areas ranging in color from pale pink to black. This is suggestive of a collection of melanoma clones under vigorous immunologic attack. According to the above concepts, immunologic destruction of melanoma cells releases toxic melanin precursors which would have a synergistic effect on neighboring cells. One would expect that melanoma cells under the duress of cytotoxic attack might be prone to misrepair of DNA, leading to mutation. If a cell mutated so that an early step in melanin synthesis became nonfunctional, it would have an immediate proliferative advantage over its neighbors. That is, it would still be under immunologic stress and the influence of extracellular melanin precursors, but it would not carry the extra burden of intracellularly produced toxins. One would therefore predict several alternative consequences of a vigorous host response to a CMM: (1) the tumor regresses completely; (2) most of the tumor regresses, leaving an amelanotic clone; (3) the tumor regresses, but metastasizes to a less hostile environment before total destruction. The third alternative explains the detection of metastatic melanoma with unknown primary. Kopf[270] suggested that examination of such a patient's skin with a Wood's lamp may reveal a lightly pigmented area which, on biopsy, exhibits dermal melanophages characteristic of a regressed primary CMM. The alternatives cited also dictate the predictions that amelanotic metastasis with unknown primary would not be uncommon, and amelanotic metastases would be more frequent than amelanotic primary CMM. Nathanson[271] described a patient with an actively regressing primary CMM who had several metastatic subcutaneous nodules that were diagnosed as amelanotic melanoma. Sober et al.[272] reported that amelanotic primary CMMs probably account for less than 5% of diagnosed cases, and that amelanotic metastases are much more frequent. Hinds and Kolonel[273] reported 333 cases of invasive CMM in residents of Hawaii from 1960 to 1977. Doctor Hinds kindly referred my inquiries to W. Rellahan, Ph.D., Administrator, Hawaii Tumor Registry. The latter informed me that of the 333 reported cases, nine (2.7%) were amelanotic. An interesting fact derived from this thorough computer-based study is that five of the nine amelanotic tumors developed melanotic metastases.

Lentigo maligna, a precancerous lesion of melanocytes, is often treated by excision. Reports of its recurrence as amelanotic lentigo maligna lend support to the previous comments. Su and Bradley[274] described a seven-year follow-up of a patient. After excision of her lentigo maligna, she had a foreign-body reaction to catgut sutures. Over the next seven years, the excision site gradually evolved into a hypopigmented, erythematous macule. Biopsy at the end of that period confirmed the presence of amelanotic lentigo maligna. The foreign-body reaction after surgery probably stimulated the host's immune response to the extent that abnormal melanocytes not removed by surgery were either killed or rendered incapable of unusual metabolic activity. Perhaps a few amelanotic cells survived the vigorous host defense and slowly developed into a lesion of amelanotic lentigo maligna. It is pertinent that a biopsy revealed a moderate inflammatory infiltrate in the upper dermis, suggestive of constant immunologic attack. A patient described by Burket[275] developed an erythematous macule of long duration at the site of removal of a pigmented compound nevus. Upon examination 13 years after surgery, two nodules in the center of the amelanotic lesion were detected. Shave biopsy of the more elevated nodule revealed amelanotic melanoma. It is of interest that the less elevated nodule, which was not biopsied, regressed within one week after the other nodule was shaved. Apparently, the biopsy procedure produced an inflammatory response which was sufficient to eliminate the lesser nodule.

An interesting analysis of cases of malignant melanoma (MM) with unknown primary was described by Baab and McBride.[276] Of 2,446 cases of histologically proven MM, 98 (4%) were of unknown primary. The male/female ratio was 71/27 (2.6/1), and 27 of the 98 (28%) had a family history of cancer. Surprisingly, only one of the 27 had a family history of melanoma.

The remarkable survival of Lynch's patient with FAMMM syndrome[260] merits discussion. This person's surveillance system for melanoma must be exceedingly high, perhaps as a consequence of the familial malignant melanoma gene. On nine separate occasions over an interval of 18 years, a CMM escaped the host's defense; yet with the aid of the surgeon, no adverse sequelae (metastasis or recurrence) ensued. The patient's urine should be examined for the presence of MSP. The levels of MSP in urines tested to date are so low that a qualitative fluorescence inhibition technique must be employed to detect it. The individual with FAMMM syndrome may be continuously rejecting aberrant melanocyte clones and thus may be a convenient source of MSP. Although this protein appears to be a cytoplasmic rather than a membrane antigen (therefore, possibly not cytotoxic), its concurrent association with vitiligo, halo nevus, and CMM renders it of interest. The patient's serum should also be examined for cytotoxic, melanoma-specific antibodies.

Spontaneous Regression of Metastatic Malignant Melanoma in Patients with XP.
Four cases have been reported. Lynch et al.[186] described spontaneous regression of metastatic MM in two siblings with XP. Ronchese[277] reported an unusual sequence of events occurring in a patient with XP. In 1942, numerous subcutaneous MMs "healed as if they were nonmalignant" after electrocoagulation; in 1956, a metastatic MM of the brain regressed after treatment with x-rays. Lastly, at the time of the report (1966), large melanotic freckles had been fading in

color for two or three years. Ronchese cited a Japanese report of a previous case of spontaneous regression of MM in a patient with XP.

Burnet[278] has been developing the concept of intrinsic mutagenesis for several years. Chu et al.[279] discussed theoretical and experimental aspects of theories proposed by Burnet and by others, and developed a unifying theory encompassing the major elements of several of them. Burnet proposed that intrinsic mutagenesis is a necessary prerequisite for survival and evolutionary advance of a species, and that such mutations occur because of the error proneness of key enzymes involved in the replication and repair of nucleic acids. Knudsen's[83] two-hit theory of carcinogenesis is consistent with increased cancer rate in hereditary disorders associated with cancer: the first event is genetic; the second, somatic. The precipitating event is therefore a somatic mutation, in accord with Burnet's hypothesis. I agree with Burnet's basic concepts, but am inclined to place different emphasis on some parts of his theory. The following concepts should therefore be interpreted as my understanding of his views, tempered with my background in skin metabolism.

A freckle is viewed as a self-limiting clone of mutant melanocytes, induced by sunlight. There is a wide range in tendency to freckle among humans: upon exposure to sunlight, some individuals develop a uniform tan without freckling; others sunburn easily and develop numerous freckles. Patients with XP represent the extreme: although they consciously avoid sunlight, they develop innumerable deeply pigmented, confluent freckles. Irradiation of skin results in an increase in the number of functioning melanocytes and increased melanin production in each melanocyte. These responses, along with the known ability of UVR to damage DNA, suggest that sunlight exposure triggers increased DNA repair and replication in melanocytes. In terms of fidelity of DNA synthesis without mutation, then, one can rank humans in the following order: non-frecklers are better than frecklers who, in turn, are much better than XP patients. Thus, the response of XP cells to environmental stress such as UVR (or to endogenous stress) is much more likely to create a mutation leading to carcinogenesis. It must be stressed that although XP cells exhibit reduced DNA repair, kinetic studies reveal the defect is in reduced rate of repair, rather than inability to repair. Also, as stressed by Burnet, in order for a malignant clone to develop, the initiating mutant must have undergone sufficient DNA repair to have physiologically functional template capacity. Thus, carcinogenesis may be viewed as the consequence of a nonlethal somatic mutation, and the increased induction of cancer in XP patients is the result of reduced fidelity of DNA synthesis and repair. As pointed out by Burnet, the experimental methods employed to date have provided much information about quantitative and kinetic aspects of DNA repair in XP cells, but little data are available concerning fidelity of repair.

Application of the above concepts to explain spontaneous regression of metastatic melanoma in XP patients seems straightforward. If the previous discussion of immunologic and nonimmunologic control of melanocyte prolifera-- tion is valid, then there is a relatively high probability that an XP melanoma cell will undergo another mutation which triggers antocatalytic processes that destroy the entire tumor mass. It is difficult to visualize how a single mutated melanoma cell can cause destruction of a tumor, except by invoking production of a "transforming factor" which adversely influences the metabolism of neighboring cells. The probability of such an event occurring is admittedly low, but much greater than that in a melanoma cell of a patient without XP. Thus, the presumed genetic flaw in XP (decreased fidelity of DNA synthesis) which causes increased incidence of CMM may improve the host's chance of coping with metastic tumors.

The spontaneous bleaching of large, deeply pigmented freckles of Ronchese's patient is intriguing; the author stated he had never seen or heard of such regression before. The response must be localized, since there was no indication of vitiligo. This patient was 48 years old at the time of the latest report in 1966 and had been closely followed for over 20 years.[277] When first seen at age 25 in 1943, she had a history of XP since age 2 and had been treated with UVR for a period of six years. (Our present knowledge, of course, precludes this type of therapy.) For ten years prior to 1943, her condition had progressively worsened. The 1966 report, and the earlier ones cited there, present a fascinating photographic record of progressive darkening and enlargement of melanotic freckles until some time after 1962, when numerous pigmented areas became markedly lighter or disappeared. Perhaps this phenomenon is not as unusual as it seems; perhaps the symptoms of XP lessen with time, if the patient lives long enough. With the present atmosphere of early detection of XP and rigorous avoidance of UVR, many patients will attain the age of Ronchese's patient. Clinicians treating individuals with XP should periodically photograph skin areas of interest to provide documentation if freckles begin to fade. Biochemical studies of cells in a regressing freckle may provide valuable information concerning cellular transformation and differentiation.

Comment. Perhaps the speculative concepts of this and the preceding section will stimulate productive cogitation by the reader. There may be an important clue in the spontaneous bleaching of freckles in an older XP patient; the more knowledgeable reader may be able to interpret this phenomenon constructively.

Psoriasis

Psoriasis, a multifactorial[280] hereditary disorder, is characterized by nonmalignant epidermal hyperplasia. Since aberrant cells never invade the dermis, psoriatic lesions develop into thickened epidermal plaques. Psoriasis often occurs at flexion points (knees and elbows) and on the eyelids. This is consistent with observations that mechanical stretching of skin causes epidermal hyperplasia.[281]

The Koebner phenomenon occurs in patients with psoriasis: physical trauma of a skin area induces epidermal proliferation and development of a psoriatic lesion. Although a few biochemical abnormalities have been reported, uninvolved epidermis of psoriatics is very similar to that of persons without skin disease. Psoriasis appears to be the ideal human model for the study of cellular proliferation: epidermal slices are easy to collect, the uninvolved epidermis of an experimental subject affords a suitable control, and scratching will elicit new lesions.

The introduction of PUVA therapy constitutes an extensive human experiment in control of cellular proliferation and should receive exhaustive biochemical investigation. A fascinating aspect of PUVA is that it turns off epidermal cells, but turns on melanocytes; patients quickly acquire a deep natural tan on uninvolved epidermis. A unique marker for increased melanocyte metabolism, urinary 5-S-cysteinyldopa, is elevated within two days after start of PUVA therapy, before increased pigmentation is apparent.[282]

Fine et al.[283] reported a possible link between psoriasis and cancer. A glycoprotein, EDC1, is present in high concentrations in plasma and urine of patients with seven different types of metastatic cancer, and is not detectable in body fluids of normal humans. Of 24 untreated psoriatics, 55% of urine specimens and 75% of plasma samples were positive for EDC1 by radioimmunoassay. Plasma and urine levels of the "tumor marker" were directly correlated with disease severity. It has not been resolved whether EDC1 is the result of cellular proliferation or the cause of it.

Psoriasis may also be linked to melanocyte metabolism, although the association may be indirect. De Moragas and Winkelmann[284] described two patients with psoriasis and concurrent vitiligo; the psoriatic lesions were strictly confined to vitiliginous areas. The presence of vitiligo did not interfere with therapy; the Goeckerman treatment (coal tar and UV irradiation; see below) readily cleared the lesions. Because areas of vitiligo contain no protective melanin, it was suggested that UVR exerted the paradoxical effect of eliciting psoriasis via a Koebner reaction. Vitiligo itself has been elicited by a Koebner response to scratching.[285] Chapmen[286] reported a case of coexistence of psoriasis and vitiligo in which the psoriatic lesions were not confined to depigmented areas. In fact, some lesions included both pigmented and vitiliginous epidermis. Although psoriasis is the most thoroughly studied skin disorder, the literature contains few references to melanocyte metabolism in psoriatic lesions. A number of reports described PUVA-induced changes in psoriatic and uninvolved epidermis. Presumably, lack of comments about melanocytes in lesions before therapy indicates the cells exhibit no unusual features.

Hereditary Resistance to Cancer. For many years, Lynch et al.[287,288] have been encouraging investigators to look for negative associations of hereditary disorders and cancer. If negative association exists, a likely candidate is psoriasis (at least for reduced incidence of skin cancer). It has been repeatedly noted in print that although the skin of many psoriatics has been subjected to chronic insults of therapeutic regimens, patients do not have an increased incidence of skin cancer. For example, the Goeckerman treatment has been widely used for several decades. It involves repeated application of crude coal tar, followed by exposure to UV-B, over an interval of several weeks. Yet, despite the presence of numerous aromatic hydrocarbons in coal tar and the cocarcinogenic action of UV-B, it is universally accepted that the treatment does not cause skin cancer. (However, see discussion of the report by Stern et al.[289] below.)

The above observation, and the report that psoriatics in Australia have a greatly reduced incidence of solar keratoses, led Shuster and colleagues to a hypothesis explaining the resistance of psoriatic skin to the effects of polycyclic aromatic hydrocarbons.[290,291] These carcinogen precursors require metabolic activation by aryl hydrocarbon hydroxylase (AHH), an inducible enzyme present in many tissues including epidermis. The authors observed that baseline activity of AHH in explants of psoriatic epidermis was 54% that of normal tissue and was not significantly induced by benzathracene, whereas activity in normal epidermis was induced twofold. The implications for reduced induction of skin cancer in psoriatics are obvious, but a more general phenomenon may be operative:[290] the fact that uninvolved epidermis of psoriatics had intermediate AHH baseline activity and inducibility suggests the enzyme defect may be present in other tissues. This raises the possibility that psoriatics may have a decreased incidence of noncutaneous cancer. For example, if AHH is involved in induction of lung cancer, psoriatic smokers may be less prone to develop such tumors. It is significant that Guirgis et al.[292] observed that benz(a)pyrene-induced AHH activity of lymphocytes from patients with lung cancer was elevated. Shuster et al. suggested that the ancestral psoriasis gene may have persisted because of the selective advantage afforded by resistance to cancer.

Jacobs et al. have initiated a long overdue epidemiological study of the incidence of cancer in psoriatics. In a preliminary retrospective study[293] they encountered one basal cell carcinoma in 100 psoriatics, whereas a nonpsoriatic control group had five BCCs, one SqCC, and one Bowen's disease (intraepidermal SqCC). Since then, the study has been expanded to a larger patient sample. The low incidence of carcinoma and the preponderance of BCC over SqCC (as is observed in nonpsoriatics) are still evident (P.H. Jacobs, personal communication). Stern et al.[26] reported the incidence of skin tumors in 1,182 psoriatics before PUVA therapy. They also observed a high proportion of BCCs (70%), but reported the relative rate to be similar to that of the general population. However, there may be unrecognized bias in the patient sample; those accepted for PUVA often have severe psoriasis and have been unsuccessfully treated with a number of drastic regimens. In a current report, Stern et al.[289] reported that patients treated with high doses of tar and/or UV-B had an increased relative rate of cutaneous carcinoma, before receiving PUVA therapy. Thus, it appears that the tendency to somewhat lower risk of skin cancer in psoriatics may be overcome by vigorous therapy.

Cutaneous Carcinoma after PUVA Therapy. Stern et al.[26] reported the initial results of a 16-center project to monitor the occurrence of cutaneous carcinoma in psoriatics after PUVA therapy. Several important observations have already been made in this two-year prospective study; those germane to the present subject will be noted. (1) Patients with a prior risk factor for skin cancer (treatment with ionizing radiation or previous cutaneous carcinoma) had a higher than expected incidence of SqCC after PUVA treatment. (2) The normal BCC/SqCC ratio of three was reversed to less than one. (3) Of the 48 carcinomas, 30 occurred more than one year after start of treatment, and in that interval, SqCCs outnumbered BCCs four to one (24 vs 6). Halprin[294] presented arguments that the study of Stern et al., and their interpretation of their data, were in error. His citing of anecdotal data, and his failure to estimate the size of the at-risk population he obtained them from, were adequately rebutted by Stern et al.[295] However, one argument requires comment. Halprin stated that since the induction period for cancer in humans is 20 years or more, it "test one's scientific incredulity" to suggest that PUVA treatment could induce cancer within two years. He overlooked the facts that cells may exhibit dose-rate responses to irradiation and that the UV-A doses employed in PUVA are enormous. In terms of the short induction period of SqCC, one might visualize the following scenario. A keratinocyte in a psoriatic lesion is transformed before or during PUVA therapy, but initially has little or no proliferative advantage over the rapidly growing psoriatic tissue. As the lesion regresses, the tumor clone attains a growth advantage. Depending on the balance between rates of cell division and death, the clone will grow to a clinically detectable tumor in some unpredictable length of time. There is no a priori reason to believe this interval must be 20 years or more, and the ethics of experimentation with humans forbid a controlled assessment of the induction period. Consequently, it is imperative that Stern and colleagues determine whether post-PUVA SqCCs are indeed occurring at sites of former psoriatic lesions. Since many patients accepted for PUVA therapy have involvement of 30% of their body or more, the spurt of SqCCs appearing after one year of start of treatment may represent survival of transformed clones which would have been controlled if the lesions had not been cleared (see the following section: "Why is the Incidence of Cutaneous Carcinoma Reduced in Psoriatics?").

In my opinion, Stern and his colleagues are conducting their prospective study of PUVA-treated patients in a thoroughly scientific manner. They stressed the need for careful risk/benefit analysis for each psoriatic before conducting therapy, and pointed out that continued monitoring of their large treatment sample will provide quantitative information concerning PUVA doses and increased risk of cancer in patients with different skin types. As noted above, they might also consider addressing another important question, are the post-PUVA SqCCs appearing in previously uninvolved skin or in sites of former lesions? My guess is the latter. Ideally, the extent and distribution of a patient's lesions should be recorded or photographed before therapy. Testimony of patients already in the study is not ideal but would provide corroborative information.

Before leaving this subject, one should consider a potentially important aspect of PUVA therapy which has been overlooked to date. Induction of cutaneous carcinomas entails some morbidity, but these tumors are usually not life threatening, especially if the patient is under close surveillance for their early detection. However, PUVA stimulation of melanocyte metabolism raises the specter of CMM. This has been my concern since the PUVA regimen was first announced but, upon reflection, there may be room for some optimism. When a patient is subjected to multiple PUVA treatments, his uninvolved skin quickly acquires a deep, natural tan; psoriatic lesions do not become pigmented until they are nearly resolved. Since melanin absorbs broadly through the UV region and into the visible,[16] uninvolved skin quickly acquires protection, not only from PUVA but from sunlight. When a patient's lesions have cleared, he is placed on a reduced PUVA schedule to prevent recurrence. Thus, if a uniform deep tan is maintained, the patient will continue to have yearlong protection from the carcinogenic action of sunlight. It is encouraging that only one CMM has appeared in PUVA-treated patients during the four-year interval that SqCCs have been detected (R.S. Stern, personal communication).

The above considerations are reassuring, but only time will provide a measure of the incidence of post-PUVA cutaneous malignant melanoma. In an electron microscopic study, Zelickson et al.[296] observed melanocyte proliferation, ultrastructural changes, and invasion of the dermis by melanocytes during PUVA therapy. Extension of melanocytes into the dermis was observed 6 months after cessation of therapy, and abnormal structural features were still present after 15 months.

After this section was written, I became aware of a current report by Bridges and Strauss[297] who suggest that PUVA may act as a tumor promotor by compromising the patient's immune response. They based their concept on reports that PUVA induces tumor susceptibility in mice (see "Biological Effects of Ultraviolet Radiation: Effect of Ultraviolet Radiation on Host Resistance to Cancer") and causes rapid appearance of cutaneous carcinomas in XP patients (see "Xeroderma Pigmentosum: Cumulative Actinic Damage — Implications for Black Patients with XP"). The reader may wish to study this report in detail, but a couple of points require clarification. Firstly, action of PUVA as a suppressor of immune response could act in concert with the mechanisms outlined above. If the former predominated, one might expect post-PUVA SqCCs in psoriatics to appear mainly in the skin areas that had never been sites of lesions. If both immune and nonimmune effects are important, SqCCs might be distributed more uniformly. An important point must be made about the use of psoralens and natural exposure to sunlight vs PUVA. The latter usually involves whole-body exposure in a light box containing lamps which emit an extremely high dose of UV-A. It is impossible to obtain a UV-A dose from sunlight equivalent to that of PUVA; the UV-B solar component would produce a severe burn long before significant UV-A exposure was attained. Patients with XP have never been treated with PUVA and never will; by the time PUVA was developed, we were well aware of the sensitivity of XP skin to carcinogenic radiations. Oral and topical psoralens, plus exposure to sunlight, have been employed (cosmetically and therapeutically) for several decades to produce a natural tan in human skin. There is no evidence that these mild treatments induce carcinomas in normal human skin. Consequently, the exaggerated tumorigenic response of XP patients to psoralen and low-dose UV-A is not analogous to the response of psoriatic skin to PUVA. In fact, psoralen and sunlight may very well act as a tumor promotor in XP patients; their exposed skin contains numerous precancerous lesions, ready to develop into malignant tumors.

Why is the Incidence of Cutaneous Carcinoma Reduced in Psoriatics? This question is posed in a positive sense, because the ongoing studies of Jacobs and colleagues support this position. One may propose several reasons why a transformed clone would have a poor chance of survival in a psoriatic lesion. (1) It has no growth advantage over the surrounding psoriatic tissue. (2) Population pressure of underlying psoriatic cells would rapidly push a squamous clone away from its nutrient supply (the dermis), to eventual death and incorporation into the psoriatic plaque. (3) Initiation of a malignant clone in uninvolved epidermis could trigger a Koebner response. This concept is not new; Burgener[298] proposed it in 1939. (4) Psoriatic plaques on extensive areas of skin will shield dividing epidermal cells from UVR.

To better understand carcinoma in psoriasis, one should address the question of the ratio of BCC to SqCC. Why do BCCs predominate in humans? To answer this question requires knowledge about the nature of induction and growth of BCCs and SqCCs. Since such information is scanty, there is room for speculation and development of rational scenarios. One may begin by pointing out that the terminology is operational: the cells in a BCC look like basal cells, and SqCCs look like keratinizing squamous tissue. In considering the probability of induction of epidermal cancer by an exogenous agent such as UVR, it seems likely that the dividing basal cells are far more apt to undergo mutation than keratinocytes. If a basal cell underwent a heritable mutation that prevented it from entering the differentiation pathway, that cell and its progeny would remain in the mitotic cycle, and the clone would consequently gain a proliferative advantage over neighboring basal cells. Thus, a BCC arises. Induction of a SqCC may be viewed as a multistep process. The initial event is again mutation of a basal cell to yield a slight proliferative advantage by some unstated mechanism. The progeny of this mutated cell would be capable of differentiating and migrating to the skin surface, but would retain some capacity to divide. The cells remaining in the basal layer, because of a slightly higher than normal proliferation rate, would spread out and replace normal basal cells. The result, after an appropriate growth period, would be a clone of abnormal cells distributed in a cone-shaped volume, with the base at the basal layer and the apex at the skin surface. This clone of cells will constitute the familiar skin lesion, actinic keratosis (see Pinkus, reference 299, for a lucid discussion of this and other processes involved in the induction of skin cancer). A keratotic cell would then require a second hit to develop into an invasive SqCC. Since these cells divide infrequently, the probability of a second hit will be low. An important aspect of this model is that the partially differentiated keratotic cell has migratory capability (keratinocytes migrate to the skin surface by both active and passive processes). Consequently, when a second mutation imparts an additional growth advantage, the transformed cell and its progeny will invade the dermis and even metastasize. Other types of SqCC may require somewhat different induction mechanisms. These can be accommodated with the concept that for some interval after a basal cell enters the differentiation pathway, the process is reversible (e.g., after wounding, suprabasal keratinocytes near the wound edge may undergo mitosis). The interested reader is referred to a report by Bullough[300] for a thorough discussion of cell cycle kinetics and epidermal homeostasis.

The simplistic models outlined above provide no new information, but may be helpful in understanding several observations:

1. The ratio of occurrence of BCC to SqCC is three or more. Since induction of a BCC requires a single hit in a population of dividing cells, such an event will occur relatively frequently. The first step in development of a SqCC may occur with equal probability, but will produce a precancerous clone which requires a second low-probability event for malignant transformation.
2. The induction period for human skin cancer is generally considered to be 20 years or more. The growth of BCCs is often very slow. Even though a large proportion of tumor cells are capable of dividing, cell death apparently nearly equals cell production. Thus, a transformed basal cell may require a period of years to grow to a clinically detectable BCC. On the other hand, a mutated basal cell and its progeny may exist for a long time as a precancerous lesion before a second hit induces a SqCC.
3. Low doses of UVR may produce BCC, whereas high doses are required for SqCC.[301] Vitaliano and Urbach[302] studied the relative importance of

risk factors in cutaneous carcinoma. For BCC, ability to tan was more important than age; the converse was true for SqCC. Their data suggested that increasing exposure to UVR has a greater effect on development of SqCC than on that of BCC. They cited a report to the effect that the BCC/SqCC ratio in northern cities (low UV exposure) is 10 to 1; whereas in southern rural areas (high exposure), it is 2 or 3 to 1. The proposed models for induction of BCC and SqCC suggest that low doses of UVR are sufficient to induce BCC and the first step for SqCC, and high doses increase the probability of occurrence of the second required event for induction of SqCC. Fleming et al.[303] reported that although skin cancer is rare in blacks, SqCCs were severalfold more frequent than BCCs. This observation is consistent with the conclusion by Vitaliano and Urbach that ability to tan is an important factor in preventing development of BCC. However, it must be noted that 61% of the SqCCs were in unexposed skin, indicating an etiologic factor other than UVR for blacks. It should be noted that the preceding comments relate to the differential carcinogenic effects of UV-B; Stern et al.[26] provided analogous information concerning UV-A (PUVA). The median number of PUVA treatments of psoriatics before development of the first tumor was significantly higher for SqCC than for BCC (96 treatments vs 25, respectively).

The above considerations may help to explain the reversal of the BCC/SqCC ratio in post-PUVA psoriatics. Instead of the single layer of dividing cells of normal epidermis, psoriatic tissue has two or three layers of dividing cells. Thus, the probability of an initial hit on a suprabasal cell is relatively high. Such a mutated cell will have little or no proliferative advantage over psoriatic keratinocytes, and at best may produce a local clone of cells which are eventually forced outward and incorporated into the psoriatic plaque. However, if a clone is viable during PUVA therapy, the combination of psoralen and high-dose UV-A will greatly increase the probability of a second event which leads to SqCC, and simultaneous resolution of the psoriatic lesion will improve the tumor's proliferative advantage. These considerations will not apply to the same degree to BCCs. Resolution of psoriatic plaques may render preexisting BCCs clinically apparent, but induction of new tumors by PUVA may not be noticeable for several years. The fact that SqCCs do not predominate over BCCs until one year after start of PUVA therapy provides an estimate of the actual induction time after the second event occurs in a precancerous clone.

If one accepts the premise that impaired ability to repair DNA increases the probability of carcinogenesis, the clinical histories of five XP patients (ages 5 to 29 years) may be pertinent.[197] By age 5, they all developed carcinomas which were mainly early SqCCs of the face. These patients had very few BCCs. In general, patients with XP develop so many tumors that clinicians may not give thought to the BCC/SqCC ratio. If this ratio is indeed reversed in XP patients, it would be consistent with the concept that defective DNA repair in altered keratinocytes renders them susceptible to UV carcinogenesis. On the other hand, the only reported tumors of the black patient of Hananian and Cleaver[204] and of the two Korean patients of Suh et al.[304] were BCCs. Bartholdson et al.[305] reported that two of their patients developed mainly BCCs. However, these persons were undergoing periodic treatment with 5-FU to remove actinic keratoses (possible precursors of SqCCs).

Do SqCCs occur in psoriatic lesions? Reports of such occurrences are rare.[306] The older literature is not helpful because ionizing radiation and inorganic arsenic, known carcinogens for skin and other tissues, were used to treat psoriasis. Lagerholm and Skog[306] reported the occurrence of "psoriasis cancer" in three patients. One patient had received arsenic; one had had grenz-ray treatment for ten years; the third had used a petrolatum base ointment which may have contained aromatic carcinogens. The authors concluded there was no evidence at that time (1968) for the existence of genuine psoriasis cancer. Perhaps some readers have knowledge of the occurrence of SqCCs in psoriatic lesions; if so, they are reportable. Of particular interest would be detection of such tumors in patients without prior treatment for psoriasis, with detailed histories to rule out undue prior exposure to environmental carcinogens. One might expect to find some SqCCs in mild psoriatic lesions of long duration.

Additional Comments. In a current abstract,[307] Roenigk and collaborators described the initial results of a multicenter study similar to that of Stern et al.[26] Four years after initiation of PUVA treatment of 690 patients, 10 had developed 13 skin carcinomas; 6 of these persons had had x-ray treatment. However, the ratio of BCC/SqCC (10/3) was not reversed in this study. In view of this new communication, foregoing comments about psoriasis, PUVA, and skin cancer must be viewed with the reservation that they may require revision as new information appears. To further complicate the picture, a current report[308] describes the occurrence of multiple BCCs in two patients after PUVA therapy.

Maddin and Wood[309] described the occurrence of multiple keratoacanthomas and SqCCs at psoriatic treatment sites of four patients. The patients had received treatment with tar and with grenz rays, and tumors appeared in areas of maximum involvement of psoriasis. Although there was no clinical or histologic evidence that the tumors actually occurred at sites of former psoriatic plaques, a couple of points are of interest: (1) one patient developed numerous keratoses, keratoacanthomas, and SqCCs, but no BCCs or MMs; (2) his tumors were so numerous that excision and grafting on both legs was required, and new tumors appeared on the graft sites.

Albinism

To properly examine the implications of albinism and skin cancer will require an exhaustive review of the literature to ferret out data concerning specific topics that have not been stressed to date. Rather than do this, I will present comments and questions related to subjects discussed in the two preceding sections, in hopes of encouraging readers to conduct their own inquiries. Much of the basic information presented is from a thorough review by Witkop et al.[310]

In contrast to vitiligo, which is characterized by absent or nonfunctional melanocytes, albino epidermis contains normal numbers of viable melanocytes; their only apparent biochemical flaw is a greatly reduced ability to produce fully developed packets of melanin (melanosomes). Total albinos may be assigned to one of two broad classes, tyrosinase positive or negative (ty-pos or ty-neg), depending on whether or not their hair bulbs synthesize melanin when incubated with tyrosine. Tyrosinase catalyzes the first steps in melanin synthesis, the hydroxylation of tyrosine to dihydroxyphenylalanine (dopa), and the oxidation of dopa to dopaquinone. Hair bulbs from ty-pos individuals exhibit normal tyrosinase activity and kinetic properties,[311] indicating the block in melanin synthesis is at some other step. One might ask the question, Since ty-neg individuals do not produce the intracellular quinones which may control melanocyte proliferation, are they more prone to develop CMM? One may also ask, Do albinos develop mostly amelanotic melanoma? Before addressing the latter question, one should consider the fact that ty-pos albinos develop freckles, whereas ty-neg persons apparently do not.[310] The freckles of ty-pos patients may be amenable to interpretation by Burnet's theory of intrinsic mutagenesis; their failure to develop in ty-neg persons may mean the mutation causing that disorder is not susceptible to back mutation. If the latter is true, all CMMs developing in ty-neg individuals must be amelanotic. If these persons do develop melanotic tumors, perhaps they constitute a unique human model for studying the relationship between melanin synthesis and induction of CMM.

Another question (and a possible answer) is, Why don't melanocytes in hair bulbs and the retina transform into MM?[310] Perhaps because they are shielded from UVR. The cornea and ocular lens of an albino provide as much photoprotection to the retina as do those of a normal individual; the hair bulb is located deep in the dermis.

Finally, why do ty-pos Cuna Indians develop many SqCCs and few BCCs?[312] Does this reversed BCC/SqCC ratio reflect an association between melanin synthesis and transformation of keratinocytes?

Neurofibromatosis

This autosomal disorder is characterized by abnormal growths of neural crest derivatives, resulting in multiple peripheral neurofibromas and tumors of the central nervous system. Malignant change may occur, and rapid, space-filling growth of neoplasms in critical body sites is also a hazard. Two basic forms of the disease have been proposed: (1) the peripheral or disseminated type (von Recklinghausen's disease), characterized by early onset and rapidly growing neurofibromas and intracranial tumors; (2) the central form, distinguished by later age of onset, mainly CNS involvement, and bilateral acoustic neuromas.

Nerve growth factor (NGF) has had a long and controversial history, and will not be discussed in detail. Yu et al.[313] have reviewed this topic. A puzzling feature of NGF is that, despite extensive investigation, its only known sources are the submaxillary gland of the adult male mouse and snake venom. Sensitive bioassays or radioisotope methods are required to detect NGF in other biological materials. Since radioassays are based on the purified beta subunit of mouse NGF, they detect moieties with structural features similar to that factor. On the other hand, bioassays detect NGF-like activity and provide no information concerning the structure of the component(s) eliciting the biologic response. These considerations may explain the difficulties encountered in attempting to assign a physiologic role for NGF in man or to elucidate possible relationships with disease states.

Schenkein et al.[314] used a bioassay to demonstrate increased nerve growth stimulating activity in sera of 19 of 24 patients with disseminated neurofibromatosis. They noted that the relationship of this activity to NGF remained to be determined. Siggers et al.[315] found no increased NGF in disseminated neurofibromatosis by radioimmunoassay, which suggests that the bioassay activity constitutes a different type of growth promotor. On the other hand, sera of patients with central neurofibromatosis had somewhat elevated immunoreactive NGF. A significant observation was that two of three family members below the usual age of onset of bilateral acoustic neuroma (the hallmark of central disease) had elevated serum NGF, whereas three members above the age of onset had normal levels. Fabricant et al.[316] reported increased competitive binding of sera from patients with disseminated disease, measured by radioreceptor assay, whereas sera of persons with the central form had low or normal binding activity. They also verified that patients with central neurofibromatosis had elevated immunoreactive NGF, as did some unaffected members of the kindreds. The authors suggested the latter could represent carriers of the central neurofibromatosis gene. It would be of interest to know how many of these individuals were young enough to still be at risk for development of the disease.

Comment. Measurement of immunoreactive NGF levels in sera of family members of patients with central neurofibromatosis may be of value in the prognosis for young members and in genetic counseling of persons of reproductive age. In this context, the factor may be a marker for the central neurofibromatosis gene, but is not directly associated with its phenotypic expression.

The state of knowledge concerning NGF and patients with disseminated neurofibromatosis is confusing, and perhaps detailed comment should be reserved until assays based on human NGF are established. One is confronted with the curious anomaly that sera of patients have increased NGF-like activity (via bioassay) that does not crossreact with antiserum to the beta unit of mouse NGF, yet competes with the same NGF unit for receptors on melanoma cells (the test cells in radioreceptor assay). Thus, three relevant components may be present: a growth factor different from mouse NGF, an immunoreactive NGF (patients have normal levels), and a material which binds to NGF receptors. The first and third components could be identical, an idea consistent with the concept that receptor binding capability implies functional activity. However, this relationship is not absolute; receptor sites can be blocked without eliciting a biologic response. In particular, since proinsulin and NGF exhibit amino acid homologies and structural similarities,[317] one wonders if the hormone is immunoreactive or binds NGF receptors. In fact, insulin and proinsulin have been reported to inhibit binding of NGF to target tissues.[318] Fabricant et al. purified serum samples by chromatography on Sephadex G-75; it is not clear if insulin or proinsulin would elute in the fraction tested for competitive binding activity. If one or both components do appear in the test fraction, two key questions must be addressed: (1) Do insulin and proinsulin crossreact with NGF antiserum? (2) What is the insulin/proinsulin status of patients with disseminated neurofibromatosis? It appears there are no reports relative to these questions. It may be pertinent that Gabbay et al.[319] reported a kindred with familial hyperproinsulinemia. Eighteen members of four generations had no symptoms of deranged glucose metabolism or other manifestations of serious disease.

EPILOGUE

As promised in the introduction, this report is wide ranging; hopefully, readers with a variety of backgrounds will find specific sections of interest. Because of the variety of topics covered, no attempt will be made to summarize the foregoing discussions. Instead, this section will be used to present ideas arising after the main body of the report was written and to provide new information.

The high doses of UV-A involved in PUVA therapy for psoriasis were mentioned repeatedly. It may be useful to indicate the magnitude of these doses. Depending on the patient's skin type (degree of pigmentation, tendency to burn) the starting dose may be 0.5 to 3.0 J/cm^2, two or three times per week.[320] Exposure is gradually increased to levels of 10 to 20 J/cm^2, and mean total doses to clear psoriatic lesions may range from 208 to 368 J/cm^2.[321] In terms of joules per square meter, these values are indeed enormous, but are tempered by the fact that the natural tan acquired during therapy shields the patient's skin from much of the incident radiation. To gain some perspective, the whole-body UV-A dose employed by Roberts et al.[31] to render mice susceptible to tumors was 65 J (see "Biological Effects of Ultraviolet Radiation: Effect of Ultraviolet Radiation on Host Resistance to Cancer").

Haseltine et al.[322] reported the presence of a DNA repair enzyme in *M. luteus* which requires revision of our current concepts of excision repair of pyrimidine dimers. This "pyrimidine dimer DNA glycosylase" catalyzes cleavage of the N-glycosidic bond of the 5' pyrimidine of a dimer, creating an apyrimidinic site which is susceptible to the action of an AP endonuclease. One of their control experiments may have broad application. When UV-irradiated DNA was subjected to the action of dimer DNA glycosylase, then to photomonomerization conditions, thymine was released. Depending on the specificity of the enzyme, this procedure may be useful in the study of UV induction of cytosine-thymine dimers (see "Xeroderma Pigmentosum: Nature of UV-induced Dimers").

In contrast to other cancer-linked genodermatoses, XP does not appear to be associated with internal cancers. As noted earlier, this lack of association may not be surprising because XP may not be a disorder of familial cancer: the skin tumors arising in persons with XP may simply reflect a consequence of an inherited inability to cope with UV-induced DNA damage. This view conflicts with the conventional outlook that since XP cells exhibit impaired ability to repair DNA damaged by chemical carcinogens, there should be an increased incidence of internal cancers as well as UV-induced skin neoplasms. Kraemer, after a thorough review of the literature, listed 12 cases of internal neoplasms in patients with XP.[323,324] He noted several problems in assessing the incidence of internal cancer in XP; the fact that many patients die at an early age is especially pertinent. An association of XP with internal cancer might be assumed from the epidemiological study of Swift and Chase,[194] who observed excess deaths from lung, stomach, and prostate cancers in relatives of XP patients. However, this relationship is tenuous, since there were no reported cases of such malignancies in XP homozygotes. Also, the excess deaths were not concentrated in families belonging to a specific classical XP group or to XP variant (M. Swift, personal communication). The pigmented xerodermoid family described by Hofmann et al.[139] is of special interest, because of late onset of cutaneous symptoms of XP and the presence of familial cancer. Three unaffected siblings of the proband and one affected brother died of internal carcinoma, as did the son of another affected brother. It is imperative that extensive pedigrees for other late onset cases of XP be obtained. If the association with familial cancer proves valid, one may conclude that although pigmented xerodermoid may be biochemically indistinguishable from XP variant, it represents a unique type of DNA repair disorder.

Earlier (see "Xeroderma Pigmentosum: Clinical Implications of XP in Blacks") it was noted that high levels of melanin in blacks with XP delay the onset of cutaneous symptoms and thereby preclude diagnosis until serious UV-induced damage has occurred. One may note two important corollaries (K.H. Kraemer, personal communication): (1) melanin affords considerable protection against UVR, but cannot compensate entirely for reduced DNA repair; (2) about half of the cases of XP in Caucasians have delayed onset of skin changes and, therefore, are diagnosed later in life.

Lastly, one might speculate about the possible significance of uracil-DNA glycosylase in DNA repair in XP cells (see "Xeroderma Pigmentosum: Is Defective DNA Repair Responsible for Carcinogenesis in XP?"). If XP lymphocytes had reduced levels or inducibility of the enzyme, it would be imperative to immediately test lymphocytes from heterozygotes. This analysis might finally yield the long-awaited, convenient test for heterozygosity in XP. While this report was in press, E.C. Friedberg informed me of two reports of uracil-DNA glycosylase activity in XP cells. Sekiguchi et al.[325] observed normal activity in XP-A cells, and Kuhnlein et al.[326] reported similar enzyme levels in fibroblasts belonging to groups A and D. The latter also observed that XP variant cells from two patients had about one-half normal activity, and fibroblasts from a mother of one of the patients had intermediate activity.

Acknowledgment. While responsibility for the accuracy of statements in this report is solely mine, I received much help from the following: J.E. Cleaver, E.C. Friedberg, P.H. Jacobs, K.H. Kraemer, R.S. Stern, M. Swift, J.E. Trosko, and M.H. Wade.

NOTES ADDED IN PROOF

A current report by Shiraishi et al.[327] provides important information about Bloom's Syndrome (see Other Genodermatoses Associated with Cancer). They observed that fusion of fresh lymphocytes from a patient with those of normal subjects or a BS heterozygote resulted in a normal frequency of sister chromatid exchanges (SCE) in BS nuclei. Normalization of SCE indices occurred after the first mitosis of fuzed cells. and the frequency of SCE in normal or BS heterozygote lymphocytes was not increased by fusion with BS cells.

Cohen et al.[328] recently described a study which helps allay the fear that PUVA therapy may stimulate melanocytes and thereby increase the probability of induction of melanoma (see Genodermatoses Associated with Cancer, Psoriasis). Cultured Cloudman murine melanoma cells or human fibroblasts were irradiated with UV-A in the presence of 4, 5', 8-trimethylpsoralen. In each instance, the cells were blocked in the G_2 phase of their cycle. The authors noted that melanin synthesis in Cloudman melanoma cells is stimulated by melanocyte stimulating hormone, and surface receptors for the hormone are present only in the G_2 phase. Thus, a mechanism is provided for stimulation of melanogenesis by PUVA without increased proliferation of melanocytes.

REFERENCES

1. Cleaver, J.E.: Defective repair replication of DNA in xeroderma pigmentosum. *Nature* 218:652–656, 1968.
2. de Weerd-Kastelein, E.A., Keijzer, W., and Bootsma, D.: Genetic heterogeneity of xeroderma pigmentosum demonstrated by somatic cell hybridization. *Nature* 238: 80–83, 1972.
3. Mulvihill, J.J., Miller, R.W., and Fraumeni, J.F., Jr. (Eds.): Genetics of human cancer, *Prog. Cancer Res. Ther.* 3, 1977.
4. Schimke, R.N.: *Genetics and Cancer in Man.* New York: Churchill Livingstone, 1978.
5. Evans, H.J., and Lloyd, D.C. (Eds.): *Mutagen-induced Chromosome Damage in Man.* Edinburgh: University Press, 1978.
6. Wolf, P.L. (Ed.): *Tumor Associated Markers.* New York: Masson, 1979.
7. Ruddon, R.W. (Ed.): *Biological Markers of Neoplasia: Basic and Applied Aspects.* New York: Elsevier, 1978.
8. Hanawalt, P.C., Friedberg, E.C., and Fox, C.F. (Eds.): *DNA Repair Mechanisms.* New York: Academic Press, 1978.
9. Symposium on Skin Carcinogenesis. *Bull. du Cancer* 65 (2, 3), 1978.
10. Helm, F.: *Cancer Dermatology.* Philadelphia, PA., Lea & Febiger, 1979.
11. International Conference on UV Carcinogenesis. *NCI Monog.* 50, 1978.
12. Seiji, M., and Bernstein, I.A. (Eds.): *Biochemistry of Cutaneous Differentiation.* Baltimore, MD: University Park Press, 1977.
13. Jarrett, A. (Ed.): *The Physiology and Pathophysiology of the Skin.* New York: Academic Press. Vol. 1: The Epidermis, 1973. Vol. 2: The Nerves and Blood Vessels, 1973. Vol. 3: The Dermis and the Dendrocytes, 1974. Vol. 4: The Hair Follicle, 1977. Vol. 5: The Sweat Glands, Skin Permeation, Lymphatics, Nails, 1978. Vol. 6: Mucous Membranes, in press, 1980.
14. Montagna, W., and Parakkal, P.F.: *The Structure and Function of Skin* (3rd ed.). New York: Academic Press, 1974.
15. Johnson, J.A., and Fusaro, R.M.: The role of the skin in carbohydrate metabolism. *Adv. Metab. Disorders* 6:1–55, 1972.
16. Kaidbey, K.H., Agin, P.P., Sayre, R.M., and Kligman, A.M.: Photoprotection by melanin – a comparison of black and Caucasian skin. *J. Am. Acad. Dermatol.* 1: 249–260, 1979.
17. Owens, D.W., and Knox, J.M.: Influence of heat, wind and humidity on ultraviolet radiation injury. *NCI Monog.* 50:161–167, 1978.
18. Sobell, H.M., Lozansky, E.D., and Lessen, M.: Structural and energetic considerations of wave propagation in DNA. *Cold Spring Harbor Symp.* 48:11–19, 1978.
19. Gefter, M.L.: DNA replication. *Ann. Rev. Biochem.* 44:45–78, 1975.
20. Smerdon, M.J., and Lieberman, M.W.: Distribution of UV-induced DNA repair synthesis in human chromatin. In: *DNA Repair Mechanisms* (P.C. Hanawalt, E.C. Friedberg, and C.F. Fox, Eds.). New York: Academic Press, 1978, pp. 327–332.
21. Crick, F.: Split genes and RNA splicing. *Science* 204:264–271, 1979.
22. Giannelli, F.: Xeroderma pigmentosum and the role of DNA repair in oncogenesis. *Bull. Cancer (Paris)* 65:323–334, 1978.
23. Smith, K.C.: Molecular changes in the nucleic acids produced by ultraviolet and visible radiation. In: *Sunlight and Man* (T.B. Fitzpatrick, et al., Eds.). Tokyo: University of Tokyo Press, 1974, pp. 57–66.

24. Hariharan, P.V., and Cerutti, P.A.:   Excision of damaged thymine residues from gamma-irradiated poly (dA-dT) by crude extracts of *Escherichia coli. Proc. Nat. Acad. Sci. USA* 71:3532-3536, 1974.
25. Epstein, J.H.: Photocarcinogenesis: a review. *NCI Monog.* 50:13-25, 1978.
26. Stern, R.S., Thibodeau, L.A., Kleinerman, R.A., Parrish, J.A., Fitzpatrick, T.B., and 22 participating investigators: Risk of cutaneous carcinoma in patients treated with oral methoxsalen photochemotherapy for psoriasis. *New Engl. J. Med.* 300:809-813, 1979.
27. Kripke, M.L.: Antigenicity of murine skin tumors induced by ultraviolet light. *J. Natl. Cancer Inst.* 53:1333-1336, 1974.
28. Kripke, M.L., and Fisher, M.S.: Immunologic aspects of tumor induction by ultraviolet radiation. *NCI Monog.* 50:179-183, 1978.
29. Fisher, M.S.: A systemic effect of ultraviolet irradiation and its relationship to tumor immunity. *NCI Monog.* 50:185-188, 1978.
30. Rosdahl, I.K.: Local and systemic effects on the epidermal melanocyte population in UV-irradiated mouse skin. *J. Invest. Dermatol.* 73:306-309, 1979.
31. Roberts, L.K., Schmitt, M., and Daynes, R.A.: Tumor susceptibility generated in mice treated with subcarcinogenic doses of 8-methoxypsoralen and long-wave ultraviolet light. *J. Invest. Dermatol.* 72:306-309, 1979.
32. Lee, J.A.H., and Merrill, J.M.: Sunlight and the aetiology of malignant melanoma: a synthesis. *Med. J. Aust.* 2:846-851, 1970.
33. Dermer, P.: Light sources. In: *Photobiology Course,* Chicago, IL: Am. Acad. Dermatol. Mtg., Dec. 1 and 2, 1979.
34. Harm, W.: Biological determination of the germicidal activity of sunlight. *Rad. Res.* 40:63-69, 1969.
35. Cleaver, J.E.: DNA damage and repair in light-sensitive human skin disease. *J. Invest. Dermatol.* 54:181-195, 1970.
36. Trosko, J.E., Krause, D., and Isoun, M.: Sunlight-induced pyrimidine dimers in human cells in vitro. *Nature* 228:358-359, 1970.
37. Andrews, A.D.: Sensitivity of xeroderma pigmentosum lymphoblasts to ultraviolet B (290-320 nm) and ultraviolet A (320-400 nm) light. *J. Invest. Dermatol.* 74:255-256, 1980 (Abstr.).
38. Smith, K.C.: Multiple pathways of DNA repair and their possible roles in mutagenesis. *NCI Monog.* 50:107-114, 1978.
39. Hewitt, R.R., and Meyn, R.E.: Applicability of bacterial models of DNA repair and recovery to UV-irradiated mammalian cells. *Adv. Rad. Biol.* 7:153-179, 1978.
40. Sutherland, B.M.: Human photoreactivating enzymes. In: *Research in Photobiology,* (A. Castellani, Ed.). New York: Plenum Press, 1977, pp. 307-315.
41. Sutherland, B.M., Oliver, R., Fuselier, C.O., and Sutherland, J.C.: Photoreactivation of pyrimidine dimers in the DNA of normal and xeroderma pigmentosum cells. *Biochem.* 15:402-406, 1976.
42. Sutherland, B.M., and Oliver, R.: Culture conditions affect photoreactivating enzyme levels in human fibroblasts. *Biochem. Biophys.* Acta 442:358-367, 1976.
43. Grossman, L., Braun, A., Feldberg, R., and Mahler, I.: Enzymatic repair of DNA. *Ann. Rev. Biochem.* 44:19-43, 1975.
44. Waldstein, E.: Enzymology of nucleotide excision repair. In: *DNA Repair Mechanisms* (P.C. Hanawalt, E.C. Friedberg, and C.F. Fox, Eds.). New York: Academic Press, 1978, pp. 219-224.

45. Cleaver, J.E.: Xeroderma pigmentosum: A human disease in which an initial stage of DNA repair is defective. *Proc. Nat. Acad. Sci. USA* **63**:428-435, 1969.
46. Kuhnlein, U., Penhoet, E.E., and Linn, S.: An altered apurinic DNA endonuclease activity in group A and group D xeroderma pigmentosum fibroblasts. *Proc. Nat. Acad. Sci. USA* **73**:1169-1173, 1976.
47. Deutsch, W.A., and Linn, S.: DNA binding activity from cultured human fibroblasts that is specific for partially depurinated DNA and that inserts purines into apurinic sites. *Proc. Nat. Acad. Sci. USA* **76**:141-144, 1979.
48. Cleaver, J.E., Williams, J.I., Kapp, L., and Park, S.D.: Cell survival. Excision repair and DNA replication in eucaryotic cells. In: *DNA Repair Mechanisms* (P.C. Hanawalt, E.C. Friedberg, and C.F. Fox, Eds.). New York: Academic Press, 1978, pp. 85-93.
49. Lehmann, A.R.: Postreplication repair of DNA in mammalian cells. *Life Sci.* **15**:2005-2016, 1974.
50. Pawsey, S.A., Magnus, I.A., Ramsay, C.A., Benson, P.F., and Giannelli, F.: Clinical, genetic and DNA repair studies on a consecutive series of patients with xeroderma pigmentosum. *Quart. J. Med.* **48** (190):179-210, 1979.
51. Lavin, M.F.: A model for postreplication repair of UV damage in mammalian cells. In: *DNA Repair Mechanisms* (P.C. Hanawalt, E.C. Friedberg, and C.F. Fox, Eds.). New York: Academic Press, 1978, pp. 509-512.
52. Higgins, N.P., Kato, K., and Strauss, B.: A model for replication repair in mammalian cells. *J. Mol. Biol.* **101**:417-425, 1976.
53. Witten, E.M., and Wermundsen, I.E.: Targeted and untargeted mutagenesis by various inducers of SOS function in *Escherichia coli. Cold Spring Harbor Symp.* **43**:881-886, 1979.
54. McCormick, J.J., and Maher, V.M.: Mammalian cell mutagenesis as a biological consequence of DNA damage. In: *DNA Repair Mechanisms* (P.C. Hanawalt, E.C. Friedberg, and C.F. Fox, Eds.). New York: Academic Press, 1978, pp. 739-749.
55. Boiteux, S., Villani, G., Spadari, S., Zambrano, F., and Radman, M.: Making and correcting errors in DNA synthesis: In vitro studies of mutagenesis. In: *DNA Repair Mechanisms* (P.C. Hanawalt, E.C. Friedberg, and C.F. Fox, Eds.). New York: Academic Press, 1978, pp. 73-84.
56. Zajdela, F., and Latarjet, R.: Inhibition of skin carcinogenesis in vivo by caffeine and other agents. *NCI Monog.* **50**:133-140, 1978.
57. Zajdela, F., and Latarjet, R.: Ultraviolet light induction of skin carcinoma in the mouse; influence of cAMP modifying agents. *Bull. Cancer (Paris)* **65**:305-313, 1978.
58. Lynch, H.T., Frichot, B.C., and Lynch, J.F.: Cancer control in xeroderma pigmentosum. *Arch. Dermatol.* **113**:193-195, 1977.
59. Cleaver, J.E.: Repair processes for photochemical damage in mammalian cells. *Adv. Rad. Biol.* **4**:1-75, 1974.
60. Hanawalt, P.C.: DNA repair schemes in bacteria and in human cells. In: *Research in Photobiology*, (A. Castellani, Ed.). New York: Plenum Press, 1977, pp. 285-292.
61. Paterson, M.C.: Use of purified lesion-recognizing enzymes to monitor DNA repair in vivo. *Adv. Rad. Biol.* **7**:1-53, 1978.
62. Cleaver, J.E., Bootsma, D. and Friedberg, E.: Human diseases with genetically altered DNA repair processes. *Genetics* **79**:215-225, 1975.
63. Gospodarowicz, D.: Humoral control of cell proliferation: the role of fibroblast growth factor in regeneration, angiogenesis, wound healing and neoplastic growth. *Prog. Clin. Biol. Res.* **9**:1-19, 1976.
64. Ehmann, U.K., Cook, K.H., and Friedberg, E.C.: Studies on the molecular mechanisms of nucleotide excision repair in UV-irradiated human cells in culture. In:

DNA Repair Mechanisms (P.C. Hanawalt, E.C. Friedberg, and C.F. Fox, Eds.). New York: Academic Press, 1978, pp. 315-318.

65. Scudiero, D., Henderson, E., Norin, A., and Strauss, B.: The measurement of chemically-induced DNA repair synthesis in human cells by BND-cellulose chromatography. *Mutat. Res.* 29:473-488, 1975.

66. van Zeeland, A.A.: Introduction of T4 endonuclease V into frozen and thawed mammalian cells for the determination of removal of UV-induced photoproducts. In: *DNA Repair Mechanisms* (P.C. Hanawalt, E.C. Friedberg, and C.F. Fox, Eds.). New York: Academic Press, 1978, pp. 307-310.

67. Meyn, R.E., and Fletcher, S.E.: The kinetics of postreplication repair in mammalian cells as studied by the alkaline elution technique. In: *DNA Repair Mechanisms* (P.C. Hanawalt, E.C. Friedberg, and C.F. Fox, Eds.). New York: Academic Press, 1978, pp. 513-516.

68. Lehmann, A.R.: Replicative bypass mechanisms in mammalian cells. In: *DNA Repair Mechanisms* (P.C. Hanawalt, E.C. Friedberg, and C.F. Fox, Eds.). New York: Academic Press, 1978, pp. 485-488.

69. D'Ambrosio, S.M., and Setlow, R.B.: On the presence of UV-endonuclease sensitive sites in daughter DNA of UV-irradiated mammalian cells. In: *DNA Repair Mechanisms* (P.C. Hanawalt, E.C. Friedberg, and C.F. Fox, Eds.). New York: Academic Press, 1978, pp. 499-503.

70. Meneghini, R., and Menck, C.F.M.: Pyrimidine dimers in DNA strands of mammalian cells synthesized after UV irradiation. In: *DNA Repair Mechanisms* (P.C. Hanawalt, E.C. Friedberg, and C.F. Fox, Eds.). New York: Academic Press, 1978, pp. 493-497.

71. Edenberg, H.J.: Inhibition of DNA replication by ultraviolet light. *Biophys. J.* 16:849-860, 1976.

72. Doniger, J.: The mechanism of postreplication repair in mammalian cells. In: *DNA Repair Mechanisms* (P.C. Hanawalt, E.C. Friedberg, and C.F. Fox, Eds.). New York: Academic Press, 1978, pp. 505-508.

73. Edenberg, H.J.: DNA replication in ultraviolet-irradiated mammalian cells. In: *DNA Repair Mechanisms* (P.C. Hanawalt, E.C. Friedberg, and C.F. Fox, Eds.). New York: Academic Press, 1978, pp. 489-492.

74. Park, S.D., and Cleaver, J.E.: Postreplication repair: questions of its definition and possible alteration in xeroderma pigmentosum cell strains. *Proc. Nat. Acad. Sci. USA* 76:3927-3931, 1979.

75. Sutherland, B.M.: Photoreactivation: evaluation of pyrimidine dimers in ultraviolet radiation-induced cell transformation. *NCI Monog.* 50:129-132, 1978.

76. Linn, S., Kuhnlein, U., and Deutsch, W.A.: Enzymes from human fibroblasts for the repair of AP DNA. In: *DNA Repair Mechanisms* (P.C. Hanawalt, E.C. Friedberg, and C.F. Fox, Eds.). New York: Academic Press, 1978, pp. 199-203.

77. Linn, S.: Enzymology of base excision repair. In: *DNA Repair Mechanisms* (P.C. Hanawalt, E.C. Friedberg, and C.F. Fox, Eds.). New York: Academic Press, 1978, pp. 175-178.

78. Lindahl, T., and Andersson, A.: Rate of chain breakage at apurinic sites in double-stranded deoxyribonucleic acid. *Biochem.* 11: 3618-3623, 1972.

79. Day, R.S.: Studies on repair of adenovirus 2 by human fibroblasts using normal, xeroderma pigmentosum, and xeroderma pigmentosum heterozygous strains. *Cancer Res.* 34:1965-1970, 1974.

80. Coppey, J., Moreno, G., and Nocentini, S.: Herpes virus production as a marker of repair in ultraviolet irradiated human skin cells of different origin. *Bull. Cancer (Paris)* 65:335-340, 1978.

81. Chang, K.S.S.: Susceptibility of xeroderma pigmentosum cells to transformation by murine and feline sarcoma viruses. *Cancer Res.* 36:3294-3299, 1976.

82. Whittemore, A.S.: Quantitative theories of oncogenesis. *Adv. Cancer Res.* 27:55-58, 1978.

83. Knudson, A.G., Jr.: Mutagenesis and embryonal carcinogenesis. *NCI Monog.* 51:19-24, 1979.

84. Burnet, F.M.: Cancer: somatic-genetic considerations. *Adv. Cancer Res.* 28:1-29, 1978.

85. Merkin, L.: The aetiology of cancer: clues from spontaneous recovery. *Medical Hypotheses* 4:136-140, 1978.

86. Lynch, H.T., Lynch, J., and Lynch, P.: Management and control of familial cancer. In: *Prog. Cancer Res. Ther.* (J.J. Mulvihill, R.W. Miller, and J.F. Fraumeni, Eds.). 3: 235-256, 1977.

87. Fraumeni, J.F., Jr.: Clinical patterns of familial cancer. In: *Prog. Cancer Res. Ther.* (J.J. Mulvihill, R.W. Miller, and J.F. Fraumeni, Eds.). 3:223-233, 1977.

88. Anderson, D.E.: Familial cancer and cancer families. *Sem. Oncol.* 5:11-16, 1978.

89. Murphy, E.A.: A statistician's viewpoint of familial cancer. In: *Prog. Cancer Res. Ther.* (J.J. Mulvihill, R.W. Miller, and J.F. Fraumeni, Eds.). 3:217-221, 1977.

90. Albert, S., and Child, M.: Familial cancer in the general population. *Cancer* 40: 1674-1679, 1977.

91. Meisner, L.F., Gilbert, E., Ris, H.W., and Haverty, G.: Genetic mechanisms in cancer predisposition. *Cancer* 43:679-689, 1979.

92. Sasazuki, T., McDevitt, H.O., and Grumet, F.C.: The association between genes in the major histocompatibility complex and disease susceptibility. *Ann. Rev. Med.* 28: 425-452, 1977.

93. Holliday, R.: The relationship between cellular aging and genetic defects. In: *DNA Repair Mechanisms* (P.C. Hanawalt, E.C. Friedberg, and C.F. Fox, Eds.). New York: Academic Press, 1978, pp. 769-777.

94. Hecht, F., and McCaw, B.K.: Chromosome instability syndromes. In: *Prog. Cancer Res. Ther.* (J.J. Mulvihill, R.W. Miller, and J.F. Fraumeni, Eds.). 3:105-123, 1977.

95. Mitelman, F., and Levan, G.: Clustering of aberrations to specific chromosomes in human neoplasms. III. Incidence and geographic distribution of chromosome aberrations in 856 cases. *Hereditas* 89:207-232, 1978.

96. Harnden, D.G.: Cytogenetics of human neoplasia. In: *Prog. Cancer Res. Ther.* (J.J. Mulvihill, R.W. Miller, and J.F. Fraumeni, Eds.). 3:87-104, 1977.

97. Minna, J.D.: Genetic analysis of malignancy using somatic cell hybrids. In: *Prog. Cancer Res. Ther.* (J.J. Mulvihill, R.W. Miller, and J.F. Fraumeni, Eds.). 3:343-354, 1977.

98. Fialkow, P.J.: Clonal origin and stem cell evolution of human tumors. In: *Prog. Cancer Res. Ther.* (J.J. Mulvihill, R.W. Miller, and J.F. Fraumeni, Eds.). 3:439-453, 1977.

99. Knudson, A.G., Jr.: Genetics and etiology of human cancer. *Adv. Human Genet.* 8:1-66, 1977.

100. Herrmann, J., and Elejalde, B.R.: Clinical genetics and pediatric neoplasms: pathogenetic and etiologic perspectives. *NCI Monog.* 51:7-18, 1979.

101. Purtilo, D.T., Paquin, L., and Gindhart, T.: Genetics of neoplasia – impact of ecogenetics on oncogenesis. *Am. J. Pathol.* 91:609-688, 1978.

102. Mulvihill, J.J.: Genetic repertory of human neoplasia. In: *Prog. Cancer Res. Ther.* (J.J. Mulvihill, R.W. Miller, and J.F. Fraumeni, Eds.). 3:137-143, 1977.

103. Lynch, H.T., and Frichot, B.C.: Skin, heredity and cancer. *Sem. Oncol.* 5:67-84, 1978.

104. Reed, W.B., Boder, E., and Gardner, M.: Congenital and genetic skin disorders with tumor formation. *Birth Defects* 10(4):265-284, 1974.

105. Schimke, R.N.: Cancer of the skin. *Genetics and Cancer in Man.* New York: Churchill-Livingstone, 1978, pp. 37-46.

106. McEvoy, B.F.: Genodermatoses associated with malignancies. In: *Cancer Dermatology* (F. Helm, Ed.). Philadelphia, PA: Lea & Febiger, 1979, pp. 39-55.

107. Salamon, T.: Maligne tumoren innerer organe und dermatosen. *Dermatol. Monatsschr.* 163:700-705, 1977.

108. Swift, M.: Fanconi's anaemia in the genetics of neoplasia. *Nature* 230:370-373, 1971.

109. Swift, M.: Malignant disease in heterozygous carriers. *Birth Defects* 12(1):133-144, 1976.

110. Setlow, R.B.: Repair deficient human disorders and cancer. *Nature* 271:713-717, 1978.

111. Cleaver, J.E.: Human diseases with in vitro manifestations of altered repair and replication of DNA. In: *Prog. Cancer Res. Ther.* (J.J. Mulvihill, R.W. Miller, and J.F. Fraumeni, Eds.). 3:355-363, 1977.

112. Friedberg, E.C., Ehmann, U.K., and Williams, J.I.: Human diseases associated with defective DNA repair. *Adv. Rad. Biol.* 8:85-174, 1979.

113. Arlett, C.F., and Lehmann, A.R.: Human disorders showing increased sensitivity to the induction of genetic damage. *Ann. Rev. Genet.* 12:95-115, 1978.

114. Robbins, J.H.: New forms of diseases with DNA repair defects. *Photochem. Photobiol.* 30:739-741, 1979.

115. Arlett, C.F., and Harcourt, S.A.: Cell killing and mutagenesis in repair-defective human cells. In: *DNA Repair Mechanisms* (P.C. Hanawalt, E.C. Friedberg, and C.F. Fox, Eds.). New York: Academic Press, 1978, pp. 633-636.

116. Lehmann, A.R., Kirk-Bell, S., Arlett, C.F., Harcourt, S.A., de Weerd-Kastelein, E.A., Keijzer, W., and Hall-Smith, P.: Repair of ultraviolet light damage in a variety of human fibroblast cell strains. *Cancer Res.* 37:904-910, 1977.

117. Cleaver, J.E., Bodell, W.J., and Park, S.D.: Repair deficient and hypersensitive diseases of man. In: *Radiation Research,* (S. Okada, et al., Eds.). Tokyo, Japan: Maruzen Co., 1979, pp. 476-482.

118. Johnson, B.E.: Formation of thymine containing dimers in skin exposed to ultraviolet radiation. *Bull. Cancer (Paris)* 65:283-297, 1978.

119. Jung, E.G.: Xeroderma pigmentosum; heterogeneous syndrome and model for UV carcinogenesis. *Bull. Cancer (Paris)* 65:315-321, 1978.

120. Takebe, H., Fujiwara, Y., Sasaki, M.S., Sato, Y., Kozuka, T., Nikaido, O., Ishizaki, K., Arase, S., and Ikenaga, M.: DNA repair and clinical characteristics of 96 xeroderma pigmentosum patients in Japan. In: *DNA Repair Mechanisms* (P.C. Hanawalt, E.C. Friedberg, and C.F. Fox, Eds.). New York: Academic Press, 1978, pp. 617-620.

121. Bootsma, D.: Xeroderma pigmentosum. In: *DNA Repair Mechanisms* (P.C. Hanawalt, E.C. Friedberg, and C.F. Fox, Eds.). New York: Academic Press, 1978, pp. 589-601.

122. Friedberg, E.C.: Xeroderma pigmentosum. *Arch. Pathol. Lab. Med.* 102:3-7, 1978.

123. Robbins, J.H.: Significance of repair of human DNA: Evidence from studies of xeroderma pigmentosum. *J. Natl. Cancer Inst.* 61:645-656, 1978.

124. Cleaver, J.E.: Xeroderma pigmentosum: biochemical and genetic considerations. *Ann. Rev. Genet.* 9:19-38, 1975.

125. Robbins, J.H., Kraemer, K.H., Lutzner, M.A., Festoff, B.W., and Coon, H.G.: Xeroderma pigmentosum. An inherited disease with sun sensitivity, multiple cutaneous neoplasms, and abnormal DNA repair. *Ann. Int. Med.* 80:221-248, 1974.

126. Robbins, J.H., and Moshell, A.N.: DNA repair processes protect human beings from premature solar skin damage: evidence from studies on xeroderma pigmentosum. *J. Invest. Dermatol.* 73:102-107, 1979.

127. Weichselbaum, R.R., and Little, J.B.: Familial retinoblastoma and ataxia telangectasia. *Cancer* 45:775-779, 1980.

128. Kleijer, W.J., de Weerd-Kastelein, E.A., Sluyter, M.L., Keijzer, W., de Wit, J., and Bootsma, D.: UV-induced DNA repair synthesis in cells of patients with different forms of xeroderma pigmentosum and of heterozygotes. *Mutat. Res.* 20:417-428, 1973.

129. Kraemer, K.H., Coon, H.G., Petinga, R.A., Barrett, S.F., Rahe, A.E., and Robbins, J.H.: Genetic heterogeneity in xeroderma pigmentosum: complementation groups and their relationship to DNA repair rates. *Proc. Nat. Acad. Sci. USA* 72:59-63, 1975.

130. Kraemer, K.H., de Weerd-Kastelein, E.A., Robbins, J.H., Keijzer, W., Barrett, S.F., Petinga, R.A., and Bootsma, D.: Five complementation groups in xeroderma pigmentosum. *Mutat. Res.* 33:327-339, 1975.

131. Arase, S., Kozuka, T., Tanaka, K., Ikenaga, M., and Takebe, H.: A sixth complementation group in xeroderma pigmentosum. *Mutat. Res.* 59:143-146, 1979.

132. Giannelli, F., and Pawsey, S.A.: DNA repair synthesis in human heterokaryons. III. The rapid and slow complementing varieties of xeroderma pigmentosum. *J. Cell Sci.* 20:207-213, 1976.

133. de Weerd-Kastelein, E.A., Keijzer, W., Sabour, M., Parrington, J.M., and Bootsma, D.: A xeroderma pigmentosum patient having a high residual activity of unscheduled DNA synthesis after UV is assigned to complementation group A. *Mutat. Res.* 37: 307-312, 1976.

134. Ramsay, C.A., Coltart, T.M., Blunt, S., Pawsey, S.A., and Giannelli, F.: Prenatal diagnosis of xeroderma pigmentosum. *Lancet* 2:1109-1112, 1974.

135. Andrews, A.D., Barrett, S.F., and Robbins, J.H.: Relation of DNA repair processes to pathological aging of the nervous system in xeroderma pigmentosum. *Lancet* 1: 1318-1320, 1976.

136. Andrews, A.D., Barrett, S.F., and Robbins, J.H.: Xeroderma pigmentosum neurological abnormalities correlate with colony-forming ability after ultraviolet radiation. *Proc. Nat. Acad. Sci. USA* 75:1984-1988, 1978.

137. Giannelli, F., and Pawsey, S.A.: DNA repair synthesis in human heterokaryons. II. A test for heterozygosity in xeroderma pigmentosum and some insight into the structure of the defective enzyme. *J. Cell Sci.* 15:163-176, 1974.

138. Baden, H.P., Parrington, J.M., Delhanty, J.D.A., and Pathak, M.A.: DNA synthesis in normal and xeroderma pigmentosum fibroblasts following treatment with 8-methoxypsoralen and long wave ultraviolet light. *Biochem. Biophys. Acta* 262:247-255, 1972.

139. Hofmann, H., Jung, E.G., and Schnyder, U.W.: Pigmented xerodermoid: first report of a family. *Bull. Cancer (Paris)* 65:347-350, 1978.

140. Robbins, J.H., Kraemer, K.H., and Andrews, A.D.: Inherited DNA repair defects in H. sapiens: their relation to UV-associated processes in xeroderma pigmentosum. In: *Biology of Radiation Carcinogenesis*, (J.M. Yuhas, R.W. Tennant, and J.D. Regan, Eds.). New York: Raven Press, 1976, pp. 115-127.

141. Tanaka, K., Sekiguchi, M., and Okada, Y.: Restoration of ultraviolet-induced unscheduled DNA synthesis of xeroderma pigmentosum cells by the concomitant treatment with bacteriophage T4 endonuclease V and HVJ (Sendai virus). *Proc. Nat. Acad. Sci. USA* 72:4071-4075, 1975.

142. Tanaka, K., Hayakawa, H., Sekiguchi, M., and Okada, Y.: Specific action of T4 endonuclease V on damaged DNA in xeroderma pigmentosum cells in vivo. *Proc. Nat. Acad. Sci. USA* 74:2958-2962, 1977.

143. Mortelmans, K., Friedberg, E.C., Slor, H., Thomas, G., and Cleaver, J.E.: Defective thymine dimer excision by cell-free extracts of xeroderma pigmentosum cells. *Proc. Nat. Acad. Sci. USA* 73:2757-2761, 1976.

144. Lehmann, A.R., Kirk-Bell, S., Arlett, C.F., Paterson, M.C., Lohman, P.H.M., de Weerd-Kastelein, E.A., and Bootsma, D.: Xeroderma pigmentosum cells with normal levels of excision repair have a defect in DNA synthesis after UV irradiation. *Proc. Nat. Acad. Sci. USA* 72:219-223, 1975.

145. Day, R.S.: Caffeine inhibition of the repair of ultraviolet-irradiated adenovirus in human cells. *Mutat. Res.* 33:321-325, 1975.

146. Fujiwara, Y., and Tatsumi, M.: Replicative bypass repair of ultraviolet damage to DNA of mammalian cells: caffeine sensitive and caffeine resistant mechanisms. *Mutat. Res.* 37:91-109, 1976.

147. Fujiwara, Y.: Replicative repair in xeroderma pigmentosum (XP) variants. In: *DNA Repair Mechanisms* (P.C. Hanawalt, E.C. Friedberg, and C.F. Fox, Eds.). New York: Academic Press, 1978, pp. 519-522.

148. Sutherland, B.M., Rice, M., and Wagner, E.K.: Xeroderma pigmentosum cells contain low levels of photoreactivating enzyme. *Proc. Nat. Acad. Sci. USA* 72:103-107, 1975.

149. Sutherland, B.M., and Oliver, R.: Low levels of photoreactivating enzyme in xeroderma pigmentosum variants. *Nature* 257:132-134, 1975.

150. Sutherland, B.M., and Oliver, R.: Inheritance of photoreactivating enzyme deficiencies in human cells. *Photochem. Photobiol.* 24:446-452, 1976.

151. Bacchetti, S., van der Plas, A., and Veldhuisen, G.: A UV-specific endonucleolytic activity present in human cell extracts. *Biochem. Biophys. Res. Comm.* 48:662-669, 1972.

152. Hariharan, P.V., and Cerutti, P.A.: Excision of ultraviolet and gamma ray products of the 5,6-dihydroxy-dihydrothymine type by nuclear preparations of xeroderma pigmentosum cells. *Biochem. Biophys. Acta* 447:375-378, 1976.

153. Bacchetti, S., and Benne, R.: Purification and characterization of an endonuclease from calf thymus acting on irradiated DNA. *Biochem. Biophys. Acta* 390:285-297, 1975.

154. Ciarrocchi, G., and Linn, S.: A cell-free assay measuring DNA synthesis in human fibroblasts. *Proc. Nat. Acad. Sci. USA* 75:1887-1891, 1978.

155. Smith, C.A., and Hanawalt, P.C.: Phage T4 endonuclease V stimulates DNA repair replication in isolated nuclei from ultraviolet-irradiated human cells, including xeroderma pigmentosum fibroblasts. *Proc. Nat. Acad. Sci. USA* 75:2598-2602, 1978.

156. Helene, C.: Mechanism and diversity of photoreactivation. In: *DNA Repair Mechanisms* (P.C. Hanawalt, E.C. Friedberg, and C.F. Fox, Eds.). New York: Academic Press, 1978, pp. 123-128.

157. Helene, C.: Excited state interactions and photochemical reactions in protein-nucleic acid complexes. In: *Research in Photobiology*, (A. Castellani, Ed.). New York: Plenum Press, 1977, pp. 31-39.

158. Setlow, R.B., and Carrier, W.L.: Pyrimidine dimers in ultraviolet-irradiated DNA's. *J. Mol. Biol.* 17:237-254, 1966.

159. Wang, S.Y., and Varghese, A.J.: Cytosine-thymine addition product from DNA irradiated with ultraviolet light. *Biochem. Biophys. Res. Comm.* 29:543-549, 1967.

160. Feldberg, R.S.: Non-dimer UV damage in DNA and poly d(A-T). In: *DNA Repair Mechanisms* (P.C. Hanawalt, E.C. Friedberg, and C.F. Fox, Eds.). New York: Academic Press, 1978, pp. 39–42.

161. Takebe, H., Furuyama, J-I., Miki, Y., and Kondo, S.: High sensitivity of xeroderma pigmentosum cells to the carcinogen 4-nitroquinoline-1-oxide. *Mutat. Res.* 15: 98–100, 1972.

162. Robbins, J.H., Andrews, A.D., and Moshell, A.N.: DNA repair nucleotide sequences which prevent premature death of neurons in humans: evidence from studies on xeroderma pigmentosum. In: *DNA Repair Mechanisms* (P.C. Hanawalt, E.C. Friedberg, and C.F. Fox, Eds.). New York: Academic Press, 1978, pp. 609–612.

163. Andrews, A.D., Barrett, S.F., Yoder, F.W., and Robbins, J.H.: Cockayne's syndrome fibroblasts have increased sensitivity to ultraviolet light but normal rates of unscheduled DNA synthesis. *J. Invest. Dermatol.* 70:237–239, 1978.

164. Arlett, C.F., Harcourt, S.A., and Broughton, B.C.: The influence of caffeine on cell survival in excision-proficient and excision-deficient xeroderma pigmentosum and normal human cell strains following ultraviolet-light irradiation. *Mutat. Res.* 33: 341–346, 1975.

165. Day, R.S.: Xeroderma pigmentosum variants have decreased repair of ultraviolet-damaged DNA. *Nature* 253:748–749, 1975.

166. Day, R.S., Giuffrida, A.S., and Dingman, C.W.: Repair by human cells of adenovirus-2 damaged by psoralen plus near ultraviolet light treatment. *Mutat. Res.* 33:311–320, 1975.

167. Aaronson, S.A., and Lytle, C.D.: Decreased host cell reactivation of irradiated SV40 virus in xeroderma pigmentosum. *Nature* 228:359–361, 1970.

168. Hall, J.D., and Tokuna, S.: Enhanced transformation of xeroderma pigmentosum variant cells by ultraviolet light-irradiated simian virus 40. *Cancer Res.* 39:4064–4068, 1979.

169. Lynch, H.T., Anderson, D.E., Smith, J.L., Jr., Howell, J.B., and Krush, A.J.: Xeroderma pigmentosum, malignant melanoma, and congenital ichthyosis. *Arch. Dermatol.* 96:625–635, 1967.

170. Hashem, N., Bootsma, D., Keijzer, W., Greene, A., Coriell, L., Thomas, G., and Cleaver, J.E.: Clinical characteristics, DNA repair, and complementation groups in xeroderma pigmentosum patients from Egypt. *Cancer Res.* 40:13–18, 1980.

171. Epstein, J.H., Fukuyama, K., Reed, W.B., and Epstein, W.L.: Defect in DNA synthesis in skin of patients with xeroderma pigmentosum demonstrated in vivo. *Science* 168:1477–1478, 1970.

172. Epstein, W.L., Fukuyama, K., and Epstein, J.H.: Ultraviolet light, DNA repair and skin carcinogenesis in man. *Fed. Proc.* 30:1766–1771, 1971.

173. Jung, E.G.: New form of molecular defect in xeroderma pigmentosum. *Nature* 228:361–362, 1970.

174. Robbins, J.H., Levis, W.R., and Miller, A.E.: Xeroderma pigmentosum epidermal cells with normal UV-induced thymidine incorporation. *J. Invest. Dermatol.* 59: 402–408, 1972.

175. Robbins, J.H., and Burk, P.G.: Relationship of DNA repair to carcinogenesis in xeroderma pigmentosum. *Cancer Res.* 33:929–935, 1973.

176. Taichman, L.B., and Setlow, R.B.: Repair of ultraviolet light damage to the DNA of cultured human epidermal keratinocytes and fibroblasts. *J. Invest. Dermatol.* 73: 217–219, 1979.

177. Kitano, Y.: Keratinization of human epidermal cells in culture. *Int. J. Dermatol.* 18:787–796, 1979.

178. Stanley, J.R., Foidart, J-M., Murray, J.C., Martin, G.R., and Katz, S.I.: The epidermal cell which selectively adheres to a collagen substrate is the basal cell. *J. Invest. Dermatol.* 74:54–58, 1980.

179. Berger, D.S.: Specification and design of solar ultraviolet simulators. *J. Invest. Dermatol.* 53:192–199, 1969.

180. Norman, A., Ottoman, R.E., Chan, P., and Klisak, I.: Unscheduled DNA synthesis in some spontaneous human tumors. *Mutat. Res.* 15:358–360, 1972.

181. Sirover, M.A.: Induction of the DNA repair enzyme uracil-DNA glycosylase in stimulated human lymphocytes. *Cancer Res.* 39: 2090–2095, 1979.

182. Study group: Malignant and benign neoplasms of the skin. In: Analysis of research needs and priorities in dermatology. *J. Invest. Dermatol.* 73(5), Part II: 443–451, 1979.

183. Robbins, J.H., Kraemer, K.H., and Flaxman, B.A.: DNA repair in tumor cells from the variant form of xeroderma pigmentosum. *J. Invest. Dermatol.* 64:150–155, 1975.

184. Setlow, R.B., and Regan, J.D.: Defective repair of N-acetoxy-2-acetylaminofluorene-induced lesions in the DNA of xeroderma pigmentosum cells. *Biochem. Biophys. Res. Comm.* 46:1019–1024, 1972.

185. Bootsma, D., Mulder, M.P., Pot, F., and Cohen, J.A.: Different inherited levels of DNA repair replication in xeroderma pigmentosum cell strains after exposure to ultraviolet irradiation. *Mutat. Res.* 9:507–516, 1970.

186. Lynch, H.T., Frichot, B.C., Fisher, J., Smith, J.L., Jr., and Lynch, J.F.: Spontaneous regression of metastatic malignant melanoma in two sibs with xeroderma pigmentosum. *J. Med. Genet.* 15:357–362, 1978.

187. Lynch, H.T., Frichot, B.C., and Lynch, J.F.: Familial atypical multiple mole-melanoma syndrome. *J. Med. Genet.* 15: 352–356, 1978.

188. der Kaloustian, V.M., de Weerd-Kastelein, E.A., Kleijer, W.J., Keijzer, W., and Bootsma, D.: The genetic defect in the de Sanctis Cacchione syndrome. *J. Invest. Dermatol.* 63:392–396, 1974.

189. Cleaver, J.E.: Repair of damaged DNA in human and other eucaryotic cells. In: *Nucleic Acid-Protein Interactions. Nucleic Acid Synthesis in Viral Infection*, (D.W. Ribbons, J.F. Woessner, and J. Schultz, Eds.). Vol. 2. Amsterdam: North-Holland, 1971, pp. 87–112.

190. Maher, V.M., Ouellette, L.M., Mittlestat, M., and McCormick, J.J.: Synergistic effect of caffeine on the cytotoxicity of ultraviolet irradiation and of hydrocarbon epoxides in strains of xeroderma pigmentosum. *Nature* 258:760–763, 1975.

191. Ahmed, F.E., and Setlow, R.B.: DNA repair in xeroderma pigmentosum cells treated with combinations of ultraviolet radiation and N-acetoxy-2-acetylaminofluroene. *Cancer Res.* 39:471–479, 1979.

192. Lambert, W.C., Okordudu, A.O., Amari, N.M., and Lambert, M.W.: A method for detecting defective DNA endonucleases in genodermatoses. *J. Invest. Dermatol.* 74:255, 1980 (Abstr.).

193. Peck, G.L.: Retinoids in dermatology. *Arch. Dermatol.* 116:283–284, 1980.

194. Swift, M., and Chase, C.: Cancer in families with xeroderma pigmentosum. *J. Nat. Cancer Inst.* 62:1415–1421, 1979.

195. Reed, W.B.: Treatment of psoriasis with oral psoralens and longwave ultraviolet light. *Acta Dermatovener.* 56:315–317, 1976.

196. Carter, V.H., Smith, K.W., and Noojin, R.O.: Xeroderma pigmentosum. Treatment with topically applied fluorouracil. *Arch. Dermatol.* 98:526–527, 1968.

197. Reed, W.B., Landing, B., Sugarman, G., Cleaver, J.E., and Melnyk, J.: Xeroderma pigmentosum: clinical and laboratory investigation of its basic defect. *J. Am. Med. Assoc.* 207:2073–2079, 1969.

198. Gleason, M.C.: Xeroderma pigmentosum—five-year arrest after total resurfacing of the face. *Plastic Reconstr. Sug.* **46**:577–581, 1970.

199. Epstein, E.H., Burk, P.G., Cohen, I.K., and Deckers, P.: Dermatome shaving in the treatment of xeroderma pigmentosum. *Arch. Dermatol.* **105**:589–590, 1972.

200. Bellows, R.A., Lahav, M., Lepreau, F.J., and Albert, D.M.: Ocular manifestations of xeroderma pigmentosum in a black family. *Arch. Ophthalmol.* **92**:113–117, 1974.

201. Reese, A.B., and Wilber, I.E.: The eye manifestations of xeroderma pigmentosum. *Am. J. Ophthalmol.* **26**:901–911, 1943.

202. Loewenthal, L.J.A., and Trowell, H.C.: Xeroderma pigmentosum in African negroes. *Brit. J. Dermatol.* **50**:66–71, 1938.

203. Freedman, J.: Corneal transplantation with associated histopathologic description in xeroderma pigmentosum occurring in a black family. *Ann. Ophthalmol.* **11**: 445–448, 1979.

204. Hananian, J., and Cleaver, J.E.: Xeroderma pigmentosum exhibiting neurological disorders and systemic lupus erythematosus. *Clin. Genet.* **17**:39–45, 1980.

205. Plotnick, H.: Xeroderma pigmentosum and mucocutaneous malignancies in three black siblings. *Cutis* **25**:311–313, 1980.

206. Targowsky, I., and Loewenthal, L.J.A.: Xeroderma pigmentosum. Report of a case in a Bantu child. *So. Afr. Med. J.* **30**:984–986, 1956.

207. Bell, E.T., and Rothnem, T.P.: Xeroderma pigmentosum with carcinoma of the lower lip in two brothers aged sixteen and thirteen years. *Am. J. Cancer* **30**:574–576, 1937.

208. Fialkow, P.J.: Clonal origin of human tumors. *Biochim. Biophys. Acta* **458**:283–321, 1976.

209. Reed, W.B.: The genetics of the photodermatoses. *Birth Defects* **7** (8):129–139, 1971.

210. Takebe, H.: Genetic complementation tests of Japanese xeroderma pigmentosum patients, and their skin cancers and DNA repair characteristics. In: *Fundamentals in Cancer Prevention*, (P.N. Magee, S. Takayama, T. Sugimura, and T. Matsushima, Eds.). Baltimore, MD: University Park Press, 1976, pp. 383–395.

211. German, J.: DNA repair defects and human disease. In: *DNA Repair Mechanisms* (P.C. Hanawalt, E.C. Friedberg, and C.F. Fox, Eds.). New York: Academic Press, 1978, pp. 625–631.

212. Paterson, M.C., and Smith, P.J.: Ataxia telangiectasia: an inherited human disorder involving hypersensitivity to ionizing radiation and related DNA-damaging chemicals. *Ann. Rev. Genet.* **13**:291–318, 1979.

213. Paterson, M.C., Smith, B.P., Knight, P.A., and Anderson, A.K.: Ataxia telangiectasia: an inherited human disease involving radiosensitivity, malignancy and defective DNA repair. In: *Research in Photobiology*, (A. Castellani, Ed.). New York: Plenum Press, 1977, pp. 207–218.

214. Lehmann, A.R., and Stevens, S.: The production and repair of double strand breaks in cells from normal humans and from patients with ataxia telangiectasia. *Biochim. Biophys. Acta* **474**:49–60, 1977.

215. Hutchinson, F.: Current knowledge of the formation and repair of DNA double-strand breaks. In: *Molecular Mechanisms for Repair of DNA*, (P.C. Hanawalt and R.B. Setlow, Eds.) Part B. New York: Plenum Press, 1975, pp. 699–702.

216. Cole, A., Shonka, F., Corry, P., and Cooper, W.G.: CHO cell repair of single-strand and double-strand DNA breaks induced by γ- and α-radiations. In: *Molecular Mechanisms for Repair of DNA*, (P.C. Hanawalt and R.B. Setlow, Eds.). New York: Plenum Press, 1975, pp. 665–676.

217. Dunlap, B., and Cerutti, P.: Apyrimidinic sites in gamma-irradiated DNA. *FEBS Lett.* 51:188–190, 1975.

218. Little, J.B.: Biological consequences of x-ray induced DNA damage and repair processes in relation to cell killing and carcinogensis. In: *DNA Repair Mechanisms* (P.C. Hanawalt, E.C. Friedberg, and C.F. Fox, Eds.). New York: Academic Press, 1978, pp. 701–711.

219. Hutchinson, F.: DNA strand break repair in eukaryotes. In: *DNA Repair Mechanisms* (P.C. Hanawalt, E.C. Friedberg, and C.F. Fox, Eds.). New York: Academic Press, 1978, pp. 457–463.

220. Sheridan, R.B., and Huang, P.C.: Ataxia telangiectasia: further considerations of the evidence for single strand break repair. *Mutat. Res.* 61:415–417, 1979.

221. Cerutti, P.A., and Remsen, J.F.: Gamma-ray excision repair in normal and diseased human cells. In: *Biology of Radiation Carcinogenesis,* (J.M. Yuhas, R.W. Tennant, and J.D. Regan, Eds.). New York: Raven Press, 1976, pp. 93–101.

222. Remsen, J.F., and Cerutti, P.A.: Excision of gamma-ray induced thymine lesions by preparations from ataxia telangiectasia fibroblasts. *Mutat. Res.* 43:139–145, 1977.

223. Sheridan, R.B., and Huang, P.C.: Apurinic and/or apyrimidinic endonuclease activity in ataxia telangiectasia cell extracts. *Mutat. Res.* 52:129–136, 1978.

224. Taylor, A.M.R., Rosney, C.M., and Campbell, J.B.: Unusual sensitivity of ataxia telangiectasia cells to bleomycin. *Cancer Res.* 39:1046–1050, 1979.

225. Ahmed, F.E., and Setlow, R.B.: Excision repair in ataxia telangiectasia, Fanconi's anemia, Cockayne's syndrome, and Bloom's syndrome after treatment with ultraviolet radiation and N-acetoxy-2-acetylaminofluorene. *Biochim. Biophys. Acta* 521:805–817, 1978.

226. Taylor, A.M.R.: Unrepaired DNA strand breaks in irradiated ataxia telangiectasia lymphocytes suggested from cytogenetic observations. *Mutat. Res.* 50:407–418, 1978.

227. Chen, P.C., Lavin, M.F., and Kidson, C.: Identification of ataxia telangiectasia heterozygotes, a cancer prone population. *Nature* 274:484–486, 1978.

228. Paterson, M.C., Anderson, A.K., Smith, B.P., and Smith, P.J.: Enhanced radiosensitivity of cultured fibroblasts from ataxia telangiectasia heterozygotes manifested by defective colony-forming ability and reduced DNA repair replication after hypoxic γ-irradiation. *Cancer Res.* 39:3725–3734, 1979.

229. Swift, M., Sholman, L., Perry, M., and Chase, C.: Malignant neoplasms in the families of patients with ataxia telangiectasia. *Cancer Res.* 36:209–215, 1976.

230. Daly, M.B., and Swift, M.: Epidemiological factors related to the malignant neoplasms in ataxia-telangiectasia families. *J. Chron. Dis.* 31:625–634, 1978.

231. Boder, E.: Ataxia telangiectasia: some historic, clinical and pathologic observations. *Birth Defects* 11(1):255–270, 1975.

232. Biggar, W.D., and Good, R.A.: Immunodeficiency in ataxia telangiectasia. *Birth Defects* 11(1):271–276, 1975.

233. Berkel, A.I., Ersoy, F., Epstein, L.B., and Spitler, L.E.: Transfer factor therapy in ataxia telangiectasia. *Clin. Exp. Immunol.* 29:376–384, 1977.

234. Bar, R.S., Levis, W.R., Rechler, M.M., Harrison, L.C., Siebert, C., Podskalny, J., Roth, J., and Muggeo, M.: Extreme insulin resistance in ataxia telangiectasia. Defect in affinity of insulin receptors. *New Engl. J. Med.* 298:1164–1171, 1978.

235. Waldmann, T.A., and McIntire, K.R.: Serum-alpha-fetoprotein levels in patients with ataxia telangiectasia. *Lancet* 2:1112–1115, 1972.

236. Simons, M.J., and Hosking, C.S.: A.F.P. and ataxia telangiectasia. *Lancet* 1:1234, 1974.

237. Keller, R.H., Guirgis, H., Lynch, H., and Tomasi, T.B., Jr.: Alpha-fetoprotein (AFP) in cancer-prone families. *Clin. Res.* 24:331A, 1976 (Abstr.).

238. Swift, M., Caldwell, R.J., and Chase, C.: Reassessment of cancer predisposition of Fanconi anemia heterozygotes. *JNCI* 65:863–867, 1980.

239. Dosik, H., Steier, W., and Lubiniecki, A.: Inherited aplastic anaemia with increased endoreduplications: a new syndrome or Fanconi's anaemia variant? *Brit. J. Haematol.* 41:77–82, 1979.

240. Teebor, G.W., and Duker, N.J.: Human endonuclease activity for DNA apurinic sites. *Nature* 258:544–547, 1975.

241. Regan, J.D., Carrier, W.L., Smith, D.P., Waters, R., and Lee, W.H.: Pyrimidine dimer excision in human cells and skin cancer, *NCI Monog.* 50:141–143, 1978.

242. Fujiwara, Y., Tatsumi, M., and Sasaki, M.S.: Cross-link repair in human cells and its possible defect in Fanconi's anemia cells. *J. Mol. Biol.* 113:635–649, 1977.

243. Fornace, A.J., Little, J.B., and Weichselbaum, R.R.: DNA repair in a Fanconi's anemia fibroblast cell strain. *Biochim. Biophys. Acta* 561:99–109, 1979.

244. Hirsch-Kauffmann, M., Schweiger, M., Wagner, E.F., and Sperling, K.: Deficiency of DNA ligase activity in Fanconi's anemia. *Hum. Genet.* 45:25–32, 1978.

245. Auerbach, A.D., and Wolman, S.R.: Carcinogen-induced chromosome breakage in Fanconi's anaemia heterozygous cells. *Nature* 271:69–71, 1978.

246. German, J., Bloom, D., and Passarge, E.: Bloom's syndrome. V. Surveillance for cancer in affected families, *Clin. Genet.* 12:162–168, 1977.

247. Vincent, R.A., Hays, M.D., and Johnson, R.C.: Single-strand DNA breakage and repair in Bloom's syndrome cells. In: *DNA Repair Mechanisms* (P.C. Hanawalt, E.C. Friedberg, and C.F. Fox, Eds.). New York: Academic Press, 1978, pp. 663-666.

248. Selsky, C., Weichselbaum, R., and Little, J.B.: Defective host-cell reactivation of UV-irradiated herpes simplex virus by Bloom's syndrome skin fibroblasts. In: *DNA Repair Mechanisms* (P.C. Hanawalt, E.C. Friedberg, and C.F. Fox, Eds.). New York: Academic Press, 1978, pp. 555-558.

249. Tice, R.R., Rary, J.M., and Bender, M.A.: An investigation of DNA repair potential in Bloom's syndrome. In: *DNA Repair Mechanisms* (P.C. Hanawalt, E.C. Friedberg, and C.F. Fox, Eds.). New York: Academic Press, 1978, pp. 659-662.

250. Tice, R., Windler, G., and Rary, J.M.: Effect of cocultivation on sister chromatid exchange frequencies in Bloom's syndrome and normal fibroblast cells. *Nature* 273: 538-540, 1978.

251. Schonberg, S. and German, J.: Sister chromatid exchange in cells metabolically coupled to Bloom's syndrome cells. *Nature* 284:72-74, 1980.

252. Rudiger, H.W., Bartram, C.R., Harder, W., and Passarge, E.: Rate of sister chromatid exchanges in Bloom's syndrome fibroblasts reduced by co-cultivation with normal fibroblasts. *Clin. Genet.* 17:82, 1980 (Abstr.).

253. Wade, M.H., and Chu, E.H.Y.: Effects of DNA damaging agents on cultured fibroblasts derived from patients with Cockayne's syndrome. In: *DNA Repair Mechanisms* (P.C. Hanawalt, E.C. Friedberg, and C.F. Fox, Eds.). New York: Academic Press, 1978, pp. 667-670.

254. Schmickel, R.D., Chu, E.H.Y., Trosko, J.E., and Chang, C.C.: Cockayne's syndrome: a cellular sensitivity to ultraviolet light. *Ped.* 60:135-139, 1977.

255. Kraemer, K.H., Coon, H.G., and Robbins, J.H.: Cell-fusion analysis of different inherited mutations causing defective DNA repair in xeroderma pigmentosum fibroblasts. *J. Cell Biol.* 59:176A, 1973 (Abstr.).

256. Takebe, H., Miki, Y., Kozuka, T., Furuyama, J., Tanaka, K., Sasaki, M.S., Fujiwara, Y., and Akiba, H.: DNA repair characteristics and skin cancers of xeroderma pigmentosum patients in Japan. *Cancer Res.* 37:490-495, 1977.

257.   Friedberg, E.C.: Xeroderma pigmentosum. *Arch. Pathol. Lab. Med.* 102:3-7, 1978.

258.   Chu, E.H.Y., Schmickel, R.D., Wade, M.H., Chang, C.C., and Trosko, J.E.: Ultraviolet light sensitivity and defect in DNA repair in fibroblasts derived from two patients with Cockayne's syndrome. *Am. J. Hum. Genet.* 27:26A, 1975 (Abstr.).

259.   Rook, A.: Genetics in dermatology. In: *Textbook of Dermatology,* (A. Rook, D.S. Wilkinson, and F.J.G. Ebling, Eds.; 2nd ed.). London: Blackwell, 1972, pp. 91-126.

260.   Lynch, H.T., Fusaro, R.M., Pester, J., and Lynch, J.F.: Familial atypical multiple mole melanoma (FAMMM) syndrome: genetic heterogeneity and malignant melanoma. *Brit. J. Cancer,* 42:58-70, 1980.

261.   Poste, G., and Fidler, I.J.: The pathogenesis of cancer metastasis. *Nature* 283:139-146, 1980.

262.   McBurney, E.I.: Vitiligo. Clinical picture and pathogenesis. *Arch. Int. Med.* 139:1295-1297, 1979.

263.   Hertz, K.C., Gazze, L.A., Kirkpatrick, C.H., and Katz, S.I.: Autoimmune vitiligo. Detection of antibodies to melanin-producing cells. *New Engl. J. Med.* 297:634-637, 1977.

264.   Lerner, A.B., and Nordlund, J.J.: Vitiligo. What is it? Is it important? *J. Am. Med. Assoc.* 239:1183-1187, 1978.

265.   Lerner, A.B., and Nordlund, J.J.: Should vitiligo be induced in patients after resection of primary melanoma? *Arch. Dermatol.* 113:421, 1977.

266.   Chavin, W., Jelonek, E.J., Jr., Reed, A.H., and Binder, L.R.: Survival of mice receiving melanoma transplants is promoted by hydroquinone. *Science* 208:408-410, 1980.

267.   Cooke, K.B., Bennett, C., and Staughton, R.C.D.: Melanoma specific protein: occurrence in the urine of patients with halo naevus and vitiligo. *Brit. J. Dermatol.* 98:663-668, 1978.

268.   Bennett, C., and Copeman, P.W.M.: Melanocyte mutation in halo naevus and malignant melanoma? *Brit. J. Dermatol.* 100:423-426, 1979.

269.   Sober, A.J., Mihm, M.C., Jr., Fitzpatrick, T.B., and Clark, W.H., Jr.: Malignant melanoma of the skin, and benign neoplasms and hyperplasias of melanocytes in the skin. In: *Dermatology in General Medicine,* (T.B. Fitzpatrick et al., Eds.; 2nd ed.). New York: McGraw-Hill, 1979, pp. 629-654.

270.   Kopf, A.W.: Editorial comment on metastatic melanoma with unknown site of origin. In: *Year Book of Dermatology 1976,* (F.D. Malkinson and R.W. Pearson, Eds.). Chicago, IL: Year Book Med. Pub., p. 213.

271.   Nathanson, L.: Spontaneous regression of malignant melanoma: a review of the literature on incidence, clinical features, and possible mechanisms. *NCI Monog.* 44:67-77, 1976.

272.   Sober, A.J., Fitzpatrick, T.B., and Mihm, M.C., Jr.: Primary melanoma of the skin: recognition and treatment. *J. Am. Acad. Dermatol.* 2:179-197, 1980.

273.   Hinds, M.W., and Kolonel, L.N.: Malignant melanoma of the skin in Hawaii, 1960-1977. *Cancer* 45:811-817, 1980.

274.   Su, W.P.D., and Bradley, R.R.: Amelanotic lentigo maligna. *Arch. Dermatol.* 116:82-83, 1980.

275.   Burket, J.M.: Amelanotic lentigo maligna. *Arch. Dermatol.* 115:496, 1979.

276.   Baab, G.H., and McBride, C.M.: Malignant melanoma. The patient with an unknown site of primary origin. *Arch. Surg.* 110:896-900, 1975.

277.   Ronchese, F.: Spontaneous bleaching of melanotic freckles. *Arch. Dermatol.* 94:739-741, 1966.

278.   Burnet, F.M.: Intrinsic mutagenesis, an interpretation of the pathogenesis of xeroderma pigmentosum. *Lancet* 2:495-498, 1974.

279. Chu, E.H.Y., Trosko, J.E., and Chang, C.C.: Mutational approaches to the study of carcinogenesis. *J. Toxicol. Environ. Health* 2:1317-1334, 1977.

280. Farber, E.M., and Nall, M.L.: The natural history of psoriasis in 5,600 patients. *Dermatologica* 148:1-18, 1974.

281. Squier, C.A.: The stretching of mouse skin in vivo: effect on epidermal proliferation and thickness. *J. Invest. Dermatol.* 74:68-71, 1980.

282. Agrup, G., Hansson, C., Rorsman, H., Rosengren, A.M., Rosengren, E., and Tegner, E.: 5-S-cysteinyldopa excretion after treatment with 8-methoxypsoralen and UVA light. *J. Invest. Dermatol.* 70:25-26, 1978.

283. Fine, R.M., Chawla, R.K., Kutner, M., and Rudman, D.: Accumulation of urinary cancer-related glycoprotein, EDC1, in psoriasis. *J. Invest. Dermatol.* 73:264-265, 1979.

284. de Moragas, J.M., and Winkelmann, R.K.: Psoriasis and vitiligo. *Arch. Dermatol.* 101:235-237, 1970.

285. Sweet, R.D.: Vitiligo as a Koebner phenomenon. *Brit. J. Dermatol.* 99:223-224, 1978.

286. Chapman, R.S.: Coincident vitiligo and psoriasis in the same individual. *Arch. Dermatol.* 107:776, 1973.

287. Lynch, H.T., Lemon, H.M., and Krush, A.J.: A note on "cancer-susceptible" and "cancer-resistant" genotypes. *Nebr. State Med. J.* 51:209-211, 1966.

288. Lynch, H.T., and Guirgis, H.A.: Cancer resistance. *Nebr. Med. J.* 59:156-161, 192-196, 1974.

289. Stern, R.S., Zierler, S., and Parrish, J.A.: Skin carcinoma in patients with psoriasis treated with topical tar and artificial ultraviolet radiation. *Lancet* 1:732-735, 1980.

290. Shuster, S., Chapman, P.H., and Rawlins, M.D.: Psoriasis and cancer. *Brit. Med. J.* 1:941-942, 1979.

291. Chapman, P.H., Rawlins, M.D., and Shuster, S.: Activity of aryl hydrocarbon hydroxylase in psoriatic skin. *Lancet* 1:297-298, 1979.

292. Guirgis, H.A., Lynch, H.T., Mate, T., Harris, R.E., Wells, I., Caha, L., Anderson, J., Maloney, K., and Rankin, L.: Arylhydrocarbon hydroxylase activity in lymphocytes from lung cancer patients and mormal controls. *Oncol* 33:105-109, 1976.

293. Jacobs, P.H., Farber, E.M., and Nall, M.L.: Psoriasis and skin cancer. In: *Psoriasis.* (E.M. Farber, A.J. Cox, P.H. Jacobs, and M.L. Nall, Eds.). New York: Yorke Medical Books, Div. of Dun-Donnelley Publishing Corp., 1977, pp. 350-352.

294. Halprin, K.M.: Psoriasis, skin cancer and PUVA. *J. Am. Acad. Dermatol.* 2:334-337, 1980.

295. Stern, R.S., Parrish, J.A., and Fitzpatrick, T.B.: Response to ref. 294, *J. Am. Acad. Dermatol.* 2: 337-339, 1980.

296. Zelickson, A.S., Mottaz, J.H., and Muller, S.A.: Melanocyte changes following PUVA therapy. *J. Am. Acad. Dermatol.* 1: 422-430, 1979.

297. Bridges, B., and Strauss, G.: Possible hazards of photochemotherapy for psoriasis. *Nauture* 283: 523-524, 1980.

298. Burgener, J.: Gibt es ein "echtes" psoriasiskarzinom? *Dermatologica* 80: 86-97, 1939.

299. Pinkus, H.: The border line between cancer and noncancer. In: *Year Book of Dermatology 1966-1967,* (A.W. Kopf, and R. Andrade, Eds.). Chicago, IL: Year Book Med. Pub., pp. 5-34.

300. Bullough, W.S.: The epidermal chalone mechanism. *NCI Monog.* 38: 99-107, 1973.

301. Madison, J.F.: Basal cell epitheliomas after repeated fluoroscopic examinations of the chest. *Arch. Dermatol.* 116:323-324, 1980.
302. Vitaliano, P.P., and Urbach, F.: The relative importance of risk factors in nonmelanoma carcinoma. *Arch. Dermatol.* 116:454-456, 1980.
303. Fleming, I.D., Barnawell, J.R., Burlison, P.E., and Rankin, J.S.: Skin cancer in black patients. *Cancer* 35:600-605, 1975.
304. Suh, M.S., Hahm, J.H., and Kook, H.I.: Two cases of xeroderma pigmentosum. *Korean J. Dermatol.* 16:261-265, 1978.
305. Bartholdson, L., Lilja, J., Mobacken, H., and Waldenstrom, J.: Xeroderma pigmentosum–biochemical and therapeutic aspects. *Scand. J. Plast. Reconstr. Surg.* 11: 173-177, 1977.
306. Lagerholm, B., and Skog, E.: Squamous cell carcinoma in psoriasis vulgaris. *Acta Dermatovenereol.* 48:128-136, 1968.
307. Roenigk, H.H., Jr., and 12 cooperating investigators: Skin cancer in the PUVA-48 cooperative study of psoriasis. *J. Invest. Dermatol.* 74:250, 1980 (Abstr.).
308. Brown, F.S., Burnett, J.W., and Robinson, H.M., Jr.: Cutaneous carcinoma following psoralen and long-wave ultraviolet radiation (PUVA) therapy for psoriasis. *J. Am. Acad. Dermatol.* 2:393-395, 1980.
309. Maddin, W.S., and Wood, W.S.: Multiple keratoacanthomas and squamous cell carcinomas occurring at psoriatic treatment sites. *J. Cutan. Pathol.* 6:96-100, 1979.
310. Witkop, C.J., Jr., Quevedo, W.C., Jr., and Fitzpatrick, T.B.: Albinism. In: *The Metabolic Basis of Inherited Disease*, (J.B. Stanbury, J.B. Wyngaarden, and D.S. Fredrickson, Eds.; 4th ed.). New York: McGraw-Hill, 1978, pp. 283-316.
311. King, R.A., Olds, D.P., and Witkop, C.J.: Characterization of human hairbulb tyrosinase: properties of normal and albino enzyme. *J. Invest. Dermatol.* 71: 136-139, 1978.
312. Keeler, C.E.: Albinism, xeroderma pigmentosum and skin cancer. *NCI Monog.* 10:349-359, 1963.
313. Yu, M.-Y.W., Lakshmanan, J., and Guroff, G.: Chemical control of neuronal growth– the nerve growth factor. In: *Essays in Neurochemistry and Neuropharmacology*, (M.B.H. Youdim, W. Lovenberg, D.F. Sharman, and J.R. Lagnado, Eds.). Vol. 3, New York: Wiley 1978, pp. 33-48.
314. Schenkein, I., Bueker, E.D., Helson, L., Axelrod, F., and Dancis, J.: Increased nerve-growth-stimulating activity in disseminated neurofibromatosis. *New Engl. J. Med.* 290:613-614, 1974.
315. Siggers, D.C., Boyer, S.H., and Eldridge, R.: Nerve-growth factor in disseminated neurofibromatosis. *New Engl. J. Med.* 292:1134, 1975.
316. Fabricant, R.N., Todaro, G.J., and Eldridge, R.: Increased levels of a nerve-growth-factor cross-reacting protein in "central" neurofibromatosis. *Lancet* 1:4-7, 1979.
317. Frazier, W.A., Angeletti, R.H., and Bradshaw, R.A.: Nerve growth factor and insulin. *Science* 176:482-488, 1972.
318. Hogue-Angeletti, R.A., Bradshaw, R.A., and Frazier, W.A.: Nerve growth factor: structure and mechanism of action. *Adv. Metab. Disorders* 8:285-299, 1975.
319. Gabbay, K.H., DeLuca, K., Fisher, J.N., Jr., Mako, M.E., and Rubenstein, A.H.: Familial hyperproinsulinemia. *New Engl. J. Med.* 294:911-915, 1976.
320. Epstein, J.H., and 29 co-investigators: Current status of oral PUVA therapy for psoriasis. *J. Am. Acad. Dermatol.* 1:106-117, 1979.
321. Melski, J.W., Tanenbaum, L., Parrish, J.A., Fitzpatrick, T.B., Bleich, H.L., and 28 participating investigators: Oral methoxalen photochemotherapy for the treatment of psoriasis: a cooperative clinical trial. *J. Invest. Dermatol.* 68:328-335, 1977.

322. Haseltine, W.A., Gordon, L.K., Lindan, C.P., Grafstrom, R.H., Shaper, N.L., and Grossman, L.: Cleavage of pyrimidine dimers in specific DNA sequences by a pyrimidine dimer DNA-glycosylase of *M. luteus. Nature* **285**:634–641, 1980.

323. Kraemer, K.H.: Oculo-cutaneous and internal neoplasms in xeroderma pigmentosum: implications for theories of carcinogenesis. In: *Carcinogenesis: Fundamental Mechanisms and Environmental Effects,* (B. Pullman, and P. Ts'o, Eds.). Dordrecht: Reidel: in press.

324. Kraemer, K.H.: Xeroderma pigmentosum. In: *Clinical Dermatology* is published in loose-leaf format to allow updating; and is arranged in Sections. Section 19 is Environmental Dermatoses. Unit 19-7 is Xeroderma Pigmentosum, in Section 19. (D.J. Demis, R.L. Dobson, and J. McGuire, Eds.). New York: Harper and Row, in press.

325. Sekiguchi, M., Hayakawa, H., Makino, F., Tanaka, K., and Okada, Y.: A human enzyme that liberates uracil from DNA. *Biochem. Biophys. Res. Communs.* **73**: 293–299, 1976.

326. Kuhnlein, U., Lee, B., and Linn, S.: Human uracil DNA N-glycosidase: studies in normal and repair defective cultured fibroblasts. *Nuc. Acids Res.* **5**:117–125, 1978.

327. Shiraishi, Y., Matsui, S., and Sandberg, A.A.: Normalization by cell fusion of sister chromatid exchange in Bloom Syndrome lymphocytes. *Science* **212**:820–822, 1981.

328. Cohen, S.R., Burkholder, D.E., Varga, J.M., Carter, D.M., and Bartholomew, J.C.: Cell cycle analysis of cultured mammalian cells after exposure to a 4, 5′, 8-trimethylpsoralen and long-wave ultraviolet light. *J. Invest. Dermatol.* **76**:409–413, 1981.

11

Genetic Counseling and Cancer-associated Genodermatoses

Henry T. Lynch, M.D., Patrick M. Lynch, J.D., and Jane Lynch, R.N.

INTRODUCTION

Genetic counseling is a term which is used by the laity, by medically and non-medically trained geneticists, and by physicians. Yet its meaning to each group may vary significantly. For example, the average concerned layman with or at risk for a hereditary disorder fervently hopes that he will learn something about the disease in his family which will lighten the burden to either himself or his loved ones. He is often fearful about its consequences.

The nonmedically trained geneticist may have a command of the mechanisms of inheritance of the specific disease or trait and can often communicate this effectively to his counselees. However, by the nature of his training and background, he often lacks comprehension of the disorder's pathogenesis, diagnosis, therapy, and prognosis. The physician, on the other hand, may handle the medical aspects of the disorder capably only to be confused about mechanisms of its inheritance and unable to communicate risk factor information to his patient. Meeting the emotional needs of the patient, communicating accurately the mode of genetic transmission, and providing a clear understanding of the medical problems thus remain unrealized goals in many cases. These needs are ideally met by a team comprised of family physicians, psychologists, psychiatrists, geneticists, and other specialists, depending upon the particular disorder.[1,2]

Regardless of whether genetic counseling is provided by a team or by a medically qualified geneticist, the patient should be provided an empathetic listening ear,[3,4] particularly when dealing with potentially fatal hereditary diseases, including cancer-associated genodermatoses. The patient must be given every opportunity to discuss underlying anxieties, apprehensions, and fears, ideally in a nondirective setting. An impersonal approach, on the other hand, may restrict free exchange of the patient's underlying feelings. Such a stereotyped approach has unfortunately been considered by some to represent effective genetic counseling. McKusick[5] has taken strong issue with this prevailing attitude:

> Too long genetic counseling has, by default, fallen to the province of the college professor, who is informed that the diagnosis is Humpty Dumpty's disease, who looks up the usual mode of inheritance of H-D disease in a book, and on the basis of this and the specific pedigree gives advice. Genetic counseling, like other medical prognoses, should be an integral part of the practice of clinical medicine. The physician is in the best position to meet [the needs of genetic counseling] ... [and] with improved education in medical genetics, sound genetic counseling should become the rule in medical practice.

In other words, the patient's problem must be viewed within the fame of reference of those *psychological, social,* and *medical* concerns reflected in any serious hereditary disorder, including certain of the cancer-associated genodermatoses.

FAMILY HISTORY

The family history of cancer is a subject which is given short shrift in clinical practice. This is regrettable in that the family history can provide the physician a powerful tool for early diagnosis, management, and cancer control. A well-documented family history can aid significantly in the identification of patients who are genetically susceptible to cancer of specific target organs and tissues. In the case of the cancer-associated genodermatoses, the clinician has readily at hand a most invaluable marker, namely cutaneous signs, a subject discussed in detail throughout this book. Early cancer diagnosis of high risk patients is the logical consequence of a targeted surveillance program. Prophylactic surgery such as bilateral subcutaneous mastectomy in Cowden's disease may be indicated.[6-12]   It is important to appreciate the fact that genetic counseling and management may be appropriately extended to the entire family unit.

Use of Family History in Genetic Counseling of
Cancer-associated Genodermatoses[6]

In the following paragraphs, we shall discuss examples of the use of family history and related medical-genetic factors in counseling kindreds with cancer-associated genodermatoses. Cases will be drawn from experiences in genetic counseling of families with xeroderma pigmentosum and malignant melanoma.

Methodologies for compiling family histories on a consecutive series of oncology clinic patients have been previously described.[13]   Details of the patient's genealogy and family cancer history include current ages, ages at death, and ages at cancer diagnosis (when applicable) for first degree relatives and selected second degree relatives (grandparents, aunts, and uncles). In our clinic, the histories are obtained by registered nurses. These nurses were provided an orientation program, emphasizing fundamentals of human genetics as these apply to the cancer problem. Training in interview techniques fostered efficiency in obtaining family histories, thereby allowing the clinic physicians to devote more time to pedigree analysis, hereditary cancer syndrome identification, and in turn, genetic counseling.

XERODERMA PIGMENTOSUM: GENETIC COUNSELING IMPLICATIONS

A midwestern family with xeroderma pigmentosum (XP) has been the subject of several reports[14-17] and is discussed elsewhere in this book (Chapter 9, Figure 9-28). Skin fibroblasts from members of this family were used by Cleaver in his initial studies of defective DNA repair in XP.[18]

The family was originally referred upon diagnosis of metastatic malignant melanoma in the XP-affected proband who, at the time, was 17 years old. Details of his cancer history, including spontaneous regression of metastatic malignant melanoma in him and a similarly affected sister, had been previously noted. Their parents' first knowledge of the disease in the family occurred when their second born child, a daughter, then age 13, was treated for what appeared to them to be a cold sore on her lip, following exposure to the sun while swimming. When the lesion did not heal normally, she was referred to a surgeon who quickly suspected XP. Aware of the clinical-genetic significance of XP, he examined two other affected siblings and established the diagnosis. Assuming responsibility for total management of the family, the surgeon explained the carcinogenic role of sunlight exposure, advising total restriction of exposure to sunlight for the three affected children. The effort to provide a "normal" environment sheltered from sunlight exposure sternly tested the parents' ingenuity. When the family was seen initially for genetic counseling, both parents expressed an interest in the natural history of XP as well as in its inheritance in their family. It was apparent that there existed misconceptions about the genetic transmission of XP. For example, the parents thought that the disorder would most likely be passed on by their unaffected children. They repeated in detail their grave concerns and fears, including those of their adult daughters who had rejected the thought of marriage and children. The parents were provided with an opportunity to express their worries and fears, and were reassured that it was not unusual for patients to entertain such concerns.

The next phase of genetic counseling was to acquaint the family, in lay terminology, with the fundamentals of genetic transmission. Particular emphasis was given to the derivation of probabilities for "passing on genes," stressing the rarity of the XP gene and the unlikelihood of a mating between unrelated gene carriers. The parents were told that since both of them were carriers, the prior probability of each child being affected was 25%, even though five of their seven children were affected. They were shown how this result was still simply a matter of probability.

This family has been followed closely by us for 14 years. The XP-affected daughters (Figure 9-28, II-1, II-2) were able to work through their emotional concerns about this disease; they have married, had normal children, are happy, and seem to be well adjusted. The proband is also married, raising a family, and is successfully engaged in a career as an architect.

The youngest affected siblings, identical twins, have been protected from solar radiation exposure virtually since birth. They are now age 18 and remain free of cancer.[16] The successful outcome in this family can be attributed to genetic counseling coupled with strong supportive help from several family physicians.

FAMILIAL MELANOMA: EDUCATIONAL IMPLICATIONS AND GENETIC COUNSELING

Considerable attention has been devoted to the familial atypical multiple mole-melanoma (FAMMM) syndrome in Chapter 9. Genetic counseling in the FAMMM syndrome readily fosters cancer control since the phenotype is so highly correlated with ultimate transformation of FAMMM moles into frankly malignant melanoma. One of these melanoma-prone kindreds (Chapter 9, Figure 9-1) has been followed over a 16-year span. Genetic counseling in this kindred required extensive education about this otherwise relatively unknown disease. In fact, the high cancer frequency in the kindred necessitated efforts at cancer control at a time when the significance of the FAMMM phenotype had not yet even been recognized. More recently, high risk relatives have been shown examples of moles in various stages of evolution, including transition to frankly evident malignant melanoma. These educational illustrations have reportedly been of some value in achieving relatively early diagnoses of melanoma. All relatives with the FAMMM phenotype have been provided a wallet-sized laminated card listing the signs of cutaneous malignant melanoma. In addition, the natural history of this disease has been discussed with patients and their spouses. Spouses are taught to critically inspect the skin of their mates and children for evidence of early changes in the subject moles.

Patients not available for personal counseling were contacted in order to determine whether there existed evidence of the phenotype. Affected patients were then advised of their risk for eventually developing malignant melanoma, and their physicians were provided details about the diagnosis, natural history, and prognosis of this syndrome. Because of this, two of the proband's geographically distant sisters, who manifested the FAMMM phenotype and who developed cutaneous malignant melanoma, were diagnosed while the lesions were still quite early.

At the age of 9 years, the proband's daughter was diagnosed with the syndrome and is being meticulously followed. Our plan for this family is to have all members with the cutaneous phenotype seen by a dermatologist at least four times a year. Biopsies of any suspicious lesions are obtained. Between office visits, they are encouraged to see a physician immediately upon recognition of any change in existing moles.

GENERAL COMMENTS

While the cancer risk in XP may occur very early in life, and that of the FAMMM syndrome may be as early as in the 20s, the more frequently encountered dominant disorders such as von Recklinghausen's neurofibromatosis, Type III MEN, and von Hippel-Lindau's syndrome may show either early or late onset. Hence, a given patient may have procreated prior to any realization of personal cancer risk. If a parent has had cancer or is known to be at an exceedingly high risk for harboring the deleterious gene, he or she may have strong guilt feelings about the possibility of having transmitted the disease to his offspring. This may be compounded by an acute concern for continued personal well-being. The parent may know that he carries the genetic trait because of the presence of cutaneous stigmata such as café au lait spots or neurofibromas in von Recklinghausen's neurofibromatosis or the multiple mucosal neuromas of Type III MEN. As in the discussion of the XP family, these concerns weigh heavily on the patient contemplating marriage. They may also affect career goals and influence how these should be pursued in light of the cancer risk. This is unlike the situation involving recessive disorders where, although the risk to children may be high, the heterozygous parent is usually in no danger of manifesting the disease.

Genetic counseling in cancer is further complicated by the stereotyped image of cancer in the general population. Family members may manifest anxiety, fatalism, denial, and even accusation directed toward the spouse, parents, or family members "responsible" for transmitting the disease. In certain situations, the patient's peer group may compound an already discouraging situation. For example, in cosmetically disfiguring disorders, such as dominantly inherited neurofibromatosis or multiple mucosal neuroma syndrome, the community may adopt a repugnant response, not only against the afflicted patients but against relatives of a particular patient. In short, the counselor must be fully aware of community reaction as a factor in the psychological response of the family.

More than a decade ago, some simple principles were suggested for genetic counseling.[1] These still appear to be applicable to genetic counseling in general and to the cancer issue in particular. They are repeated here in order to embellish the philosophy and objectives of genetic counseling as perceived by the authors:

1. Genetic counseling is an integral part of the management of the patient with genetic disease, the responsibility for which ideally should be assumed by the family physician.
2. The counselor must never make decisions for the patient regarding marriage, children, and other important personal issues. These decisions are the patient's responsibility and only he/she should exercise this right.
3. The genetic counselor must take meticulous care to insure the accuracy of diagnosis in hereditary disease in that ramifications of such a diagnosis may profoundly affect the entire family unit.
4. The counselor must look beyond the individual patient and be concerned with eliciting support for the medical welfare of other affected members of the kindred.
5. The genetic counselor must constantly remember that the presence of hereditary disease in the family may promote strong emotional reaction among unaffected as well as affected members of the kindred; the counselor must do everything possible to alleviate this emotional stress.
6. The genetic counselor must strive to effectively dispel unfavorable impressions and irrational responses by members of the community against individuals with certain "grotesque" mental and physical hereditary disorders. The physician will usually be in a favorable position in the community to institute a positive educational program toward this goal.
7. The genetic counselor must study all aspects of the natural history of hereditary diseases, so that when needed, he or she may effectively mobilize paramedical personnel and community resources to help the patient and the family.
8. Care must be taken to exclude extragenetic factors as being of etiologic importance. Should a nongenetic factor be the major cause of disease, as in rubella syndrome, parents must be reassured and thoroughly informed that the disorder in their midst is not genetic.
9. Hearsay evidence of disease in relatives of the affected proband should be verified whenever possible; effort extended in this direction will be highly rewarding in the long run.
10. The genetic counselor will be in a favorable position to study variations in known hereditary disorders as well as to uncover "new" hereditary diseases. The counselor should make every effort to report scientific observations to his or her colleagues.

REFERENCES

1. Lynch, H.T.: Dynamic Genetic Counseling for Clinicians. Springfield, IL: Charles C. Thomas, 1969.
2. Kessler, S. (Ed.): Genetic Counseling. Psychological Dimensions. New York: Academic Press, 1979.
3. Lynch, H.T., Krush, T.P., Krush, A.J., and Tips, R.L.: Psychodynamics of early hereditary deaths. *Am. J. Dis. Child.* **108**:605-610, 1964.
4. Tips, R.L., and Lynch, H.T.: The impact of genetic counseling upon the family milieu. *JAMA* **184**:183-186, 1963.
5. McKusick, V.A.: Genetics in medicine and medicine in genetics. *Am. J. Med.* **4**:594-599, 1963.
6. Lynch, H.T., Harris, R.E., Organ, C.H., Jr., and Lynch, J.F.: Management of familial breast cancer. I. Biostatistical-genetic aspects and their limitations as derived from a familial breast cancer resource. *Arch. Surg.* **113**:1053-1058, 1978.
7. Lynch, H.T., Harris, R.E., Organ, C.H., Jr., and Lynch, J.F.: Management of familial breast cancer. II. Case reports, pedigrees, genetic counseling, and team concept. *Arch. Surg.* **113**:1061-1067, 1978.
8. Lynch, H.T., Harris, R.E., Bardawil, W.A., Lynch, P.M., Guirgis, H.A., Swartz, M.J., and Lynch, J.F.: Management of hereditary site-specific colon cancer. *Arch. Surg.* **112**:170-174, 1977.
9. Lynch, H.T., Harris, R.E., Organ, C.H., Jr., Guirgis, H.A., Lynch, P.M., Lynch, J.F., and Nelson, E.J.: The surgeon, genetics, and cancer control: the cancer family syndrome. *Ann. Surg.* **185**:435-440, 1977.
10. Lynch, H.T., Organ, C.H., Jr., Harris, R.E., Guirgis, H.A., Lynch, P.M., and Lynch, J.F.: Familial cancer: implications for surgical management of high-risk patients. *Surgery* **83**:104-113, 1978.
11. Lynch, H.T.: Cancer Genetics. Springfield, IL: Charles C. Thomas, 1976, 639 pp.
12. Lynch, H.T., Lynch, J.F., and Lynch, P.M.: Management and control of familial cancer. In: *Genetics of Human Cancer* (J.J., Mulvihill, R.W., Miller, and J.F., Fraumeni, Jr., Eds.). New York: Raven Press, 1977, pp. 235-256.
13. Lynch, H.T., Follett, K.L., Lynch, P.M., Albano, W.A., Mailliard, J.L., and Pierson, R.L.: Family history in an oncology clinic. Implications for cancer genetics. *JAMA* **242**:1268-1272, 1979.
14. Lynch, H.T., Anderson, D.E., Krush, A.J., and Mukerjee, D.: Cancer, heredity and genetic counseling. Xeroderma pigmentosum. *Cancer* **20**:1796-1801, 1967.
15. Lynch, H.T., Anderson, D.E., Smith, J.L., Jr., Howell, J.B., and Krush, A.J.: Xeroderma pigmentosum, malignant melanoma, and congenital ichthyosis. *Arch. Dermatol.* **96**:625-635, 1976.
16. Lynch, H.T., Frichot, B.C., III, and Lynch, J.F.: Cancer control in xeroderma pigmentosum. *Arch. Dermatol.* **113**:193-195, 1977.
17. Lynch, H.T., Frichot, B.C., III, Fisher, J., Smith, J.L., Jr., and Lynch, J.F.: Spontaneous regression of metastatic malignant melanoma in two sibs with xeroderma pigmentosum. *J. Med. Genet.* **15**:357-362, 1978.
18. Cleaver, J.E.: Xeroderma pigmentosum. A human disease in which an initial state of DNA repair is defective. *Proc. Natl. Acad. Sci. USA* **63**:428-435, 1969.

Index